Third Edition

Manual of School Health

A Handbook for School Nurses, Educators, and Health Professionals

KEETA DeSTEFANO LEWIS, RN, MSN, PhD, FNASN
Healthlink
Child Health Consultant
Napa, California

BONNIE J. BEAR, RN, BSN, MA
School Health Consultant
San Diego, California

SAUNDERS

ELSEVIER

2013 → Tmro

SAUNDERS
ELSEVIER

11830 Westline Industrial Drive
St. Louis, Missouri 63146

MANUAL OF SCHOOL HEALTH: A HANDBOOK   ISBN: 978-1-4160-3778-1
FOR SCHOOL NURSES, EDUCATORS,
AND HEALTH PROFESSIONALS

Notices

The web sites listed in this book do not imply endorsement. An attempt has been
made to list important and informative health resources, but as with any electronic site, locations may change; therefore data need to be reviewed for correctness and the date the data were updated.

Knowledge and best practice in this field are constantly changing. As new research and experience broaden our knowledge, changes in practice, treatment and
drug therapy may become necessary or appropriate. Readers are advised to check
the most current information provided (i) on procedures featured or (ii) by the manufacturer of each product to be administered, to verify the recommended dose or
formula, the method and duration of administration, and contraindications. It is the
responsibility of the practitioner, relying on their own experience and knowledge of
the patient, to make diagnoses, to determine dosages and the best treatment for each
individual patient, and to take all appropriate safety precautions. To the fullest extent of the law, neither the Publisher nor the Authors assume any liability for any
injury and/or damage to persons or property arising out of or related to any use of
the material contained in this book.

The Publisher

Previous editions copyrighted 2002, 1986.

International Standard Book Number: 978-1-4160-3778-1

Acquisition Editor: Linda Thomas
Developmental Editor: Carlie Bliss Irwin
Publishing Services Manager: Deborah L. Vogel
Project Manager: Pat Costigan
Design Direction and Cover Design: Maggie Reid

Printed in the United States of America.

Last digit is the print number: 9   8   7   6   5   4   3   2   1

REVIEWERS

Jeffrey Anshel, OD
Optometrist
President, Corporate Vision
    Consulting
Carlsbad, California

Bonnie R. Bernstein, PhD
Psychologist
San Diego Unified School District
San Diego, California

Beverly J. Bradley, PhD, RN, FNASN
Assistant Clinical Professor (Retired)
University of California, San Diego,
    School of Medicine
Past President, American School
    Health Association
Reno, Nevada

Shirley Carstens, RN, MS, FNASN
School Nurse (retired)
Past President, National Association
    of School Nurses
Tacoma, Washington

Mark Chenven, MD
Vice President Clinical
    Operations, Vista Hill
Associate Clinical Professor,
    Department of Psychiatry
University of California, San Diego
San Diego, California

Gayle Coonce, MA, CCC-SP
Director of Special Education
La Mesa–Spring Valley School
    District
La Mesa, California

Ann Dexheimer, MA
Deaf/Hard of Hearing Specialist
Fremont Unified School District
Fremont, California

Janice Doyle, RN, MSN, NCSN
Lead Nurse, Bethel School District
Affiliate Clinical Faculty
Pacific Lutheran University, School
    of Nursing
Tacoma, Washington

Diane Durando, RN, PHN
School Nurse
Buchanan High School
Clovis, California

Joshua D. Feder, MD
Child and Family Psychiatry
Solano Beach, California

Cathy D. Gangstad, MPA
President, Learning Consortium, Inc.
Bellevue, Washington

Alan B. Goldsobel, MD
Allergy and Asthma Associates of
    Northern California
Associate Clinical Professor of
    Pediatrics
Stanford University Medical Center
San Jose, California

Jeffrey A. Hall, OD
Optometrist
Lake Murray San Carlos Optometric
    Center
San Diego, California

Joan Havard, MED, CCC/A
Clinical Audiologist
Speech, Language, and Hearing
    Specialist
Santa Clara County Office of
    Education
Santa Clara, California

Frank P. Hochman, MD
Private Practice
Past President, Society of Hearing
    Impaired Physicians
Pleasanton, California

Susie Horn-Sosna, RN, MSN
Resource Nurse
San Diego Unified School District
San Diego, California

Meri Jackson, RN, CNP
School Nurse Specialist (Retired)
Past President, California School
    Nurses Organization
Cayucos, California

Christopher A. Kearney, PhD
Professor of Psychology
University of Nevada
Las Vegas, Nevada

**Lisa Lewis-Javar, RN,
    SANE-P, FNC**
Forensic Nurse Specialist
Program Coordinator, SANE-SART,
    Napa/Solano Counties
Clinical Nurse Specialist/Medicine,
    Kaiser Permanente
Napa, California

**Patsy L. Maloney, RN, BC, EdD,
    MA, MSN, CNAA-BC**
Associate Professor and Director of
    Continuing Nursing Education
Pacific Lutheran University, School
    of Nursing
University Place, Washington

Maryann Martone, PhD
Professor-in-Residence, Department
    of Neurosciences
University of California, San Diego
La Jolla, California

**Maureen Ward Moffatt, RN,
    MSN**
School Nurse
San Diego Unified School District
San Diego, California

**Susan E. Proctor, RN, MPH,
    DNS, FNASN**
Professor Emeritus and Former
    School Nursing Program
    Coordinator
Division of Nursing
California State University,
    Sacramento
Past Executive Editor, *Journal of
    School Nursing*
Sacramento, California

Steven J. Rawiszer
Hearing Conservation Specialist
Department of Health Care Services
Children's Medical Services Branch
Sacramento, California

Pat Summers, RNC, BSN, MS
Special Education Itinerant Nurse
San Diego Unified School District
San Diego, California

Tania Ware, RN, BS, MA
Special Education Itinerant Nurse
San Diego Unified School District
San Diego, California

**Vickie A. Whitson, RN, BSN,
    SANE-A, FNC**
Sexual Assault Nurse Examiner
Napa/Solano Counties, SANE-SART
Clinical Nurse Specialist/
    Ophthalmology, Kaiser
    Permanente
Vallejo, California

INSPIRATION

WONDROUS MOMENTS OF THOUGHT
*Wondrous moments of dancing thoughts
nestled as a perfumed bouquet
adorn a living sculpture of caring and sharing;
Gentle hands from which touch the flesh, the Soul,
all being of nature and creation,
dismissing the word* disease *from human language, and
challenging healing with self-assured daring.
No measure of purpose
or yardstick of hope can embody
the golden kindness of nurses
and to life's cause their bearing.*
BG

DEDICATION

To our families

Lisa and Art Javar, DaNaii and Danté; John and Candi Lewis;
Rob and Thi My Scheinecker, Elise and Sophiane.

Bryan and Laura Bear, Jacob, John, and Amanda; Kevin Bear; Lisa
and Russell Holcomb, Jenna.

And our departed husbands who inspired us to unselfishly touch others
with our messages.

To our dear friends
who believe in us and deeply share the importance of our work.

FOREWORD

You are in for a treat. This book is the third edition of what has become an essential worksite companion for many thousands of school nurses! I have known the authors for many years; both are dedicated and knowledgeable school nurses. I first became acquainted with this book following its inaugural appearance in 1986. In my role as nursing faculty, I recommended the early edition to school nursing students as a valuable "at-your-elbow" resource in practice. This newest edition moves beyond being valuable: it is an indispensable *ally* for the practicing school nurse. It is with considerable pride that I offer some introductory words to this third edition.

As spectacular as was the second edition in 2002, the third edition is even more cutting-edge in its identification and coverage of urgent, contemporary issues. The authors have surveyed the practice frontier and incorporated several new or expanded perspectives into this third edition. Among these:

- The research from neuroscientists is infused into the Brain Findings sections throughout the revision.
- The new dermatology color insert provides color photos and three-dimensional dermatological illustrations of various conditions.
- Tuberculosis is added to the discussion of chronic conditions, and coverage of Lyme disease is expanded.
- Rapidly changing trends and treatments in asthma and diabetes mellitus are greatly expanded within the discussion on chronic conditions.
- "Mental Health Disorders" is the new title for the chapter previously titled "Affective and Behavioral Disorders." Content on obsessive-compulsive disorder (OCD) is expanded, and new information on both autism and Asperger's is presented, complete with illustrations of relevant brain areas.
- School-appropriate testing methods are included in Appendix A.
- The latest substance abuse federal data and trends, always vital and dynamic topics, are included.
- The chapter on violence readdresses rape and date rape as sexual assault and provides the latest information and trends.
- The chapter on special education is expanded, and the nursing role is examined in light of the latest IDEA authorizations.
- The "Twenty-first Century Health Challenges" chapter expands the discussion of backpack syndrome, with new ideas on treatment and management.
- An entirely new chapter on emergency and disaster preparedness issues is included.

Throughout the entire text, you will notice two additions:

- The inclusion of many new web sites for use by both the nurse and parents.
- The infusion of additional nursing management techniques throughout.

It is a privilege to present this book to its current and future readers.

Susan E. Proctor, RN, MPH, DNS, FNASN
Professor Emeritus and Former School Nursing Program Coordinator
Division of Nursing
California State University, Sacramento
Past Executive Editor, *Journal of School Nursing*

FOREWORD

He who has health has hope, and he who has hope has everything. —Arabic proverb

It's been five years since the last edition of this *Manual*. Yet, as before, events and interactions that occur at our schools' health offices remain remarkably prophetic and reflective of the best and worst attributes characterizing our next generation of adults. Most of what is experienced there foretells an optimistic future. This generation of students, for example, is in many ways more mature and aware than the generations that preceded it. But not all is rosy. Most school health professionals daily find students and families who have no access to health and mental health services, a problem that is too often disproportionately found among those most needing those services. We encounter students who take health and safety risks that jeopardize their future success, if not their very lives. We all know families whose financial and social stresses overwhelm their innate ability to provide a stable upbringing for their children. Unprecedented idleness and huge food portion sizes are increasingly typical for today's school-age population, predisposing these youngsters to life-shortening health conditions that may make this the first generation to live fewer years than their parents. Not least, American children of today are exposed to intense levels of impending alarm, as adults around them anticipate and prepare for risks of terror and natural disasters—increasing their levels of anxiety, resulting in emotional and physical sequelae for some. All these problems, predictably and appropriately, find their way into our schools' health and counseling offices.

Despite this, our schools' health offices have become neither gloomy nor desperate. On the contrary, school health and mental health professionals emanate confidence and hope. Attesting to this, students and their families flock to school health offices. And educators and administrators continue to refer them there. Signs of progress in medical technologies, pharmaceuticals, and evidence-based preventive health strategies abound in the field of medicine, and school nurses are generally early adopters. Modern methods of communication and evidence-based health educational practices are being exploited so that we can promote health, education, and social understanding with unparalleled results.

The pace of change does not allow school health professionals to remain complacent. Given that we encounter problems that are extraordinary in either their medical complexity or social profundity, school health professionals must know where to find resources that can help address these problems. There are tangible signs that we are making headway. Terms such as *disaster preparedness, cultural literacy, tolerance, sexual orientation, universal precautions, medically fragile, asset building, fully-integrated, technology-dependent, individualized plan, specialized health care procedure, crisis response,* and *coordinated school health* are reflections of the tools school health practitioners have used and of how we have evolved as professionals to meet today's problems.

Contemporary problems seep into our midst without invitation. In comparison, contemporary solutions take longer and require preparation and planning. To remain worthy of the trust and hope bestowed on us by educators, school administrators, students, families, and community members, we must keep abreast of change. There are several challenges that school health professionals must face as we plow forward to meet these changes. We cannot, and should not, embrace everything simply because it is new and available. For example, schools are convenient and efficient places to perform many sorts of health screens, but are all health screens effective uses of our time? Which screens have been tested, much less proven, to be effective as public health strategies? Another example of a modern challenge for school-based health professionals is that we are often the first to become aware of health education topics that need to be taught if our schools are to face health and safety risks that are arising in our communities. But is this awareness on our part translated into development of evidence-based curricula and, eventually, wide-scale adoption? And if so, how long is the lag time?

School health professionals are well positioned and well trained to witness effects, both positive and negative, of new medications, particularly those designed to improve students' mental health and attention. Do our informed impressions of these innovative pharmacotherapies consistently find their way back to primary care providers and to medical and mental health specialists who prescribe them? Lastly, there is a constant tug between those who believe schools can and should meet our students' health and social needs and those who feel that if society needs to increasingly burden the educational system to achieve primary health goals, then the health system is broken and needs to fix itself. School health professionals are at the vortex of this argument.

School nurses, school counselors, school doctors, and others cannot anticipate all upcoming societal problems or solutions that will inevitably present themselves at the front doors of our school offices over the coming years. Our best efforts must be directed toward utilizing reliable reference materials, keeping open minds, and recognizing that there are no easy solutions to complex problems. This *Manual*, by providing nonjudgmental perspective and succinct, well-organized facts, serves as an important basis for covering the issues that face our students and therefore our society. From first-aid to vision screening, and from topics like commercialization of our schools to topics addressing students' feelings of isolation, this *Manual* updates those of us who are among the first to be exposed to trends and dangers facing children and youth. Topics addressed within this edition of the *Manual* help us to maintain high levels of competence and to gain significant footholds on the contemporary challenges posed to us as school health professionals.

Howard L. Taras, MD
Division of Community Pediatrics—School Health
University of California, San Diego
La Jolla, California

PREFACE

The third edition of the *Manual of School Health* discusses new innovations and technology that influence treatments and the way nurses provide care to school-age children in the twenty-first century. With the continuing support from school nurses, administrators, and health professionals working with the school-age population, a more comprehensive and inclusive edition has been developed. The authors are keenly aware of the responsibility and accountability this support places on our shoulders.

It is our core belief that the family is the unit of care and that involving the family is essential to the success of all health care, interventions, and academic planning that occurs in the school setting. All school employees, administrators, and teaching staff are encouraged to include the parent(s) in the school experience of their children.

A school nurse is often the first to detect current trends and behaviors in the pediatric population such as violence and substance abuse. This opportunity for early detection puts the nurse in a position to advocate for appropriate health care versus punitive action alone. Knowledge of hundreds of diagnoses and treatment modalities is necessary for the school nurse to be current and proactive in providing a full range of services and being a child/family advocate.

Easy-to-use data for determining early signs and symptoms and making timely referrals to primary care, public health, and/or mental health agencies for diagnosis, management, and follow-up are included. Biotechnology provides information and new treatments that are helping individuals who in the past would not have had access to this support. Such students are often medically fragile or depend on technology that has affected nursing practice in schools. Current trends in the school environment such as commercialism of schools, computer ergonomics, and consequences of heavy backpack use are addressed.

SPECIAL FEATURES

Information found most relevant to the needs of the school-age population is summarized in this manual. School-age is defined as from birth through 21 years, thus including not only kindergarten through high school students but also children in infant and toddler programs and childcare and those in special education programs—our most vulnerable children.

- *Color plates* of skin conditions have been added, along with drawings of the layers of skin lesions for easy identification and understanding.
- The *Brain Findings* subsections are related to growth, development, behaviors, learning, and health.
- *Growth and Developmental Characteristics* encompasses typical parameters plus brain findings, prenatal, psychosexual, moral, and spiritual development.

- *Mental Health Disorders* is focused on disorders listed in the *DSM-IV TR.*
- *Violence* is included as associated to school, home, others, and self.
- *Sub stance Abuse* includes club drugs, date rape drugs, and inhalants, with the major contribution being the Neurobiology of Addiction.
- *Twenty-first Century Health Challenges* are the contemporary issues facing students, staff, parents, and the school nurse.
- A new chapter is devoted to *Emergency and Disaster Preparedness.*
- *Web sites* provide access to additional data and related agencies and organizations.
- *Appendixes* contain resources such as Centers for Disease Control and Prevention growth measurements charts and information on widely used assessment tools for students needing special education services.
- In the *Appendixes* there is also information on valuable tools for school health assessments, interventions, and management.
- The *school nursing role* is a focus throughout.
- *Key points* provide summaries of pertinent health care elements to be addressed at the school site and/or for individualized health care plan/individual educational plan (IHCP/IEP) development.
- Numerous and diverse *tables* and *boxes* provide additional concise information applicable to specific situations and assessment procedures.
- School *Exclusion and Readmission* policies provide appropriate suggestions if local or state guidelines are not already in place.
- More than 25 illustrations are easy to follow and offer a visual complement to the text.
- The *Glossary* defines concepts and key terms for quick, accurate understanding.
- *End sheets* on the inside front and back covers provide another avenue of fast reference information.

This edition includes the following chapters, in summary.

Chapter 1, *Growth and Development Characteristics,* outlines the basics for understanding normal child development, from birth through 21 years of age, in all areas of growth. This assists nurses in identifying and diagnosing deviations from the norm. New technology has provided information now presented in Brain Findings, which makes that section essential in appreciating the brain's complexities. Tanner Stages of Development have been added to this chapter.

Chapter 2, *Vision and Hearing,* concerns the most common paths to learning and two integral parts of child assessment. Major characteristics of vision and hearing conditions and tests are covered, along with a glossary of terms. Illustrations of the eye, ear, and parts of the brain that are associated with the two sensory systems can be found. The impact of noise-induced hearing loss is discussed, as well as the increased use of amplification in the classroom to overcome extraneous or environmental noise.

Chapter 3, *Acute Conditions,* includes necessary information in a concise format for the nurse's daily work. *Exclusion and Readmission* information is provided for the school nurse, ancillary school staff, and parents. School nurses can share these references with parents to enhance their understanding.

Chapter 4, *Chronic Conditions,* is a compilation of diseases or conditions the school nurse faces on a routine basis. Information in *Management/Treatment* can be used to develop the IHCP and/or the IEP. The *Concerns/Emergencies* and *Effects on Individual* sections present collateral data for the IHCP. Tuberculosis (TB) was added due to the increasing number of students taking prophylactic medication. Growth charts for students with Down syndrome and Turner's syndrome are included for easy access.

Chapter 5, *Mental Health Disorders,* is concerned with the impact on the student of disorders of mental health. The increased incidence of depression makes it incumbent upon the nurse to understand the disease, medication, and other treatments necessary for the student to function at school. Psychotropic charts have been added to provide a summary of the most commonly used medications.

Chapter 6, *Substance Abuse,* has been expanded to cover a matter that continues to have a profound effect on many students. Prescription and over-the-counter drug abuse is increasing and is discussed in the chapter along with the most commonly abused substances. Tables on drugs and withdrawal symptoms will help the nurse in management, treatment, and teaching. The Substance Abuse Assessment Procedure table makes for easy and quick screening.

Chapter 7, *Violence,* to self, to others, and by others, reflects behaviors seen in the students with whom school nurses work. The chapter contains updated information about self-mutilation, suicide, date rape, harassment, bullying, and gangs, along with child abuse and other issues related to violence.

Chapter 8, *Adolescent and Gender-Specific Issues,* reflects usual concerns such as sexually transmitted infections and acne as well as some emergent issues such as cosmetic-related skin care concerns, tattooing, and body piercing. Several tables present convenient ways to compare facts about different conditions and effectiveness of various methods of contraception. Boxes and tables about tattooing and body piercing are provided, specifically, a table titled Healing Times for Body Piercing.

Chapter 9, *Special Education,* includes the history of the law up to the current Individuals with Disabilities Education Act (IDEA). Definitions of the 13 disabling conditions, Specialized Health Care procedures, and a glossary of terms are covered. Assessment Tools can be found in Appendix A.

Chapter 10, *Twenty-first Century Health Challenges,* includes a wide variety of contemporary financial arrangements and school policies that can have health consequences. Commercialism of schools by corporations happens through a variety of methods (e.g., closed-circuit TV, book covers, school supply items with logos, and food sponsorships). School start-time for adolescents is becoming a controversial topic and warrants research; sleep time patterns change in adolescence, and sleep deprivation can impair cognitive and motor functioning, which is discussed in this chapter.

Chapter 11, *Emergency and Disaster Preparedness,* which covers contemporary perspectives, is new and is of primary interest to school nurses, professionals, and parents. Organizational and personnel planning for emergency situations and bioterrorism and pandemic flu is provided in this chapter. Hints for helping children cope and their common reactions to disaster are noted.

Chapter 12, *First Aid,* is necessary for any school manual and is especially helpful for ancillary school and health personnel. Lists of necessary supplies for the school nurse office are included.

ACKNOWLEDGMENTS

With this third edition of the *Manual of School Health,* the opportunity comes again for us to express our gratitude for the eager support for this book and the incredible encouragement we have received for this endeavor. This book would not exist without this continued support and encouragement.

The first edition, published in 1986, was uniquely accepted by school nurses, community health nurses, educators, other professionals, and staff working with all ages of school children and—not least—by parents and grandparents. We continue to recognize the awesome responsibility and accountability we have in making this a fine, useful, and unique manual.

Helen Thomson and Keeta Lewis, both school nurses, co-authored the first edition. We appreciate and honor Helen's unique contribution to the original work. We also offer a continued "thank you" to Thomas Eoyang, our first editor, who believed in the *Manual of School Health* and launched it in 1986.

We are indebted to many nurses, educators, and other health care experts who took time to share their knowledge and expertise with us to review materials, provide ideas, references, and resources, and encourage us. A special thanks goes to Maryann Martone, a University of California, San Diego, neuroscientist, who lent her help to make clear some of the nuances in the realm of the brain, making the knowledge understandable to the reader. Drs. Joshua Feder and Mark Chenven, child psychiatrists, helped to clarify some of the current issues with children in the spectrum of autism. Dr. Terry Erwin, Smithsonian scientist, gave us suggestions and sensible evidence when we were working on the Chronic Conditions and Acute Conditions chapters. Dr. B.J. Krell, professor, wrote a loving tribute to nurses everywhere that is found in the Inspiration. Beverly Bradley carefully reviewed and provided additional information, materials, and resources regarding the adolescent. Susan Proctor is still the "shero" of the book and remains one of our strongest and most loving supporters. Many others, listed in the reviewer information, helped with sections of the review process, for which we are eternally grateful.

We are indebted to Linda Thomas, managing editor, Carlie Irwin, developmental editor, and Jeanne Robertson, illustrator. We were especially blessed by having Linda as our direct editor. She moved us along when there were innumerable new technology and research articles and data that needed to be read and condensed into a concise format. This process was time consuming, and Linda was always there, consistent and confident. We offer deep gratitude and love to our dear friend Virginia Means for her manuscript preparation and support of us and the book. She reviewed every page and challenged us many times in positive ways and helped to make this a successful project.

Finally, we wish to express our deepest love and gratitude to our dear families and friends. They put up with us while we obsessed over the revising of the book and used any time we could free up to work on the book. They willingly gave us the freedom to dedicate ourselves fully to this undertaking. They are our inspiration.

The two of us took turns flying back and forth between our California homes, from Napa to San Diego, to make a great book even greater. We have shared, endured, and learned a lot together, and it has made us still the "best of friends." We are happy the revision is complete and ready to be shared with all of you. Thank you for your loyalty.

Keeta DeStefano Lewis
Bonnie J. Bear

CONTENTS

CHAPTER 1

Growth and Development Characteristics

Chapter Outline

*T*he nurse often encounters concerns regarding the development of an infant, child, adolescent, or young adult. Increasingly, school nurses are working with this wide age range in a variety of school settings. These concerns center on cognition, communication, psychomotor domains, emotional/social skills, psychosexual status, and moral, spiritual, and physical traits. To assess, evaluate, treat, seek consultation, or make a referral, the nurse needs knowledge of normal growth and development in all domains. This chapter is a guide for facilitating this process, and it covers the life cycle from the time of conception through young adulthood. Developmental characteristics for individual age groups are presented in a systematic and sequential form for easy reference.

Embryonic growth (conception to 6 weeks) and fetal development (7 weeks to 9 months) are the first points of discussion. These growth periods are crucial to later development. The period of infancy through early childhood (birth to 5 years) is of utmost importance because brain growth and physical development change rapidly during this critical time. Any deviation from the norm must be detected so that early intervention and remediation can begin.

By elementary age (6 to 12 years), most major developmental problems have been identified. However, many problems are so subtle that they remain undetected until later developmental stages. As children enter the school environment, they face increased physical and mental demands. Numerous health, emotional, and developmental problems can occur during this age span. The nurse plays an important role in early detection, appropriate nursing care, and referral.

Adolescents (13 to 18 years) are in transition from childhood to adulthood. This period is characterized by many rapid physical, emotional, and sexual changes. In addition, it is imperative that this age group successfully achieves numerous developmental tasks. These challenging tasks and the rapid succession of changes can contribute to stress-related illness, dysfunctional family life, interpersonal conflicts, and antisocial behavior. The risk-taking adolescent too often becomes identified with an unhealthy lifestyle and a myriad of teenage issues and concerns that are well known to the school nurse. Young adult development (19 through 21 years) is summarized in this chapter, concluding with the reaching of maturity and achievement of developmental tasks of the young adult.

PRENATAL AND POSTNATAL DEVELOPMENT

Brain Findings

The ectoderm, endoderm, and mesoderm layers separate at approximately day 10 to 13 of gestation. The neural plate forms from the ectoderm and eventually becomes the brain and spinal cord. By about 3 weeks, the nervous system consists of a hollow tube, called the *neural tube.* The neural tube differentiates into the brain and spinal cord. As the tube develops, groups of cells termed the *neural crest* pinch off; these will eventually give rise to the neurons in the peripheral nervous system (PNS). Differentiation of the *hindbrain,* the *midbrain,* and the *forebrain*—the three major divisions of the brain—begins by the third week of gestation.

Continued

Growth and Development Characteristics

Neurodevelopment of the human brain is defined as the production of nerve cells (both neurons and glia), their migration, differentiation, and establishment of connections (the "wiring diagram" of the nervous system). Neurodevelopment occurs in a predetermined genetic pattern. Production, position assignment, and migration of brain neurons occur mostly during embryonic and early postnatal life.

Brain development occurs in a sequential and hierarchical pattern. The brain organizes from the lower (brainstem and areas of the midbrain) to the higher, most complex areas (limbic and cortical areas). The brainstem and midbrain are the first to develop and are necessary for survival by regulating body functions, such as respiratory and cardiovascular function, appetite, and sleep cycles. Some structures such as the cerebellum (Figure 1-1) continue to produce new neurons well into the postnatal period.

The limbic areas (emotion regulation and experience processing) and cortical areas (executive and cognitive function) develop during the first 3 years of life, but the prefrontal lobes and neocortex continue to develop throughout childhood and adolescence. Development, organization, and functionality of the various areas take place at different times throughout the life span (Perry, 2002; Davies, 2004).

STRUCTURES OF THE BRAIN

The *cerebral cortex,* also called the *neocortex,* is the outer covering of the brain. The brain has two *hemispheres,* and each hemisphere has four major *lobes* that can be further subdivided into many specialty areas. Further division also occurs, including cortical and subcortical structures, such as the hypothalamus. Figure 1-1 and Figure 1-2 present the basic structural areas of the brain.

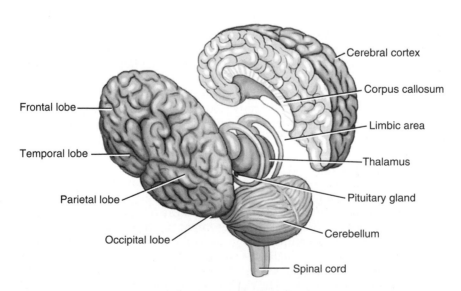

FIGURE 1-1 Structure of the brain.

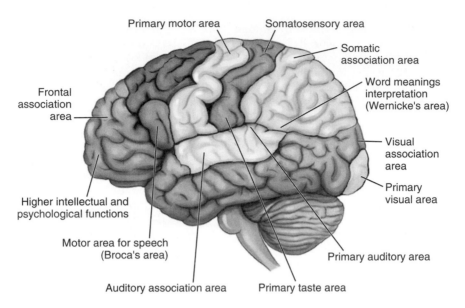

Primary motor area

Somatosensory area

Somatic association area

Word meanings interpretation (Wernicke's area)

Frontal association area

Visual association area

Primary visual area

Higher intellectual and psychological functions

Motor area for speech (Broca's area)

Primary auditory area

Auditory association area

Primary taste area

FIGURE 1-2 Mapping of the brain, including thought, movement, and sensory functions.

The four lobes are *frontal, occipital, parietal,* and *temporal.*
- The *frontal lobes* are responsible for thinking, conceptualizing, planning, emotional regulation, social interaction, abstract thinking, decision making, and memory.
- The *occipital lobes* are the primary centers for visual processing.
- The *parietal lobes* are concerned with functions of calculation, orientation, movement, and particular types of recognition, somatic interpretation, and integration.
- The *temporal lobes* are responsible primarily for sound, hearing, speech comprehension (left side generally), and the formation of long-term memory.
- The fibrous *corpus callosum* connects the two hemispheres and allows them to pass information back and forth.

At 7 months of gestation, *convolutions* begin to form in the outer layer of the brain to accommodate for the restricted space; this formation is one of the factors responsible for the eventual power of the brain. These convolutions allow the cortex to increase its surface area without an increase in skull size. Gyri—bumps, bulges, or convolutions—and sulci, shallow grooves or fissures between convolutions, form anatomical landmarks that can be identified on MRI scans, which helps demarcate areas of the cortex associated with different functions (M. Martone, personal communication, July 15, 2006).

The *motor cortex* is located at the junction of the frontal and parietal lobes, below the area where a set of headphones might sit across the top of the head. The motor cortex plays a critical role in controlling muscle movements, as do the cerebellum and basal ganglia, a compilation of associated subcortical cell groups in the forebrain. All movement areas of the body have a corresponding area in the motor cortex. The right side controls muscles on the left side of the body, and the left side controls muscles on the right side.

The *premotor cortex* is dedicated to initiation and sequencing of movements and is part of the frontal lobe.

The *somatosensory cortex,* a strip across the top of each hemisphere, is adjacent and posterior to the motor cortex and is associated with the processing of incoming sensory stimulation: pain sensation, touch, pressure, temperature, and proprioception (body position in space).

The *angular gyrus* is located on the margins of the temporal, parietal, and occipital lobes, up and behind Wernicke's area. This area is associated with vision, spatial skills, and language and is believed to act as a bridge between the language process and visual word recognition(meaning).

The brain is basically hollow. Fluid-filled canals and caverns inside the brain make up the *ventricular system (VS).* The fluid is called *cerebrospinal fluid (CSF),* and it fills the lateral, third, and fourth ventricles and the cerebral aqueduct. This is of importance to the nurse because of the incidence of hydrocephalus in children caused by a blockage in the ventricular system.

During the first 7 months of gestation, neurons generate at an awesome speed and migrate to designated places; approximately 50% are pruned away before birth. This is a normal process called *apoptosis,* or *programmed cell death* (Diamond and Hopson, 1998; Bear, Connors, and Paradiso, 2007). This usually is thought to contribute to the efficiency of the brain. Unfinished apoptosis may contribute to the dramatic abilities of autistic savants and may also be one factor affecting their other deficits (Carter, 1999). Conversely, overpruning may lead to the cognitive impairment in a child with Down syndrome. This pruning of cells and connections occurs from 7 months gestation and continues throughout childhood and adolescence (Diamond and Hopson, 1998; Huttenlocher and Dabholkar, 1997).

Language areas for general processing are located in the left hemisphere in approximately 96% of the population. There are two major language areas:
- *Wernicke's area* is located in the frontal lobe near the junction of the temporal lobe and is associated with comprehension of speech. This area is also near the auditory cortex, which receives sound signals from the ears.
- *Broca's area* is located at the posterior of the frontal lobe in the left hemisphere and is associated with generating speech. It also is near the motor cortex area that controls muscles of the lips and mouth.

OTHER AREAS OF THE BRAIN

The *thalamus* lies beneath the cortex and acts as a relay station that transmits incoming sensory signals, such as pain, to the appropriate part of the cortex for further processing. All sensory systems, except the sense of smell, send signals to the thalamus.

The *cortex* controls the *hypothalamus,* which is a subcortical brain structure that lies below the thalamus. In turn, the hypothalamus controls the *pituitary gland,* which is often referred to as the *head gland,* because it controls the other glands of the body. The hypothalamus, together with the pituitary gland, is involved in activities vital to survival, such as the maintenance of blood glucose levels, body temperature, body rhythms, heart rate, thirst, activity and rest, sexual desire, and reproductive and menstrual cycles. The hypothalamus works to maintain homeostasis, the "set point" in the body, by regulating the balance between the sympathetic and parasympathetic branches of the autonomic nervous system.

The *hippocampus,* a structure shaped like a ram's horn, is located deep within the temporal lobe near the amygdala and hypothalamus. It is associated with conscious long-term memory, spatial ability, learning, and motivation. Damage to the hippocampus causes severe memory problems.

The *amygdala* consists of two almond-shaped structures located at the anterior end of each hippocampus. They coordinate autonomic and endocrine responses with states of emotions, such as anger or fear, and emotional behavior, and they are involved in the regulation and storage of emotional memory. The *nucleus accumbens* is a small, hook-like structure linked to pleasure, cravings, and reward.

The *ventral tegmental area (VTA),* located at the front of the brainstem, relays messages of pleasure from their nerve cells to nerve cells in the nucleus accumbens through neurotransmitters, chemicals involved in transmission of nerve impulses between synapses, such as dopamine. This pleasure circuit also includes the prefrontal cortex and is called the *mesolimbic dopamine system,* which is associated with acts of pleasure—such as eating and sexual activity—and addiction.

To understand the brain, scientists delineate the parts by shape and function and name the structures and areas; however, the purpose of particular structures of the brain, or which areas are involved in any given brain activity, are not always clearly understood.

OTHER FETAL DEVELOPMENT

Until approximately 6 weeks, the embryo is basically gender neutral. Genetic predetermination and the absence or presence of male hormones begins the sexual design for development. At 6 weeks, a male embryo begins to convert gonadal lumps into testes that produce testosterone; at 8 weeks, external genitalia are present; and at 12 weeks, a female embryo begins to develop ovaries. At 25 weeks, the fetus weighs approximately 1 pound and responds to the maternal voice and to light and smells, which suggests that learning occurs *in utero.*

Human *deoxyribonucleic acid (DNA)* contains approximately 30,000 to 40,000 *genes* that determine characteristic development—such as eye color, hair color, and body size—and they predispose an individual to certain diseases, disorders, or traits, such as temperament. Genetic endowment, along with the environment, plays a decisive role in development. Both nature and nurture are required for the neurodevelopment of the mature, efficient human brain.

The *intrauterine environment* can influence development in a positive or negative way. Factors such as early and significant exposure to alcohol, nicotine, cocaine, or poor nutrition and stress all play a role in fetal development.

EARLY CHILDHOOD: BIRTH TO 5 YEARS

Newborn: Birth to 1 Month
Brain Findings
Basic connectivity of the newborn brain has been established, although it does not function the same as an adult brain. After birth, the infant demonstrates utilization of networks of neurons by moving arms and legs,

Continued

opening and closing eyes, and by crying and breathing. The brain's early developmental task is to continue forming and reinforcing some connections and pruning others. This process is a function of genetic predisposition and experience with the outside environment. If experience does not occur during a critical period, synaptic connections do not develop, and the potential ability is gone. For example, cataracts impair visual acuity, and if they are not detected and surgically removed by 2 years of age, visual acuity does not develop, and the synapses in the visual cortex are pruned away and the child is forever blind.

A. Brain weight at birth is approximately 400 g.
B. At birth, the cortex is approximately 1 mm thick—about one half the thickness of an adult brain.
C. Synapses form in the newborn's brain at the rate of approximately 3 billion per second at given times.
D. Each neuron can be connected to as many as 15,000 other neurons and, with some, many more thousands of synapses are made.
E. The brain uses about 20% oxygen; and in the cerebral cortex, from birth to about 4 years of age, glucose usage is twice that of an adult's brain.
F. The brain's capacity is not fixed at birth and is most plastic during infancy. The more complex areas of the brain, such as the cortex, are more plastic; the life sustaining areas of the brain, such as the brainstem, are less plastic.
G. The brain does not grow uniformly but has peaks that correspond to the learning of various skills.
H. The brain constitutes approximately 12% of body weight at birth and approximately 2% to 3% of body weight in adulthood.
I. Brain growth is reflected in the head circumference; growth charts (see Appendix B) indicate that brain growth occurs more rapidly in the first year of life than at any subsequent age. The brain reaches one half its eventual size by 12 months.
J. Neurons are still being produced postnatally, and the neurons are increasing in size and complexity (M. Martone, personal communication, July 15, 2006). A significant part of the increase in brain weight observed at this time can be attributed to the development of glial cells, primarily those that produce myelin.
K. The newborn's head is approximately one fourth of the total body length (see Head and Body Proportions in Figure 1-3 on page 8).

I. Physical and Anatomical Traits

NOTE: A child continues to follow own unique growth curve, which is more important than conformity to averages.

A. Undifferentiated, almost immobile at birth with many primitive reflexes (e.g., sucking, grasping, rooting, squinting).
B. Weight gain 5 to 7 oz weekly (150 to 210 g).
C. Height growth 1 in (2.5 cm) monthly.
D. Head circumference larger than chest circumference; median head circumference at birth 13.5 in (35 cm), chest 13 in (33 cm). Head circumference increases over 3 in (8 cm) during first 6 months of life. Figure 1-3 presents head and body proportions throughout development.
E. Chubby appearance. At 1 month muscles are firmer than at birth.

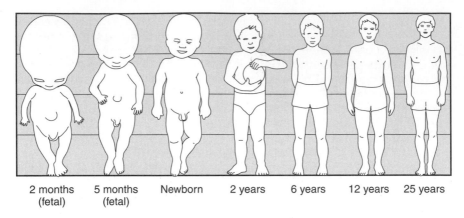

| 2 months (fetal) | 5 months (fetal) | Newborn | 2 years | 6 years | 12 years | 25 years |

Figure 1-3 Head and body proportions from prenatal development to 25 years.

F. Posterior fontanel may be closed at birth; if open, will close around 2 months.

G. Anterior fontanel closes around 14 months.

H. Obligatory nose breathing.

I. Visual acuity approaches 20/100.

II. Gross and Fine Psychomotor Traits

A. Asymmetric posture with head to one side, one arm extended, and the other flexed toward the shoulder (asymmetric tonic neck reflex [ATNR] posture).

B. Extremities extend and abduct with fanning of fingers, followed by flexion and adduction of the extremities. Results from a sudden horizontal lowering of infant (Moro/startle reflex).

C. Head is unsteady when infant is pulled to a sitting position.

D. Movement of arms and legs is symmetrical bilaterally and generally smooth.

E. Both hands clenched, grasp reflex strong.

F. Momentarily grasps rattle placed in hand; grasp reflex.

G. Follows object to midline, but focuses best on objects 8 to 15 inches away.

H. Prefers black-and-white geometric designs.

III. Cognitive and Language Traits

A. Involuntary reflexive behavior.

B. Makes comfort sounds during feeding, gurgling, or crying sounds.

C. Alerts to high-pitched voices.

D. Cries when unhappy. Small, throaty noises may turn into cooing by the end of first month.

E. Arms flex and fists clench after sudden loud noise (Moro/startle reflex). Head turns toward voice or other soft auditory stimuli in alert state.

IV. Emotional and Social Traits

A. Inward orientation, asocial but symbiotic; newborn appears joined to the mother.

B. Unable to discern self, non-self, or others.
C. Detectable temperament differences: active, irritable, quiet, alert.
D. May recognize parents' voices, especially the mother's.
E. Derives simple physical pleasure from being held, cuddled, and rocked.
F. Regards face intently when engaged verbally.
G. Reacts to social overtures by reducing general activity.
H. Social smile begins about 2 months.

V. Psychosexual Traits
A. Orality: primary source of pleasure centered on mouth, lips, and tongue.
B. Male babies have penile erections before and after birth.
C. Sensual feeling triggered by kicking, rocking, or rubbing genitals gives sensory pleasure that may not be erotic as in later stage of sexuality.
D. Sucking and rooting reflexes during breast feeding or bottle feeding are the precursors of sexual pleasures.

VI. Moral and Spiritual Traits
A. Premoral, amoral, primordial.
B. Egocentric, narcissistic.

INFANCY: 2 TO 12 MONTHS
3 Months (12 Weeks)

Brain Findings

Visual cortex synapse formation peaks while brain is enhancing the connections that allow the eyes to focus on objects, thereby developing depth perception.

At approximately two months of age, the infant begins to lose startle and rooting reflexes. The mastering of purposeful movements begins for more coordinated movements, reflecting the development of the motor cortex and higher motor centers (M. Martone, personal communication, July 25, 2006).

Expression of genetic predisposition is influenced by environmental factors, including physical, mental, social, and emotional influences.

Development of subcortical and limbic areas is influenced by early experiences of trauma or ongoing abuse and may result in extreme depression, anxiety, or inability to develop empathy or form appropriate attachments.

Brain development at all stages is highly susceptible to chemical, structural, hormonal, and environmental influences, including drugs, poor nutrition, physical trauma, radiation, and poverty.

I. Physical and Anatomical Traits
A. Posterior fontanel closed.
B. Has gained approximately 5 lb (2.3 kg).
C. Length increased 3.75 in (9 to 10 cm).
D. Head circumference has grown approximately 2 in (5 cm).
E. Chest circumference has increased 2.75 in (7 cm).
F. Establishes sleep–wake cycles.

II. Gross and Fine Psychomotor Traits
A. Asymmetrical tonic neck reflex (ATNR) begins to disappear, and head usually is held in midline.

B. On abdomen, can lift head 90 degrees with weight supported on forearms.
C. Tightens muscles when pulled to a sitting position in an attempt to control head.
D. Turns head and eyes to a moving object within visual range.
E. Puts hands and objects in mouth.
F. Grasp reflex is inactive.
G. Hands generally open or loosely closed.
H. Holds rattle for a short time if placed in hand.
I. Regards one or both hands.
J. Follows object with eyes to 180 degrees.
K. Can sit with head erect for short periods with support.
L. Lifts head while lying in supine position.
M. Makes precrawling attempts.
N. Attempts to grasp objects but misses.

III. Cognitive and Language Traits
A. Reflexive behavior generally replaced by voluntary movements.
B. Most recognize common objects: bottle, mobiles, and toys.
C. Babbling.
D. Responds to a familiar face by cooing, chuckling noise, or laughter.
E. Vocalizing accompanies smiling.
F. Crying is more related to specific needs or wants and becomes differentiated.
G. Vocal responses are reflexive in display: yawn, gurgle, sneeze, coo, cry, laughter, squealing.
H. Single vowel sounds are predominant: "aaah," "ooo."
I. Actively interested in environment; curious, visually searches to locate sounds.
J. Uses subtle engagement (hands open, relaxed) and disengagement (frowning, hiccups, sneezing) cues.

IV. Emotional and Social Traits
A. Beginning separation of self from others.
B. Can be attentive, calm, and alert.
C. Displays recognition signs at sight of mother.
D. Longer period of wakefulness without crying.
E. Stops crying at sight of parent.
F. Smiles often to others, may laugh.
G. Demands attention by fussing, enjoys attention.
H. Freezes in the presence of strangers.

V. Psychosexual Traits
A. Remains the same as newborn.

VI. Moral and Spiritual Traits
A. Remains the same as newborn.

6 Months (24 Weeks)

I. Physical and Anatomical Traits
A. Since birth, weight has doubled; infant has grown an average of 6 in.
NOTE: Between 6 and 12 months, average weight gain is 3 to 5 oz weekly (90 to 150 g) and height growth is ½ in (1.25 cm) monthly.

B. Head circumference has increased 3 in (8 cm).

C. Beginning of tooth eruption, generally lower central incisors.

D. Growth rate slower than first 6 months.

E. By 4 to 7 months has full color vision.

II. Gross and Fine Psychomotor Traits

A. Raises chest and upper part of abdomen off surface with weight on hands.

B. Rolls over from stomach to back (supine) and, in another month, from back to stomach (prone).

C. Sits alone but may need to lean forward on hands.

D. Holds on to feet and pulls them to mouth.

E. Begins weight bearing when held.

F. Rocks on hands and knees.

G. Will drop one cube if another is presented.

H. Can transfer cube from hand to hand and manipulate objects.

I. Holds own bottle.

J. Grasps and explores small objects.

K. Begins pincer grasp and self-feeding.

L. Drinks from a cup when cup is held to lips.

III. Cognitive and Language Traits

A. May look in response to name.

B. Response may vary to angry or happy voices.

C. Responds and imitates differences in intonation (melody pattern).

D. Imitates simple actions or movements; hands on head, waves or responds to "bye-bye."

E. Babbling sounds are one-syllable utterances, consonants, and vowels: "da," "ma."

F. Recognizes vowel sounds basic to speech.

G. Responds to voice by turning head or vocalization.

H. Variety of vocal responses to show feeling. May squeal to show pleasure.

I. Talks to people as well as to toys.

J. Smiles and laughs aloud.

K. Experiments with vocalization.

IV. Emotional and Social Traits

A. May withdraw from strangers.

B. Shows displeasure at removal of toy.

C. Holds arms out to be picked up.

D. Smiles at mirror images.

E. Laughs aloud when stimulated, such as person hiding head in towel.

F. Begins to show distress if mother leaves.

G. Other family members, beyond mother, become important or trusted.

V. Psychosexual Traits

A. Can wean infant from pleasures derived from the breast or bottle.

B. Biting and oral aggression; exploration begins.

VI. Moral and Spiritual Traits

A. Beginning to value caregiver over others and to show likes and dislikes based on voluntary choices associated with less distress or discomfort.

B. Definite ability to delay personal gratification to get beyond primary narcissism.

9 Months (36 Weeks)

Brain Findings

Between 7 and 12 months, linkage occurs among concepts, feelings, and language.

At approximately 8 or 9 months, the hippocampus becomes more functional in forming, storing, and recalling some types of memories. This is the beginning of cause-and-effect behavior. Infants can be taught that their behavior (e.g., touching an object) will result in a certain outcome (e.g., hearing a pleasant sound).

In certain time periods, such as during nonlinear brain development, various types of learning are more efficient; at 1 month, increased activity in subcortical and cortical regions makes visual and auditory stimulation important, because regions are associated with control of sensorimotor functions; at 8 months, frontal lobe shows increased metabolic activity, and this is an important time for strengthening or weakening caregiver attachment and self-regulation, because the frontal lobe is associated with the ability to think, plan, regulate, and express emotion.

I. Physical and Anatomical Traits

A. Rapid weight gains begin to decrease, with a gain of 3.3 lb (1.5 kg) between 6 and 9 months.

B. Gains 3 to 5 oz per week; grows 1 cm a month.

C. Eruption of upper lateral incisors.

II. Gross and Fine Psychomotor Traits

A. Sits well without support.

B. Pulls self to standing position.

C. Stands holding on to furniture; cruises.

D. Bounces actively when held in standing position.

E. Gets to sitting position alone.

F. Pivots while seated.

G. Crawls on hands and knees, purposefully creeping; can crawl backward.

H. Drinks from a cup.

I. Pincer grasp is developing; bangs two blocks together.

J. Attempts to grasp third cube.

K. Hand preference may be noticeable.

L. Mouthing is prominent.

III. Cognitive and Language Traits

A. Produces four or more sounds.

B. Combines two or more syllables but without specific meaning: "da-da," "ba-ba."

C. Will imitate sounds such as clicking of tongue or a cough but does not form words.

D. Responds to own name.

E. Understands "bye"; comprehends "no-no."

F. Understands simple commands.

G. Has one word with specific reference.

H. Imitates animal sounds.

I. All vowels and many consonants present.

    J. More adept with nonverbal communication and gestures.

    K. Listens intently to conversations.

IV. Emotional and Social Traits

    A. Can maintain object constancy; internalizing caring and familiar family members.

    B. Able to trust others; increasing interest in pleasing others.

    C. Interacts in a purposeful, reciprocal manner.

    D. Can ascertain moods and imitate them (e.g., crying when someone cries).

    E. Separation anxiety issues; fear of going to bed and being alone; nighttime rituals important.

    F. Distressed by new and strange situations and people.

    G. Powerful urge toward independence in feeding and locomotion.

    H. Responds to simple requests.

    I. Plays peekaboo and pat-a-cake.

    J. Shows displeasure if activity is inhibited.

V. Psychosexual Traits

    A. No change from 6-month infant.

VI. Moral and Spiritual Traits

    A. May show signs of inhibition or suppression when admonished for inappropriate conduct.

    B. Has sense of awe for caretakers as powerful or preferred people.

TODDLER: 1 TO 3 YEARS

Brain Findings

The number of neurons remains relatively stable while neurons are undergoing vigorous growth and remodeling during the first 3 years. The brain's neuroplasticity is reflected by change in response to experience. Prime times for growth occur in specific brain areas at different times. For example, optimal development of the brain systems responsible for attachment is dependent upon the positive interaction between caregiver and infant during the first year of life. Unhealthy early bonding of caregiver and infant can lead to a fragile, neurological, and emotional foundation for later development of relationships (Perry, 2002).

The brain can compensate or alter itself after insults dependent on timing, intensive intervention, and the nature of the insult. The plasticity of the young brain is more acute than the adult brain.

Animal research supports the fact that more synaptic growth occurs when living in enriched environments versus impoverished environments, which can lead to thinning of neuronal networks (Diamond and Hopson, 1998). Brain functions remain dynamic through practice and use, although current knowledge does not prove that more stimulation will necessarily create smarter children with denser brain systems (Nelson, 2000).

12 Months (48 Weeks)

I. Physical and Anatomical Traits

    A. Weight has tripled since birth.

    B. Head circumference has increased approximately 5 in (12 cm) since birth.

C. Anterior fontanel almost closed.

D. Has grown an average of 10 in (25 cm) since birth.

E. Chest is equal to or slightly greater in circumference than the head.

F. Has total of six to eight deciduous teeth.

II. Gross and Fine Psychomotor Traits

A. Stands without support.

B. Walks holding on to furniture and when both hands are held.

C. Most children walk alone between 12 and 15 months.

D. When sitting, can twist around to pick up an object.

E. Begins to throw things on floor.

F. Neat pincer grasp. Finger feeds.

G. Beginning to use spoon with assistance, much spilling.

H. Can hold crayon.

I. Starts sequential play by separately placing several cubes into container.

J. Waves with wrist.

K. Turns pages of a book many at a time.

III. Cognitive and Language Traits

A. Recognition of personal name.

B. Begins to look where parent points, recognizes objects by name.

C. Understands simple requests (e.g., "give it to me").

D. Discriminates simple geometric forms (e.g., circle).

E. Egocentric pretend play.

F. Actively searches for a hidden object.

G. Generally uses several words in addition to "mama" and "dada."

H. Most words are nouns.

I. Squeals and makes noise for attention and pleasure.

J. Can wave bye-bye and plays pat-a-cake.

K. Vocalizes when spoken to.

L. Expressive jargon: imitates animal sounds, shakes head for no, 25% of language intelligible to an unfamiliar person.

IV. Emotional and Social Traits

A. Reacts to restrictions with frustration.

B. Able to show emotions of fear, anger, affection, and jealousy.

C. May develop attachments to security blanket or favorite toy.

D. Smiles at, pats, or even kisses mirror image.

E. Differences between boys and girls are seen in the way they assert themselves; boys are more assertive.

F. Gives toy to person on request.

G. Plays peekaboo by covering face.

H. Crying usually indicates distress.

I. Rolls ball to another.

V. Psychosexual Traits

A. Gender-specific stereotyped play begins as part of parents' socialization process.

VI. Moral and Spiritual Traits

A. Parents and caretakers are the primary role models for conduct.

B. Infant behavior conforms to approval and disapproval of caring and supervising adults.

18 Months (72 Weeks)

I. Physical and Anatomical Traits
A. Anterior fontanel closed.
B. Gains 4.4 to 6.6 lb per year.
C. For girls, five times their current weight is approximately their future adult weight.
D. For girls, two times their current height is approximately their future adult height.
E. Decreased growth rate results in reduced food intake.
F. Body proportions change: arms and legs grow at faster rate than head.
G. Trunk long and legs short.
H. First four molars have erupted.
I. Some girls physiologically able to control urinary and anal sphincters.

II. Gross and Fine Psychomotor Traits
A. Runs clumsily, falls often.
B. Walks backward.
C. Walks up stairs with one hand held.
D. Creeps downstairs.
E. Seats self on chair.
F. Begins to jump with both feet.
G. Pulls and pushes toys; throws ball overhand.
H. Proficient with finger foods.
I. Takes off some garments occasionally (e.g., shoes, socks, pants).
J. Builds tower of three or four cubes.
K. Uses spoon to feed self without rotation.
L. Turns pages of a book (two or three at a time).
M. Scribbles spontaneously; makes strokes imitatively.
N. Picks up small beads and puts in receptacle.

III. Cognitive and Language Traits
A. Vocabulary increases rapidly, may learn as many as 12 words a day. Correlation reported between highly verbal parent/caregiver and development of language.
B. Uses words to make needs known.
C. May combine two words spontaneously for elementary sentences: "All gone," "Big boy."
D. May repeat end of adult sentences.
E. Remains in jargon phase.
F. Can follow two-directional commands.
G. Favorite words may be *no* and *mine.*

IV. Emotional and Social Traits
A. Solitary play declines and parallel play begins, but still possessive of own toys.
B. Increases pretend play.
C. Frustration may trigger temper tantrums.
D. Siblings and peers become more important for bonding.
E. Beginning to test limits.

V. Psychosexual Traits
 A. Stereotypical gender dress and play is usually promoted by parents.
 B. Aware of being wet or dry; will sit on toilet to imitate adults.
VI. Moral and Spiritual Traits
 A. Comprehension of adult's moral code consists of simple good/bad distinctions.
 B. Verbal sanctions and corporal punishment inhibit nonconformity or oppositional behavior.

24 Months (2 Years)
I. Physical and Anatomical Traits
 A. For boys, five times current weight is approximately their future adult weight.
 B. For boys, two times current height is approximately their future adult height.
 C. Weight gain 4 to 6 lb (1.8 to 2.7 kg) per year.
 D. Height gain of 4 to 5 in (10 to 12.5 cm) per year.
 E. Chest circumference now exceeds head circumference.
NOTE: Head circumference is approximately 19 in (48.5 cm). Little growth takes place after this time; average adult head size is only 19.6 in (50 cm).
 F. Protuberance of abdomen with slight lordosis of the spine.
 G. Wide-spaced gait.
 H. Dry at night (50% of children).
 I. Usually bowel trained but still has occasional accidents.
 J. Most toddlers have 20/60 vision.
II. Gross and Fine Psychomotor Traits
 A. Throws overhand.
 B. Picks up objects from floor without falling.
 C. Walks up and down stairs alone, 2 feet per step.
 D. Runs without falling.
 E. Kicks ball.
 F. Puts on coat with assistance; washes and dries hands.
 G. Uses a straw.
 H. Holds small glass in one hand and drinks with moderate spilling.
 I. Inserts spoon in mouth and does not turn it upside down.
 J. Helps remove clothes.
 K. Puts on shoes, socks, and pants.
 L. Builds a tower of six to seven cubes.
 M. Aligns two or more cubes for a train.
 N. Turns book pages one at a time.
 O. Imitates vertical and circular pencil strokes.
 P. Cuts crudely with scissors.
 Q. Unscrews lids and can turn doorknob.
III. Cognitive and Language Traits
 A. Uses more words than jargon.
 B. Vocabulary consists of 300 words or more; talks incessantly.
 C. Sentences comprise two- to three-word combinations.
 D. May form plurals by adding "s" (doll-dolls).
 E. Uses negative two-word phrases: "no go."
 F. Uses pronouns: "I," "me," "you," "mine."

G. Speech emerges as a way to communicate ideas, needs, and wants (e.g., toilet, food, drink).
H. Can follow two-directional command.
I. Refers to self by given name.
J. Jargon decreases; language 65% intelligible.
K. Difficulty discerning reality and fantasy.
L. Trial-and-error learning; can comprehend simple designs.
M. Knows five body parts, including mouth, nose, tongue, eye, and ear.

IV. Emotional and Social Traits

A. Fear of darkness, ghosts, monsters, and bodily injury.
B. Greater autonomy and independence.
C. Initiates activity rather than just imitating.
D. Time of discovery, curiosity, and social interactions.
E. May become bossy, self-willed, and manipulative.
F. Able to explain feelings and desires using gestures and simple phrases.
G. Generally trusts adults; can be very affectionate.
H. Plays more with siblings and peers; learns simple rules.
I. Shows signs of possessiveness and jealousy.
J. Can regress to more infantile ways with distress or insecurity.
K. Occasionally seeks solitude and quiet when emotionally confused or upset.
L. Parallel play.
M. Reacts strongly to separation from parents.
N. Resists going to bed.
O. Extreme use of "no."
P. World revolves around self.

V. Psychosexual Traits

A. With toilet training, more touching and play with genitalia/anus.
B. Interest in urine and feces.
C. Adults caring for and supervising toddler should teach modesty and model privacy relating to body parts without negativity.
D. Beginning self-control of urination and defecation.

VI. Moral and Spiritual Traits

A. Behavior viewed by adults as immature, naive, stubborn or willful, and defiant.
B. Parents begin socializing toddler in basic rules of conduct, imposing restrictions to teach simple concepts of right and wrong.

30 Months (2½ Years)

I. Physical and Anatomical Traits

A. Birth weight has quadrupled.
B. Has complete set of 20 primary teeth.
C. Daytime bladder control with occasional accidents when absorbed in play.

II. Gross and Fine Psychomotor Traits

A. Jumps in place with both feet off floor.
B. Walks on tiptoes.
C. Balances on one foot for 1 second.
D. Walks backward.
E. Builds tower of eight cubes.

    F. Adds chimney to train alignment.
    G. Imitates horizontal and vertical pencil strokes.
    H. Holds pencil or crayon with thumb and fingers.
    I. Uses fork held in fist.
    J. Unbuttons large buttons.
    K. Removes pull-down clothing.
    L. Dresses and undresses with help.

III. Cognitive and Language Traits
    A. Increased curiosity and simple questions (i.e., why? how come?).
    B. Very one-sided reasoning; cannot understand an issue from two angles.
    C. Conversational with parent; communicates with sentences using two or more ideas.
    D. Vocabulary consists of 450 words or more.
    E. Can understand simple time concepts.
    F. Refers to self by use of pronoun "I."
    G. Knows first and last name.
    H. Dysfluencies are common (i.e., stuttering).
    I. Uses prepositions.

IV. Emotional and Social Traits
    A. Parallel play increases.
    B. Shows sympathy or pity to familiar people.
    C. Tends to be impetuous, contrary.
    D. Dawdling, defiant, or ritualistic.

V. Psychosexual Traits
    A. Knows own sex and begins to notice sex differences.
    B. Self-regulation of bowel and bladder continues.
    C. Pleasure can be associated with excretory function.

VI. Moral and Spiritual Traits
    A. Concepts of right and wrong, or good and bad, are limited.
    B. Obedience is based on fear of sanction or punishment and desire to please.

PRESCHOOLER: 3 TO 5 YEARS

Brain Findings

Normal brain development and learning is a process of making or eliminating synapses (i.e., primarily a building of new cells or clearing away of unused brain cells, apoptpsis). Repeated activation of the cells strengthens neuronal pathways, whereas inactive cells are likely to be pruned.

    The 3-year-old brain has approximately 1000 trillion synapses and is two and a half times more active than an adult's brain and remains that way throughout approximately the first decade of life (Shore, 1997). From birth to approximately 10 years of age, the use of glucose by the cerebral cortex is about twice that of the adult's brain (Chugani, 1998).

3 Years (36 Months)

I. Physical and Anatomical Traits
    A. Protuberant abdomen and lordosis disappear, and child grows thinner.
    B. Develops individual body characteristics as a result of genetics and lifestyle.

    C. Average weight gain 4 to 6 lb (1.8 to 2.7 kg).

    D. Average height gain 2 to 2.5 in (5 to 6.25 cm).

    E. Eruption of deciduous teeth complete.

II. Gross and Fine Psychomotor Traits

    A. Walks and runs without looking at feet.

    B. Jumps off bottom step.

    C. Pedals tricycle.

    D. Catches and kicks a ball.

    E. Broad jumps.

    F. Hangs by hands.

    G. Balances on one foot momentarily.

    H. Goes up stairs, alternating feet but comes down two feet per step.

    I. Eats with fork held in fingers and feeds self well.

    J. Minimal spilling when using cup, glass, or spoon.

    K. Pours from pitcher or bottle.

    L. Prepares simple meals, such as cold cereal.

    M. Snips with scissors.

    N. Builds tower of 9 to 10 cubes.

    O. Imitates a bridge with cubes.

    P. Can copy a circle or cross.

    Q. Makes a circle containing facial features

III. Cognitive and Language Traits

    A. Understands *cold, hungry,* and *tired.*

    B. Names one or two colors but recognizes others.

    C. Uses *why, what,* and *where* questioning.

    D. Continues to talk, even when no one is listening.

    E. Sense of quantity (big or little) emerging.

    F. Vocabulary consists of 900 words; understands 1200 to 2000 words.

    G. Language 90% to 100% intelligible.

    H. Uses consonants *m, n, p, f, h, w* and diphthong *ng.*

    I. Speech is simple; uses three- to four-word sentences.

    J. Uses plurals.

    K. Sentences may not be syntactically correct.

    L. Uses past tense, personal pronouns *I, you, she* and most prepositions, such as *under, on, in front of.*

    M. Hesitation and repetition may be common.

    N. Refers to self as *I.*

    O. Knows first and last name, sex, and often home street name.

    P. May recite favorite nursery rhymes, begins to sing songs.

IV. Emotional and Social Traits

    A. Less jealous of younger siblings.

    B. More interest in playing with others and associative play.

    C. Common coping skills are temper tantrums, crying, negativism, affection seeking, and regression.

V. Psychosexual Traits

    A. Recognizes gender of others.

    B. Learns gender roles and has more sense of privacy and modesty.

    C. Boys identify more with father and male figures.

    D. Has a generalized idea about birth; baby comes out of mommy's stomach.

VI. Moral and Spiritual Traits

A. Some capable of feeling ashamed or guilty in specific situations, but not yet generalized.

B. Will pray with simple words and gestures as imitative behavior.

C. Aware of dangers regarding body safety and pets being disabled or dying.

4 Years (48 Months)

I. Physical and Anatomical Traits

A. Growth rate is similar to previous year.

B. Birth length has doubled.

C. Legs make up 44% of body length.

D. In past year, has gained approximately 4 to 6 lb (1.8 to 2.7 kg) and 2 to 2.5 in (5 to 6.25 cm).

II. Gross and Fine Psychomotor Traits

A. Goes down stairs one foot per step.

B. Skips on one foot, hops on one foot.

C. Catches a ball with extended arms and hands.

D. Enjoys stunts or aerobatics.

E. Puts on shoes and socks without help.

F. Imitates square and diamond with pencil.

G. Draws three parts of a stick man.

H. Laces shoes but may not tie a bow.

I. Washes and dries hands and face.

J. Buttons and unbuttons.

K. Manages front snaps and belts.

L. Removes and puts on pullover garments.

M. Knows front from back of clothing.

III. Cognitive and Language Traits

A. Recalls recent past.

B. Comprehends *big* and *little*.

C. Follows two- or three-directional commands.

D. Asking *why* questions at peak level.

E. Confuses fact with fiction while telling a story; exaggerates.

F. Vocabulary consists of 1500 words or more.

G. Uses consonants; uses four- and five-word sentences.

H. Language almost complete in structure and form. Sentences include adjectives, adverbs, conjunctives, nouns, verbs, and prepositions.

I. Often uses boastful, bossy, and sometimes profane language.

J. May count correctly.

K. Speech should be totally intelligible; however, some sounds may not be complete.

IV. Emotional and Social Traits

A. Very independent, may run away from home.

B. Mood swings.

C. More aggressive physically and verbally with family members.

D. Enjoys associative play (e.g., simple board games).

E. Can make and honor an agreement.

F. Able to control emotions (e.g., crying, laughing).

G. Converses with imaginary playmate or companion.

H. Emotional reaction to dreams, scary or happy.

V. Psychosexual Traits
    A. Stronger identification with parent of opposite sex.
    B. More curiosity and interest in genital area.

VI. Moral and Spiritual Traits
    A. Less egocentrism and more social awareness but still egocentric; displays wishful thinking.
    B. Obeys out of fear of punishment and desire to please.
    C. Concrete sense of justice about possessions or personal hurt and simple fairness constructs.
    D. Animistic beliefs: objects have feelings, consciousness, and thoughts like humans.
    E. Primitive sense of bad or good (e.g., monsters, ghosts, angels).

5 Years (60 Months)

I. Physical and Anatomical Traits
    A. Girls are slightly ahead of boys in skeletal growth.
    B. Hand dominance is developed; about 90% are right-handed.

II. Gross and Fine Psychomotor Traits
    A. Skips on alternate feet.
    B. Jumps rope and jumps over objects.
    C. Tandem walks forward.
    D. Can walk on a balance beam.
    E. Catches a ball with both hands.
    F. Hops two or more times on each foot.
    G. Prints some numbers, letters, and possibly name.
    H. When appropriate, chooses fork over spoon.
    I. Washes and dries self without supervision.
    J. Needs occasional supervision in dress and hygiene.
    K. Manages zipper in back.
    L. Ties shoelaces.
    M. Combs hair with help.
    N. Brushes and rinses teeth.
    O. Wipes self independently and flushes toilet after use.

III. Cognitive and Language Traits
    A. Draws six or more parts of a stick figure.
    B. Knows the names of coins (penny, nickel, etc.).
    C. Follows a three- and four-directional activity.
    D. Knows opposites, such as large and small.
    E. Understands concepts of same and different.
    F. Knows time-associated words, such as days of the week and months.
    G. May know own right and left hand, but cannot identify on others.
    H. Vocabulary consists of 2200 words.
    I. Uses consonants "t," "v," "l," and "th."
    J. Uses sentences consisting of five to eight words.
    K. Language is generally complete in terms of structure and form.
    L. Uses different forms of sentences, including complex sentences and conditional clauses.
    M. Recognizes object pronouns (her, him, them).

IV. Emotional and Social Traits
    A. Less rebellious and quarrelsome than at age 4.
    B. Takes increased responsibility for actions; more trustworthy.

    C. Eager to please.

    D. Capable of expressing emotions through drawings, drama, game playing.

    E. Able to verbalize motivation and meaning of different emotions.

    F. Expresses sorrow or hurt if encouraged or instructed.

    G. Shows preferences for specific playmates and fondness for certain family members.

V. Psychosexual Traits

    A. Strongly identifies with interests and activities of same-sex parent.

    B. Dramatic play enacting parent role in same sex behavior (e.g., playing house).

    C. Transition of negative feelings toward parent of opposite sex to positive feelings.

    D. Engages in gendered play on occasion, pretending to be married or have babies.

    E. Greater interest in sexual body parts and questions about birth.

    F. Aware of adult sexual organs.

VI. Moral and Spiritual Traits

    A. Able to tell right from wrong; knows when behavior is good or bad, according to adult standards.

    B. Internalizing adult standards and values, beginning of social conscience.

    C. Begins to question parents' thinking and principles.

    D. Can play games by rules but may cheat to avoid losing.

    E. May notice prejudice and bias in outside world.

    F. May have been trained to express spirituality through rituals of singing, reciting sacred words, or praying.

    G. Increased questions and imagination about ultimate life concerns (e.g., death, suffering, higher power, creation, wonders of nature).

ELEMENTARY/LATENCY CHILD: 6 TO 12 YEARS

Brain Findings

The brain forms trillions of synapses and organizes them into networks of neural pathways, or "maps." When continuously used, these networks become a relatively permanent part of the brain's circuitry; however, if not repeatedly used, they can be eliminated.

    The prefrontal cortex undergoes a growth spurt and makes an overabundance of new synapses. The pruning of these synapses occurs in different parts of the brain at different times and is part of the maturational process. The relatively short attention span during prepubescent years is related to the fact that the *reticular activating system (RAS)* only becomes fully myelinated at or after puberty. This region of the brain is found in the *medulla oblongata* and is involved in maintaining attention and overall level of arousal.

    The *hypothalamus* activates, controls, and integrates the endocrine system. The cerebral centers trigger the endocrine system to initiate major body changes from puberty through adulthood. The *endocrine system*

Continued

includes the *pituitary, thyroid, parathyroid* and *adrenal glands, ovaries, testes,* and *islets of Langerhans* in the pancreas. Figure 1-4 shows the endocrine system and the developing characteristics of puberty.

EARLY ELEMENTARY: 6 TO 8 YEARS

I. Physical and Anatomical Traits

A. Binocular vision well developed.

B. Begins to lose primary teeth.

C. Permanent teeth appear at the rate of four per year.

D. Considerable variation in height and weight.

NOTE: From 6 to 12 years, height and weight growth shows a sex-related difference. Girls tend to gain slightly less weight each year than boys. Growth in height is similar for both sexes; however, boys tend to be a little taller until approximately age 12.

E. Larger and stronger muscles; good coordination related to posture, locomotion, and activity.

II. Gross and Fine Psychomotor Traits

A. Constant activity; difficulty sitting still.

B. Roller skates.

C. Hops on alternating feet

D. Clumsy and awkward movements.

E. Tandem walks backward.

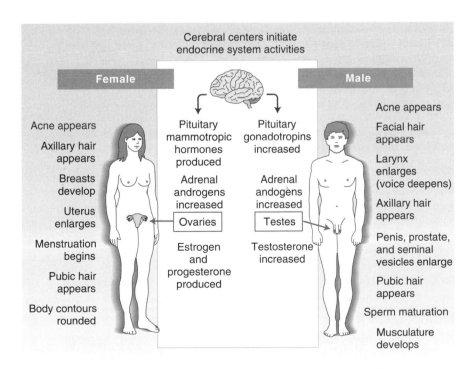

FIGURE 1-4 The endocrine system and developing characteristics of puberty.

F. Dexterity increases but still has imprecise small-muscle coordination.
G. Clumsy pencil manipulation.
H. Some reversals of letters.
 I. Knows right from left.

III. Cognitive and Language Traits
A. Drawing of a person includes neck, hands, and clothes.
B. Few articulation errors.
C. Corrects own grammar.
D. Majority of 5- to 17-year-olds use the computer and over half use the Internet.

IV. Emotional and Social Traits
A. Capable of a wide range of emotional states, ideas, and thinking.
B. Identified with a primary temperament style of relating.
C. Capable of emotional self-regulation and control appropriate to different situations.
D. Understands family group in terms of birth order, parental pair, and sibling group.
E. Definite acceptance of an affinity to a racial, ethnic, and religious group.
F. Shares and cooperates more.
G. Often jealous of younger siblings.
H. Imitates adults.
 I. Behavior is unpredictable, agreeable, and loving one minute, disliking everything and everyone the next.
J. Demanding of others.
K. Compulsive about winning and does not lose gracefully.
L. Needs and enjoys company of peers but tattles on others.
M. Likes active games and rough play.
N. Difficulty making decisions.
O. Tells tales.

V. Psychosexual Traits
A. Knows gender differences, identifies with sex roles, and has a primary sexual orientation as to preference and affinity.
B. Experiences sensual pleasure and sexual arousal through masturbation or manipulation of genitals.
C. Capable of discerning socially acceptable mores or customs regarding toileting, physical touch, and dress codes.

VI. Moral and Spiritual Traits
A. Parents viewed as the ultimate or primary authorities for good conduct.
B. Internalized hierarchy of values about reality enables simple moral decisions.
C. Greater respect for law rather than mere fear of law.
D. Able to find personal security with simple faith in higher power and to associate a personal worth in the care of the higher power for self and others.

MIDDLE ELEMENTARY: 8 YEARS

I. Physical and Anatomical Traits
A. Growth rate approximately 2 in (5 cm) per year.
B. Arms grow longer in proportion to body.
C. More limber; bones grow faster than ligaments.
D. Continues to lose baby teeth; has 10 to 11 permanent teeth.

II. Gross and Fine Psychomotor Traits
   A. Gradual increase in rhythm and smoothness of movements; strength and endurance increase.
   B. Constantly on the go: jumping, skipping, chasing, and so on.
   C. Long-distance throwing.
   D. Fine motor control smoother and speed increased.
   E. Uses common tools (e.g., hammer and saw).
   F. Helps with household tasks; assumes responsibility for certain household chores.
   G. Likely to overdo; hard to quiet down after recess.
   H. Writes in cursive.
   I. Uses knife for cutting.
   J. Prepares for bathing and can carry out task when reminded.
   K. Clips, cuts, and files fingernails and toenails.
   L. Styles hair with a comb.

III. Cognitive and Language Traits
   A. Concentration, memory, and recall are substantial, allowing for learning and academic gains.
   B. Understands abstract vocabulary; uses compound and complex sentences.
   C. Ability increases for developing creative aptitudes in art and music.
   D. Special interests (e.g., coin, baseball or other card collecting, computer technology) become emerging hobbies.
   E. Reads for enjoyment; likes pictorial magazines.

IV. Emotional and Social Traits
   A. Relationships with parents and family are strengthened with domestic life (e.g., chores, games, leisure activities, camping, and organized sports).
   B. Involved with peers in group activities but has one or two best friends at school or in the neighborhood.
   C. Prefers certain friends and groups
   D. Dramatic and emotionally expressive.
   E. Likes to compete and play games; enjoys school.
   F. Dislikes doing things alone.
   G. More critical of self and more sensitive to criticism from others.
   H. Likes to select own clothes.
   I. Still likes to be tucked in at bedtime.
   J. Social manners are better but still need improvement.
   K. Friendly and gregarious.
   L. Argues; wheels and deals.
   M. Concerned with parental approval and disapproval.
   N. Prefers immediate reward for work (preferably money).

V. Psychosexual Traits
   A. Prefers same-sex friends and companions.
   B. Girls may begin puberty with release of sex hormones; boys may experience onset 2 or 3 years later.
   C. Usually both boys and girls are modest and self-conscious about their bodies but curious about sex differences; body-image issues emerge.

VI. Moral and Spiritual Traits
   A. Sense of morality determined by family value system and rules.
   B. Likes reward systems and seeks recognition for good behavior.

C. Influenced by authority figures and seeks role models, heroes, and so on.

D. Learning to distinguish natural from supernatural (e.g., can see cause and effect in a natural realm, fantasy and reality, wishing and faith).

E. Receptive to religious training, understanding dogma and performing rituals.

MIDDLE ELEMENTARY: 10 YEARS

I. Physical and Anatomical Traits

A. Because of slowing height growth and an increase in weight gain, tendency toward obesity at this age.

B. High energy level.

II. Gross and Fine Psychomotor Traits

A. Able to engage in complex physical activities; can excel in competitive organized sports.

B. Almost equal to fine motor skills of an adult.

C. Makes things and does small repair work.

D. Does simple paintings and drawings.

E. Takes responsibility for care of hair but may need reminding.

F. Can wink alternately.

III. Cognitive and Language Traits

A. Good reality testing with distinct boundaries between fantasy and wishful thinking.

B. Seeks to be logical; able to engage in elementary levels of inductive and deductive reasoning.

C. Can be multilingual or proficient in more than one language.

IV. Emotional and Social Traits

A. Parents and siblings remain as primary reference groups but peers become more significant.

B. Other adults at school, church, temple, and youth organizations become role models, mentors, and ego ideals.

C. Respects parents; tends to idolize both and enjoys their company.

D. Exhibits sharp outbursts of anger, which are brief and explosive, but does not bear grudges.

E. Can tolerate frustration.

F. Tends to be "cliquey," especially girls.

G. Likes belonging to clubs (scouts) and forms own.

H. Girls have "best friends" and like small, intimate groups.

J. Tends toward hero worship.

K. Still separates into like-sex groups for games and activities.

L. Cries when angry.

V. Psychosexual Traits

A. Masculine and feminine roles learned with more confidence and mastery. Figure 1-4 depicts the developing characteristics of puberty for both males and females.

B. Most girls are either preparing for menstruation or have developed secondary sex characteristics (e.g., breast enlargement).

C. Boys are conscious of body build and are more interested in the opposite sex, especially the more mature girls.

D. Refer to Figure 1-5 for Tanner's stages of development for girls and boys.

VI. Moral and Spiritual Traits
A. Opposes cheating.
B. More aware of different value systems and ethical orientations given the wider exposure to neighbors, school, Internet, movies, and community organizations.

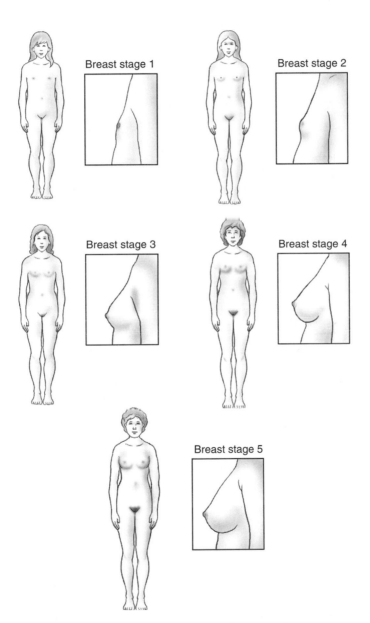

FIGURE 1-5 Tanner Stages of Development. **A,** Female breast development stages.

Continued

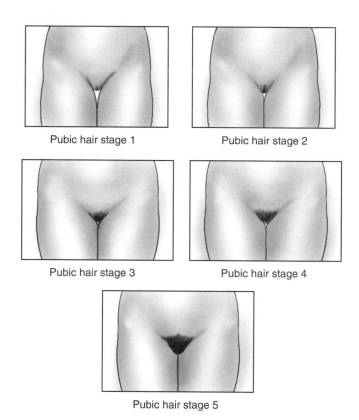

Pubic hair stage 1

Pubic hair stage 2

Pubic hair stage 3

Pubic hair stage 4

Pubic hair stage 5

FIGURE 1-5, **cont'd** Tanner Stages of Development. **B,** Female pubic hair stages.

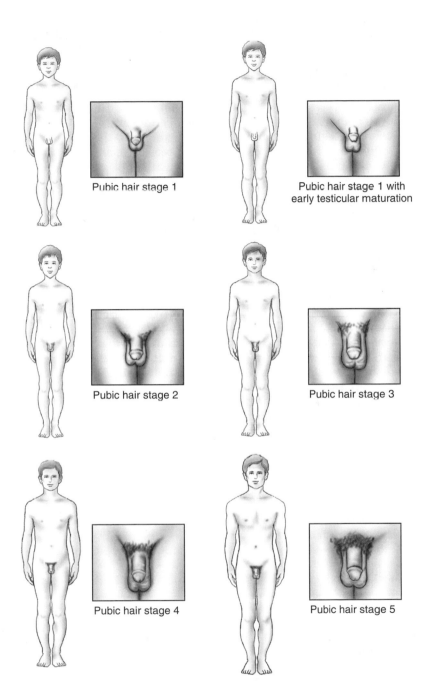

Pubic hair stage 1

Pubic hair stage 1 with early testicular maturation

Pubic hair stage 2

Pubic hair stage 3

Pubic hair stage 4

Pubic hair stage 5

FIGURE 1-5, cont'd Tanner Stages of Development. **C,** Male breast development and pubic hair stages.

C. Maintains law-and-order approach to morality.

D. Generally concerned about being good, obeying authorities, and treating others with fairness and kindness.

LATE ELEMENTARY: 12 YEARS

I. Physical and Anatomical Traits

A. Onset of puberty or sex-hormone activation, which somewhat determines body size, energy level, and somatic integrity.

B. Menarche begins between 9 and 15 years in girls. Usually cannot reproduce for 1 to 2 years after menarche because of anovulation.

C. Boys attain puberty between 12 and 16 years.

D. Girls tend to be larger than boys.

E. Body lines begin to soften and round out in girls.

F. Posture more similar to an adult.

G. Between 12 and 14 years, all permanent teeth have erupted except for third molars and wisdom teeth.

II. Gross and Fine Psychomotor Traits

A. Participates intensely in activity, then suddenly reaches saturation point and collapses.

B. Enjoys gross motor activities, but now capable of more refined motor activities.

III. Cognitive and Language Traits

A. Vocabulary and speech patterns more conforming to peer terminology and slang.

B. Enjoys conversation, especially with peers and friends.

IV. Emotional and Social Traits

A. Hormonal changes influence emotionality, leading to mixed feelings, moodiness, or outbursts.

B. Desires more independence from parents, challenging authority and testing limits.

C. Concerned about peer acceptance and having close peer relationships; may have a best friend.

D. Girls are prone to segregate into twosomes; girls enjoy talking about boys.

E. Earning money is a good motivator.

V. Psychosexual Traits

A. More intense curiosity about sexual anatomy, reproduction, and gender behavior.

B. Secondary sex characteristics become apparent (e.g., increased size of genitals and coarseness of pubic hair).

C. Usually more self-conscious with a need for privacy and a desire for modesty.

D. Enjoys group activities that involve both sexes; may show interest in opposite sex.

VI. Moral and Spiritual Traits

A. Interpersonal issues regarding privacy, dress, speech, public manners or etiquette, and respect for adults have an ethical meaning in terms of right or wrong, good or bad.

B. Beginning of doubt or questioning about the family's religious practices, relevance of spirituality, and general philosophical outlook on life.

Growth and Development Characteristics

ADOLESCENCE: 13 TO 19 YEARS

Brain Findings

In early adolescence, the elimination of synapses seems to be the dominant process. In late adolescence, approximately one half of all synapses have been discarded, which is part of a natural process that makes the brain more efficient. The overabundance of connections appears to make room for a complex system of neural pathways. Repeated experiences strengthen synaptic networks, which tend to become permanent.

Prefrontal cortex is not fully developed, whereas the emotional area is actively developing; this may be thought of as the emotional area overriding the prefrontal area, or emotional response versus logic and reasoning. This may help explain why adolescents are often more emotional and impulsive than adults.

Tendencies to act impulsively and misjudge dangerous situations also may be related to a genetic predisposition, or it may be the result of brain chemical differences found in individuals. These tendencies are strongly influenced by environmental factors—such as dysfunctional family life, drugs, alcohol, violent television and movies, or electronic games that romanticize gunplay—and are a function of the prefrontal cortex. During adolescence, many of the changes in the brain are not established by genetics but by experience.

Parietal lobes continue to mature through the middle-teen years and are believed to integrate information from sensory signals that are visual, auditory, and tactile.

Sex hormones change the brain's structural arrangement, including emotional centers, and may precipitate thoughts about sex. Testosterone production increases during puberty, which influences the activity of the amygdala and may produce feelings of fear and anger. This is more pronounced in the male but may account for increased aggressiveness and irritability in both sexes. Increased levels of estrogen influences the growth of the hippocampus, and this structure may develop to become proportionally larger in females. Estrogen and testosterone surges may have a profound influence on moodiness and sex drive.

Myelination of axons in brain regions related to regulation of emotion, judgment, and impulse control occurs earlier in female adolescents. Male myelination may not catch up until about age 30.

EARLY ADOLESCENCE: 13 TO 15 YEARS

I. Physical and Anatomical Traits

   A. Height and weight vary according to genetic endowment, nutrition, sleep patterns, and exercise.
   B. Growth decelerates in girls; stature reaches 95% of adult height.
   C. Marked increase in muscle mass in boys related to androgen.
   D. Self-conscious about deformities, disabilities, or disease.
   E. Personal hygiene practices governed by adult exhortations and peer pressure.
   F. Requires an average of 9¼ hours of sleep (Howard, 2006; Parker, Zuckerman, and Augustin, 2005). Deprivation can interfere with learning, behavior, and safe driving.

G. Insomnia is experienced by 10% to 20% of adolescents (Behrman, Kliegman, and Jenson, 2000). Adolescents need to start school later, instead of earlier, than other ages to ameliorate the disruption of circadian rhythms that occurs at the onset of puberty (Howard, 2006).

II. Gross and Fine Psychomotor Traits

A. Capable of wide range of endurance; coordination of body mastery dependent on temperament, physical aptitude for sports, and adult expectations (parents, teachers, youth workers).

B. Has limited cooking and sewing skills.

III. Cognitive and Language Traits

A. Usually has an identifiable level of learning and academic achievement as low, average, or high.

B. Most of the intellectual growth influence is centered at school or associated with teachers as an ego ideal.

C. Concerned with philosophical, political, and social problems.

D. Has idealistic and rich fantasy life.

IV. Emotional and Social Traits

A. Pushes for more independence and disengagement from parents.

B. Is capable of emotional intensity and wide range of feelings yet marked by insecurity and less than predictable self-control.

C. Social orientation to the peer group, usually relates to older youth; very aware of degrees of popularity or acceptance, which is accompanied by a fear of rejection.

D. Begins to take initiative toward establishing a stable boyfriend/ girlfriend relationship.

V. Psychosexual Traits

A. Most youth will come into puberty and seek an acceptable feminine or masculine orientation.

B. Some youth experiment with sex, but most cope with sexual impulses, fantasies, and genital gratification through masturbation.

C. Learning about the facts of life and sexual knowledge is accelerated with peer information most influential.

D. Exploration of body appeal and physical attraction to opposite sex.

VI. Moral and Spiritual Traits

A. More inward and introspective about life. Generally concerned about being a responsible youth with care, tolerance, honesty, and industry.

B. Able to foresee future implications of current behavior.

C. Able to project a persona of goodness; critical about being phony or hypocritical regarding values and beliefs.

MIDDLE ADOLESCENCE: 15 TO 17 YEARS

I. Physical and Anatomical Traits

A. Most growth spurts have occurred.

B. Height growth usually ceases at 16 to 17 years for girls.

C. Adult cardiovascular rhythms are developed by age 16.

D. By age 17, muscle mass is two times greater in boys than girls, resulting in strength two to four times greater in boys.

II. Gross and Fine Psychomotor Traits

A. Similar to the 13- to 15-year-old youth.

III. Cognitive and Language Traits
A. Has capacity for hypothetical reasoning and increased abstract thinking.
B. Shows interest in political and social issues.
C. Is able to make decisions with conceptual ability to foresee long-term consequences.
D. Is idealistic and has a rich fantasy life.

IV. Emotional and Social Traits
A. Is capable of the emotional intensity and wide range of feelings of an adult.
B. Has distinctive feelings of omnipotence and exceptionality, which promotes greater risk-taking behavior.
C. Views self from the standards of an adult in terms of maturity and responsibility.
D. Greatest need is to distinguish oneself from parents and have one's own identity or degree of separateness.
E. Usually relates upward for a reference group and friendship.

V. Psychosexual Traits
A. Generally pursues close, affectionate, and sexual relationships with the opposite sex.
B. Faces peer pressure to be sexually active but is pressured by adults to be sexually conservative.
C. Sexual feelings may be felt toward same-sex and/or opposite-sex peers, causing gender orientation confusion and concern.
D. Can be very secretive about sexual behavior with a great need to present a sophisticated persona of sexual adequacy.

VI. Moral and Spiritual Traits
A. Is capable of wise moral judgment about self-care, relationships, and lifestyle.
B. Is capable of formal operational thinking that allows for exploring the deeper meaning of religious symbols and rituals.
C. Can be sensitive to issues of fairness, justice, charity, and authority or power.
D. May become very religious and invested in transcendental spirituality, or may reject religion and be indifferent to spiritual reality.
E. Can identify passionately with religious leaders, such as Moses, Jesus, Malcolm X, Muhammad, and Mother Theresa.

LATE ADOLESCENCE: 17 TO 19 YEARS

I. Physical and Anatomical Traits
A. Physically mature with reproductive growth almost complete.
B. Height growth usually ceases at 18 to 20 years for males.

II. Gross and Fine Psychomotor Traits
A. Is well developed with coordination and agility.
B. Possesses the dexterity and precision movements similar to an adult.

III. Cognitive and Language Traits
A. Is capable of formal cognitive operations, including abstract thinking, complex problem solving, and prepositional reasoning.
B. Is capable of advanced reasoning skills and rigorous thinking.

    C. Can articulate ideologies and engage in philosophical discourse.

    D. Can be aware of intellectual strengths and usually has a realistic perspective on success at higher learning beyond high school.

IV. Emotional and Social Traits

    A. Physical and emotional separation from parents more complete.

    B. Generally can distinguish emotional states and has acceptable emotional self-regulation.

    C. Emotional disturbances or disorders may be diagnosed and treated similar to an adult.

    D. Peer orientation has become at least as significant as relating to adult family members and other adults.

    E. Usually has close association with a peer group with common ethnic, civic, occupational, or religious interests.

    F. Concerned about having special friendships and being in an intimate relationship.

V. Psychosexual Traits

    A. Strong erotic and affectionate feelings are being integrated for loving relationships with the opposite sex or same sex; capable of forming intimate relationships.

    B. Conscious of sexual maturity and experience with a personal need to enjoy adult sexuality according to legal and social norms.

VI. Moral and Spiritual Traits

    A. More social pressures to go beyond an egocentric orientation to life with a caring and tolerant code of ethics.

    B. Development of a personal value system.

    C. More emphasis on subjective and internal aspects of religious life and less active participation in organized and institutional religion.

    D. Membership in a religious cult often associated with psychosocial stress and identity diffusion.

    E. Interpersonal and personal wrongdoing capable of being adjudicated as an adult criminal.

    F. Capable of having a credo for life that conforms to the highest universal and transcendent principles and precepts.

YOUNG ADULT: 19 TO 21 YEARS

Brain Findings

The brain has tripled in weight from that at birth. The increase in weight is primarily a function of the increase in support cells, such as glial and myelin cells. Maturation continues throughout the twenties, and learning takes place throughout life.

NOTE: With all maturational growth completed, young adults must find personal success and social support with the developmental tasks listed below:

- Acceptance of the physical/biological endowment, temperament, and gender identity that represents their unique, personal self.
- Emancipation from family dependence to become an emotionally, financially, and legally responsible adult.
- Completion of the necessary education and training to secure a meaningful occupation.

- Establishment of caring and committed peer relationships for the fulfill-ment of sexual and affectionate love and companionship needs.
- Accomplishment of lifestyle decisions about marriage, parenthood, and family life.
- Adoption of a personal system of values for social, moral, and legal well-being.
- Maintenance of a realistic yet fulfilling philosophy of life and a spiritual frame of reference to cope with the ultimate issues of aging, disease, exis-tential anxiety, suffering, death, and immortality.

ADOLESCENT GENDER DEVELOPMENTAL CHARACTERISTICS

MALE

- Appearance of facial hair; fuller eyebrows.
- Muscle development and strength increase steadily.
- Face elongates; mouth and jaw become fuller; voice deepens.
- Shoulders rapidly increase in breadth.
- Axillary, body, and pubic hair appear.
- Growth of penis, testes, and testicles increases.
- Skin color on scrotum darkens.
- Erections increase and nocturnal emissions occur.
- Spermatozoa produced.
- Androgen hormone produced.
- Reproductive organs mature at about 12 to 18 years.
- Between ages of 12 and 16 years, gains 4 to 12 in (10 to 30 cm) in height and 15 to 65 lb (7 to 30 kg) in weight.
- Height growth usually ceases at about 18 to 20 years.

FEMALE

- Voice becomes fuller and slightly deeper.
- More subcutaneous fat.
- Axillary and perineal hair appear.
- Breasts develop a more rounded shape; nipples enlarge and protrude; areo-las enlarge.
- External genitalia enlarge.
- Pelvis enlarges and hips widen.
- Ovulation and menstruation begin.
- Estrogen hormone produced.
- Reproductive organs mature at about 10 to 16 years.
- Between 10 and 14 years, girls gain 1 to 8 in (5 to 20 cm) in height and 15 to 55 lb (7 to 25 kg) in weight.
- Height growth usually ceases at 16 to 17 years.

GENDER DEVELOPMENT

MALE AND FEMALE

- Accelerated growth begins earlier in girls.
- Skeletal system growth exceeds growth of supporting muscles.
- Large muscles develop faster than small muscles.
- Body odor becomes evident.

- Attains maximum growth; ossification takes place.
- Skin texture coarsens, pores enlarge, and sebaceous glands become more active, which often causes acne.
- Rapid growth of neck, arms, legs, hands, and feet in comparison to trunk occurs.
- Extremities reach adult size before the trunk does.
- Jaw becomes fuller as adult size is reached; mandible in boys is wider and lower.
- Gonadotropic hormones present in urine.

WEB SITES

Centers for Disease Control and Prevention, Child Development
   http://www.cdc.gov/ncbddd/child/devtool.htm
Dana Foundation and the Dana Alliance
   http://www.dana.org
Developmental Pediatrics Online
   http://www.dbpeds.org
Federal Interagency Forum on Child and Family Statistics
   http://www.childstats.gov
Society for Neuroscience
   http://www.sfn.org
Zero to Three
   http://www.zerotothree.org

BIBLIOGRAPHY

American Academy of Pediatrics: Developmental surveillance and screening of infants and young children, *Pediatrics* 108 (1):192-196, July 2001 (available online): http://aappolicy.aappublications.org/cgi/content/full/pediatrics%3b108/1/192.

Bear MF, Conors BW, Paradiso MA: *Neuroscience: exploring the brain,* Baltimore, 2007, Lippincott Williams & Wilkins.

Behrman RE, Kliegman RM, Jenson HB: *Nelson textbook of pediatrics,* Philadelphia, 2000, WB Saunders.

Blum D: *Sex on the brain: the biological differences between men and women,* New York, 1997, Penguin Putnam.

Carper J: *Your miracle brain,* New York, 2000, HarperCollins.

Carter R: *Mapping the mind,* Los Angeles, 1999, University of California Press.

Chess S, Thomas A: *Temperament and development,* New York, 1986, Brunner/Mazel.

Chugani HT: Biological basis of emotions: Brain systems and brain development, *Pediatrics* 102:1225-1229, 1998.

Coles R: *The moral intelligence of children,* New York, 1997, Random House.

Coles R: *The spiritual life of children,* Boston, 1990, Houghton Mifflin.

Damon W: The moral development of children, *Sci Am* 281:72-78, 1999.

Damon W: *The moral child: nurturing children's natural moral growth,* New York, 1988, Free Press.

Davies D: *Child development: a practitioner's guide,* New York, 2004, Guilford Press.

Diamond MC: *Enriching heredity: the impact of the environment on the anatomy of the brain,* New York, 1988, Free Press.

Diamond MC, Hopson J: *Magic trees of the mind: how to nurture your child's intelligence, creativity, and healthy emotions from birth through adolescence,* New York, 1998, Penguin Putnam.

Dixon SD, Stein MT: *Encounters with children,* Philadelphia, 2006, Mosby.
Elkind D: *The development of the child,* New York, 1978, Wiley.
Erikson E: *The life cycle completed,* New York, 1985, WW Norton.
Fowler JW: *Stages of faith: the psychology of human development and the quest for meaning,* San Francisco, 1981, Harper & Row.
Freud A: *Normality and pathology in childhood: assessment of development,* New York, 1965, International Universities Press.
Gardner H: *Multiple intelligences: the theory in practice,* New York, 1993, Basic Books.
Gesell A, Armatruda CS: *Developmental diagnosis,* New York, 1947, Haber.
Glaser D: Child abuse and neglect and the brain—a review, *J Child Psychol Psychiatry* 41(1):97-116, 2000.
Greenfield SA: *The human brain: a guided tour,* New York, 1997, Basic Books.
Greenspan SI: *First feelings: milestones in the development of your baby and child,* New York, 1985, Viking Press.
Havighurst RJ: *Human development and education,* New York, 1953, David McKay.
Havighurst RJ: *Developmental tasks and education,* New York, 1952, Longman Publishers.
Hockenberry MJ, Wilson D, Winkelstein ML: *Wong's essentials of pediatric nursing,* St Louis, 2005, Mosby.
Hooper J, Teresi D: *The 3-pound universe,* New York, 1986, Dell.
Howard PJ: *The owner's manual for the brain,* Austin, Tex, 2006, Baird Press.
Huttenlocher PR, Dabholkar AS: Regional differences in synaptogenesis in human cerebral cortex, *J Comp Neurobiol* 387 (2):167-178, 1997.
Kagan J: *The nature of the child,* New York, 1984, Basic Books.
Kohlberg L: *The philosophy of moral development,* San Francisco, 1981, Harper & Row.
Kotulak R: *Inside the brain: revolutionary discoveries of how the mind works,* Kansas City, Mo, 1996, Andrews and McMeel.
LeDoux J: *The emotional brain,* New York, 1996, Simon & Schuster.
Maslow AH: *Motivation and personality,* New York, 1970, Harper & Row.
Moir A, Jessel D: *Brain sex: the real difference between men and women,* New York, 1991, Dell.
Nelson CA: Neural plasticity and human development: the role of early experience in sculpting memory systems, *Dev Science* 3:135-136, 2000.
Osborn LM, DeWitt TG, First LR et al, editors: *Pediatrics,* Philadelphia, 2005, Mosby.
Perry BD: Childhood experience and the expression of genetic potential: what childhood neglect tells us about nature and nurture, *Brain Mind* 3:79-100, 2002.
Pert C: *Molecules of emotion,* New York, 1997, Scribner.
Piaget J: *The origins of intelligence in children,* New York, 1952, International Universities Press.
Schaefer CE, DiGeronimo TF: *Ages and stages: a parent's guide to normal child development,* New York, 2000, John Wiley & Sons.
Siegel D: *The developing mind: toward a neurobiology of interpersonal experience,* New York, 1991, Guilford Press.
Shore R: *Rethinking the brain: new insights into early development,* New York, 1997, Families and Work Institute.
Squires J, Potter L, Bricker D: *The ages and stages questionnaires: a parent-completed, child-monitoring system,* Baltimore, Md, 1995, Paul H. Brookes.
Swedo S, Leonard HL: *Is it just a phase? How to tell common childhood phases from more serious disorders,* New York, 1998, Golden Books.
Sylwester R: *A celebration of neurons: an educator's guide to the human brain,* Alexandria, Va, 1995, Association for Supervision and Curriculum Development.
Wahlstrom K: Changing times: findings from the first longitudinal study of later high school start times, *Natl Assoc Secondary Sch Principals Bull* 86 (633):1-19, 2002.

CHAPTER 2

Vision and Hearing

Chapter Outline

*V*ision and hearing problems are the "quiet debilitators." Often defects in these two important senses are so subtle that they are unnoticed until educational or significant medical implications emerge. Because vision and hearing problems generally begin in a child's critical years of development, early detection and diagnosis are vital so that medical treatment and rehabilitation can begin sooner, physical or behavioral complications can be avoided or minimized, and long-term educational implications can be eliminated or reduced. Such measures ensure that the child will have a fuller and more productive life.

Ideally, the first visual and hearing screening should occur when the newborn is in the nursery. Universal newborn hearing screening is becoming the standard so infants will receive early, optimal intervention for language development. Tests for the infant and very young child do not obtain acuities or thresholds; testing relies on elicitation of responses from various forms of stimuli. The younger the child, the more general the screening procedure.

Any nurse who works with infants and young children can play a major role in early detection of a vision or hearing deficit. The nurse has the opportunity to observe behavior, listen to parental concerns, and, in many instances, perform developmental, hearing, and vision screening. The school nurse is often the first person to observe and screen an older child with a vision and hearing problem.

Once the nurse suspects a vision or hearing problem, an appropriate referral should be initiated. Depending on the circumstances, the referral is made to the attending physician or one or more specialists, such as an ophthalmologist, optometrist, otolaryngologist, or audiologist.

Various vision and hearing problems occur in children and young adults. This chapter addresses the more common problems and presents major characteristics of vision and hearing development, a list of high-risk conditions that impair infants, screening methods, and certain testing procedures. Useful glossaries and acronyms of vision and hearing terms are listed at the end of their respective sections.

Information regarding vision, hearing, and brain development has been added to this chapter. Technology and research have prompted a new awareness of the importance of early vision and hearing deprivations. Torsten Wiesel and David Hubel won the Nobel Prize in 1981 for two very significant discoveries. They found that even with an intact brain, if an individual does not process visual experiences early in life, he/she will not be able to see due to the absence of cortical stimulation. They demonstrated that organization of the adult visual cortex is dependent on early visual experiences; and after that sensitive time period has passed, significant deficits occur in the visual cortex; e.g., cataracts prevent seeing visual experiences; therefore, if not removed early infant will be blind.

Other discoveries demonstrated that if words are not heard by age 10, the individual will never totally learn his/her native language as the brain cells will migrate to other functioning areas (Kotulak, 1996). The developing postnatal brain differs from that of an adult; thus, this period of early critical experiences is essential for brain development in the sensory systems.

Figures 2-1 to 2-4 illustrate the basic structures of the eye and ear and the pathways and mechanics that enable vision, hearing, and the understanding of a language.

The cross-section depicts the lens in each eye, focusing light on the retina and inverting the image. Receptors in the retina convert the image into nerve impulses that travel along the optic nerve to the optic chiasm, where half of the nerves from each eye cross over to the other side of the brain, continuing on alternate pathways to the visual cortex. What is seen in the right half of the visual field is transmitted to the left hemisphere of the brain, and what is seen in the left half of the visual field is transmitted to the right hemisphere. Each hemisphere is aware of what the other perceives as visual information flows back and forth.

The visual cortex lies within the occipital lobes. Other visual association areas are located in various areas of the cerebral hemispheres; these areas interpret visual images. See Figures 1-1 and 1-2, pages 3-4.

Sound is perceived in both the left and right sides of the auditory cortex in the brain from impulses received by both ears. The left hemisphere translates sound impulses into meaning and is the language-processing center of the brain. The auditory cortex receives incoming impulses; the angular gyrus links vision to Wernicke's area, whereas Wernicke's area supplies the meanings of words, and Broca's area controls the mechanics of speech.

MAJOR CHARACTERISTICS OF VISUAL DEVELOPMENT

Cortical neuronal dendritic growth and synaptic information begins in the twenty-fifth week of gestation. This growth is extremely active around birth and continues into the first 2 years of life. In human infants, the maturity of the visually evoked potential has been correlated with the degree of dendrite information (Hoyt, Jastrzebski, and Marg, 1983). Vision depends on human experiences to enhance neuronal connections.

The visual development for the full-term, healthy infant is described in the following text.

I. Prenatal
   A. The lens of the eye begins to develop about the twenty-seventh day of embryonic growth with differentiation of the lens capsule.

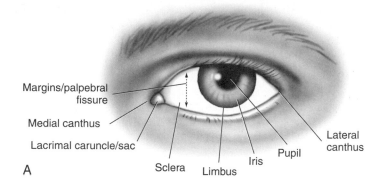

Margins/palpebral fissure
Medial canthus
Lacrimal caruncle/sac
Lateral canthus
Pupil
Iris
Sclera   Limbus
A

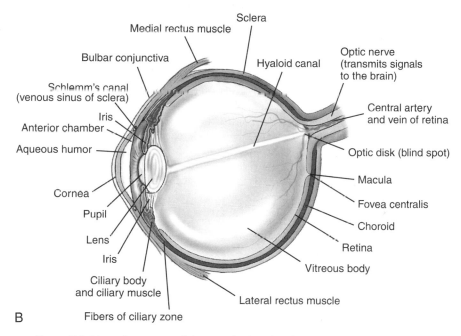

Sclera
Medial rectus muscle
Bulbar conjunctiva
Hyaloid canal
Optic nerve (transmits signals to the brain)
Schlemm's canal (venous sinus of sclera)
Iris
Anterior chamber
Central artery and vein of retina
Aqueous humor
Optic disk (blind spot)
Cornea
Macula
Pupil
Fovea centralis
Lens
Choroid
Iris
Retina
Ciliary body and ciliary muscle
Vitreous body
Lateral rectus muscle
B   Fibers of ciliary zone

FIGURE 2-1 Normal structure of the eye. **A,** Anterior view. **B,** Cross-sectional view.

B. Eyes are completely formed by the fifteenth week of gestation.
C. Cortical neuron dendrite growth and synaptic information begins in the twenty-fifth week of gestation.
D. Eyelids are fused with a thin membrane until the end of the twenty-eighth week.
E. Pupils respond to light between the twenty-ninth and thirty-first weeks.
F. Premature infants are normally myopic because of the elongated anterior-posterior diameter of the globe.

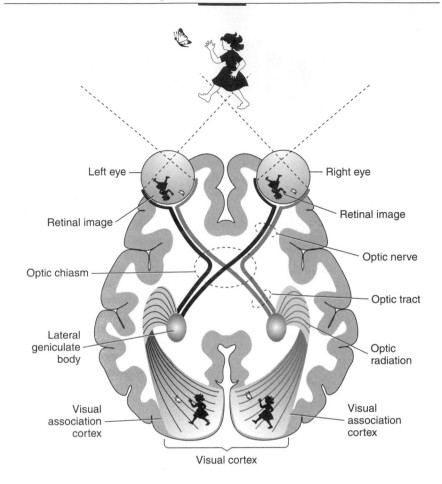

FIGURE 2-2 Visual pathway.

II. Birth to 4 Weeks
NOTE: Some techniques devised for assessing visual acuity in infants use the evoking of optokinetic nystagmus, visually evoked potentials (VEPs), and preferential looking. These methods often indicate an infant's visual acuity to be much better than previously reported.

    A. Cortical neuronal dendrite growth and synaptic information is remarkably active around birth.

    B. Some neural pathways that relay information from the retina to the brain may be immature.

    C. Pupils usually are constricted for several weeks.

    D. Measurable color discrimination is possible by 2 weeks; the infant needs brighter colors and larger objects than do adults.

    E. Visual acuity is 20/400 to 20/600, regardless of type of visual testing, because of the short diameter of newborn eye, retinal immaturity, and incomplete myelination of the optic nerve.

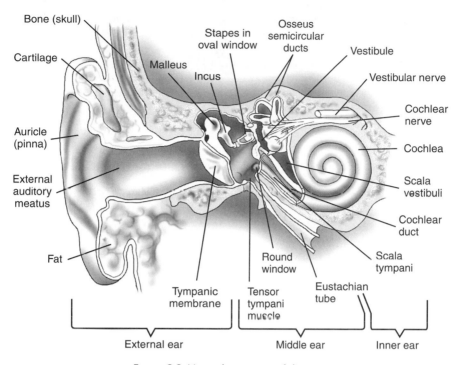

Bone (skull)

Cartilage

Malleus

Incus

Stapes in oval window

Osseus semicircular ducts

Vestibule

Vestibular nerve

Cochlear nerve

Cochlea

Auricle (pinna)

Scala vestibuli

External auditory meatus

Cochlear duct

Fat

Round window

Scala tympani

Tympanic membrane

Tensor tympani muscle

Eustachian tube

External ear

Middle ear

Inner ear

FIGURE 2-3 Normal structures of the ear.

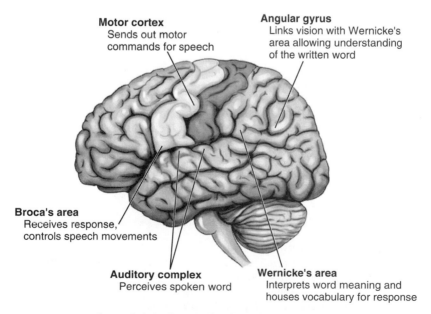

Motor cortex
Sends out motor commands for speech

Angular gyrus
Links vision with Wernicke's area allowing understanding of the written word

Broca's area
Receives response, controls speech movements

Auditory complex
Perceives spoken word

Wernicke's area
Interprets word meaning and houses vocabulary for response

FIGURE 2-4 Auditory processing of sounds in the brain.

    F. Eye's size is approximately ½ to ¾ the size of an adult eye; however, the cornea is almost adult size at birth, thus babies appear to have "huge" eyes.

    G. Newborn can fixate on moving object in range of 45 degrees.

    H. Eyes move independently.

    I. Newborn sees and responds to illumination; after exposure to bright light will refuse to open eye.

    J. Newborn blinks, squints, or may sneeze when exposed to bright lights.

    K. Newborn fixates on contrasts (e.g., black and white).

    L. Eye and head movements are not coordinated (doll's-eye reflex present).

    M. Newborn is generally hyperopic or farsighted because of immaturity of the lens of the eye and spherical nature of the globe.

    N. Large-angle or severe strabismus at birth should be evaluated immediately.

    O. Box 2-1 lists high-risk conditions for visual impairment for a newborn.

III. 1 Month (4 Weeks)

    A. Infant fixates on face and objects about 8 to 12 in (acuity 20/100 to 20/200) and can follow object.

    B. Vision is hyperopic or farsighted.

    C. Infant can fixate on large moving object in range of 90 degrees.

    D. Tear glands start to function.

    E. Intermittent alignment deviations may be present; (normal).

    F. Infant watches parents intently when they speak.

IV. 2 Months (8 Weeks)

    A. Visual acuity is 20/60 to 20/200, depending on type of visual testing.

    B. Lateral peripheral vision is equal to adult or older child—90 degrees each eye.

    C. Myelination completed around 2½ months.

    D. Blinking, protective reflex, present between 2 and 5 months.

    E. Binocular vision and convergence on near objects begins at 6 weeks.

    F. Follows moving object with eyes; movement may be jerky.

Box 2-1	*High-Risk Conditions for Visual Impairment of the Newborn*

Perinatal	*Postnatal*
Family history	Premature or low birth weight
Maternal rubella	Retinopathy of prematurity (ROP)
Syphilis, gonorrhea	Meningitis/encephalitis
Chlamydia	Herpes infections
Toxoplasmosis	Histoplasmosis
Cytomegalovirus	Disorders: albinism, cataracts, hydrocephalus, retinoblastoma, sickle cell disease
Herpes infections	Trauma: birth

V. 3 Months (12 Weeks)
  A. Infant regards hand.
  B. Convergence established.
  C. Saccades are well developed.
  D. Doll's-eye reflex has disappeared.
  E. Infant can follow moving object from side to side (range of 180 degrees).
  F. Smooth pursuit well developed.
  G. Infant briefly able to fixate on near objects.
  H. Infant reaches toward toy.
  I. Infant charmed with bright objects, color preference for bright yellows and reds.
  J. Visualmotor coordination emerges.
  K. Eyes parallel most of the time.

VI. 4 Months (16 Weeks)
  A. Visual acuity 20/60 to 20/200, depending on type of testing.
  B. Binocular vision fairly well established.
  C. Differentiation of fovea complete.
  D. Color vision closer to that of an adult.
  E. Tears are present.
  F. Infant fixates on 1-in cube.
  G. Infant recognizes familiar objects (e.g., feeding bottle).
  H. Infant observes mirror images.
  I. If strabismus is suspected, referral should be made by 4 to 6 months of age.

VII. 6 Months (24 Weeks)
  A. Visual acuity 20/20 to 20/150, depending on type of testing.
  B. Stereoscopic vision well developed by 3 to 7 months.
  C. Color of iris can be determined.
  D. Infant adjusts position to view objects.
  E. Infant watches falling toy.
  F. Eye-hand coordination is developing.
  G. Smooth eye movements apparent in all directions.
  H. Color preference for bright reds and yellows is developing.
  I. No deviation from parallelism exists.

VIII. 9 Months (36 Weeks)
  A. Ability to discern fine details is at adult level by age 6 to 9 months.
  B. Depth perception development begins between the seventh and ninth month.
  C. Ability to fuse two retinal images begins to mature.
  D. Can fixate on and follow object in all directions.
  E. Infant attentive to environment.
  F. Infant observes activities of people and animals with sustained interest within distance of 10 to 12 ft.

IX. 1 Year (12 Months)
  A. Visual acuity 20/20 to 20/60, depending on type of testing.
  B. Cornea is adult in size (12 mm), and eye muscles are reaching adult level of functioning; can fixate and follow object in all directions.
  C. Macula will mature by the end of first year.

D. Toddler tracks rapidly moving objects.

E. Toddler recognizes familiar people at 20 ft or more.

F. Toddler can place peg into small hole and stack blocks.

X. 1½ Years (18 Months)

A. Convergence well established.

B. Toddler fixates on small objects.

C. Toddler sees and points to distant interesting object outdoors.

XI. 2 Years (24 Months)

A. Toddler has potential for 20/20 acuity.

B. Optic nerve myelination completed by 7 months to 2 years.

C. Eye is 85% of adult size.

D. Accommodation well developed.

E. Toddler fixates on small object for 60 seconds.

F. Toddler recognizes fine details in picture books.

XII. 3 Years (36 Months)

A. Visual acuity is 20/20 as measured by VEPs; in some 3 year olds, by subjective measures.

B. Convergence smooth.

C. Child copies geometric designs: circle, cross.

XIII. 4 Years (48 Months)

A. Visual acuity 20/20.

B. Tear (lacrimal) glands are completely developed.

C. Child can distinguish shapes and letters.

XIV. 5 Years

A. Visual acuity 20/20.

B. Depth perception developed.

XV. 7 to 10 Years

A. Eye achieves full globe size between 5 and 7 years.

B. Hyperopia continues until approximately age 7 years.

C. By 9 years, the visual system is mature enough to resist effects of abnormal visual stimulation.

D. Continuation of synapse development in visual cortex to approximately 10 years.

E. Amblyopia likely if causative/contributing factors are not detected and treated.

XVI. 12 Years

A. Eye growth is complete between 10 and 12 years.

REFRACTIVE ERRORS

ASTIGMATISM

I. Definition

A. Astigmatism is a refractive error in which light rays are refracted different at two or more points, because of the irregularity of the cornea, producing a distorted image. May occur along with myopia or hyperopia.

II. Etiology

A. Astigmatism may be caused by an irregularly shaped or defective curvature of the cornea or lens, which creates unequal refraction of incoming light rays in different meridians. This prevents the eye from focusing clearly on an image. Astigmatism may be congenital or acquired.

III. Signs, Symptoms, and History
Dependent on severity of refractive error in each eye:
A. Higher astigmatism.
  1. Blurred vision.
  2. Squinting; eye rubbing.
  3. Tilting or turning of the head.
  4. Reading material held close to eyes.
B. Lower astigmatism.
  1. Tired eyes.
  2. Blurred vision.
  3. Frontal headache.
C. Mild astigmatism.
  1. There may be no symptoms.

IV. Effects on Individual
A. Safety concerns; susceptibility to accidents because of blurry vision.
B. Difficulty with near and/or distance activities, such as close schoolwork and chalkboard activities, depending on associated visual error. Child may tire quickly with reading assignments and seem easily distracted.
C. May have same clinical manifestations as myopia.

V. Management/Treatment
A. Correction for refractive errors that creates a uniform surface (cornea or lens) through which light rays may pass, such as lenses (glasses or contacts). It is corrected with a combination of plus and minus lenses to fit the individual curvature of the astigmatic eye (Anshel, 2007).
B. Rescreen at appropriate intervals.
C. Be cautious of a child who does not like to wear the new glasses. Astigmatism corrections usually require an adaptation period. Check with prescribing doctor if doubt exists.

VI. Additional Information
A. Most people's eyes are not perfectly symmetrical; thus, they may have small amounts of astigmatism. Astigmatism is common in infants. High astigmatism can result in amblyopia.

MYOPIA

I. Definition
A. Commonly called *nearsightedness*, myopia is the inability to see objects at distance. Myopia is a refractive error in which parallel light rays from a distant object focus in front of the retina, causing images at a distance from the individual to appear blurred. Figure 2-5 illustrates the distortion caused by myopia, as well as hyperopia and astigmatism, and corrections for each condition.

II. Etiology
A. Myopia may be caused by an elongated anterior-posterior diameter of the eyeball or a cornea curve that is too severe, thereby refracting the light rays too much. Heredity plays a role in myopia.

III. Signs, Symptoms, and History
   A. Blurred distance vision.
   B. Unusual posturing.
   C. Squints at distant object to sharpen vision.
   D. Rubs eyes frequently.
   E. Headache, but rare.
   F. Dizziness.
   G. Nausea after close work, but rare.
   H. Holds book close to face (severe or high myopia); however, this behavior is normal behavior between 4 and 7 years. It is also a first sign of a problem.
   I. Depending on classroom seating, unable to see whiteboard or chalkboard or at home, television.
   J. Fails distance vision testing.
IV. Effects on Individual
   A. Difficulty participating in sports or playground activities.
   B. Safety concerns; may walk into objects, inability to read road signs.
   C. May miss whiteboard or chalkboard instructions if not sitting at front of classroom.
   D. Academic performance *may* be affected if myopia severe or/and seating cannot be changed.
V. Management/Treatment
   A. Correction, if indicated, with concave (minus) lens to focus rays on retina: either fitted glasses or contact lens may be used; or corneal surgery in older children to reduce corneal curvature (see Figure 2-5).
   B. Surgery: laser techniques to reduce curvature of the cornea. These surgeries can be performed as early as 18 years, but typically should not be done before the eye has stopped growing.
   C. Recheck periodically with and without prescribed glasses to see if error remains corrected.
VI. Additional Information
   A. Growth produces visual changes, so child may need new eyeglasses every 1 or 2 years. Generally stabilizes around the mid-teen years.

HYPEROPIA
I. Definition
   A. Commonly called *farsightedness,* hyperopia is the inability to see objects clearly at close range. Hyperopia, also termed *hypermetropia,* is a refractive error in which parallel light rays focus behind the retina, causing images close to the individual to appear blurred. In middle age, hyperopia is confused with *presbyopia* which is caused by the decreased elasticity of the crystalline lens.
II. Etiology
   A. Hyperopia may be caused by insufficient length of the eyeball or by a lens that is too flat (unresponsive) to bend light rays adequately, thereby causing an image to focus beyond the retina, or by an inadequately curved cornea.

III. Signs, Symptoms, and History

A. Blurred vision at close range.

B. Tired eyes when focusing for prolonged periods of time.

C. Pain in the eyes.

D. Frontal headaches.

E. Eye strain after long periods of reading or writing.

F. Lines appear to run together while reading.

NOTE: Symptoms A to F intensified when individual is tired or ill.

G. Light sensitivity.

H. May fail visual screening.

I. Esotropia or an inward (medial) deviation of one or both eyes from parallelism.

J. Fails near vision testing.

IV. Effects on Individual

A. Schoolwork may suffer, and child may be unable to keep up with classmates.

B. Teachers may expect only poor academic achievement.

C. Student is more easily irritated because of constant eyestrain.

D. Student may be nervous during school visual tasks (e.g., reading, computer work).

E. Student may develop poor self-esteem if vision is affecting academic achievement or performance in playground activities.

V. Management/Treatment

A. Correction with use of convex (plus) lenses (glasses or contacts) to focus rays on retina (see Figure 2-5).

B. Correction may be necessary in children with only a moderate degree of hyperopia and no other symptoms or a strabismus.

C. Recheck periodically, with and without prescribed glasses, to determine whether error remains corrected.

VI. Additional Information

Most infants are hyperopic, and children continue to be so until they reach about 5 to 7 years, when normal development elongates the eyeball. These children can accommodate to objects at close range. If the child is truly hyperopic, the continual muscular effort of accommodation may cause eyestrain to result in strabismus (esotropia) or amblyopia. Hyperopia is measured in plus diopters rather than as a Snellen notation.

ANISOMETROPIA

I. Definition

A. Anisometropia is present when a different refractive power is present in each eye. In many states, difference in visual acuity of two or more lines following distance or near vision testing is cause for a referral. Anisometropia makes it difficult for the two eyes to function together.

II. Etiology

A. When refractive errors in the eyes differ, the muscle relaxation or contraction of one eye attempts to correct the vision for the better eye but the vision in the other eye may worsen. The condition may be congenital or acquired as a result of disease or asymmetrical changes that occur with age.

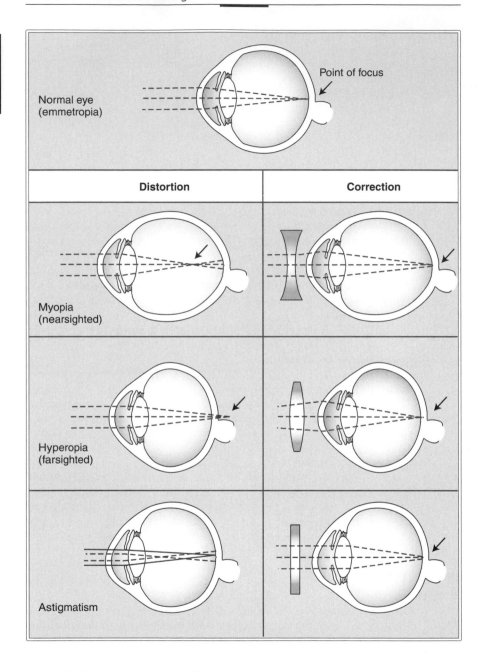

FIGURE 2-5 Refractive errors displaying point of focus, distortion of globe, and lens correction. *Arrow* indicates point of focus, or fovea. Astigmatism could have both convex and concave surfaces and not necessarily flat.

III. Signs, Symptoms, and History
  A. Dependent on severity of the refractive error in each eye.
  B. Clinical manifestations may be the same as those of myopia or hyperopia.

IV. Effects on Individual
  A. A child's brain may ignore the visual image from the weaker eye (cortical suppression); if suppression is prolonged, amblyopia can result.
  B. Eyes generally appear normal and remain straight; screening is necessary to detect anisometropia.

V. Management/Treatment
  A. Corrective lenses improve the vision in each eye, allowing them to function as a unit.
  B. Any deviation in parallelism (strabismus) should be identified and corrected.

VI. Additional Information
  A. This condition should be identified and treated as soon as possible because it can lead to amblyopia in children younger than 7-9 years.

COLOR DISORDERS

COLOR DEFICIENCY/ABSENCE

I. Definition
  A. Color deficiency or absence is the inability to distinguish between the primary colors red, green, and blue. In color deficiencies, photochemical receptors in the cones are diminished while in color absence, there is an actual lack of one or more of three receptors. Color vision is a function of central vision in the fovea cones of the eye. When stimulated by light, the cones transmit impulses to the brain. The cones facilitate discernment of color and detail while the rods are sensitive to movement and light; helps one adjust to darkness. Deficiencies or absences range from mild to severe. Color blindness, or the complete absence of all three photochemical receptors in the cones, is rare but limits vision to black, white, and gray shades.

II. Etiology
  A. Color disorders are a defect inherited as an X-linked recessive trait that primarily affects the male population. The gene for color vision may not be faulty, but the gene that chemically triggers the color vision gene to function may be defective. Occasionally, a color disorder may be acquired from injury, disease (sickle cell anemia, diabetes), or certain drugs (antibiotics, chlorpromazine [Thorazine]); however, most incidences are about 4% hereditary. In any given classroom, about 4% of the students may have color disorders. Approximately one half the populations of a group of children are male; therefore, about 4% of a given class will be color-affected. Deficiencies/absences in the green photochemical receptors are the most common; blue receptors are the least common. Color disorders can affect many areas of life, including education, safety, and some occupational choices.

CHAPTER 2

Vision and Hearing

III. Signs, Symptoms, and History
A. Unable to discriminate colors, particularly reds and greens.
B. Difficulty learning primary colors.
C. Family history of a color disorder.
D. Child fails pseudoisochromatic screening or other acceptable color vision testing.

IV. Effects on Individual
A. At early age, unable to follow directions about coloring materials.
B. Teacher and student may become frustrated because of student's inability to learn colors and perform other color-related tasks.
C. Child may become frustrated and be identified as nonachiever in classroom.
D. Child may be teased by other children.
E. Child has difficulty matching and coordinating colors for personal dress.
F. Child may be perceived as a difficult student or not intelligent.
G. Student must seek guidance and counseling regarding career goals in relationship to color confusion.

V. Management/Treatment
A. Color screen all boys upon first entrance to school. Rescreen if results are questionable. Check state law and district policy if testing limited to boys only.
B. No known complete correction. However, a variety of methods to allow the individual to distinguish various colors are available: use of light and filters; red or green overlay on colored text; X-Chrom lens (one red contact in one eye), ColorMax lenses, (lens coated to filter certain colors). The efficacy of these methods needs further investigation.
C. Parents, teachers, and other professionals must be aware of the color disorder. They must further understand that the student could say that grass is green and a tree trunk is brown but yet not perceive color accurately and is only repeating what he or she is told, thus compensating for the disorder by masking the problem.
D. Student usually learns to distinguish colors by own system of assigning brightness or location. Teacher and parent can help student to articulate this process for the child to maximize learning.
E. Provide guidance for adolescents regarding driving issues and color difficulties that may be related to high school and college course work, vocational plans, and possible military goals.
F. Career plan limitations depend on degree of deficiency.
G. Color difficulties that could affect college education and career plans include interior decorator, commercial pilot, law enforcement, firefighter, some electrical and chemical engineering, cosmetology.
H. Color-affected children may have trouble with colored marker writing on whiteboards and do better with black-white contrasts.

VI. Additional Information
A. All cases of color deficiency/absence differ; some individuals see all colors if shown one at a time but are unable to identify colors when they are mingled. Still others (e.g., green color confusion) may see gray, white, or yellow in daylight, and others report the green traffic

light at night looks the same as street lights, rendering this a useless traffic cue.

B. The color-defective male inherits the deficiency from his mother. Heterozygous females (carriers) have one recessive gene for color deficiency and one dominant gene for normal color vision. The male Y chromosome does not carry a color discrimination gene. Color deficiency results when genes cross over during meiosis, causing an alteration in the red or green cone pigments. The crossover may result in a hybrid, the loss of a gene, or duplication of the gene (does not cause problem). If a female has X genes for color blindness from her father and normal X genes from her mother, she is a carrier, half her sons will be color defective and half her daughters carriers. If the chromosome inherited from her mother is defective for color vision and she also inherits a defective X chromosome from her father, she herself will be color-defective. If she marries a normal male, all her daughters will be carriers and all her sons affected. If she marries a color-defective male, all her children, both male and female, will be affected.

CLASSIFICATIONS OF COLOR BLINDNESS

Three basic groups of anomalous trichromatism or dichromatism exist; monochromatism is rare.

1. *Protanomaly/protanopia:* Bold red is seen as black or as nonexistent. Affected individuals seem to need an abnormal amount of red or have no sense of red color vision. Red-orange and yellow-green may be seen as brown. May say red and green are the same color but will see two different browns. Red deficiency, protanomaly, is 1% of male population while protanopia, red absence, also has a 1% prevalence rate (Proctor, 2005).

2. *Deuteranomaly/deuteranopia:* Difficulty with green; deuteranomaly is the most common form of color deficiency (5%). Often have problems with red-green discrimination. Can identify color if contrasted with another color in good light. Can choose red and green from package of colored papers, but if handed a red or green crayon and asked for the color, they may be puzzled. Red-green weakness produces trouble along the "tomato line" in the white light spectrum. The prevalence of deuteranomaly, green deficiency, and deuteranopia, green pigment absence, are found in about 1% of the male population (Proctor, 2005).

3. *Tritanomaly/tritanopia:* Problems with blue, yellow, or both colors. Often acquired but not inherited. May see blue and yellow as white; see mint green or pink as equal to light blue. Tritanomaly, blue deficiency, is 1/100 of 1% of the male population while tritanopia, blue absence, is 1/10 of 1% (Proctor, 2005).

NOTE: Traffic lights in most areas in the United States may not be a problem because of the consistent placement of colors. Also, the red and green in the traffic lights are not pure colors. However, persons with severe red-green color disorders often have trouble with traffic lights at night.

Color Vision Screening Tests

Pseudoisochromatic Plates for the Older Child and Adult Pseudoisohromatic plates are the most commonly used screening tests used in the United States schools. The plates have colored mosaic figures or numbers on heavy cardstock paper. Natural sunlight or fluorescent lighting is recommended for the best viewing; and the student can identify the shapes by either using a cotton tipped applicator, clean small paintbrush, or by identifying the image seen on the paper. Follow the instructions included with the test material. Several brands of plates are sold. The American Optical Hardy-Rand-Rittler (AO H-R-R) plate is again available. The test detects the kind of color deficiency and provides a severity rating such as mild, moderate or severe. Other tests are the Ishihara, Good-Lite Color Test, and the Dvorine. For young children, the Color Vision Testing Made Easy (CVTME) is available.

Other newer tests are: Farnsworth F-2 test (the latest of many Farnsworth color tests), and Quantitative Color Vision Test PV-16, by Lea Hyvärinen who created the Lea Symbols.

Color names are used to represent human feeling, moods, and thoughts, such as "I feel blue," "she is white as a ghost," or "draw the colors of the rainbow." Colors also signal danger, such as red or yellow in nature. Human beings use colors for verbal communications, to learn from color-coded materials, as adjectives or nouns in language, or to enjoy and remember their environment and joy in nature.

BINOCULAR DISORDERS

STRABISMUS

I. Definition

A. Strabismus is an abnormal deviation of ocular alignment. When the optic axes are not directed simultaneously to the same object, the eyes are gazing in different directions and not in alignment. Strabismus is often used as a connotation for a *heterotropia* or *tropia*. The terms are used interchangeably.

II. Etiology

A. Numerous causes of strabismus exist; the most common is extraocular muscle imbalance. With disorders of binocularity, the eyes do not function equally either in tandem or in perception of images. The underlying causes are refractive errors; anisometropia; extrinsic muscular dysfunction; or, less commonly, organic disease. Amblyopia may develop when the brain suppresses vision in the deviating eye due to diplopia, (double vision) intolerable to the developing cortex.

III. Signs, Symptoms, and History

A. Parents of a newborn state that the child's eyes cross.

B. Complaints of diplopia; younger children are unable to describe or express this symptom.

C. Tilts head when reading.

D. Closes one eye to see or rubs eyes.

E. Frequently blinks or squints eye.

F. Absence of red reflex and/or fails *Brückner* test.

IV. Effects on Individual

A. May appear clumsy and awkward because of unequal vision and poor depth perception.

B. Poor self-esteem if the strabismus is apparent to others.

C. Awkward writing skills.

D. Young child has difficulty doing puzzles, block building, and other fine motor tasks that affect development of preacademic skills.

E. Unable to see moving objects or prints easily.

V. Management/Treatment

A. Restore normal visual acuity in each eye by patching, glasses, or vision therapy.

B. Eyeglasses, surgery, or a combination of surgery and eyeglasses.

C. Botulinum toxin injections temporarily weaken the stronger muscle, which allows the weaker muscle to strengthen. May need to be repeated to achieve orthotropia (absence of strabismus).

VI. Additional Information

A. There are four types of strabismus: (1) *esotropia*, an inward or medial deviation of one or both (rare) eyes; (2) *exotropia*, an outward or lateral deviation of one or both (rare) eyes; (3) *hypertropia*, an upward or superior deviation of an eye; and (4) *hypotropia*, a downward deviation of an eye. Esotropia, convergent strabismus, may be nonparalytic or paralytic. Nonparalytic (comitant) esotropia is the most common type in infants and children. The angle of deviation in the deviating eye is constant in all areas of gaze. The two types of nonparalytic esotropia are nonaccommodative and accommodative.

B. Nonaccommodative esotropia manifests early in life, often at birth but generally by the first year. The condition can be congenital or acquired. The cause is related to abnormalities of the eye or its development rather than refractive error. Treatment is surgery.

C. The onset of accommodative esotropia is usually between 18 months and 4 years of age. The deviation is usually greater for near than for far, is often monocular, but may be alternating. The child is commonly hyperopic. Accommodative esotropia is the most common of the esotropias. If treatment is delayed, amblyopia may develop depending upon the severity of the hyperopia. Treatment is eyeglasses first.

D. Paralytic (noncomitant) esotropia results from birth injury or congenital anomaly and is seen much less frequently than comitant esotropia. The angle of deviation in the deviating eye varies in all directions of gaze. May require surgery.

E. *Exotropia* (divergent strabismus) is less common in infants and children than esotropia. The prevalence increases with age. Exotropia may be intermittent, constant or alternating. The onset of intermittent exotropia generally is not noted before the age of 2 or 3 years. Exotropia may be secondary to high, uncorrected myopia. There is usually a greater exotropia for distance; fusion occurs for near vision. Intermittent exotropia may progress to constant exotropia. Treatment consists of eyeglasses, vision therapy or surgery. Constant exotropia is less common than intermittent exotropia. The condition may be present at birth or progress from intermittent to constant exotropia. The onset may occur later in life if the condition is related to loss of vision in one eye. Constant exotropia is usually monocular but may be alternating. Myopia of varying degrees of severity is often associated with constant exotropia. The treatment is eyeglasses, vision therapy or surgery.

F. *Hypertropia* is a vertical deviation of one eye and may be paralytic or nonparalytic. In paralytic hypertropia, the amount of deviation varies according to the direction of the gaze. Hypertropia is treated with prismatic lenses (glasses). In nonparalytic hypertropia, the angle of deviation is always the same and does not depend on the direction of the gaze. The treatment is eyeglasses, vision therapy, or surgery.

G. *Pseudostrabismus* is the appearance of strabismus as a result of prominent epicanthal folds or a wide-bridged nose. A small portion of the medial aspect of the eye, particularly the white sclera, is covered, creating an illusion of strabismus. The cover/uncover and corneal light reflex tests (Hirschberg test) differentiate between true and pseudostrabismus. As children grow, the flat nasal bridge develops, lifting the excessive epicanthal skin, which corrects the condition.

H. *Hypertelorism* is a disproportionate growth of the facial bones. As a primary deformity, it may cause wide-spaced separation of the eyes. The eyes appear exotropic even though they are perfectly straight. Testing for deviations determines whether the eyes are normal.

AMBLYOPIA

I. Definition

A. Amblyopia is a visual condition associated with reduced visual acuity in one eye as a result of suppressed cortical response in the occipital lobe. In children, vision in one eye is suppressed to avoid seeing double. Unfortunately, the condition often is called *lazy eye.* Except in unusual circumstances; i.e., organic causes, so-called functional amblyopia occurs in an otherwise normal eye.

II. Etiology

A. The four primary causes of amblyopia are: (1) uncorrected strabismus (usually esotropia), (2) anisometropia (unequal refractive errors in each eye), (3) high, uncorrected hyperopia and (4) physical occlusion, such as ptosis, cataract, or deprivation, such as prolonged enclosure in dark places. Heredity plays a role; can be functional or organic. Organic causes can include optic atrophy, macular scar, or anoxic occipital brain damage. Amblyopia is usually a result of changes in the occipital lobe and less likely from specific damage to the eye (e.g., deterioration of fovea/macular degeneration). Functional amblyopia is referred to as those conditions in which the visual acuity deficit may be reversible with occlusion therapy (patching of unaffected eye) and treatment of refractive errors provided that treatment is initiated early enough. Classifications include: strabismic amblyopia, (unilateral distortion of form caused by amblyopia, usually anisometropia), ametropic amblyopia (significant bilateral refractive errors), deprivation amblyopia (impaired clarity of image formed on retina in infancy), and occlusion amblyopia (prolonged occlusion of normal eye).

III. Signs, Symptoms, and History

A. Eyes may cross or wander.

B. Child shuts or covers one eye.

C. Avoids close work.

    D. Squints.

    E. Two-line difference or more between eyes in acuity testing at near or far distance.

    F. May have no symptoms, making adequate screening critical.

IV. Effects on Individual

    A. If condition remains untreated, there is loss of central vision in weaker eye.

    B. Child may be considered clumsy or lacking in motor development because of poor depth perception.

    C. During correction, child may become upset when good eye is patched. Patching may cause skin irritation caused by adhesive materials, however, there are nonabrasive materials available.

V. Management/Treatment

    A. Refractive amblyopia needs early correction of visual acuity. Treatment of the underlying refractive error or alignment deviation, occlusion therapy or both.

    B. With strabismic amblyopia, force use of the weaker eye by covering the better eye (occlusive therapy). Later in treatment, patching may be alternated because amblyopia may be induced in the better eye if eye is covered for too long.

    C. Other amblyopic corrections include eye drops to blur vision in the good eye as an alternative to patching, or, as a last resort, surgical correction.

VI. Additional Information

    A. Disease or damage of the remaining good eye will cause low vision or lateral blindness. Strabismic amblyopia should be corrected in the first two years of life. Refractive amblyopia should be corrected during the first 5 to 6 years of life; thereafter, treatment becomes more difficult. If left untreated, the condition can cause profound and irreversible visual loss in the affected eye. Success depends on compliance to treatment and degree of condition. Close follow-up by preschool nurse or personnel and vision specialist is critical. Childhood amblyopia is the most frequent cause of visual loss in adults.

OTHER VISUAL CONDITIONS

ALBINISM

I. Definition

    A. Albinism refers to a group of genetic conditions that affect the pigment cell system (melanocyte) causing reduction or absence of normal pigmentation of the eye, hair, and skin. The altered gene does not allow the production of normal amounts of pigment called *melanin*. Albinism causes alteration in vision as a result of ocular changes.

II. Etiology

    A. Several different types of albinism exist and are caused by alterations at six different genes. The two main categories of albinism are (1) oculocutaneous albinism (OCA), in which the degree of melanotic pigment of the eyes, skin, and decreased visual acuity varies and (2) ocular albinism (OA), in which the melanin pigment is normal or only slightly diluted in the skin and hair. OCA is more common than OA.

Albinism can be inherited as autosomal recessive and X-linked OA; rarer forms are associated with a variety of other anomalies. The incidence of albinism is listed in "Additional Information."
  B. The altered gene prevents normal melanin pigment development. Melanin pigment absorbs ultraviolet light to protect the skin and other areas from sunlight. Melanin is present in the retina and the fovea of the retina; and if it is not present, these structures do not develop appropriately.
  C. The nerve connections between the retina and certain parts of the brain are altered if melanin is not present during development.

III. Signs, Symptoms, and History
  A. Decreased visual acuity, farsightedness, nearsightedness, and astigmatism common.
  B. Nystagmus, strabismus, and photophobia may be present.
  C. Iris color usually blue-gray or light brown.
  D. Iris pigment is reduced; iris is translucent to light but develops and functions normally in these children.

IV. Effects on Individual
  A. Children with albinism can function well in a mainstream classroom environment provided that they have specific attention to their special visual needs.
  B. Infant and preschool services (birth to age 5) are available through federally mandated services, Individuals with Disabilities Education Act (IDEA).
  C. May use a head tilt and commonly hold the written page close to eyes while reading.
  D. Often hyperactive with short attention span; personal safety at risk.
  E. Psychosocial and self-esteem are issues of concern.

V. Management/Treatment
  A. Symptomatic treatment with routine, on-going, low-vision care.
  B. Usually do not tan but burn easily in the sun.
  C. Need sunscreen, hats, dark glasses to prevent overexposure to sun and other special clothing for outdoor play.
  D. Benefit from written materials that have a black-on-white high contrast, large-type textbooks, audiotapes, computers, and various optic devices.
  E. Optic devices can include handheld monocular, video enlargement machine (closed circuit television), telescopic lenses mounted over eyeglasses, and other types of magnifiers.
  F. Provide copies of the teacher's board notes which can be helpful for older students.

VI. Additional Information
  A. Approximately 1 in 17,000 people has a type of albinism. In the United States, approximately 18,000 people are affected.

CATARACTS
I. Definition
  A. In a cataract, the crystalline lens located behind the pupil becomes cloudy or opaque. Cataracts may be monocular, binocular, complete, or partial and can be on or in the lens or capsule. Cataracts impair vision and may cause blindness.

II. Etiology

A. Cataracts may be congenital, hereditary, or caused by an infectious process or metabolic condition. They also can result from trauma, inflammation, radiation, degeneration, and long-term administration of corticosteroids. The many types of cataracts are classified by morphology (size, shape, location) or etiology (cause or time of appearance).

III. Signs, Symptoms, and History

A. Blurred vision.

B. Absence of red reflex.

C. Gradual, progressive, painless loss of vision.

D. Occasional double vision in affected eye.

E. Gray opacity in lens.

F. Nystagmus (late symptom).

G. Amblyopia may result from uncorrected congenital and infantile cataracts.

H. Strabismus.

IV. Effects on Individual

A. May need frequent change of prescriptive lenses.

B. Fear of blindness.

C. Apprehension regarding hospitalization and surgery.

D. Hinders normal school activities.

V. Management/Treatment

A. For child with congenital monocular cataract, surgery is necessary as soon as possible after birth and before 2 months if vision is to be normal.

B. Surgical removal of lens (aphakia).

C. Intraocular lens implants are most common.

D. Sometimes eyeglasses or soft contact lens are prescribed to compensate for refractive power lost after lens has been removed.

VI. Additional Information

A. *Aphakia* is the term used when the lens has been removed during surgery. The absence of the lens causes an increase in the size of the image with glasses; however, this abnormal magnification is less with contact lenses. Contact lenses are the treatment of choice for congenital cataract in infants younger than 1 year of age. After 2 years of age, intraocular lens implantation (IOL) should be considered. The visual field is also considerably affected.

CONGENITAL BLINDNESS

I. Definition

A. Congenital blindness is a visual acuity for distance of 20/200 (6/60 m) or less in the better eye or peripheral vision of less than 200 in the better eye; also known as *legal blindness*.

II. Etiology

A. The following factors may contribute to blindness:

1. Familial factors such as a genetic disease.
2. Intrauterine insult (e.g., rubella or toxoplasmosis).
3. Perinatal factors such as prematurity or oxygen toxicity.
4. Postnatal factors such as trauma or infection (e.g., measles).
5. Inflammatory disorders (e.g., juvenile arthritis).

III. Signs, Symptoms, and History

A. No eye-to-eye contact with caregiver.
B. Inability to follow large moving objects.
C. Abnormal eye movements.
D. Unresponsiveness to visual stimuli.
E. Does not move around.
F. Fixed pupils.
G. Strabismus.
H. Constant nystagmus.

IV. Effects on Individual

A. Develops "blindisms" to compensate for inadequate stimulation (e.g., body rocking, finger flicking, arm twirling).
B. May have continuous falls, bumps, and bruises if environment is not made safe.
C. Delayed motor and speech skills.
D. Curtailed social play because of child's fear of falling or running into unknown obstacles.
E. Unable to observe others who may be role models.
F. Delayed development of social behaviors.
G. Misses important visual cues.
H. General delay in all developmental milestones because they are in some way related to sight (e.g., crawling is guided in movement by sight, social smile is learned by observation, development of eating skills and use of utensils rely heavily on sight).
I. Older child's self-concept may be harmed because peers may laugh if dress is inappropriately matched; facial expression is lacking, which may be misunderstood as lack of interest or sullenness.

V. Management/Treatment

A. Early diagnosis important.
B. Surgical repair, if indicated.
C. Eyeglasses.
D. Special training for parent(s) and child.
E. Early orientation and mobility instruction.
F. Speech and language therapy, as needed.
G. Early stimulation program.
H. Referral to available resources and counseling services.

VI. Additional Information

A. For education purposes, a child who loses vision before the age of 5 or 6 is classified as having a congenital vision defect. These children have difficulty with visual imagery and memory of color. The child who becomes blind at an older age retains concepts of reading, writing, and colors and may easily transfer this knowledge to learning the Braille system. Educational implications differ greatly for both groups. Technology has opened new and challenging avenues for individual or group learning.

GLAUCOMA

I. Definition

A. Glaucoma is defined as increased intraocular pressure that may cause atrophy of the optic nerve, damage to the retina, and eventual blindness. Several types of glaucoma exist. There are three types of pediatric glaucoma; congenital glaucoma, associated with infants at birth; infantile glaucoma which appears within the first 3 years; and juvenile glaucoma diagnosed from 3 to teens or young adults.

II. Etiology

A. Glaucoma can be a congenital defect resulting from inadequate development of the aqueous filtering mechanism of the anterior chamber angle. It also can be acquired by an injury resulting in scar tissue blocking the drainage of aqueous humor or a disease process.

III. Signs, Symptoms, and History

A. Earlier symptoms are excessive tearing (epiphora), photophobia, eye pain, and redness of eye.

B. Pupil large and fixed.

C. Eyeball enlarges because young eye is distensible.

D. Sclera is blue tinged.

E. Cornea is thinned, cloudy, and bulging.

F. Blinking, headache.

G. Usually bilateral.

H. Congenital glaucoma symptoms are visible early in life.

IV. Effects on Individual

A. Limited peripheral vision causes clumsiness and bumping into objects.

B. Discomfort affects general well-being and behavior when intraocular pressure increases.

C. Limited vision affects motor skills.

D. Parents overindulge and overprotect child, thus stunting child's physical, social, and emotional growth.

V. Management/Treatment

A. Surgery is necessary to increase the outflow of fluids to the eye. A second surgery may be necessary, but pressure reducing medications are used first. Surgery is reserved as a last option.

VI. Additional Information

A. In early stages, corneal haziness is reversible once the ocular pressure has been reduced. Juvenile glaucoma occurs between 3 and 20 years of age and follows a course similar to that of adult glaucoma. It is usually related to another disease process. The "puff test" for measuring intraocular pressure may be used as early as 4 years of age. This test is administered as play, instructing the child to keep eyes open wide until the puff comes.

NYSTAGMUS

I. Definition

A. Nystagmus is an involuntary repetitive movement of one or both eyeballs. It can be a rhythmic oscillation in any direction and at any speed or frequency. Nystagmus often is associated with defective vision or systemic neurological disease.

II. Etiology

A. Nystagmus is congenital or acquired. It may be ocular or systemic (neurological). Congenital nystagmus may be caused by organic eye disease. Corneal opacity, congenital cataract, albinism, total color blindness, or congenital anomalies of the optic nerve may cause ocular nystagmus. Neurological nystagmus is secondary to lesions in the brain. Momentary, transient nystagmus may be seen with fatigue and is generally of no consequence.

III. Signs, Symptoms, and History
A. Eyes move repetitively and uncontrollably in any direction at different speeds with no purpose.
B. In congenital nystagmus, eye movement can be in all directions of gaze.
C. In ocular nystagmus, searching movement is pendular of equal speed and amplitude.
D. In neurological nystagmus, movements are horizontal, rotary, or jerky.

IV. Effects on Individual
A. May become self-conscious or embarrassed by response of others to condition.
B. May avoid eye contact.
C. Head posturing to obtain null point (eye position that stabilizes nystagmus, such as face turn, chin elevation or depression, and head tilt that minimizes nystagmoid eye movements).

V. Management/Treatment
A. Complete assessment necessary.
B. Treatment of underlying cause.

VI. Additional Information
A. Intermittent nystagmus in an infant until approximately age 3 months is normal. Continuous nystagmus from birth is not normal and should be evaluated. Congenital nystagmus generally is not diagnosed until the child is 2 or 3 months old.

TESTING PROCEDURES

Vision is the main sensory modality for educational activities. Therefore, *consistent* visual assessment during the school-age years is important. Early detection and correction of visual problems may prevent deficits in academic performance and permanent vision loss. The screening and testing methods presented in this section can be used for a comprehensive school vision screening program. Box 2-2 defines terms related to vision impairment.

Box 2-2   *Vision Impairment*

Partial vision is defined as visual acuity between 20/70 and 20/200 in the better eye with correction.

Legal blindness is defined as distant visual acuity of 20/200 in the better eye and/or a visual field not greater than 20 degrees (tunnel vision).

The definition for legal blindness in the United States is a legal term versus an educational term. It allows particular educational and governmental eligibilities; such as access to special educational schools, designated funding sources, tax status and other benefits.

DISTANCE VISION

I. **Optotype Charts: Sloan, Lea Symbols, and others; and Optotype Slides on Computer Software** (Box 2-3 lists tests used for different age groups.)
   A. Screening criteria.
      1. These tests are used for preschool (ages 3-4 years), kindergarten or first grade (age 5 or 6 years), second grade (age 7 years), and children with special needs, as required. Some children may be difficult to test at these ages with a distance optotype chart because of developmental level rather than a visual problem. Table 2-1 lists visual screening recommendations for each age group.
   B. Equipment and preparation.
      1. Self-illuminating 10- or 20-ft (3- or 6-m) distance chart, wall-mounted chart, or optotypes on computer screen, Lea Symbols (younger children), or Sloan letters (older children) preferable to other optotypes including picture charts (Proctor, 2005). Single optotypes on a line should be avoided and used only for training purposes.
      2. Window cards may be used for occluding background figures for younger children only when exposed to multiple optotypes first with or without matching and unable to succeed.
      3. Eye occluder. Adhesive patch best for young children. Otherwise, a two-sided "flipper" apparatus-occluder.
      4. Rescreening and referral forms.
      5. Shadows and glare should be eliminated in testing situation.
      6. Position chart at eye level. Optotype chart should have capability of height adjustment for different aged children.
   C. Screening procedure.
      1. Have student stand or sit at recommended distance from chart (10 or 20 ft). If student is standing, the toe of the foot should be on the line; and, if student is sitting, place back legs of chair on marked line.
      2. Give screening instructions and how student is to respond; demonstrate, if necessary, with single large optotype.

Box 2-3 *Distance Acuity*

Preschool Children

- Lea Symbols
- HOTV
- Illiterate E charts
- Other acceptable optotype charts
- Photorefractor systems
- Portable autorefractors
- Hand held refractors-small versions of table refractor

Special Education Children

- Photorefractor systems
- Portable autorefractors

- Faye symbol chart
- Lea Symbols
- HOTV
- STYCAR test

School-Age Children

- Sloan letters
- Lea numerals
- Photorefractor systems
- Portable autorefractors
- Computer software screening programs
- Others

Table 2-1	*Visual Screening Recommendations*
Age	**Screening**
Birth-3 mo	Inspection and observation Red reflex/Brückner test Corneal light reflex (Hirschberg)
6 mo-1 yr	Inspection and observation Red reflex/Brückner test Corneal light reflex (Hirschberg) Blink reflex Fixate and follow bilaterally Alternate occlusion
Toddler (1-3 yr)	Inspection and observation Visual acuity test (age appropriate test) Red reflex/Brückner test Corneal light reflex (Hirschberg) Blink reflex Cover-uncover and alternate cover
Preschool (3-5 yr)	Inspection and observation Visual acuity test (age appropriate test) Red reflex/Brückner test Corneal light reflex (Hirchberg) Blink reflex Cover-uncover and alternate cover
School-age-adolescent	Inspection and observation Visual acuity test (age appropriate test) Peripheral vision/visual fields Fixation Cover-uncover and alternate cover

3. Show student how to use occluder to cover one eye or have assistant occlude one eye. Tell student to keep both eyes open while using occluder. This is an important concept.
4. If student wears glasses or contact lenses, screen with glasses/contacts in place to determine baseline acuity. Then repeat testing without glasses or contacts.
5. *Evaluate each eye separately*, right eye first and then left eye.
6. Begin at 20/40 line and proceed downward to ascertain best vision. If visual acuity difficulties are suspected, begin screening at 20/200 line and proceed downward. Continue until student is able to read correctly three of four symbols on the short line or four of six symbols on the longer line.

NOTE: Check individual state for passing criteria, since each state varies.

7. Observe for blinking, tilting of head, squinting, rubbing of eyes, or complaints of blurring.
8. When screening young children, attempt full line first; if unsuccessful, use matching technique or window cards to expose only one symbol at a time.

D. Failure criteria.
1. The failure criteria in 3-year-olds vary from state to state. Generally, a visual acuity of 20/50 or less in either eye is of concern. This indicates inability to correctly identify one more than half the symbols on the 40-ft line on the chart at a distance of 20 ft (6 m).
2. Any 3-year-old with a two-line difference in visual acuity between the eyes in the passing range (e.g., 20/20 in one eye, 20/40 in the other eye) fails the distance acuity examination, should be rescreened, and referred, depending upon findings.
3. In all other ages and grades, visual acuity of 20/40 or poorer indicates inability to identify correctly one more than half the symbols on the 30-ft line of the chart at a distance of 20 ft (Prevent Blindness America recommendations). As with younger children, this acuity score varies from state to state.
4. Each state generally has its own standards and criteria; the National Association of School Nurses provides vision guidelines; *To See or Not to See: Screening the vision of children in school* by Susan E. Proctor (2005).
5. The accepted standard for normal acuity in adults and older children is 20/20 (Neff, 1991). If the individual can only read the 20/100 line, this indicates he/she sees at 20 feet what an individual with normal visual acuity would see at 100 feet. Charts or tests scaled for 10 feet (3 m) use 10 as the numerator instead of 20.
E. Rescreening.
1. All students/children who fail initial screening should be rescreened (use the same screening procedure); although recreening is not universally required in all states.
NOTE: Check testing criteria in own state, since the criteria vary.
F. Action.
1. If a child fails the second screening, notify parents and send a written referral for a complete professional eye examination by an ophthalmologist or optometrist.
NOTE: Check state criteria before referral, since the criteria vary. The referral should indicate test results, screening dates, observations of the child, and any teacher comments. Follow up with parents regarding results of the professional examination and implications for the school setting. Any other visual testing should be considered and referral made if deviations from the norm, even when visual acuity is normal, especially if the student is having academic/school difficulty.
G. Photorefractive imagers, portable autorefactors.
1. See page 75 for information on photorefractive imagers and portable autorefactors.

COLOR VISION

I. **Screening criteria: color plates, sorting tests, or pegs, depending upon state law**
A. All males by or before age 6 or according to individual state mandates.
II. **Screening information**
A. See individual test instructions. Various older child and adult pseudoisochromatic plate tests are available, such as Ishihara, Dvorine, and AO. The Hardy Rand Rittler (HRR) plates are well developed.

Young child plates are available. One brand is "Color Vision Testing Made Easy." Pseudoisochromatic plates consist of printed plates of letters, numbers, winding paths or pictures (young child plates), composed of colored dots of different sizes that differ systematically in hue from background dots. The child must identify the designs. Each figure color and background dot is so similar that the test figure does not stand out plainly enough for the color-deficient person to identify. Adult and older-child-screening plates can be used with some children as young as 4 years.

B. Pseudoisochromatic tests are easy to administer; the manufacturer's instructions should be followed exactly, especially with regard to illumination (e.g., daylight, fluorescent lighting). The most common error is administering the test under incorrect illumination. Proper illumination is as important as the ink used in printing the plates. The tests are designed for use under average daylight, which can also be provided by a daylight lamp or fluorescent lighting. If plates are displayed under ordinary (incandescent) light, a color deficiency may not be identified because incandescent bulbs contain too much yellow.

NOTE: Be aware of state standards, since some color perception tests are illegal to use in particular states. The color vision testing slide housed in some vision testing machines use incandescent light which distorts accurate assessment of color perception.

C. Of the color plates mentioned, only the HRR is diagnostic, identifying the type and degree of the defect. The others are screening tests that determine whether the child has normal color vision. Ishihara plates are frequently used in schools and are similar to other plates; the Ishihara consists of numbers imbedded in circles of colored dots. In screening, the number of plates missed does *not* indicate the severity of the defect. Test plates should be protected from unnecessary light exposure and handling. Ink fades with time, and fading is increased by exposure to light. Keep plates clean and untouched. A soft, dry paintbrush or cotton-tipped swab should be used for tracing the symbols on the plates; and plates should not be touched by hands or fingers.

III. Failure criteria
A. According to test instructions.

IV. Rescreening
A. No rescreening is necessary. Rescreen young children to rule out other factors (e.g., illness, fatigue, fear).

V. Action
A. Notify and educate parent(s) if a deficiency exists and educate staff and the child, as appropriate, about the deficiency.

BINOCULAR VISION

I. Cover/Uncover Test (Figure 2-6)
A. This test determines the presence or absence of a heterotropia or strabismus. Heterotropia (strabismus) is a misalignment of the eyes that is manifest during binocularity and may be unilateral, alternating, or intermittent depending on the vision. The test should be done at near and far distances.

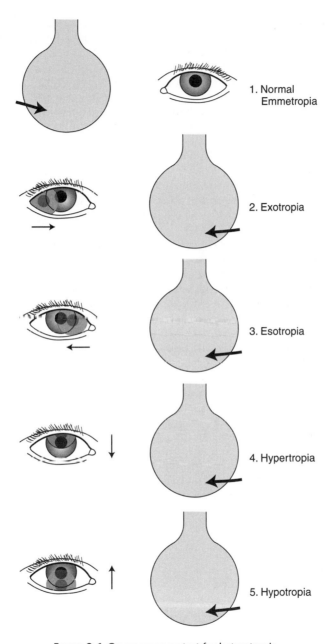

1. Normal Emmetropia

2. Exotropia

3. Esotropia

4. Hypertropia

5. Hypotropia

FIGURE 2-6 Cover-uncover test for heterotropia.

B. Screening procedure.
   1. Observe for refixation movement of the uncovered eye while uncovering the covered eye.
   2. As student fixates on target at near (13 in [33 cm]) and far (20 ft [6 m]) distances, cover left eye and observe right eye. If right eye shows no fixation movement, no deviation is present.
   3. If right eye moves to fixate, deviation is present.
   4. Repeat procedure, covering right eye and observing left eye.

NOTE: The Cover/Uncover Test may miss intermittent deviations which will be detected by administering the Alternate Cover Test (Figure 2-7).

C. Screening results.
   1. When one eye is covered and there is no movement of uncovered eye, it is probable that no deviation exists. However, the alternate Cover Test should still be performed to rule out an intermittent strabismus.
   2. When one eye is covered and other eye moves inward, exotropia is likely since the eye was pointed outward from the target while both eyes were open.
   3. When one eye is covered and other eye moves outward, esotropia is likely since the eye was pointed inward from the target while both eyes were open.
   4. When one eye is covered and other moves downward, hypertropia is indicated since the eye was pointed upward while both eyes were open.
   5. When one eye is covered and other eye moves upward, hypotropia is indicated since the eye was pointed downward while both eyes were open.

II. Alternate Cover Test

A. This test can determine the presence or absence of both heterotropia (strabismus) or heterophoria. It is the only traditional school-appropriate test that will detect hetrophoria. Heterophoria is a latent tendency for the eyes to deviate during conditions of monocularity and is normally controlled by fusional mechanisms which facilitate binocular vision and avoid diplopia. The eye can deviate under stress, fatigue, illness, or when normal fusion is interfered with, such as covering the eye. However, heterophorias are of lesser consequence than are heterotropias because monocularity is not a normal state.

B. Screening procedure.
   1. Hold the occluder with the handle upward and briskly move the occluder over the bridge of the nose, keeping one eye covered at all times to disrupt fusion. Observe for a refixation shift of the covered eye as it is being uncovered.
   2. Both the student's eyes should be open; student screening should be done while child is viewing *near* (13 in [33 cm]) and *far* (20 ft [6 m]) distances. Heterophorias are controlled by the fusion mechanism only when both eyes are open and, therefore, if present, do not significantly impact quality of life. Fusion is disrupted when one eye is covered.

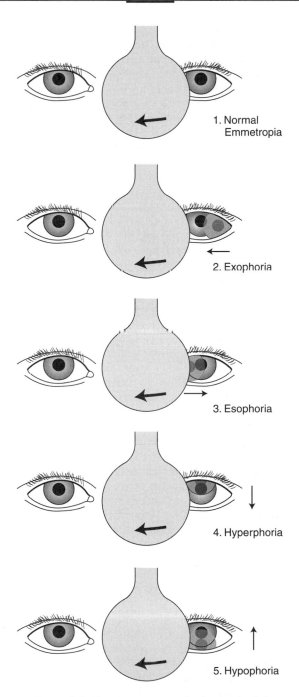

FIGURE 2-7 Alternate cover test for heterophoria.

3. As the student fixates on a distant or near object, cover one eye with the occluder, holding the occluder with the handle up, and then quickly uncover the eye.
4. As occluder is removed, observe whether the eye under cover has deviated. Perform this procedure on both eyes.
5. If covered eye moves in any direction to fixate when occluder is removed, a heterophoria is present.

C. Screening results.

1. When eye is uncovered and there is no movement, no deviation is present.
2. When eye is uncovered and moves inward to fixate, exophoria is indicated since the eye was drifting outward when covered.
3. When eye is uncovered and moves outward to fixate, esophoria is indicated since the eye was drifting inward when covered.
4. When eye is uncovered and moves downward to fixate, hyperphoria is indicated since the eye was drifting upward when covered.
5. When eye is uncovered and moves upward to fixate, hypophoria is indicated since the eye was drifting downward when covered.
6. Heterophorias are usually not referred for professional evaluation unless the return to alignment is slow, or the child is having learning problems. A heterophoria can progress to a heterotropia.

III. Corneal Light Reflex Test (Hirschberg Test)

This test is used to detect misalignment of the eyes (strabismus).

A. Screening procedure.

1. Direct a penlight toward student's eyes from distance of 13 in (33 cm). Student's eyes should be focused on examiner's face.
2. Observe images of corneal light reflections (CLRs) penlight makes on pupils.
3. If CLRs are approximately equally placed on both corneas, test result is negative.
4. If penlight images are not symmetrical, eyes are misaligned.

B. Screening results.

1. Symmetrical light reflection on each cornea indicates normal alignment.
2. Asymmetrical light reflection in each pupil indicates misalignment.
3. Light reflection on outer aspect of cornea or iris indicates esotropia.
4. Light reflection on inner aspect of cornea or iris indicates exotropia.
5. Notify parents and make a referral for formal evaluation.
6. Students with epicanthal folds may give false impression of misalignment (pseudostrabismus); however, light reflex test should be equal.

IV. Photorefractive Imagers (Photoscreeners)

See page 75 for information on photorefractive imagers.

NOTE: Corneal reflections appear differently placed depending upon pupil size. Focus at close range engages accommodation, narrowing the pupil and making many esotropias more important.

NEAR VISION

I. Plus Lens Test for Hyperopia

Hyperopia screening determines farsightedness with use of a plus sphere lens or other methods.

    A. Screening procedure.

        1. Place plus lens glasses on student (+2.50 diopters) for all ages (Proctor, 2005). Ask student to look at optotype chart for approximately 1 minute.

NOTE: Check state screening recommendations.

        2. Direct student to read 20/30 line of chart while standing or sitting 20 ft away (10/30 line at 10 ft if chart scaled for 10 ft).

        3. Test one eye at a time.

        4. The following materials are used to test near vision.

           a. Plus lenses (at least +2.50D).

           b. Optotype chart or appropriate slide on stereoscope.

    B. Screening results

        1. If student reads at least four of seven optotypes correctly with the plus lens, screening has been failed and should be repeated about 2 weeks later.

NOTE: Criteria may vary by state.

        2. Passing: student should be *unable* to read 20/20 or 20/30 line on the chart or slide.

        3. If student fails rescreening (e.g., can successfully read 20/30 line), refer to an eye professional.

    C. Photorefractive imagers; portable autorefactors.

See page 75 for information on photorefractive imagers and portable autorefractors.

See page 75 for information on photorefractive imagers and portable autorefractors.

INFANT, PRESCHOOL, AND SPECIAL EDUCATION SCREENING

Vision is the most important modality for learning. The learning process is not restricted to the traditional school-age years; thus, detection and treatment of visual problems in the early years is critical to a child's overall optimal development. The Prevent Blindness America organization estimates that 1 in every 20 preschool children in the United States has a vision problem, and if uncorrected, it can lead to needless decrease of vision or loss of sight. New technology and information allows newborns to be screened and tested for visual estimates and impairments. Even with this ability, almost 80% of preschool children have not had an eye examination according to Prevent Blindness America. Table 2-2 summarizes techniques used in visual assessment for infants and young children.

VISION SCREENING PROCEDURE FOR INFANTS AND YOUNGER CHILDREN

I. Rough Estimate Procedures

The following screening procedure can be used on children younger than 1 year to detect amblyopia.

    A. Screening Procedure.

        1. Try to occlude one of the infant's eyes. Notice infant's behavior.

Table 2-2	*Visual Assessment Techniques for Infants and Young Children*
Variable	**Assessment Techniques**
Testing site	Be aware of intensity and location of light source; the source should be behind the children. Darken the room or use colored lights if infant makes no visual responses in normal lighting.
Distractions	Be aware of visual and auditory distractions; minimize to prevent overstimulation (e.g., shadows, light through windows, colorful objects in room, radio, television noise, adults in conversation, children playing nearby).
Positioning	Child should be in secure position; on parent's shoulder or lap; on back or stomach, or in infant seat.
Physiological state	Observe and note if alert, sleepy, fussy, hungry state; ill or recently ill.
Social state	If infant is wary of stranger, caregiver is better person to work with child to elicit behaviors. If infant likes faces, then examiner can use own face as visual stimulus for testing.
Attention	Combine auditory and visual stimulation for attention (voice and face; shake rattle). Then elicit responses with familiar nonaudible object. If unresponsive, repeat with shiny/bright objects (tin foil, tinsel, costume jewelry) or high-contrast object, or use filtered light by placing pop bead over penlight. Some colors are seen easier than others, so vary colors of toys and objects for testing.
Observations	Observe carefully; cues are often subtle (e.g., quieting, widening of eyes, moving fingers, reaching for objects). Document all observations and history.
Reward	End with activity infant can do with ease and provide verbal praise and smile.

Modified from Chen D, Friedman C, Cavello G: *Parents and visually impaired infants: identifying visual impairment in infants (PAVII),* Louisville, Ky, 1990, American Printing House for the Blind.

    2. Occlude other eye. If infant cries or tries to push away occluder from eye, suspect reduced visual acuity in uncovered eye.
  B. Screening Results.
    1. If vision is normal or near normal, infant will not react strongly to either eye being covered. Ocular malalignment will also elicit a negative response.
    2. Refer for formal testing if reduced visual function in either eye is suspected.
  II. Optotype Tests
For children younger than 3 years of age, research shows that Lea Symbols are best; followed by HOTV then Illiterate E, and lastly, the picture cards. However, picture tests are sometimes the only tests effective with very young children. (Proctor, 2005; Vision in Preschoolers Study Group, 2005). The National Preschool Vision Screening Committee (2000) recommends testing preschoolers at 10 feet.

ALLEN CARD TEST

I. Appropriate Age
A. This test for visual acuity may be used on cooperating children 24 months and older.

II. Summary of Test
A. The test consists of seven picture cards (tree, birthday cake, horse and rider, telephone, car, house, and teddy bear) that are presented at a distance of 15 ft. The cards are first shown to the child at a close distance to determine whether the child can identify the pictures correctly. The child is given three to five trials and must identify correctly three of seven pictures to pass. The test does not allow testing of acuity better than 20/30 (this test may miss anisometropia).

BLACKBIRD PRESCHOOL VISION SCREENING SYSTEM

I. Appropriate Age
A. This screening tool can be used to assess the visual acuity in 3- to 6-year-old children, children with special needs, and other children whose eye-hand coordination has not fully developed.

II. Summary of Test
A. The test involves the story of a blackbird in flight, which is in the shape of a modified E, to engage attention. The story can be adapted according to the needs of the child being screened. A wall-mounted chart or flash cards are available. Six individual cards are used; each card has a blackbird picture of varying size on one side and a visual acuity notation on the reverse side. The cards are presented to the child from a distance of 10 or 20 ft (3 or 6 m). The child indicates, with her or his arms, the direction of the blackbird's flight. Vision screening guidelines are included for uncommunicative, non-readers, or non-English speaking children, and other difficult-to-test populations. The blackbird system is now available in Spanish. The *Blackbird Storybook Home Eye Test* is available for parents who choose to prescreen their young children at home. There is a pass-fail criterion.

LEA SYMBOLS CHART

I. Appropriate Age
A. The Lea Symbols test is suitable for children 18 months and older.

II. Summary of Test
A. Lea Symbols use four seemingly universal symbols, an apple, a circle, a house and a square. The test is available in a variety of configurations and sizes and various presentations for assessing distance and near acuity. The child is asked to name the symbol or is presented a hand-held card and asked to match. The symbols blur equally at threshold. The crowding of symbols helps to detect amblyopia. It is designed so that child never feels like a failure as they can also identify a symbol just not always correctly (symbols will look like circles/balls/rings). The distance chart's smallest lines have 15 optotypes, arranged in groups of fives. Child training materials are also available.

HOTV OR MATCHING SYMBOL

I. Appropriate Age

A. This test can be used with children from 3 years of age. It avoids the issues of eye-hand coordination and image reversal that can occur with the traditional letter chart.

II. Summary of Test

A. The test uses four letters, H, O, T, and V, in a chart that is shown to the child at 10 or 20 ft (3-6 m). The child matches the letters with demonstration cards or names the letters. This avoids eye-hand coordination and image reversal concerns that can occur with E vision charts. There are HOTV charts that have 5 optotypes minimally, in all lines.

ILLITERATE E VISION SCREENING

I. Appropriate Age

A. This test can determine visual acuity in cooperating children as young as 2½ to 3 years using the E game and is one of the most universal.

II. Summary of Test

A. The child's parent(s) are instructed to teach the test to the child at home using the E game method. The child plays the game by pointing with his/her hand the direction the legs of the E letter are facing. Once the child understands the test and is able to point consistently to the direction of the big E, then a nurse, physician, or other examiner can perform efficient and appropriate screening. This test can be incorporated into day care programs as a group activity.

STEREOACUITY TESTS

I. Appropriate Age

A. Appropriate ages are 3 years through third grade to check for depth perception which is important to determine if both eyes are working together.

II. Summary of Tests

A. Stereoacuity tests provide assessment of stereopsis, depth perception, and of binocular vision. To have depth perception, binocular vision must be present; lack of binocularity may indicate anisometropia, strabismus or amblyopia.

III. Available Information

A. Stereoacuity tests screening products have been popular for a number of years and can include: Stereo Smile II, Random Dot E Test, Stereo Fly Test, Randot Stereo Test. Polarized glasses are used with the screening tests.

PHOTOREFRACTION/PHOTOSCREENING AND PORTABLE AUTOREFRACTORS

NOTE: Photorefractive systems and portable autorefractors can be used with infants as young as 6 months. The systems are especially useful with young children or children with special needs because they are objective and require no response from the child. See page 75 for further information on photorefractive systems and portable autorefractors.

OTHER SCHOOL TESTING METHODS

I. Stereoscopes/Portables Slide-based Vision Screeners

A. Appropriate age.

    1. Portable vision screeners are generally used with older students. However, there are newer models available that provide slides appropriate for younger children or those without letter recognition.

B. Summary of test.

    1. They are used in numerous schools throughout the United States. Portable vision screeners combine many testing functions in one single piece of equipment. They are also called stereoscopes as they are able to create stereoscopic images and assess stereopsis. They are reported to test near, distance, binocular and color vision this being done by the rotation of slides mounted in a single drum. There is some controversy regarding the advantages and disadvantages of the portable vision screeners, i.e., color slides are used with an incandescent bulb making the color test invalid and plus lenses may come in a lower strength than recommended by district or state policy (Proctor, 2005). The equipment may be manually or electronically controlled.

II. Computer sofware programs

A. Appropriate age.

    1. Can be used with younger and older students, grades 3 through 12, while others utilize Lea Symbols and/or HOTV charts making them useful with preschool children.

B. Summary of test.

    1. Numerous computer software packages are available for use by the school nurse. Most of the programs test for near and distance vision, ocular alignment, and color vision. This method has advantages and disadvantages. Computer software advantages are much the same as portable stereoscopes, i.e., many visual functions can be screened during the same sitting. Some software programs can be programmed to record the results and prepare a referral letter to the parent(s). Disadvantages are the lack of research regarding the optotypes for sensitivity and specificity; and if testing for color, the lighting may not be appropriate for optimal color vision testing.

C. Available information.

    1. Software can be ordered from nursing and school health supply companies as well as vision companies and might include: Smart System II First-Test™, Vision Screen 9000, VERA Version III, and Eye-CEE System for Schools.

    2. Computer controlled vision screener is a newer developed method for vision screening. The child looks into an apparatus for the test; the computer is used as the control mechanism and records the data; e.g., VS-V Standard Vision Screener.

III. Photorefraction/Photoscreening and Portable Autorefractors

A. Appropriate age.

    1. The *Photorefractive imager* systems are cameras that can be used with infants as young as 6 months. The systems are especially useful with young children or children with special needs because they are objective and require no response from the child.

2. Portable autorefractors, handheld devices, can also be used with the younger child as a response from the child is not required.
   B. Summary of tests.
   1. Several new *camera systems* or *photorefractive imagers* also are available, known as photometer or photorefractors. All use a similar process. Photorefractors are being used in some school vision screening programs. A photograph of the eyes is taken, and the flash of light induces a red reflex and bilateral corneal light reflections (CLRs). The resulting photograph provides information regarding visual impairments. Some systems provide pass-fail results by computer interpretation rather than human interpretation; some provide a diagnosis and objective refraction information. These screening systems screen for a variety of conditions, including refractive errors such as myopia, hyperopia, astigmatism, and anisometropia as well as identifying cataracts, and other media opacities. They are most effective in identifying strabismus. Interpretation of the results must be done by a trained professional while taking the picture may be done by volunteers.
   2. *Portable Autorefractor is* another newer piece of school vision screening equipment. It is hand-held and a smaller version of refractive equipment found in a vision specialist's office. The portable refractor measures distances between the cornea and retina and can detect differences in corneal surfaces indicative of astigmatism and can provide information regarding refractive error along with the nature and exact degree. It can also detect myopia, hyperopia, presbyopia, and anisometropia accurately (Proctor, 2005).
   C. Available information.
   1. Photorefractors include brands such as Photoscreener, and Visiscreen-100. Visual function includes binocular vision (ocular alignment) and near vision (accommodation).
   2. Portable autorefractors include brands such as Sure Sight, and the Rmax Plus 2. Visual function includes distance and near vision (accommodation).

WEB SITES

Vision Service Plan (VSP) Sight for Students
   http://www.sightforstudents.org
American Academy of Ophthalmology
   http://www.aao.org
American Optometric Association
   http://www.aoa.org
Better Vision for Children Foundation
   http://www.bvcnow.org/
Lions Club International
   http://www.lionsclubs.org
National Eye Institute
   http://www.nei.nih.gov/

GLOSSARY OF VISION TERMS

Accommodation   The shape of the eye's lens increases through contraction of the ciliary muscle to focus on objects at near distances.

Acquired   Not innate or hereditary.

Acuity   Ability to discriminate details, as in reading. Measurements indicate the smallest figure or symbol recognizable in central vision. Acuity is a measure of the function of the cones in the fovea centralis.

Amblyopia   Reduced vision in one eye; not caused by refractive errors or organic defect. Contributing factors cause developmental lag in occipital lobe and retinal cones; often called *lazy eye.*

Aniridia   Lack of iris tissue, usually bilateral with reduced visual acuity and photophobia.

Anisometropia   Refractive errors of the two eyes are unequal, usually two or more lines difference as measured by acuity assessments.

Aphakia   Absence of the crystalline lens.

Astigmatism   Vision defect usually caused by uneven curvature of the cornea.

Binocular vision   Ability of the brain to fuse a retinal image from each eye into one single image resulting from clear images on both foveae and parallel alignment of the eyes.

Brückner test   Using an ophthalmoscope check child's eyes at near range, move ophthalmoscope back and forth quickly observing for pupillary reaction and red reflexes. If there is a discrepancy in the darkening of the red reflexes in one eye it may indicate strabismus.

Cataract   Any partial or complete clouding of the lens.

Central visual acuity   Ability of the eye and brain to discriminate form and shape in the direct line of vision when elicited by stimuli impinging directly on the fovea centralis area of the macula retinae.

Certified ophthalmic registered nurse   Nurse with specialized knowledge, experience, and skills to perform assessments, eye examinations, education, and assistance in eye surgeries. Services provided in ambulatory clinics, private offices, operating rooms, and hospitals.

Coloboma   Congenital notch or defect of the iris; may also involve retina, macula, or optic nerve. Visual function varies from normal to severely impaired, depending on structures involved.

Cones   Photoreceptor cells in the retina that provide detailed vision and color sensitivity.

Congenital   Present at birth.

Cornea   A clear, transparent structure covering over the iris and pupil; part of the eye's refracting system.

Cortical visual impairment   A permanent or temporary visual impairment caused by disturbance of the posterior visual pathways, the occipital lobes of the brain, or both. Ranges from severe impairment to total blindness depending on the time of onset, location, and intensity of the insult. Caused by perinatal hypoxia, metabolic disturbances, hydrocephalus, head trauma, infection, and brain defects.

Cycloplegia   Paralysis of ciliary muscle, resulting in paralysis of accommodation; usually intentionally induced by an eye examiner to facilitate examination of the structure and function of the eye.

Depth perception   Ability to perceive spatial (distance) relationships similar to stereopsis. Both eyes must be functional for stereopsis.

Dichromatism   Ability to perceive only 2 of the 160 colors the normal eye discriminates.

Diopter   Unit of measurement that expresses a lens' refractive power. Also, a measure of the degree of refractive error. Myopia is measured in minus diopters, whereas hyperopia is measured in plus diopters.

Diplopia   Perception of two images of a single object; double vision.

Distensible   Capable of being enlarged.

Doll's-eye reflex   Eyes remain stationary when head is moved. Normal reflex for first 10 days of life. Detects paresis of the abducens nerve and weakness of the lateral rectus muscle. May be localized or the result of damage to the central nervous system.

Emmetropia   Parallel light rays coming to exact focus on the retina; ideal optical condition.

Epiphora   Tearing of eye.

Esophoria   Deviation of the visual axis of an eye toward the other eye after the visual fusion stimuli has been eliminated.

Esotropia   Strabismus that manifests deviation of a visual axis toward that of the other eye, possibly resulting in diplopia, also called *cross-eye* and *convergent* or *internal strabismus.*

Exophoria   Deviation of the visual axis of one eye away from the other eye when the visual fusional stimulus is absent.

Exotropia   Strabismus that manifests permanent deviation of the visual axis of one eye away from the other, possibly resulting in diplopia; also called *wall-eye* and *divergent* or *external strabismus.*

Fixation   The act of holding or staying in a fixed position.

Fovea centralis   A small depression in the center of the macula lutea that contains elongated cones. This is the area of clearest vision because the layers of the retina spread aside, permitting light to fall directly on the cones.

Glaucoma   Degeneration of the optic nerve characterized by increased intraocular pressure and loss of vision.

Hyperopia   A refractive error in which parallel light rays focus behind the retina. Frequently called *farsightedness;* also called *hypermetropia.*

Hyperphoria   Upward deviation of the visual axis of an eye after elimination of the visual fusional stimulus; form of heterophoria.

Hypertropia   Strabismus that displays permanent upward deviation of the visual axis of an eye.

Hypophoria   Downward deviation of the visual axis of an eye after elimination of the visual fusional stimulus; form of heterophoria.

Hypotropia   Strabismus that displays permanent downward deviation of the visual axis of an eye.

Intermittent   Activity is suspended at intervals.

Iris   Eye tissue behind the cornea, which contracts or dilates to regulate the amount of light entering the eye.

Legal blindness   Correction of 20/200 or less with or without a visual field of 20 degrees or less in the better eye.

Lens   Transparent, oval, and colorless structure of the eye that undergoes accommodation to focus rays so that a perfect image is formed on the retina; sometimes called the *crystalline lens.*

Low vision   See *Partially sighted*.

Macula lutea   A part of the retina behind the lens that is responsible for central vision. The central area of the macula is called the *fovea centralis*.

Miosis   Contraction of the pupil.

Monochromatism   Total color blindness, inability to discriminate hues, a rare condition in which all colors of the spectrum appear as neutral grays varying in shades of light and dark.

Monocular   Involving only one eye.

Mydriasis   Physiological dilatation of the pupil.

Myopia   A refractive error in which parallel light rays from a distant object focus in front of the retina; often called *nearsightedness*.

Nystagmus   Involuntary repetitive movement of the eyeball. Movement can be horizontal, vertical, rotary, or mixed.

Occlusive therapy   An attempt to straighten or improve vision in an eye by patching the other eye.

Ocular hypotony   Low intraocular pressure.

Oculogyric crisis   Eyeballs become fixed in one position for minutes or hours.

Opaque   Unable to be penetrated by light rays or other forms of radiant energy.

Ophthalmologist   Medical doctor who specializes in the treatment of eye diseases and disorders; performs surgery and prescribes treatment.

Optic axis   A straight line through the center of the eye joining the central points of curvature of the anterior and posterior spheres.

Optic nerve   A bundle of nerve fibers that carry light-generated impulses from the eye to the brain.

Optic nerve atrophy   A permanent visual impairment caused by damage to the optic nerve. May be progressive, depending on etiology and cause.

Optic nerve hypoplasia   An underdevelopment of optic nerve in utero. Visual function can range from near normal to no light perception. One of the three most common causes of visual impairment in children.

Optician   A person trained in the grinding of lenses, dispensing, and fitting of glasses and sometimes contact lenses.

Optokinetic   Movement of the eyes, as in optokinetic nystagmus.

Optometrist   Professional degree is Doctor of Optometry (O.D.). Optometrists are independent primary health care providers who examine, diagnose, treat, and manage diseases and disorders of the visual system, the eyes, and associated structures. Examines the eyes for the presence of a vision problem, disease, or other abnormality; prescribes lenses, medications, and other optical aids and exercises.

Optotype   Test used to determine visual acuity, defined by Snellen.

Orientation and mobility specialist   Teacher trained to teach individuals who are visually impaired how to move safely in their environment.

Orthoptics   Technique of eye exercises for correcting defects in binocular vision.

Orthotropia   Alignment of the eyes. The normal condition when the visual axes remain parallel when the visual fusional stimuli has been eliminated either entirely or partially. Also termed parallelism.

Oscillation   Pendulum-like movement, fluctuation, or vibration.

Papillitis   Inflammation of the optic disc (papilla).

Parallelism   Ability of eyes to be directed to same target simultaneously; normal ocular alignment. Also termed orthotropia.

Partially sighted   Visual acuity better than 20/200 but worse than 20/70 in the better eye after correction.

Peripheral vision   Ability to perceive images and motion outside the direct line of vision.

Phoria   Deviation of the eyes from normal when fusion is prevented; latent; during condition of monocularity.

Photophobia   Varying degrees of intolerance to light.

Pleoptics   Eye exercises for training and stimulating an amblyopic eye.

Ptosis   Drooping of the upper eyelid. May affect vision development.

Pupil   Opening in the center of the iris that determines the amount of light that will pass to the interior of the eye. The iris controls the size of the opening.

Pursuits   Ability of the eye to smoothly follow a moving target.

Refraction   Bending of a light ray as it passes from one transparent medium into one of a different density.

Refractive error   Ocular condition in which images focus either in front of or behind the retina because of the size of the orbit or inappropriate refraction.

Retina   Innermost layer of the eye that contains the light- and movement-sensitive rods and the color- and detail-sensitive cones.

Retinoblastoma   A malignant intraocular tumor that usually occurs before age 5; generally a congenital condition.

Retinopathy of prematurity   An eye disorder in the premature infant. ROP affects immature blood vessels of the retina and is caused by conditions that stop the orderly growth of retinal blood vessels and stimulate their wild overgrowth (e.g., excessive oxygen, infection, excessive exposure to light).

Saccade   Series of quick or rapid movements of both eyes simultaneously when changing the point of fixation on a visualized object; this is normal functioning. Saccadic eye movement essential for successful reading.

Sclera: The white outer coating of the eyeball.

Scotoma   Area of lost vision in the visual field surrounded by an area of less compromised vision or normal vision.

Snellen chart   Series of letters, symbols, or numbers of decreasing size used for testing distance and near central vision acuity.

Snellen notion   Ratio that expresses visual acuity. The numerator is the distance at which the test was given; the denominator is the distance at which a person with normal vision can see the chart symbols or the smallest line read on the chart.

Stereopsis   Vision in which the visual field is perceived in three dimensions through a fusion of images from each eye.

Strabismus   Misalignment of the eyes; the two eyes are not focused on the same target. Condition is often called *squint,* which is an English term infrequently used in the United States.

Trichromatism   Ability to distinguish the three primary colors: red, yellow, and blue and mixtures; normal color vision.

Tropia   Deviation of an eye or eyes from the normal position when eyes are open and uncovered.

Uvea   Vascular or second coat of the eye that lies beneath the sclera; consists of the iris, ciliary body, and choroid.

Uveitis   Inflammation of the iris, ciliary body, choroid, or uvea.

Vision therapy   A program of techniques and other activities designed to reduce stress, guide the development of the visual system, improve visual skills, and enhance visual performance.

Visual evoked potential   A test used to gather data about the visual system. A flashing light stimulates the eye; information to the visual cortical pathways in the brain then is measured and documented in electrical activity through scalp electrodes.

ABBREVIATIONS OF VISION TERMS

A/C Anterior chamber
ACTH Adrenocorticotropic hormone
AMB Amblyopia
Ang Angles, drainage system of the eye
BRVO Branch retinal vein occlusion
CAG Closed-angle glaucoma
CD Cup to disc ratio, indication of glaucoma
CF Count fingers
CL Contact lenses
CRVO Central retinal vein occlusion
CT Cover test for strabismus
CVI Cortical visual impairment
Cyclo Cycloplegic drugs to paralyze muscles used
D Diopter
DFE Dilated fundus examination to see the retina
DR Diabetic retinopathy
DUCT Eye muscle test
DVA Distance visual acuity
EOM Extraocular muscle or test for eye movements
EP Esophoria
ERG Electroretinogram
ERRLA Equal, round, reactive to light and accommodation, pupils
ET Esotropia; eye deviates inward, toward the nose
EUA Examination under anesthesia
F Fixation, the ability to keep eye steady on a target
HM Hand motion
IOL Intraocular lens
IOP Intraocular pressure
Lens Crystalline lens
LP Light perception
MAO Monoamine oxidase
NLP No light perception
NPC Near point of convergence
NVA Near visual acuity
Ø No
OA Optic atrophy
O.D. Optometrist
OD Right eye (oculus dexter)
OKN Optokinetic nystagmus; rhythmic eye movement from moving striped target
OS Left eye (oculus sinister)

OU Both eyes (oculi uterque)
Pd Prism diopter
PD Pupillary distance from the center of one to the center of the other
PERRLA Pupils, equal, round, reactive to light and accommodation
POAG Primary open-angle glaucoma
PSC Posterior subcapsular cataract
RD Retinal detachment
Refr Refraction for farsightedness/nearsightedness
RLP Retrolental fibroplasia
ROP Retinopathy of prematurity
RPE Retinal pigment epithelium; layer of cells that nourishes the retina
S Saccade; tracking or shifting eye movement
SLE Slit lamp evaluation; instrument used for eye examination
SRX Spectacle prescription
V Version, following eye movement
VA Visual acuity
VEP Visual evoked potential; tests the central 10 degrees
VF Visual fields, peripheral vision test
WNL Within normal limits
XP Exophoria
XT Exotropia; eye deviates outward
+ Indicates possibility of farsightedness
− Indicates possibility of nearsightedness

MAJOR CHARACTERISTICS OF HEARING DEVELOPMENT

I. Prenatal
A. After the twentieth week of gestation, the fetus may respond to sound by startle, generalized body movement, quieting of activity, and/or autopalpebral reflex (involuntary eye blink).
B. Cochlea has normal functioning by twentieth week.
C. Environmental sounds have the greatest impact on auditory ability from the time the inner ear and the eighth cranial nerve become functional to central nervous system maturation; approximately 5 months' gestation to 18 to 28 months of age.
D. Inner ear reaches adult shape and size by the twentieth to twenty-second week of gestation.
E. The ears develop simultaneously with kidney formation; thus, an anomaly or dysfunction in one system may be indicative of problems in the other.

II. Birth to 1 Month
A. Hearing is more developed than vision at birth.
B. Infant distinguishes between familiar and unfamiliar sounds by 3 days of age.
C. Responds to sudden sound by crying, blinking eyes, or opening eyes widely.
D. Extends limbs and fans out fingers and toes; has startle reflex (Moro).
E. May become still if active at time of stimulation.
F. Responds to voice more than any other sound.

III. 3 Months (12 Weeks)
A. Begins to turn head to the side in attempt to locate sound source.
B. May smile in response to speech.
C. Stirs from sleep when there is a loud sound.

IV. 6 Months (24 Weeks)
A. Turns head directly to the side, then downward to locate sound made below eye level.
B. Learns to control and adjust response to sound (e.g., may delay response and listen for sound again or may not attempt localization).
C. Babbling sounds increase from birth to 32 weeks in infants with normal hearing but decrease in infants who are deaf.
D. Comprehends "no-no" and "bye-bye."
E. Imitates sounds.
F. Discriminates vowel sounds of language or languages to which they are continually exposed.
G. Hears variances in vowel and consonant sounds that establish neural connections for future speech development. Tested in laboratories by changes in sucking.

V. 12 Months (52 Weeks)
A. Locates sound in any direction and turns toward it.
B. Understands simple instructions when they are accompanied by gestures (e.g., "Give it to Mommy," "Say bye-bye.").
C. Says two or three words with meaning by 1 year.

VI. 1½ Years (18 Months)
A. Responds to verbal commands.

VII. 2 Years (24 Months)
A. Brainstem reaches maturity in the first 2 to 3 years of age.
B. Auditory cortex reaches near maturity by 2 to 3 years of age.
C. Directly locates a sound signal of 25 dB at all angles.
D. Joins words together spontaneously.
E. Developmental progression of speech and language are good indicators of normal hearing.

VIII. 36 Months and Older
A. The critical period for learning language is the first 36 months of life. The brain is developing rapidly during the first 3 years. If the auditory system is not stimulated, neural tracks and clusters do not develop, and language acquisition is negatively affected. Early detection of hearing loss is crucial for language development; babies can be fitted with hearing aids or assistive hearing devices as early as 4 weeks of age.
B. Nearly 100% of all children experience some period of hearing loss related to otitis media (OM) in the first 11 years of life. Approximately 15% of children ages 6 to 19 years have a low- or high-frequency hearing loss in one or both ears (Niskar, 1998).

HIGH-RISK CONDITIONS FOR HEARING IMPAIRMENT OF THE NEWBORN

The prevalence of significant, bilateral sensorineural hearing loss in newborns in the well-baby nursery population is approximately 1 to 2 per 1000 and an additional 1 to 2 per 1000 have milder or unilateral hearing loss (Haddad, 2004). In the neonatal intensive care unit (NICU), 2 to 4 per 100 infants have a hearing loss (American Academy of Pediatrics, 1999). Universal newborn hearing screening (UNHS) is being implemented through early hearing detection and intervention (EHDI) programs. Currently all states and the District of Columbia have implemented EHDI on either a legal or voluntary basis. Approximately 95% of newborns are being screened (ASHA, 2007), but follow-up in the community is difficult and there are sometimes delays in identifying the hearing loss and getting the infant into appropriate services. The Joint Commission on Infant Hearing (JCIH) recommends that all infants be screened before one month of age, hearing loss be identified by three months of age and early intervention services be in place by 6 months of age. Children with identified hearing loss (except those with bilateral profound impairment) who start services by 6 months of age should develop language on a level with their peers having normal hearing (Haddad, 2004; Calderon and Naidu, 2000).

Normal hearing at birth does not preclude delayed-onset hearing loss; 50% of children who ultimately are identified with a sensorineural hearing loss (SNHL) do not exhibit any risk factors at birth or they develop hearing loss after birth. Ninety percent of deaf children are born to hearing parents (Mitchell, 2004). The Joint Commission on Infant Hearing (JCIH, 2007) recommends all infants, regardless of results of newborn hearing screening, be monitored for development of auditory behaviors and communication skills at every routine well-child check. See Box 2-4 for risk factors that indicate closer supervision is required.

Box 2-4 **Risk Indicators Associated with Permanent Congenital, Delayed-Onset, or Progressive Hearing Loss in Childhood**

- Caregiver concern* regarding hearing, speech, language, or developmental delay. Family history* of permanent childhood hearing loss
- Neonatal intensive care of more than 5 days or any of the following regardless of length of stay: ECMO,* assisted ventilation, exposure to ototoxic medications (gentimycin and tobramycin) or loop diuretics (furosemide/Lasix), and hyperbilirubinemia that requires exchange transfusion
- In utero infections, such as CMV,* herpes, rubella, syphilis, and toxoplasmosis.
- Craniofacial anomalies, including those that involve the pinna, ear canal, ear tags, ear pits, and temporal bone anomalies
- Physical findings, such as white forelock, that are associated with a syndrome known to include a sensorineural or permanent conductive hearing loss.

- Syndromes associated with hearing loss or progressive or late-onset hearing loss,* such as neurofibromatosis, osteopetrosis, and Usher syndrome; other frequently identified syndromes include Waardenburg, Alport, Pendred, and Jervell and Lange-Nielson
- Neurodegenerative disorders,* such as Hunter syndrome, or sensory motor neuropathies, such as Friedreich ataxia and Charcot-Marie-Tooth syndrome.
- Culture-positive postnatal infections associated with sensorineural hearing loss,* including confirmed bacterial and viral (especially herpes viruses and varicella) meningitis
- Head trauma, especially basal skull/temporal bone fractures* that requires hospitalization
- Chemotherapy*

---

* Risk indicators that are of greater concern for delayed-onset hearing loss.
Source: Joint Commission on Infant Hearing, Year 2007 Position Statement. Available online: http://www.jcih.org/

HEARING CONDITIONS

Conductive Hearing Loss

I. Definition

A. A conductive hearing loss (CHL) is any type of interference in the transmission of sound from the external auditory canal to the inner ear; the inner ear is normal. In CHL, sounds are softer but not distorted.

II. Etiology

A. Conductive impairments are caused by conditions of the outer or middle ear and may be congenital or acquired (see "Additional Information"). The most common nongenetic cause of CHL in infants and children is otitis media (OM) in its various forms (Haddad, 2004). Young children have more horizontal, flaccid, shorter eustachian tubes, which increases their susceptibility to OM.

III. Signs, Symptoms, and History

A. About same loss of sensitivity for sounds in all frequencies.

B. Head noises localized in one or in both ears or unlocalized (tinnitus).

C. Recurring OM, frequent earaches, or draining ears.

D. Hearing loss may be intermittent if related to OM.

E. Others must speak louder than normal.

F. Individual may speak in relatively quiet voice because he or she is able to hear own voice through bone conduction; because of the air-conduction loss, person is unaware of environmental noise sounds that make hearing difficult for others.

G. Turns one ear toward speaker, if hearing less in one ear than the other.

H. Frequently needs words or sentences repeated.

I. Seems unable to follow directions well.

J. Compensates by using environmental cues.

IV. Effects on Individual

A. May cause significantly delayed language and speech development when occurring in early learning period.

B. Vocabulary develops more slowly.

C. Language deficit can cause learning problems.

D. Parent(s) may become frustrated and irritated from having to repeat information and may interpret inappropriate responses as signs of slowness.

E. Individual may develop emotional and acting-out behavior secondary to frustration and responses from others.

F. Individual subjected to parents'/teachers' discipline and anger because he/she appears to be inattentive or responses are inappropriate.

G. Peer relationships suffer.

H. Personal safety of individual may become an issue.

I. English as a second language, vision impairment, or other physical impairment compounds the effects of the hearing loss.

J. See Box 2-5 for concerns about students with a hearing loss.

Box 2-5   *Common Concerns Regarding Students with a Hearing Loss*

Characteristics associated with different types of hearing impairment:

- May be overactive as poor auditory input results in inattention leading to overcompensation or hyperactivity.
- Easily distracted from tasks when auditory input is diminished.
- May day dream when missing key points of information.
- May have external locus of control; e.g., parent, teacher, or hearing aids versus personally accepting control.
- Lower scores on achievement and verbal IQ tests.
- Progressive academic delays.
- English as a second language, vision impairment, or other physical impairment compounds the effects of the hearing loss.
- Increased need for special education or individualized classroom support.

Classroom environmental factors:

- Noise, reverberation and distance (NRD) affect ability to hear in classroom; noise masks speech and echoes smear speech.
- Distance from teacher affects decibel level of speech and limits visual cues.
- NRD affects consonants more than vowels as vowels are louder.
- Speech is garbled when consonants are lost, as English is a consonant-dependent language.
- Acoustics are also critical for students with ADHD, autism, auditory processing disorders and those with English as a second language.
- Signal-to-noise ratio is significant; need to reduce sounds in classroom so student can hear the teacher.
- Reduce classroom noise by using carpeting, sound-absorbing tiles and drapes; close doors and windows.
- Use of sound-field amplification systems in classrooms is becoming more common and benefits all children.

V. **Management/Treatment**
   A. Removal of impacted cerumen by irrigation or use of wax softeners.
   B. Medications include antibiotics; antifungals; and rarely oral steroids.
   C. Surgery (e.g., myringotomy with insertion of pressure-equalizing [PE] tubes or tympanomastoidectomy).
   D. Hearing aids.
   E. Speech therapy.
   F. Lip-reading or sign language instruction.
   G. Plastic surgery (otoplasty).
VI. **Additional Information**
   A. OM causes hearing loss between mild and moderate levels. OM is one of the most common chronic conditions of early childhood; affected children may have between 14 and 28 weeks of hearing loss annually in the first 3 years of life, which is the most critical period for language development. Pneumococcal conjugate vaccine (PCV) prevents pneumococcal bacterial infections, which cause 40% of pediatric ear infections. PCV is given at 2, 4, and 6 months of age, with a booster during the second year of life.
   B. The CHL that results from middle ear problems such as OM can cause significantly delayed speech, language, and academic skills because the loss most often occurs during a child's critical early

learning period. Early identification, referral, and treatment of middle ear disease are extremely important. Most conductive losses can be corrected through medical treatment or surgery.

C. Outer ear conditions that cause CHL include the following:
   1. Occlusion of the outer ear, from cerumen, foreign objects, tumors or malformation (e.g., mouse ear) of the pinna.
   2. Atresia (absence of a normal opening) of the external canal, either alone or in combination with other anomalies.
   3. Infection of the external canal (otitis externa), which may cause a mild conductive loss because of edema of the canal walls or accumulation of infectious debris.
   4. Perforation of the tympanic membrane from excessive pressure, necrosed (dead) tissue, trauma, or sudden pressure.
   5. Thickening of the tympanic membrane from middle ear infection.

D. Middle ear conditions that may cause CHL include the following:
   1. OM with effusion.
   2. Otosclerosis, a hereditary disease process of the inner ear that causes a growth of spongy bone in the middle ear and produces a progressive hearing loss when interference with the stapedial vibrations occurs; females are affected twice as often as males. Otosclerosis usually manifests between 10 and 30 years of age.
   3. Tympanosclerosis, new calcium plaques in the middle ear or on the tympanic membrane that occur as a result of OM and cause the conductive mechanism to lose mobility.
   4. Syndromes with craniofacial anomalies are often associated with CHL or SNHL; e.g., Pierre Robin, Crouzon, and Treacher Collins.
   5. Osteogenesis imperfecta (also called *brittle bone disease*), a hereditary condition whose major characteristics are multiple fractures, weak joints, blue sclera, thin translucent skin, and deafness. In a large percentage of cases, CHL occurs from otosclerotic changes; SNHL also has been identified.

SENSORINEURAL HEARING LOSS

I. Definition

A. SNHL is a loss of hearing caused by a pathological condition in the inner ear (cochlear) or along the nerve pathway (neural) from the inner ear to the brainstem. In SNHL, sounds (pitch or timing) are distorted, in contrast to conductive loss, in which the sounds are softer but not distorted.

II. Etiology

A. SNHL may be caused by congenital defects or acquired at any time before, during or after birth. SNHL of 26 dB or greater occurs in 13 per 1000 children in the United States including 0.5 to 1 per 1000 with a bilateral SNHL greater than 75 dB (Haddad, 2004). In sensory loss, the cochlea is damaged. In neural loss, the cochlea is normal, but auditory neuropathy, an eighth cranial nerve abnormality, is present so that sounds do not reach the brain in a normal fashion. Up to 50 % of sensorineural hearing losses are genetic in origin. SNHL may be associated with a syndrome or exist in isolation. Several genes have been implicated in SNHL not associated with a syndrome. Variants in Gap Junction Beta

2 (GJB2) also called connexin 26, cause up to 50% of nonsyndromic SNHL in some populations (Kenneson, Braun, and Boyle, 2002). These variants of GJB2 interfere with the recycling of potassium in the cochlea which is vital to sensorineural hearing function.

B. Postnatal causes include autoimmune or anatomical factors, trauma, infections, exposure to loud sounds, ototoxic medications, or the loss may be idiopathic (see "Additional Information").

C. Congenital cytomegalovirus (CMV) is the most common infectious, acquired cause of SNHL. CMV affects 1 out of 150 newborns and generally produces no symptoms, but a small number of infants (6,000 to 8,000 per year) have clinical symptoms, including 75% with SNHL (CDC, 2006). Approximately 10% of infants with asymptomatic CMV develop SNHL. The hearing loss may have delayed onset and may be progressive (Haddad, 2004).

III. Signs, Symptoms, and History

A. Individual may speak with excessive loudness because of loss of bone conduction.

B. Some difficulty in speech discrimination.

C. Better hearing in lower than in high frequencies, resulting in inability to differentiate many words that contain high-frequency consonants (e.g., fake, cake, sake).

D. Recruitment (abnormal increase in loudness).

E. Tinnitus is a generally constant ringing or buzzing noise, localized in either ear or not localized; pitch tends to be higher in SNHL than in CHL.

IV. Effects on Individual

A. Delay in speech and language development.

B. Language deficit can cause learning problems.

C. Vocabulary develops more slowly.

D. Parents can become frustrated at lack of communication and child's inability to respond appropriately.

E. May avoid social interaction with peers because of the reduced ability to understand what others are saying and poor articulation.

F. Temper tantrums or other behavior patterns may develop out of frustration.

G. Tends to have more physical complaints.

H. Poor self-concept, resulting in emotional problems.

I. Feels "different" than peers because of necessity of frequent visits to numerous helping professionals, placement in special education class, or small-group tutoring.

J. Personal safety may become an issue.

K. English as a second language, vision impairment, or other physical impairment compounds the effects of the hearing loss.

L. May affect vocational choices, although new technologies are breaking down most barriers.

M. See Box 2-5.

V. Management/Treatment

A. Hearing aids or amplification (may be used as early as 4 weeks of age).

B. Cochlear implant (electronic device surgically implanted into the cochlea with external transmitter and microphone) for those with profound loss with little or no benefit from hearing aids (see "Additional Information").

C. Prompt treatment of OM because conductive loss compounds SNHL.

D. Screen vision to rule out problems because hearing-impaired individuals rely heavily on their vision, and impairments in these senses often are associated.

E. Speech and language therapy; sign language; lip reading.

F. Auditory training.

G. Use preferential seating and control of environmental noise in classroom.

H. Make use of captioned CDs, interpreters, real time note takers.

I. Use Assistive Listening Devices (ALDs); e.g., FM systems, sound-field amplification, induction loop system, or other support systems in the classroom.

J. Few treatable causes of SNHL, such as autoimmune inner ear disease (cortisone), syphilis (penicillin and cortisone), and perilymph fistula (repair).

K. Treatment may be limited to prevention of further loss.

VI. Additional Information

A. SNHL usually is not corrected through use of medication or surgery; thus prevention is the best approach. Preventive measures include genetic counseling, early prenatal care, immunizations, control of noise levels, and identification of ototoxic drugs.

B. Prenatal (nonhereditary) causes of SNHL include rubella; influenza; Rh factor; syphilis; cytomegalovirus; anoxia; accumulation of toxic substances in the mother's bloodstream; and cerebral palsy, which has its own causes.

C. Perinatal causes include: anoxia, prematurity, and multiple births, exposure to contagious disease such as hepatitis, exposure to high noise levels, and trauma (e.g., violent contractions during birth, use of high forceps).

D. Postnatal causes include: measles, mumps, whooping cough, influenza, syphilis, excessive fever, autoimmune inner ear disease, bacterial meningitis, scarlet fever, diphtheria, encephalitis, diabetes, ototoxic drugs, accumulation of toxic substances in the blood from kidney disease, acoustic nerve tumors, head trauma, and sound trauma.

E. *Cochlear implants* act as a substitute for the hair cells of the organ of Corti and directly stimulate the nerve fibers in the cochlea. The devices may be implanted as early as 12 months of age; results are better with earlier implantation. Increased listening is the first indication of success. Development of some speech usually occurs 2 to 3 years after implantation. Cochlear implants do not restore normal hearing but increase the ability to hear environmental sounds. Binaural implants are now available and improve hearing by reducing the distraction of environmental noises. Parents who are deaf may be disinclined to consider cochlear implants for their child because this may disconnect the child from their deaf culture. Cochlear implants are contraindicated with findings of an abnormal acoustic nerve. Persons with a cochlear implant are at higher risk for pneumococcal meningitis. Centers for Disease Control and Prevention (CDC) recommend that all persons with cochlear implants receive age-appropriate vaccination against pneumococcal disease.

F. IDEA requires schools to make sure that cochlear implants are functioning adequately. Schools are not responsible for post-surgical maintenance, programming or replacement of cochlear implants.

G. An auditory brainstem implant system (ABI) can be used in teenagers and adults with neurofibromatosis type 2 when tumors (acoustic neuromas) growing on the cranial nerves must be surgically removed. Surgery requires severing the nerve, resulting in total loss of hearing. The ABI has restored at least some degree of hearing in all patients in whom the device was implanted correctly.

H. Genetic counseling is indicated when SNHL has been identified in one offspring.

MIXED CONDUCTIVE-SENSORINEURAL HEARING LOSS

I. Definition

A. Hearing loss produced by abnormalities in the middle ear and along the neural pathways.

II. Etiology

A. Recurrent OM may cause cochlear degeneration. Although otosclerosis generally is associated with a CHL, this disease may invade the inner ear and cause sensorineural impairment. A child with a diagnosed SNHL could develop a mixed loss when middle ear pathological conditions interfere with the conduction of sound waves through the middle ear.

III. Signs, Symptoms, and History

A. A child will demonstrate signs and symptoms of both types of loss. (Refer to previous sections on CHL and SNHL.)

IV. Effects on Individual

A. Delayed development of speech and language skills.

B. Learning problems resulting from language deficit.

C. Poor self-concept from reduced communication skills and poor academic achievement.

D. Social isolation because of difficulty in hearing and poor articulation.

E. See Box 2-5.

V. Management/Treatment

A. Treatment of conductive component.

B. Hearing aid; Assistive Listening Devices (ALDs) in the classroom.

C. Preferential classroom seating, as needed.

1. Seating in the center of second row is preferred so that the child is close to the teacher and able to pick up visual cues from other students; center of front row may work as well.

2. Seat away from noise sources such as air conditioners, open doors, windows, pencil sharpeners, computer centers, and aquariums.

D. Select a "buddy" to alert the student when particularly important information is presented, to take notes, or to help clarify spoken language.

E. Screen vision, since hearing-impaired individuals rely heavily on their vision; vision and hearing impairments are often associated.

NOISE-INDUCED HEARING LOSS

I. Definition

A. Noise-induced hearing loss (NIHL) is a high-frequency sensorineural hearing deficit usually involving frequencies from 3000 to 6000 Hz. It may be a temporary threshold shift (TTS) after a brief exposure to excessive sound (e.g. rock concert) or may become permanent after repeated exposure to noise. NIHL usually develops over time and is so gradual and subtle that it is not noticed until tested.

II. Etiology

A. NIHL is caused by a recurring exposure to excessive sound levels above 85 dB; it may also occur following a one-time exposure to an extremely loud, intense sound, (e.g., a bomb or gunshot). Research has demonstrated there is individual susceptibility to the effects of exposure to excessive sound (Lonsbury-Martin and Martin, 2005). Factors that may play a part include gender, race, age, smoking habits, certain diseases, and genetics. It is estimated that 12.5% of children ages 6 to 19 years in the United States have NIHL in one or both ears (Niskar et al, 2001).

III. Signs, Symptoms, and History

A. Onset is usually so gradual the loss is not detected without a hearing test.

B. Temporary loss of hearing and tinnitus or pain after exposure to loud sounds; repeated exposure may result in permanent loss.

C. Suddenly supersensitive to loud sounds.

D. Conversation becomes distorted or muffled.

E. Hearing loss is in higher frequencies (usually 3000 to 6000 Hz).

F. Hearing loss is usually symmetric, but noise from gun shots or sirens may cause asymmetric loss.

IV. Effects on individual

A. Difficulty understanding speech in noisy environments.

B. May not hear high-pitched sounds such as a distant telephone ringing.

C. May have more learning difficulties and behavioral problems than peers with normal hearing.

D. Effects similar to those of students with SNHL.

E. May have mild loss in adolescence, but can be compounded by presbycusis in later years.

V. Management/Treatment

A. Take history of exposure to excessive sounds.

B. Know which level of sounds can cause damage (See Table 2-3).

C. Educate regarding the possible long-term effects of chronic exposure to loud noise.

D. Encourage taking 15 minute "quiet" breaks when in an environment of extreme sound.

E. Advocate using protective devices when exposed to loud sounds. Look for devices with NRR (noise reduction rating) in excess of 9 dB. (See "Additional Information").

Table 2-3	*How Loud is Too Loud?*
Decibels	**Examples of sounds**
150	Firecracker
120	Ambulance siren
110	Chainsaw, rock concert
105	Personal stereo system at maximum level
100	Woodshop, snowmobile
95	Motorcycle
90	Power mower
85	Heavy city traffic
60	Normal conversation
40	Refrigerator hum

Wear ear plugs when you are involved in a loud activity.
110 Decibels—Regular exposure of more than 1 minute risks permanent hearing loss.
100 Decibels—No more than 15 minutes unprotected exposure recommended.
85 Decibels—Prolonged exposure to any noise above 85 dB can cause gradual hearing loss.
From National Institute on Deafness and Other Communication Disorders (NIDCD) WISE EARS!® 2007.

F. Discuss use of custom-made earplugs that can reduce volume without distorting the desired sounds, especially useful for musicians.

G. Stress importance of keeping volume on personal listening devices below 70% and taking breaks.

H. Recommend periodic hearing testing if routinely exposed to loud sounds.

I. Prompt parent(s) of the danger of noisy toys for young children.

J. Remind students that avoiding noise exposure stops further progression of the hearing loss.

K. Assess level of noise in school environment and advocate for reduction in noise and/or provide protection for students and faculty.

L. Promote hearing conservation programs in school. See Web Sites.

VI. Additional information

A. Typically, the use of earplugs reduces sound level to the middle ear by 15-30 dB. Ear muffs are generally more effective, especially in the 500 Hz to 1 kHz level, reducing noise by 30-40 dB. Increased protection is achieved by using both plugs and muffs.

B. Research toward finding a cure or a method to prevent NIHL is very promising. Studies using gene therapy for hair cell regeneration and/or repair are showing potential for an eventual treatment for NIHL. Conditioning may lead to the ability to adapt to excessive sounds and prevent NIHL. A number of studies are testing the prophylactic use of antioxidants to eliminate noise-induced cochlear injury by overcoming oxidative stress. Results are encouraging for a pharmacologic treatment in the near future (Lonsbury-Martin and Martin, 2005).

C. Occupational Safety and Health Administration (OSHA) protects workers through mandates for noise reduction, provision of hearing protection and hearing conservation programs. There are no such mandates on behalf of children in schools.

D. Exposure to loud sounds is especially traumatic for children with hearing aids because the sound is amplified.

E. Environmental, occupational, or household noise also causes stress-related problems, including fatigue, reduced sleep, increased frustration, difficulty in concentrating, and hypertension.

UNILATERAL HEARING LOSS

I. Definition
A. Hearing loss in one ear with normal hearing in the other ear. Prevalence of mild, moderate or severe unilateral loss is 6 to 12 children in 1000 and 0-5 in 1000 have moderate to profound unilateral loss (Lee, Gomez-Marin, and Lee, 1998).

II. Etiology
A. May be conductive or sensorineural.

III. Signs, Symptoms, and History
A. Usually have difficulty localizing sounds and voices.

B. May have difficulty hearing faint or distant speech.

C. Background noises impede speech detection.

IV. Effects on Individual
A. May become fatigued because of greater effort needed to listen.

B. May be perceived as having selective hearing or to be inattentive because of discrepancies in ability to understand speech in quiet versus noisy environment.

C. Frustration may lead to behavior problems.

D. On average, children with unilateral hearing loss are one full grade behind their peers academically.

V. Management/Treatment
A. Generally given preferential seating.

B. Hearing aid, may have a contralateral routing of signals (CROS) hearing aid.

C. May benefit from a personal or soundfield frequency modulation (FM) system.

D. Close monitoring is needed to avoid secondary complications, since a child may be thought to be noncompliant or inattentive, which may lead to behavior disorders.

AUDITORY PROCESSING DISORDER

Auditory processing disorder (APD), also known as central auditory processing disorder, is a decrease in auditory comprehension rather than a reduction in hearing acuity. APD is often confused with a hearing loss. A normal brainstem-evoked response may be present, but the child is unable to recognize or understand speech. May have normal cognitive skills but is unable to process auditory information. Condition may be mild to severe. It is a separate disorder, not the result of a cognitive, language or other related disorder; however, APD may coexist with another disorder, e.g., ADHD or autism. Treatment is individualized.

HEARING AIDS

TYPES OF HEARING AIDS

I. Conventional Analog Hearing Aid
   A. Settings programmed by the manufacturer, based on the individual's audiogram (See Box 2-6 and Table 2-4).
   B. Amplifies all sounds the same, with some minor adjustments.
   C. Appropriate for many types of loss.
   D. Least expensive hearing aid; requiring fewer repairs.

II. Analog Programmable Hearing Aid
   A. Also known as digital hybrid hearing aid.
   B. Microchip allows specific settings for diverse listening environments.
   C. Settings can be changed by pushing a button or toggle switch, or using a remote control to change channels.

III. Digital Programmable Hearing Aid
   A. Sounds in the environment are analyzed by a computer chip and converted into digital signals.
   B. Signals are adjusted to provide optimum hearing for the individual; usually self-adjusting.
   C. Greater number of programs available, more precise settings, better management of loudness, better control of feedback.
   D. Most expensive.
   E. Bone-conduction hearing aid
   F. Used for conductive hearing loss or when unable to wear hearing aid with ear mold due to continual infections or eczema.

IV. Two Types of Bone Conduction Aids
   A. Conventional type with body worn aid or behind the ear aid fitted to a headband or glasses.
   B. Bone-anchored hearing aid (BAHA) which is surgically implanted behind the ear.

V. Crossover Hearing Aid
   A. Contralateral routing-of-signal (CROS) aid is used for unilateral hearing loss.
   B. Microphone placed on the poorer ear sends the signal to a hearing aid on the better ear.
   C. May not work well in classroom due to environmental noise.

Box 2-6	*Hearing Aid Settings**

O = Off

T = Telecoil/telephone for telephone pickup, FM systems, or induction loop systems.

M = Microphone/telecoil for hearing others and own voice.

DAI = Direct audio input for connection with assistive listening devices, or other devices as TV, computer, CD player, radio, etc.

*Some hearing aids have no visible markings and work by moving a toggle switch.

Table 2-4	*Classifications of Hearing Function**
Slight (16-25)	Hears vowel sounds, difficulty hearing unvoiced consonant sounds.
Mild (26-40)	Soft or distant speech may be difficult. At 30 dB, child can miss up to 10% of speech signals. Preferential seating indicated. Auditory learning dysfunction: mild language delay, mild speech problems, inattention may manifest. Child may experience fatigue because of listening effort needed. Auditory training, FM systems, speech therapy beneficial. Without amplification, child with 35-40 dB loss can miss at least 50% of class discussion; 25 dB hearing loss is approximately amount heard with fingers in both ears.
Moderate (41-55)	Conversation speech understood at distance of 3-5 ft (face-to-face). Without amplification, child with 50 dB loss may miss 80%-100% of speech signal. May have limited vocabulary and articulation difficulties but should have good rhythm. Preferential seating, hearing aid, auditory training/FM system, and speech therapy indicated. Able to speak on telephone; can usually understand speech by hearing alone. Children rarely attend special schools or classes for deaf.
Moderately severe (56-70)	Others must speak loudly to be understood. Difficulty participating in classroom discussions. Usually cannot understand speech by hearing alone. Able to speak on telephone with amplification. Visual cues increase acquisition of speech and language. Speech should have good rhythm, tone, and articulation. Full-time amplification is essential. Preferential seating, speech and language therapy indicated. Requires resource specialist or special class depending on extent of language delay.
Severe (71-90)	May hear voices close to ear (about 1 ft). May discriminate environmental sounds. May distinguish vowels, but many consonants will be distorted. Language may not develop spontaneously and will be defective if hearing loss occurs before age 1 yr. May benefit from total communication approach, especially in early years. Auditory amplification necessary. Special education that focuses on speech, language, and auditory training needed. After sufficient training in special education, child may enter regular classroom but still requires speech therapy and support from a Deaf/Hard of Hearing Specialist.
Profound (≥91)	Some loud noises may be audible. Vision is primary method for learning and communication. Speech and language are defective; if loss is present before 1 yr, will not develop spontaneously. Requires special education or schools for deaf. Amplification is used for auditory awareness, voice control, and spatial orientation. May be considered for cochlear implant as young as 12 mo (FDA approval granted in 2000). Vibrotactile or electrotactile hearing aids may be used to support lip-reading, increase awareness of environmental sounds, and for training of speech production and reception.

*These descriptions are meant as guidelines only. They are not intended for use as labels or to influence expectations for the development of communication. The ability to develop communication in a variety of modalities varies among individuals.

EVALUATING HEARING AID FUNCTIONING

IDEA requires schools to make sure that hearing aids are working properly.

The following factors can affect the proper functioning of hearing aids:

I. Problems with Amplification
  A. Batteries; average life for behind-the-ear aids is 2-4 weeks.
  B. Wires or tubing detached.
  C. Aid turned off; volume too low.
  D. Improper mold.
  E. Wax or other material in ear or mold.
  F. Water in tubing can make hearing aid shut off suddenly.
  G. Unsuitable aid for degree of loss.
  H. Tubing: Mold may be put on wrong aid (left versus right), causing distortion in sound.
  I. Most common problem is child leaving hearing aids at home.

II. Acoustic Feedback
  A. Lower the volume of the aid.
  B. Reinsert the aid, making certain no hair is caught between ear mold and canal.
  C. Clean the ear mold/ear.

III. Whistling Noise
  A. Improperly worn.
  B. Improperly made.
  C. Worn out—crack in the tubing.
  D. Hearing may be worse, and child is turning volume up too high.
  E. Molds may need to be replaced every six to 12 months for young children. If they are loose fitting, whistling can occur.

IV. Discomfort from Earmold
  A. OM.
  B. Ear tumor.
  C. Improperly fitted mold.
  D. Ear skin or cartilage infection secondary to irritation of the tubing over the ear.
  E. Improperly worn.

CAUTION: Batteries should be kept in a childproof place and should not be changed in the presence of young children. Many hearing aids now have locks on the battery compartment.

Batteries may cause severe tissue burns, esophageal stricture or fistula if they accidentally are swallowed and become lodged in the esophagus; they must be removed. Immediate x-rays are needed to determine location. If battery has passed into the stomach, observe for discharge of the battery in the stool.

TESTING PROCEDURES

PURE TONE SCREENING

Children as young as 3 years old frequently can be conditioned for pure tone audiometric screening. Early identification of hearing and communicative problems is vital because intervention in the early years can avoid or minimize educational difficulties when the child begins academic activities.

I. Screening Criteria

A. The National Association of School Nurses (NASN) has published a manual, *The Ear and Hearing: A Guide for School Nurses* (Gregory, 1998). In the absence of state or district guidelines, pure tone audiometric screening is recommended for students as follows:
   1. Prekindergarten, kindergarten, and grades 1, 3, and 5; in higher grades as time allows.
   2. Students referred for or in special education as required by *Individuals with Disabilities Education Act* (IDEA).
   3. Requested by student, parent, or teacher.
   4. Newly enrolled students without any record of passing a hearing screening.
   5. Students who have failed hearing screening or having frequent upper respiratory infections or middle ear problems.
B. American Speech and Hearing Association (ASHA) adds screening in the second grade, eliminates screening in the fifth grade, but adds screening in seventh and eleventh grades. The upper grades are added because of the increased potential for hearing loss among adolescents due to overexposure to high levels of noise.

II. Screening Procedure

A. NASN recommends screening three frequencies (1000, 2000, and 4000 Hz). Some states may require screening four frequencies (adding 500 Hz). ASHA recommends screening at 20 dB. NASN recommends screening at 25 dB when there is no soundproof room.
   1. Select quietest room possible; let audiometer warm up, if needed.
   2. Check that earphones are plugged into correct jacks in audiometer.
   3. Put on earphones and verify that audiometer and earphones are working properly by testing all frequencies bilaterally at comfortable hearing level. Machine may need to be recalibrated if the screener cannot hear the signal at 25dB.
   4. Determine what form of signal will be most appropriate to indicate that tone has been heard (e.g., raising hand or fingers, saying "yes," or using signal light). Be certain individual understands that signal must be given the first time tone is heard, even if the tone is barely audible.
   5. Place earphones on each ear (red on right and blue on left) and adjust them for snug fit. Hair, dangling earrings, headbands, or eyeglasses may prevent a snug fit.
   6. Set hearing threshold level (HTL) at 25 dB.
   7. Starting with right ear, present tone at 1000 Hz for 1 to 2 seconds; if student does not respond, repeat the tone with a longer presentation. Proceed to 2000 and then 4000 Hz, finish at 1000 Hz.
   8. Repeat same procedures for left ear.
   9. Tone may be repeated, but not above 25 dB.
   10. Do not establish a pattern or rhythm; vary length of tone and pauses.

III. Failure Criteria

A. NASN recommends rescreening after 2 to 3 weeks if one frequency is missed in either ear. ASHA recommends rescreening at the same session, if possible, after reinstructing the student and repositioning the earphones. If testing at three frequencies, ASHA recommends 100% response; one miss is allowed if testing at four frequencies. Each state generally has its own standards and criteria.

IV. Action

A. Both NASN and ASHA recommend referral for professional evaluation after failing two sweep-check screenings. Give parent(s) a form letter that includes test results and space for the professional's report and recommendations.

B. Some states, school districts, and public funding agencies require pure tone threshold testing before making a referral.

PURE TONE THRESHOLD

I. Screening Criteria

A. ASHA recommends that only audiologists and speech-language pathologists complete threshold testing. Some states or school districts may require threshold screening after failing pure tone screening and before making referral for professional testing. A modified threshold test includes testing at 1000, 2000, and 4000 Hz and is the method described here.

B. The first six steps are the same as pure tone screening procedure.

1. Begin testing the right ear at 1000 Hz at 40 dB. Maintain each tone presented during testing for 1 to 2 seconds.

2. If there is response at 40 dB, drop back in 10-dB steps until there is no longer a response, then increase in 5-dB steps until sound is audible.

3. If there is no initial response at 40 dB, present the tone at 60 dB. If there is no response at 60 dB, stop testing at that frequency and indicate on student record "does not hear at 60 dB."

4. If the student responds at 60 dB, drop back in 10-dB steps until there is no longer a response, then increase in 5-dB steps until sound is audible.

5. Drop back 10 dB and ascend in 5-dB steps two more times to determine accuracy of threshold. Threshold is lowest level at which correct response is given two out of three times a tone is presented.

6. As you obtain thresholds for each frequency, record results numerically or in graph form (audiogram) on data sheet.

7. Impedance should be administered and results added to those obtained from pure tone audiometry.

8. When testing children, particularly younger ones, periodically remind them that signal must be given as soon as they hear the tone.

9. Conditioned play audiometry (CPA) is an effective method of testing 3- and 4-year-olds; CPA is described in the section "Infant, Preschool, and Special Education Screening" page 102.

II. Failure Criteria

A. NASN recommends that children be referred for threshold level of 30 dB or more for two or more sounds in one ear and threshold level of 35 dB or more for one tone in either ear. ASHA recommends rescreening at the same session if possible, after reinstructing the student and repositioning the earphones. Each state generally has its own standards and criteria.

III. Action

A. Notify parents of results and recommend evaluation by a physician, otolaryngologist, or audiologist. Give parent(s) a form letter that includes test results and space for the physician's report and recommendations.

IV. Additional Information

A. A screening tool developed for use by teachers is the Screening Instrument for Targeting Educational Risk (SIFTER). It consists of 15 questions relating to a student's school performance when hearing problems are suspected. Areas covered are academics, attention, communication, class participation, and school behavior. Completion of the questionnaire provides information helpful to the nurse and audiologist in completing more thorough testing; helpful as a pretest and posttest when evaluating the benefit of personal or classroom amplification; also used as in-service instrument with teachers to discuss possible effects of hearing impairment on learning.

IMPEDANCE/IMMITTANCE AUDIOMETRY

Impedance (immittance) is an objective, rapid, efficient, and noninvasive means of measuring the compliance/mobility of the tympanic membrane and air pressure of the middle ear. It is used to rule out a middle ear problem as a part of a comprehensive screening program. No special testing environment is necessary, and no response from the child is required.

In a normal ear, loud sounds cause the stapedius muscle to momentarily contract, which stiffens the ossicles and immediately lowers the membrane compliance. The muscles in both ears contract in response to a stimulus delivered in only one ear (bilateral response). This stapedial reflex generally is absent when a conductive hearing loss exists. The muscle contraction has little effect on a tympanic membrane immobilized by fluid or by fixation of the ossicle. No observable effect is present in cases of perforated membrane or discontinuity of the ossicular chain.

Impedance also determines whether the stapedial reflex is present. Some instruments also include a report of physical volume, which provides the examiner with the cavity size of the external ear canal measured in cubic centimeters. A shortened physical volume may indicate blockage or presence of a foreign object. A report of physical volume can be helpful when a child has had tubes inserted for chronic OM. When tubes are intact and functioning, the physical volume is above normal limits. If the tubes have become dislodged or are blocked by drainage or wax, the volume is normal.

I. Screening Criteria

A. Used to rule out middle ear problems; e.g., otitis media, as part of comprehensive hearing screening program.

II. Screening Procedure

A. Before testing, examine external auditory canal with an otoscope for size, obstruction, inflammation, or any abnormalities. Do not test if pain, drainage, or apparent problem is present, which indicates immediate referral to a physician.

B. Explain procedure and offer reassurance that test is not painful.

C. Use appropriate probe tip; it should be larger than meatus because objective is to obtain airtight seal.

D. To obtain best seal, ear canal must be straightened. In ages 12 months to 3 years, pinna must be pulled downward and backward. For children older than 3 years, pull the pinna upward and back, with the head tilted slightly away from examiner.

E. Apply the probe firmly to canal opening.

F. Hold probe steady until machine indicates test is completed. Remove probe.

G. Results may be in numerical or digital display or form depending on the type of instrument used.

H. A number of impedance machines are available on the market. Each machine has its own method of operation; therefore, follow manufacturer's guidelines.

I. Record results and make appropriate referral if needed.

III. Additional Information

A. To check compliance of the tympanic membrane, introduce positive pressure into the external ear canal with a probe tip. As this positive pressure (measured in millimeters of water, mm H_2O) is released, it gradually changes to negative pressure; and the membrane moves. The degree of movement is known as *middle compliance* (measured in cubic centimeters, cm^3) and is recorded by numerical digital display or on a graph. The air pressure required for the membrane to reach maximum compliance is recorded as middle ear pressure. Results of compliance and air pressure convey information regarding the state of the middle ear and function of the eustachian tube. Abnormal readings identify the possibility of middle ear disease.

B. Often young children become very fearful of the probe, regardless of how well the examiner explains what will be heard and offers assurance of no discomfort. Sometimes the child's fear is alleviated if the testers demonstrate on themselves, a doll, or a stuffed animal. (If possible, the examiner can place the probe on the child's hand because contact with the skin will cause the same humming sound as when the probe is placed in the canal.) Rather than upsetting the child and ruining the chance of a later attempt, the examiner should offer reassurance and understanding and let the child watch while others are tested. When an entire class is to be screened, demonstration of the procedure to the group before individual testing is recommended.

C. Pure tone screening is inadequate for detecting a large percentage of children with OM because the conductive hearing loss may not be significant enough for the child to fail screening standards. Pure tone screening and impedance complement each other; inclusion of both in a hearing screening program is highly recommended.

D. The complete impedance/immittance testing battery includes tympanometry, static compliance, acoustic reflex threshold measurement, ear canal physical volume test (PVT), and behavioral observation.

INFANT, PRESCHOOL, AND SPECIAL EDUCATION SCREENING

All states now have newborn hearing screening programs, with an increased number of infants identified with a hearing loss; but almost half of those identified do not receive follow-up to confirm the hearing loss and/or start early intervention services (JCIH, 2007). Infants who pass newborn screening but have a risk factor should have at least one diagnostic audiological evaluation by 24 to 30 months of age (see Box 2-4, page 84).

This section provides screening criteria and descriptions of several of the better-known tests, including the appropriate age group and source of further information. When a hearing loss is suspected, refer the child for a complete medical and audiological assessment as soon as possible.

EARLY CHILDHOOD SCREENING

I. Otoacoustic Emission (OAE) Response
  A. Appropriate age.
    1. Newborns; infants, and preschoolers who cannot follow instructions for behavioral procedures.
  B. Summary of test.
    1. Both transient evoked otoacoustic emissions (TEOAEs) or distortion product otoacoustic emissions (DPOAEs) are sensitive to hair cell dysfunction. OAE is a measurement of the inner ear (cochlear) response to a sound introduced into the external ear. This response is obtained by placing a microphone in the external ear and connecting it to a computer that provides an objective interpretation. OAE detects both sensory (cochlear or inner ear) and recurrent conductive hearing loss (CHL) and is measured in decibel sound pressure level (dBSPL).
    2. OAEs do not detect neural (eighth nerve) loss or auditory brainstem pathway dysfunction. Factors affecting quality of testing include probe fit, environmental noise, and internal (subject) noise. Newborns have a considerable amount of internal noise that decreases by 4-5 months of age.
  C. Additional information.
    1. Devices are now easier to use and available for use in the schools from school health supply companies. As the technology improves, OAEs will play an increasingly important role in hearing screening in schools.
II. Electrophysiological Procedures
  A. Appropriate age.
    1. Birth through preschool or older children who are difficult to test with behavioral test methods.
  B. Summary of test.
    1. These procedures may be called *automated auditory brainstem response (AABR), auditory brainstem response (ABR), brainstem auditory evoked response (BAER),* or *evoked response audiometry (ERA).* The child must be relaxed or sleeping to avoid muscle movements that may interfere with testing; usually requires mild sedation. Rapid clicking sounds are presented through earphones, and brain wave patterns

are recorded as measured through electrodes placed on the child's scalp. Activity of the cochlea, eighth cranial nerve, and auditory brainstem pathway are measured and can detect auditory neuropathy or neural disorders. Use of bone-conduction AABR in conjunction with the traditional air- conduction AABR discriminates CHL from SNHL and assesses the extent of conductive involvement.

2. Brainstem response procedures do not assess "hearing", but responses indicate that the auditory system up to the midbrain is responding to a stimulus.

  C. Additional information.

1. Both OAEs and ABRs can produce false-negative results; behavioral testing is recommended in high-risk infants or when language delay is noted.

III. Visual Reinforcement Audiometry (VRA)

  A. Appropriate age.

1. Approximately 6 to 24 months, or children unable to tolerate earphones.

  B. Summary of test.

1. Behavioral testing, which also may be called *conditioned orientation reflex (COR)* or *condition orienting response audiometry (CORA)* is a subjective measure of hearing. The child is seated in a sound-conditioned booth on an adult's lap. Lighted mechanical toys are flashed on simultaneously with an auditory signal (speech or warble tone) to the right or left of the child's visual field. The child responds by turning toward source of sound and is rewarded by seeing the lighted action toy. In this sound field testing environment, results provide measurement of hearing for the better ear only because the child is using both ears to respond to the sounds. When the child is able to tolerate earphones, further testing should be done to obtain ear-specific information.

IV. Conditioned Play Audiometry (CPA)

  A. Appropriate age.

1. CPA can be used for pure tone screening of children 2½ to 5 years old and children with developmental delay.

  B. Summary of test.

1. Before testing, the child is conditioned to drop blocks or other small objects into a container when a tone from the audiometer is presented. The earphones are left on the table, and the examiner plays the game with the child until the child's response is appropriate and consistent. The earphones are then securely placed on the child, and the examiner proceeds with the pure tone screening or audiogram. Sounds may be presented through loudspeakers if the child is unable to tolerate earphones.

WEB SITES

American Academy of Audiology
    http://www.audiology.org
American Society for Deaf Children
    http://www.deafchildren.org/

American Speech-Language-Hearing Association
    http://www.asha.org
National Association of the Deaf
    http://www.nad.org
National Institute on Deafness and Other Communication Disorders
    http://www.nidcd.nih.gov
The Institute for Enhanced Classroom Hearing
    http://www.classroomhearing.org
WISE EARS!® (National campaign to combat noise-induced hearing loss)
    http://www.nidcd.nih.gov/health/wise
National Hearing Conservation Association (NHCA): Crank It Down
    http://www.hearingconservation.org
Dangerous Decibels®
    http://dangerousdecibels.org

GLOSSARY OF HEARING TERMS

Adventitious   Accidental, referring to relatively sudden loss of hearing.

Agnosia   Inability to understand significance of sounds.

Air conduction   Pathway of sounds conducted to the inner ear by the outer and middle ear.

Aphasia   Partial or complete loss of expressive and receptive language; most commonly an incomplete mixture of both receptive and expressive aphasia. Causes include stroke, head trauma, or prolonged hypoxia. May be transient.

Articulation   Vocal tract movements for production of speech. Articulate speech is distinct and connected.

Assistive listening device   Any device used to enhance ability to hear by reducing background noise, amplifying sound, and overcoming negative effects of distance. Includes amplified telephones, one-to-one communicators, and frequency modulation (FM) systems.

Atelectasis of tympanic membrane   Collapse or retraction of the tympanic membrane; may or may not be associated with otitis media.

Audiogram   Graphic representation of audiometric findings.

Audiologist   One skilled in the identification, measurement, and rehabilitation of people with hearing impairments and related disorders (e.g., vestibular dysfunction, tinnitus).

Auditory perception   Ability to identify, interpret, and attach meaning to sound.

Auditory prosthesis   Device that substitutes or enhances the ability to hear.

Auditory training   Lessons to assist a person with hearing loss to maximize residual hearing.

Augmentative devices   Technical tools to assist individuals with limited or no speech, such as text telephones, communication boards, and conversion software translating text to speech.

Auricle   See Pinna.

Bel   Unit of measure expressing the ratios of acoustical or electrical power.

Bone conduction   Sounds conducted to the inner ear through mechanical vibrations in the bones of the skull.

CHAPTER 2

Vision and Hearing

Cholesteatoma   Cystic mass in middle ear composed of cholesterol and epithelial cells as a result of a congenital defect or chronic otitis media. Requires surgical removal.

Cholesterol granuloma   A serious complication of acute otitis media in which a chronic collection of infection and cholesterol crystals have formed a solid mass.

Cochlea   Spiral bony structure in the inner ear that transforms sound waves into nerve impulses that are sent to the brain; it is part of the bony labyrinth.

Cochlear nerve   One of the main divisions of the eighth cranial nerve; responsible for hearing and balance; also called *auditory nerve.*

Compliance   Inverse of stiffness.

Contralateral routing of signal   A hearing aid for persons with normal or near-normal hearing in one ear and an unaidable loss in the other ear. This device allows a person to have two-sided hearing by channeling all the signals into the "good" ear.

Decibel   A decibel (dB) is the unit of measurement of intensity in acoustics and audiometrics; one tenth of a bel.

Dysacusia   Distortion of intensity or frequency of sounds.

Dysfluency   Disruption in smooth flow of speech, e.g., stuttering.

Eustachian tube   Tube lined with mucous membrane that connects the nasopharynx and the middle ear cavity. Usually remains closed but opens during chewing, swallowing, and yawning.

Eustachian tube dysfunction   Tube does not open when needed to equalize pressure between the middle ear space and the atmospheric pressure. Most common cause is an inflammatory reaction of the membranous lining of the tube with nasal infections or allergies. Other reasons include enlargement of adenoids, developmental anomalies (e.g., cleft palate, cleft uvula), or immaturity of palatal muscles that often do not mature until after 12 months. May be acute or become chronic.

Frequency   Number of complete oscillations of a vibrating body per second. Physical attribute of sound measured in hertz (Hz).

Frequency modulation systems   These systems provide amplification of voice. They may be personal units or sound-field units for an entire classroom. The teacher wears a personal microphone for either method. Personal FM units require a receiver to be worn by the student or the placement of a boom box near the student. Sound-field units require 2-4 loudspeakers mounted on the walls or ceiling. The sound-field amplification system eliminates the identification of any one child as having special needs, and amplification has been shown to be advantageous for all students, including those with normal hearing.

Hearing threshold level   The lowest level at which the pure tone audiometer stimulates normal hearing; hearing-level dial is calibrated in dB HTL.

Hertz   Hertz (Hz) is the number of cycles per second (cps).

Impedance   Term is interchangeable with immittance. Opposition to sound wave transmission, which is made up of frictional resistance, mass, and stiffness and influenced by frequency.

Incus   An anvil-shaped bone, one of the three ossicles in the middle ear; transmits sound from the malleus to the stapes.

Induction loop system   An assistive listening device that uses electromagnetic waves for transmission. The induction loop is a cable (wire or copper foil tape) that goes around the listening area, usually at floor level. Sounds are picked up by the teacher's microphone, amplified, and sent through the wire/loop. Students pick up the sound by using the telecoil (T-switch) on their hearing aid.

Labyrinthitis   Infection or inflammation of the inner ear; affects balance and may cause temporary hearing loss.

Language   The structured, symbolic, and accepted system of interpersonal communication.

Malleus   One of the three ossicles in the middle ear, shaped like a hammer; transmits sounds from the tympanic membrane to the incus.

Mastoiditis   Infection of the mastoid process.

Meatus   Opening or passage.

Meniscus   A fluid line; when fluids are present in the middle ear, the meniscus is sometimes seen through the tympanic membrane.

Myringotomy   Surgical incision in tympanic membrane to relieve pressure by draining fluid or pus from the middle ear.

Neurofibromatosis type 1   Also called *von Recklinghausen's disease,* an inherited multisystem disorder in which nonmalignant tumors grow on the skin and nerves that may include the cochlear nerve. Symptoms of NF-1 include café-au-lait spots, axillary and inguinal freckling, bone lesions, optic gliomas, and neurofibromas. Individuals with NF-1 often have learning disabilities.

Neurofibromatosis type 2   Characterized by family history and bilateral nonmalignant tumors on the eighth cranial nerve. NF-2 may occur in the teenage years and cause hearing loss. Individuals with NF-2 often have learning disabilities.

Noise-induced hearing loss   Hearing loss caused by exposure to harmful sounds, either very loud impulse sound(s) or repeated exposure to sounds above 85-dB levels over an extended period.

Ossicular discontinuity   Disconnection of the ossicles, resulting in hearing loss. May be caused by retraction pockets, cholesteatomas, or a perforation of the eardrum.

Osteogenesis imperfecta   Hereditary disorder characterized by multiple fractures; also called *brittle bone disease.* Sixty percent of affected individuals have conductive hearing loss by adolescence or young adulthood.

Osteopetrosis   Inherited disorder with generalized increase in bone density. In severe forms, bones in the skull may become so dense that they cause compression of cranial nerves, resulting in deafness, blindness, and early death.

Otitis externa   Inflammation or infection of the external canal or auricle. Major causes are bacteria, allergies (nickel or chromium in earrings or chemicals in hair sprays or cosmetics), fungi, viruses, and trauma. Excessive swimming may wash out protective cerumen, remove skin lipids, and lead to secondary infection (also called *swimmer's ear*).

Otitis media   Acute otitis media (AOM) is fluid in the middle ear with signs or symptoms of ear infection (bulging eardrum, pain, perforated eardrum) and usually requires treatment with antibiotics. Otitis media with effusion (fluid) (OME) is otitis media without signs or symptoms of ear infection and does not usually require antibiotics.

Otoplasty   Plastic surgery of the outer ear.

Otorrhea   Malodorous discharge from the external ear. May be serous, sanguinous, purulent, or contain cerebrospinal fluid.

Otosclerosis   Formation of spongy bone in the middle ear, usually around the footplate of the stapes and oval window; a progressive conductive hearing loss results when it interferes with stapedial vibration.

Ototoxic drugs   Drugs such as a special class of antibiotics, aminoglycosides, that may have a harmful affect on the eighth cranial nerve; may cause deafness or severe hearing loss. Other such drugs include aspirin, furosemide, and quinine.

Perilymph fistula   A leak of the inner ear fluid into the middle ear; most commonly the result of head trauma.

Pinna   Projected part of the external ear (auricle); gathers sound waves from the environment.

Pressure-equalizing tubes   Tubes are inserted in the tympanic membrane to equalize pressure between the inner ear and the middle ear. Usually temporary and become dislodged, falling out in less than a year. Permanent tubes may be sutured into place when needed over long term.

Pure tone   Sound waves of only one frequency.

Pure tone average   Pure tone average (PTA) is the average hearing loss, in decibels, across all frequencies in an individual's better ear. Sometimes screened at only 500, 1000, and 2000 Hz.

Recruitment   Large increase in the perceived loudness of a signal after a relatively small increase in intensity above threshold; symptomatic of some sensorineural hearing losses.

Round window   Opening in the medial wall of the middle ear leading into the cochlea; covered by a secondary tympanic membrane.

Semicircular canals   Three bony, fluid-filled canals in the inner ear that make up the largest part of the vestibular system, which is associated with the sense of balance.

Sound-field amplification   See Frequency modulation systems.

Speech recognition threshold   Minimum hearing level at which a person can discern the presence of speech material 50% of the time. The listener does not have to identify the material as speech, but must signify awareness of the presence of sound. Sometimes called *speech detection threshold.*

Stapedius reflex threshold   Lowest intensity at which a sound causes the stapedius muscle to contract.

Stapes   One of the three ossicles, resembles a tiny stirrup. Transmits vibrations from the incus to the inner ear.

Tadoma   Method of tactile speech transmission used by deaf-blind whereby a carefully positioned hand is used to sense vibrations, movement, and airflow on the face of the speaker.

Threshold   Level at which a tone is perceived as barely audible; usual clinical criteria demand the subject be aware of the sound 50% of the time presented.

Tinnitus   Sounds in the ear; described as ringing, roaring, buzzing, and so on.

Tympanocentesis   Process of inserting a needle through the tympanic membrane to aspirate fluid from the middle ear for evaluation or treatment.

Tympanogram   A graph plotting the compliance of the tympanic membrane at specific air pressures.

Tympanosclerosis   Calcium formations in the middle ear or on the tympanic membrane; caused by otitis media; results in loss of mobility of the conductive mechanism.

Vestibular apparatus   Structures in the inner ear related to balance and sense of position; includes the vestibule and the semicircular canals.

Vibrotactile hearing aid   Sensations produced by electrical stimulation of the nerves that lead from touch receptors in the skin. Surface electrodes on the skin deliver stimulation signals to convey sounds through sense of touch. Single-channel aids are worn on the wrist, multichannel on the forearm, neck, or abdomen. May also be called *electrotactile aids*.

ABBREVIATIONS OF HEARING TERMS

AABR Automated auditory brainstem response
ABR Auditory brainstem response
AC Air conduction
AD Right ear
ALDs Assistive listening devices
AOM Acute otitis media
AS Left ear
AU Both ears
BAER Brainstem auditory evoked response
BC Bone conduction
BOA Behavioral observation audiometry
CMV Cytomegalovirus
CPA Conditioned play audiometry
dBSPL Decibel sound pressure level
DPOAE Distortion product otoacoustic emissions (two pure tone stimuli are presented at the same time)
DRF Deafness Research Foundation
EHDI Early Hearing Detection and Intervention
EOAE Evoked otoacoustic emissions
ERA Evoked response audiometry
HTL Hearing threshold level
NAD National Association of the Deaf
NBS Newborn Screening
OAE Otoacoustic emissions testing
OME Otitis media with effusion
PET Pressure-equalizing tubes
PTA Pure tone average
SDT Speech detection threshold
SRT Speech reception threshold
TEOAE Transient evoked otoacoustic emissions (elicited by brief acoustic stimuli such as clicks or tone bursts)
TM Tympanic membrane
VRA Visual reinforcement audiometry

BIBLIOGRAPHY

American Speech-Language-Hearing Association: Early detection and intervention action center. (2006). Available online: http://www.asha.org/about/legislation-advocacy/federal/ehdi/. Accessed May 21, 2007.

Anshel J: *Smart medicine for your eyes,* New York, 2007, Square One Publishing.

Bacal DA, Wilson MC: Strabismus: getting it straight, *Contemp Pediatr* 17(2): 49-60, 2000.

Bear MF, Connors BW, Paradiso MA: *Neuroscience: Exploring the brain,* Philadelphia, 2007, Lippincott Williams and Wilkins, pp 277-308.

Bryant R: Child with cognitive, sensory, or communication impairment. In Hockenberry MJ, Wilson D (editors): *Wong's nursing care of infants and children,* St. Louis, 2007, Elsevier Mosby, pp 989-1027.

Calderon R, Naidu S: Further support of the benefits of early identification and intervention with children with hearing loss. In Yoshinaga-Itano C, Sedey AL, editors: Language, speech and social-emotional development of children who are deaf and hard-of-hearing: The early years, *The Volta Review* 100:53-84, 2000.

Centers for Disease Control and Prevention (CDC) (2006). *About CMV.* Available online: http://www.cdc.gov/cmv/facts.htm. Accessed June 13, 2007.

Chen D, Friedman C, Cavello G: *Parents and visually impaired infants: identifying visual impairment in infants (PAVII),* Louisville, Ky, 1990, American Printing House for the Blind.

de Hoog M, van Zanten BA, Hop WC et al: Newborn hearing screening: Tobramycin and vancomycin are not risk factors for hearing loss, *J Pediatr* 142(1):41-46, 2003.

Evans A: Color-vision deficiency: what does it mean? *J School Nurs* 8(4):6-10, 1992.

Fligor BJ: "Portable" music and its risk to hearing health. *The Hearing Review, March 2006.* Available online: http://www.hearingreview.com/issues/articles/2006 03_08.asp. Accessed April 2, 2007.

Gregory EK: *The ear and hearing: A guide for school nurses,* Washington, DC, 1998, National Association of School Nurses.

Haddad J: Hearing loss. In Behrman RE, Kliegman RM, Jenson HB, editors: *Nelson textbook of pediatrics,* Philadelphia, 2004, WB Saunders, pp 2129-2135.

Hall JW, Chase P: Answers to 10 common clinical questions about otoacoustic emissions today, *Hearing Journal* 46(10):29-32, 1993.

Hickok G, Bellugi U, Klima E:. Sign language in the brain, *Sci Am* 284(6):58-65, 2001.

Howard PJ: *The owner's manual for the brain: everyday application from mind-brain research,* Austin, Texas, 2006, Bard Press.

Hoyt C, Jastrzebski G, Marg E: Delayed visual maturation in infancy, *Br J Ophthalmol* (67)127-130, 1983.

Hubel D, Wiesel T: Brain mechanisms of vision. *Sci Am* 241(3):150-162, 1979.

Joint Commission on Infant Hearing: Year 2007 position statement: Principles and guidelines for early hearing detection and intervention programs, *Pediatrics* 120(4):898-921, 2007.

Kenneson A, Braun KV, Boyle C: GJB2 (connexin 26) variants and nonsyndromic sensorineural hearing loss: a huGE review. *Genet Med* 4(4):258-274, 2002.

Kotulak R: *Inside the brain: revolutionary discoveries of how the mind works,* Kansas City, Mo, 1996, Andrews & McMeel.

Lee DJ, Gomez-Marin O, Lee HM: Prevention of unilateral hearing loss in children: The National Health and Nutrition Examination Survey II and the Hispanic Health and Nutrition Exam Survey, *Ear and Hearing* 19(4):329-332, 1998.

Lonsbury-Martin BL, Martin G: Noise-induced hearing loss. In Cummings CW, editor: *Otolaryngology: head & neck surgery,* Philadelphia, 2005, Elsevier Mosby, pp 2906-2923.

Mitchell RE: Chasing the mythical ten percent: parental hearing status of deaf and hard of hearing students in the United States, *Sign Language Studies* 4(2):138-163, 2004.

Mosby's Dictionary of Medicine, Nursing and Health, St. Louis, *2006.*

Motley W III, Struck M: Care of the blind child. In Osborn L et al, editors: *Pediatrics,* St. Louis, 2005, Elsevier Mosby, pp 977-988.

National Institute on Deafness and Other Communication Disorders (NIDCD): WISE EARS!® 2007, Available online: http://www.nidcd.nih.gov/health/wise/index.htm. Accessed April 2, 2007.

Niskar AS, Kieszak SM, Holmes A:. Estimated prevalence of noise-induced hearing threshold shifts among children 6-19 years of age: the Third National Health and Nutrition Examination Survey 1988-1994, *Pediatrics* 108(1):40-43, 2001.

Niskar AS, Kieszak SM, Holmes A: Prevalence of hearing loss among children 6 to 19 years of age: the Third National Health and Nutrition Examination Survey 1988-1994, *JAMA* 279(14):1071-1075, 1998.

Olitsky S, Nelson L: Disorders of the eye. In Behrman RE, Kliegman RM, Jenson HB, editors: *Nelson textbook of pediatrics,* Philadelphia, 2004, WB Saunders, pp 2083-2126.

Proctor SE: *To see or not to see: screening the vision of children in school,* Castle Rock, Colo, 2005, National Association of School Nurses.

Sato-Viacrucis K: The evolution of the Snellen E to the blackbird, *School Nurse,* Spring:18-19, 1985.

Sieving PA: Retinitis pigmentosa and related disorders. In Yanoff M, editor, *Ophthalmology,* St. Louis, 2004, Elsevier Mosby.

Sifuentes M: Approach to the deaf or hard of hearing child. In Osborn L et al, editors: *Pediatrics* St. Louis, 2005, Elsevier Mosby, pp 488-493.

Struck M. (2005). Approach to the child with vision impairment. In Osborn L et al, editors: *Pediatrics,* St. Louis, 2005 Elsevier Mosby, pp 494-499.

Vision in Preschoolers Study Group: Preschool vision screening tests administered by nurse screeners compared with lay screeners in the vision in preschoolers study, *Invest Ophthalmol Vis Sci* 46(8):2639-2648, 2005.

Vision in Preschoolers Study Group: Comparison of preschool vision screening tests as administered by licensed eye care professionals in the vision in preschoolers study, *Am Acad Ophthalmol* 111(4):637-650, 2004.

Wiesel T, Hubel D: Single responses in striate cortex of kittens deprived of vision in one eye, *J Neurophysiol* 26:1003-1017, 1963.

CHAPTER 3

Acute Conditions

Chapter Outline

Blepharitis
Conjunctivitis
Diaper Dermatitis
Diarrhea
Eczema (Atopic Dermatitis)
Erythema Infectiosum, Human Parvovirus Infection (Fifth Disease)
Fever
Frostbite
Giardiasis
Hand, Foot, and Mouth Disease
Hepatitis A
Impetigo
Kawasaki Disease
Measles (Rubeola)
Infectious Mononucleosis
Mumps (Infectious Parotitis)
Otitis Media
Pediculosis Capitis (Head Lice)
Pinworms (Enterobiasis)
Poison Ivy, Oak, and Sumac Dermatitis
Upper Respiratory Tract Infection (Common Cold)
Ringworm of the Body (Tinea Corporis)
Roseola Infantum (Exanthem Subitum)
Rubella (German Measles)
Scabies
Scarlet Fever
Shigellosis (Acute Diarrhea)
Streptococcal Pharyngitis (Strep Throat)
Sty (Hordeolum)
Tapeworm
    Beef, Pork, Fish, and Dwarf Tapeworms
Testicular Torsion
Urinary Tract Infection
Varicella-Zoster Virus (Chickenpox)

*T*he number of school-age children who come to school with an acute illness is difficult to estimate. Frequently, nurses in the school and community setting are the first called on to determine whether a health problem
exists and if further assessment is required. Thus the nurse must be aware of
signs and symptoms of individual illness, must be able to provide the necessary initial management, and must make appropriate and informative referrals for additional treatment when necessary. *Initial management* information
in this chapter gives the nurse a plan of action. After assessing the problems,
the nurse frequently must provide health care and comfort until a parent assumes responsibility or there is additional medical intervention.

Action may be necessary to protect other students and staff from exposure
to communicable disease. *Guidelines for exclusion and readmission* are provided
for the student who might have a contagious condition. Determining the
length of time for homestay and readmission is critical so as not to jeopardize
the health of others in the classroom setting. The recommendations in this
chapter are suggested when public health or school policies have not been
established.

Because this manual defines *school age* as birth through 21 years, certain
health problems included here may not be relevant to the child of traditional
school age. Early intervention with the special-needs child requires that the
nurse have knowledge of health problems associated with the very young; the
nurse must also be able to educate and support staff working with these children and their families. School nurses are often the only source of medical
care for students and their families.

BLEPHARITIS

I. Definition
   A. Blepharitis is a chronic or long-term inflammation of the eyelid mar-
      gins or the eyelash follicles. It can affect any age individual.

II. Etiology
   A. This condition may be seborrheic, staphylococcal, or a combination
      of the two; or it may be an allergic reaction. *Anterior blepharitis* affects
      the external front of the eyelid, where the eyelashes are attached.
      Most common causes are bacteria and scalp dandruff. *Posterior bleph-
      aritis* affects the inner eyelid, which is the moist part that touches
      the eye. It is caused by problems with the oil glands in this part of
      the eye, usually due to one of two skin disorders, acne rosacea and
      seborrheic dermatitis.

III. Signs, Symptoms, and History
   A. Condition is usually bilateral and chronic or recurrent.
   B. Redness and swelling.
   C. Crusting or scaling of the eyelids.
   D. Common symptoms are burning, itching, irritation, dry eyes, exces-
      sive tearing, blurred vision; eye pain is rare.
   E. Staphylococcal blepharitis: ulceration of lid margin, lashes often fall
      out; conjunctivitis and superficial keratitis are associated.
   F. Seborrheic blepharitis: greasy scaling, infrequent ulceration, lid
      margins less red.

IV. Initial Management

A. Wash hands. Cleanse the lid margins using a moistened cotton applicator, cotton ball, or cloth with diluted baby shampoo to remove scales and crusts. This is an important treatment modality, and the student can learn how to do the daily cleansing when the nurse cleans the area and teaches at the same time.

B. For seborrheic blepharitis: examine scalp, body, and eyebrows to determine if student and parent need information regarding control of seborrhea; concurrent treatment may be needed.

C. For staphylococcal blepharitis: an antistaphylococcal antibiotic is applied to the eye margins or directly into the eyes.

D. Refer student to a health care practitioner (HCP) as needed.

V. Exclusion/Readmission

A. If student is very young, exclude from school if staphylococcal infection is present.

B. Student may return to school when lesions are healed and no further crusting is present.

VI. Additional Information

A. Treatment of staphylococcal blepharitis is usually continued for a week or more after symptoms have disappeared. The student may need the antibiotic administered at school. Box 3-1 explains how to administer the eye ointment. Unless the seborrheic condition is so severe that it is limiting, the student may remain in school while under treatment.

WEB SITES

American Academy of Ophthalmology
http://www.aao.org
National Institutes of Health, National Eye Institute
http://www.nei.nih.gov/health/blepharitis/index.asp#4

CONJUNCTIVITIS

I. Definition

A. Conjunctivitis, commonly called *pinkeye,* is a contagious inflammation of the conjunctiva, the mucous membranes that line the upper and lower eyelids and extend over the sclera. The most common pediatric ocular condition, more than 50% of the time the cause is bacterial, and it is most often diagnosed in preschool children and sexually active teens.

Box 3-1	*Administering Eye Ointment*

1. Pull down the lower lid and apply a thin line of ointment along the inner margin of the lid.
2. Ointment may cause temporary blurring of vision.
3. For seborrhea, remove crusts on lids with a moist cotton applicator before applying.

II. Etiology
A. Conjunctivitis is caused by the bacteria *H. influenzae, S. pneumoniae,* and *chlamydia* and also by viruses, such as adenovirus, herpes simplex virus (HSV), herpes zoster, and enterovirus. Seasonal pollens, chemical irritants, and other allergens may also be to blame.

III. Signs, Symptoms, and History
A. Table 3-1 presents the manifestations of conjunctivitis in the school-age child.

Table 3-1	*Manifestations of Conjunctivitis in the School Age*		
	Bacterial	Viral	Allergic
Incubation	24-72 hrs	5-12 days	
Duration	2 days up to 2-3 weeks	Up to 2 wks	
Period of Communicability	Until 24 hrs of treatment	Greatest latter part of incubation period	
Signs and Symptoms			
Involvement	Generally unilateral	Generally unilateral	Commonly bilateral
Conjunctiva	Red or pink	Red or pink	Red
Discharge	Purulent, matted eyelashes	White, stringy	Watery
Tearing	Moderate	Profuse	Profuse
Photophobia	Mild	Moderate to severe	Mild
Blurred Vision	Common with discharge, clears with blinking	When keratitis present	
Chemosis (edema of conjunctiva and lining of eyelids)	Moderate	Mild	
Foreign body sensation	Unusual	Gritty sensation	Gritty sensation
Itching	Minimal or none	Minimal	Severe
Preauricular lymph node	Unusual	More common	Not present
Other			Sneezing; watery nasal discharge

IV. Initial Management
  A. Isolate from others depending on etiology.
  B. Determine if viral, bacterial, or allergic conjunctivitis, or if other serious conditions are indicated. Does student appear ill other than the eye condition? Does the student complain of headache, fever, sore throat, joint pain, nausea, or a runny nose?
  C. Obtain history of current problem. Did it just start? Has there been any exposure to chemicals, eye trauma, or allergens? Is there discharge, pain, or tenderness around the eye?
  D. Apply cool compresses.
  E. Refer to eye specialist if visual loss, moderate to severe pain, history of HSV conjunctivitis, or recurring conjunctivitis occurs.
  F. Clustering of vesicles around eye may indicate HSV.
  G. Discuss importance of proper hand-washing technique to students and staff.
  H. Contact parent or caregiver and refer to HCP if indicated.
  I. Educate school staff regarding communicable disease and precautions.
V. Exclusion/Readmission
  A. With purulent conjunctivitis, exclude from school until treatment is started.
  B. In epidemics of nonpurulent conjunctivitis, exclude only if health authority recommends.
VI. Additional Information
  A. Bacterial and viral conjunctivitis are transmitted by contact with the discharge from the conjunctiva or upper respiratory tract of infected persons or by contaminated fingers, clothing, or other articles.
  B. Treat bacterial conjunctivitis with topical antibiotic, ophthalmic solution, or ointment (e.g., erythromycin, sulfacetamide, chloramphenicol). In certain cases bacterial conjunctivitis is self-limiting, and the viral kind should clear on its own. For allergic conjunctivitis, treat with naphazoline (OTC); discuss with parent regarding referral to allergist.
  C. Differential diagnoses: Acute glaucoma, uveitis (juvenile arthritis), Lyme disease, sinusitis, herpes viral infection, orbital and eyelid inflammation, and inversion of the eyelash.

WEB SITES

American Academy of Ophthalmology, Conjunctivitis Preferred Practice Pattern
    http://www.aao.org
American Optometric Association, Care of Patient with Conjunctivitis
    http://www.aoa.org/documents/CPG-11.pdf

DIAPER DERMATITIS

I. Definition
  A. Diaper dermatitis is an inflammatory irritation of the skin that causes a breakdown of this natural barrier.

II. Etiology

    A. Diaper dermatitis is caused by prolonged exposure of the skin to urine and/or feces; a sensitivity to such things as disposable diapers, soaps, and detergents; infrequency of diaper change; inappropriate or no cleansing of the diaper area; or skin dermatoses, which are aggravated by wearing diapers; reaction to medication, such as antibiotics.

III. Signs, Symptoms, and History

    A. Mechanical.

        1. Acute or chronic erythematous, hyperpigmented area along edge of diaper or plastic pants.

        2. Erythematous skinfolds.

    B. Chemical.

        1. Erythematous macular or papular rash, which is shiny and peeling in diaper area.

        2. Erythema on buttocks and around anus.

        3. Dry erythema around head of penis.

    C. Hygienic factor.

        1. Any of the above symptoms.

        2. Noticeably poor hygiene.

IV. Initial Management

    A. Call parent; ask about changes in diet, soap, or method of treatment.

    B. Change diapers frequently; keep skin dry and clean.

    C. Use warm water and mild soap to wash genital area after every diaper change.

    D. Use ointment when skin is dry; use protection for skin irritation such as zinc oxide or petroleum jelly. Hydrocortisone may be prescribed by HCP if not a fungal infection.

    E. Wash cloth diapers well and double rinse.

    F. Dilute urine by increasing fluids.

    G. Use sitz baths; expose area to air.

V. Exclusion/Readmission

    A. Does not apply to simple diaper rash.

VI. Additional Information

    A. Differential diagnosis includes bacterial, viral, or candidiasis infections; psoriasis; atopic dermatitis; scabies; or seborrhea.

    B. Management is difficult with children who seem predisposed to diaper dermatitis. Complete healing can take several days. However, definite improvement should be observed within 48 to 72 hours after treatment has begun.

    C. Yeast and bacterial infections may be mistaken for diaper rash. If there are small, bright red, scaly spots or convex shapes, use antifungal cream. Large, fragile vesicles or pustules may indicate bacterial infection, and an antibiotic may be needed.

WEB SITE

Children's Hospital Boston

    http://www.childrenshospital.org

DIARRHEA

I. Definition

A. Diarrhea is the passage of excessive fluid and electrolytes in the stool. This condition may be acute or chronic. Chronic diarrhea is an increased frequency of unformed stool lasting longer than 2 weeks.

II. Etiology

A. The pathogenesis of diarrhea episodes includes five known causes:
   1. Inflammatory processes.
      a. Inflammatory processes include any surgical procedure or condition that has the ability to change the anatomy and functional integrity of the intestine, such as bacterial invasion (*E. coli,* celiac sprue, and irritable bowel syndrome).
   2. Motility disorders.
      a. Acute diarrhea can result from any atypical peristalsis from any source. Motility disorders may be either delayed or rapid and can be associated with infection or bacterial overgrowth.
   3. Viral and bacterial agents.
   4. Secretory diarrhea.
   5. Osmotic diarrhea.

B. Cause may be a combination of factors.

III. Signs, Symptoms, and History

A. Watery, copious bowel movement; may have foul odor or be bloody.

B. Elevated temperature, abdominal pain, and vomiting.

C. Dehydration, including decrease in urine output with increased concentration; sunken eyes; weight loss; no or few tears with crying; dry oral mucous membranes; and depressed fontanel in the infant.

D. History of exposure to contaminated food from family, school, or community sources.

E. Recent travel to high-risk area and possible correlation with change in diet.

IV. Initial Management

A. Take temperature.

B. Be aware of frequency, consistency, color of stools, and presence of blood, pus, or mucus.

C. Note any vomiting, abdominal cramping, irritability, loss of appetite, fever, or other signs of distress.

D. Give clear or electrolyte fluids in place of formula, milk, and solids as indicated.

E. Notify parent or caregiver.

F. Suggest BRAT diet: bananas, rice, applesauce, and toast or tea. Progress to regular diet on the third day, adding soft foods.

G. Practice good general hygiene.

V. Exclusion/Readmission

A. Student generally will not be dismissed for one or two loose stools unless other signs of illness exist.

B. Student must be fever-free 24 hours before returning to school.

C. If diarrhea persists, younger students must have written statement from HCP that no viral, bacteriological, or parasitic condition exists.

WEB SITES

National Institute of Diabetes and Digestive and Kidney Diseases
    http://www.niddk.nih.gov
Food Allergy and Anaphylaxis Network
    http://www.foodallergy.org

ECZEMA (ATOPIC DERMATITIS)

I. **Definition**
   A. Eczema is an acute or chronic cutaneous inflammatory condition characterized by pruritus, swelling, blistering, oozing, and scaling of the skin.
II. **Etiology**
   A. There is a strong family predisposition. The most predominant indicator is a family history of asthma, eczema, or hay fever. Infants with atopic dermatitis (AD) seem to develop allergic rhinitis and subsequent asthma. AD affects 10% to 20% of all infants and nearly half of these children will greatly improve by ages 5 to 15. Others will have some form of atopic disease the rest of their life (American Academy of Dermatology, 2005).
   B. The underlying problem is the skin's inability to retain adequate amounts of water; can be triggered by ingestion of, or contact with, a substance to which an individual is sensitive (e.g., milk, fish, eggs, or inhalation of dust, pollen, or similar substances).
III. **Signs, Symptoms, and History**
   A. Usually begins in infancy, age 2 to 3 months, or it can be delayed.
   B. Chronic lesions or red macular areas on face, neck folds, scalp, hands, behind ears, antecubital and popliteal areas.
   C. Erythematous papules, vesicles, pustules, scales, crusts, or scabs, alone or in combination; they may be dry or occur with watery discharge (see color plates, Primary and Secondary Skin Lesions).
   D. Severe itching or burning with overall dry skin.
IV. **Initial Management**
   A. Disorder can be controlled but not cured.
   B. Discuss management with student and parent or caregiver.
   C. Prevention.
      1. Teach avoidance of trigger allergens and extreme temperatures; sweating leads to itching and irritation.
      2. Moisturize frequently; avoid harsh soaps and solvents.
      3. Avoid scratchy materials, such as wool or materials that do not breathe (e.g., nylon).
      4. Reduce stress.
   D. Treatment.
      1. Keep fingernails short to prevent scratching and secondary infection.
      2. Apply cool compresses to itchy skin to help relieve itching.
      3. Colloidal bath (Aveeno, oatmeal, or cornstarch) will soothe dry, itchy skin: use 1 to 2 cups cornstarch in a bathtub of water.
      4. Limit bathing time to 5 to 10 minutes to prevent depletion of natural skin oils. Apply ointment, such as petroleum jelly, immediately to moist skin.

5. If infrequent bathing is prescribed, use a nondrying, soap-free cleanser.
6. Antihistamines may be prescribed to decrease itching, such as hydroxyzine (Atarax) and diphenhydramine (Benadryl). Can cause drowsiness, but may help some children.
7. Corticosteroids can help calm inflamed skin (e.g., hydrocortisone, desonide).

V. **Exclusion/Readmission**
   A. Does not apply.

WEB SITE

National Eczema Association
   http://www.nationaleczema.org

ERYTHEMA INFECTIOSUM, HUMAN PARVOVIRUS INFECTION (FIFTH DISEASE)

I. **Definition**
   A. Erythema infectiosum is a mild, nonfebrile erythematous skin eruption that usually occurs in children from age 2 to 13 years, but it can occur in adults. Usually seen in late winter and early spring, but it can occur anytime. It is named *fifth disease* because it was the fifth eruptive rash characterized.

II. **Etiology**
   A. Fifth disease is caused by the human parvovirus B19, transmitted in blood and respiratory secretions from an infected individual.

III. **Signs, Symptoms, and History**
   A. *Incubation period is 4 to 20 days.*
   B. *Disease is communicable until the rash appears.*
   C. Disease is usually benign and self-limiting.
   D. Prodromal phase: Rash preceded by low-grade fever (up to 102 degrees), malaise, sore throat, and headache.
   E. Secondary stage: Face has "slapped cheek" appearance, erythema, and a pallor that lasts 1 to 2 days (see color plate 1).
   F. Over the next several days, appearance of "lacy rash," a maculopapular eruption that progresses from proximal to distal surfaces of the trunk and extremities.
   G. Rash may last days or weeks.
   H. Rash may reappear months later in response to sunlight, temperature extremes, exercise, trauma, or emotional stress.
   I. Studies demonstrate that about 25% of children are asymptomatic.
   J. Lasting immunity after infection occurs.

IV. **Initial Management**
   A. Call parent regarding condition and home care.
   B. No specific management.
   C. Treat symptomatically, take temperature, and assess rash area.
   D. Educate teachers and staff of childbearing age, including those working in preschools; see "Additional Information."

V. Exclusion/Readmission
   A. Not applicable; by the time a rash appears, the individual is probably no longer contagious.
VI. Additional Information
   A. Laboratory test used for detection is B19-specific immunoglobulin M (IgM)-antibody assay. When assay is positive, it only indicates infection within the past several months.
   B. In older students and adults, arthralgias and arthritis are associated with B19 parvovirus. Affected joints in the hands may be the only symptom. Joint symptoms and rash generally occur 2 to 3 weeks after infection and can persist for many months afterward.
   C. Fifth disease may be dangerous to the fetus of pregnant women who contract the disease in the first half of pregnancy. There is a risk for an infected fetus to develop fetal anemia and hydrops fetalis (massive edema), and fetal death is possible. Alert pregnant women and students to contact their HCP regarding these risks.
   D. This disease can also precipitate an aplastic crisis in children with sickle cell disease or those with autoimmune hemolytic anemia and α-thalassemia. For those individuals with immunodeficiencies, the infection with B19 virus can lead to severe chronic anemia.

CHAPTER 3

Acute Conditions

WEB SITE

National Center for Infectious Diseases
   http://www.cdc.gov/ncidod/diseases/children/diseases.htm

FEVER

I. Definition
   A. Fever is an elevation of the body's normal temperature, which ranges from 96.8° to 99.5° F (36° C to 37.5° C) when taken *orally*. If *axillary* measurement is used, add one degree to the reading. If the temperature is taken *rectally*, subtract one degree from the reading.
   B. Fever Gradients.
      1. *Low-grade fever:* 100° to 102° F (37.7° to 38.8° C) orally.
      2. *Moderate-grade fever:* 102° to 104° F (38.8° to 40° C) orally.
      3. *High-grade fever:* above 104° F (40° C) orally (Lucile Packard Children's Hospital, 2006).
   C. Temperature can be temporarily affected by age, physical activity, ovulation, and emotional stress.

II. Etiology
   A. A fever develops in response to a disturbance in the homeostatic mechanisms of the hypothalamus, where a balance between heat production and peripheral heat loss is maintained. Pyrogens, protein substances released by leukocytes, are produced within the body whenever inflammatory and infectious processes occur.

B. In inflammatory processes—such as those that occur in tissue damage, cell necrosis, malignancy, antigen–antibody reactions, and rejection of transplanted tissues—fever is due to the action on *endogenous pyrogens,* which act on the thermoregulatory center in the hypothalamus. *Exogenous pyrogens* occur when the body is invaded by bacteria, viruses, fungi, and other types of infectious organisms (Johnson and Baltimore, 2006).

III. Signs, Symptoms, and History

A. Chilling and shivering results as the body attempts to raise the temperature.

B. This reaction produces thirst, increased respirations—4 breaths per minute per degree of temperature increase—and an increased pulse rate of about 8 to 10 beats per minute for each degree of temperature increase.

C. Rapidly rising fever may cause a febrile seizure, most commonly in infants and young children under age 5; onset of seizure is sudden. (See Chapter 4, Chronic Conditions, Seizures.)

D. Should fever persist, fluid and electrolyte losses are more severe; evidence of cellular dehydration and delirium may occur in older individuals.

IV. Initial Management

A. Observe for appearance of symptoms of disease process, such as rash, sore throat, or stiff neck.

B. Take temperature, vital signs, and assess behavior: note if the student is busy, talkative, tired, energetic, playing, or experiencing decreased appetite. Ask students to describe how they feel and what they did that morning.

C. Note any recent illnesses or medication.

D. Treat symptomatically until parent is able to pick up student from school.

E. Remind parents not to give aspirin to children under 12 due to Reye syndrome.

F. Chills raise body temperature, so when they are present, a student should be covered and protected from drafts.

G. If no chills are present, remove as much clothing as possible.

H. Apply cold compresses to the forehead.

I. Sponge with tepid water, only uncovering small areas. When skin cools, accompany sponging with rubbing to encourage circulation of blood through skin.

J. Continue sponge bath as long as necessary to lower the temperature; a quick splash may only stimulate heat production.

K. If possible, give clear fluids and ice chips by mouth.

V. Exclusion/Readmission

A. Student with a temperature of 101° F (38.3° C) or above may be dismissed from school (American Academy of Pediatrics, 2006).

B. If student appears well and fever is low-grade, consider other factors, such as recent exercise or emotional state. Retake temperature in 15 minutes.

C. Student may be readmitted to class if there has been no fever in the preceding 24 hours and no antipyretics have been taken.

VI. Additional Information
A. Oral temperature is contraindicated when seizure disorder, irrational behavior, or mouth breathing exists; when infants or toddlers are involved; or when there is disease, surgery, or structural anomaly of the oral cavity.
B. There are a variety of thermometers available, ranging from simple plastic strips to digital or infrared devices. They vary in use and levels of accuracy. Digital is more accurate than plastic strips but more expensive; electronic is safe and useful for pediatrics, and keeping the mouth closed is not required for an accurate reading; infrared are used frequently but accuracy debate continues.

WEB SITES

KidsHealth for Parents: What is fever?
http://www.kidshealth.org/parent/general/body/fever.html
Medline Plus
http://www.nlm.nih.gov/medlineplus/fever.html

FROSTBITE

I. Definition
A. Frostbite is an injury to the tissues and impaired circulation to the affected area, which can lead to cell destruction. Areas that are prone to freeze first are the cheeks, nose, ears, fingers, toes, and feet.

II. Etiology
A. In prolonged exposure to cold ranging from −2 degrees to −10 degrees, nerve, blood vessel, and other cells are temporarily frozen. Many factors can potentiate effects of cold, including fatigue, injury, immobility, dependency of the extremity, general health, duration of exposure, high altitude, and increased wind velocity. Frostbite can be mild to severe, and exposure to extremely cold chemicals—such as liquid oxygen—produces immediate frostbite.

III. Signs, Symptoms, and History
A. Exposure to cold.
B. Early signs are shivering, low body temperature, skin pain, tingling, and numbness.
C. Skin red initially, then pale, slightly yellow, or waxy white.
D. Tissue blanches early on and then may feel rock-hard or doughy.
E. Previous history of frostbite will cause increased sensitivity to cold in that area.
F. On rewarming, extent of tissue damage can be determined accurately.
G. Frostnip or superficial frostbite.
   1. Causes discomfort and redness.
   2. Skin seems to be normal within a few hours.
   3. Can be cared for at home with medical follow-up.
   4. Usually does not significantly damage tissue.
H. Deep frostbite.
   1. Erythema and swelling.
   2. Cyanosis or mottling.

3. Numbness associated with burning pain.
4. Bullae and vesicles that appear within 24 to 48 hours; however, if necrosis of tissue occurs from inadequate circulation in involved areas, blisters do not occur.
5. Gangrene.

IV. Initial Management

A. Take temperature to determine presence of hypothermia, a life-threatening condition in which body core temperature is at or below 95° F (35° C).
   1. Minor is 89.6° to 96.8° F (32° to 36° C).
   2. Moderate is 86° to 89.6° F (30° to 32° C).
   3. Severe is less than 86° F (30° C).
B. Remove wet clothing.
C. Call parent or caregiver.
D. Do not massage or rub area with snow.
E. If there is no possibility of refreezing, warm area rapidly, but do *not* use dry heat, such as a radiator or oven. Clothing, blankets, or another body surface may be used. Skin may blister, swell, and turn red, blue, or purple. An area is thawed when it is no longer numb.
F. Protect area from further trauma.
G. Keep other body areas warm by covering them with a blanket.
H. Severe frostbite must be managed by a specialist.

V. Exclusion/Readmission

A. Does not apply.

VI. Additional Information

A. Educate school staff and students; send newsletters home to parents and caregivers regarding prevention and initial management of frostbite.
B. To prevent frostbite, make sure children wear several layers of loose, protective clothing, such as face masks, hats, earmuffs, mittens, and appropriate boots. Have extra socks, mittens, and hats on hand; mittens are usually warmer than gloves. During severe cold weather, check children's cheeks and hands periodically for symptoms of frostbite. If there are suspicious signs, warm the affected area with body heat; instruct the child to tuck cold hands under their armpits or into the bends of their legs.
C. Older children and adolescents should avoid alcohol and cigarettes while they are exposed to cold. Alcohol causes peripheral vasodilation, which increases the rate of heat loss from the skin. Nicotine inhibits peripheral blood flow through vasoconstriction.

WEB SITE

eMedicine: Frostbite
http://www.emedicine.com/emerg/topic209.htm

GIARDIASIS

I. Definition

A. Giardiasis is a protozoan infection of the small intestine and duodenum. It ranges from asymptomatic infection to acute or chronic diarrhea and malabsorption. Giardia is the most commonly identified intestinal parasite in the United States (Childers, 2005).

II. Etiology
A. Giardiasis is caused by the flagellate protozoan *Giardia lamblia,* also called *Giardia intestinalis.*

III. Signs, Symptoms, and History
A. *Incubation period is 3 to 25 days with a median of 7 to 10 days.*
B. *Period of communicability can be the duration of the infection.*
C. *Transmission is by direct person-to-person contact or by contact with contaminated food and water. Can be epidemic in day care centers and custodial institutions.*
D. Acute infection usually lasts 1 to 3 weeks, but it can become chronic.
E. Usually asymptomatic in both children and adults.
F. Failure to thrive in young infants and toddlers.
G. Limited phase of acute infection with or without anorexia and weight loss, nausea, and low-grade fever.
H. Abdominal distention, cramps, flatulence, nausea, vomiting, and fatigue.
I. Initially watery stools, which later become greasy (steatorrhea), malodorous, and may float. No blood or mucus in stools.
J. May have intermittent periods of normal bowel movement and constipation.
K. Chronic infection may cause malabsorption and debilitation.

IV. Initial Management
A. Maintain good hygiene. Box 3-2 provides instructions on how to make a disinfectant solution.
B. Call parent or caregiver and refer to primary HCP.
C. Provide clear liquids; discontinue formula, milk, juices, and food.
D. Dispose of feces and diapers using sanitary precautions.
E. Use petroleum jelly on perianal area to prevent excoriation.
F. Treatment: antiprotozoal agents (e.g., metronidazole [Flagyl] and furazolidone [Furoxone]).
G. Report disease to public health authority.

V. Exclusion/Readmission
A. Exclude children and adults with acute diarrhea from day care settings.
B. Exclude children and adults from school if laboratory tests are positive and diarrhea is untreated.
C. Readmit student after diarrhea has stopped or treatment has started: check school or state guidelines and Department of Health standards, because these vary among states.

Box 3-2	*Disinfectant Solution*

One-quarter cup bleach (5.25% sodium hypochlorite) per gallon of cool water
OR
One tablespoon bleach per quart of cool water

Solution must be mixed fresh every day.

VI. Additional Information

A. Follow universal hand-washing precautions. For objects that cannot be cleaned in a dishwasher, use disinfectant solutions or bleach and water. Solutions are weakened by light, heat, and evaporation (see Box 3-2, Disinfectant Solutions).

WEB SITE

Association of State and Territorial Directors of Health Promotion and Public Health Education (ASTDHPPHE)
http://www.astdhpphe.org

HAND, FOOT, AND MOUTH DISEASE

I. Definition

A. This highly contagious viral disease is characterized by pharyngitis, fever, and exanthem, particularly on the hands and feet. More common in the summer and early autumn and in children under age 10. Hand, foot and mouth disease (HFMD) is also known as *enteroviral vesicular stomatitis with exanthema.*

II. Etiology

A. Coxsackie virus A16 is the major cause, but group B enterovirus 71 is another causative factor, is more severe, and has been associated with meningitis, encephalitis, and paralytic disease.

III. Signs, Symptoms, and History

A. *Incubation period is 3 to 5 days.*

B. *Period of communicability is during the acute phase of illness but can be longer; virus persists in feces for several weeks.*

C. *Transmission is from person to person by direct contact with nose and throat secretions or stools of infected persons.*

D. Malaise; low-grade fever of 100° to 102° F (37.7° to 38.8° C).

E. Symmetrical maculopapular eruptions on palms and soles, oral lesions, and lesions that may occur on buttocks.

F. Virus may produce vesicular lesions on palms, fingers, soles of feet, and buttocks without oral lesions. Lesions more frequent on the dorsal surfaces of hands and feet.

G. Rash may persist 1 week or longer. Rash does not itch.

IV. Initial Management

A. Ensure proper hand washing technique.

B. Isolate student from others.

C. Contact parent or caregiver and discuss communicability and disease process.

V. Exclusion/Readmission

A. Exclude student from school during the acute phase and until fever-free for 24 hours.

VI. Additional Information

A. Another viral disease caused by the Coxsackie virus A16 is vesicular pharyngitis, commonly called *herpangina* or *aphthous pharyngitis.* Herpangina is an acute, self-limiting disease with sudden onset, fever, sore throat, and small, discrete, grayish vesicular pharyngeal lesions on an erythematous base that progress to ulcers (see color plates, Primary and Secondary Skin Lesions). The ulcers heal spontaneously and the condition runs its course in less than 1 week.

1. HFMD differs from herpangina in that the oral lesions are more diffuse and can occur on the gums, sides of tongue, or buccal surfaces of the cheeks. Lesions rupture, leaving shallow ulcers.
2. Herpangina requires differentiation from herpes simplex virus (HSV); HSV has deeper, larger, more painful ulcerative lesions, usually found in the front part of the mouth.

WEB SITE

eMedicine: Pediatrics, Hand-Foot-and-Mouth Disease
   http://www.emedicine.com/emerg/topic383.htm

HEPATITIS A

I. **Definition**
   A. Hepatitis A is the most common type of hepatitis in the United States. It is an inflammation of the liver that occurs sporadically or in epidemics. About 15% of people infected with hepatitis A virus (HAV) will have prolonged or relapsing symptoms over a 6-to 9-month period (see Table 4-7, page 217).
II. **Etiology**
   A. Hepatitis A is caused by HAV. The highest rates of HAV are among children 5 to 14 years of age, with approximately one third of reported cases occurring among children under 15 years of age.
III. **Signs, Symptoms, and History**
   A. *Incubation period is 15 to 50 days, with an average of 28 days.*
   B. *Period of communicability of virus is 2 weeks prior to the onset of jaundice; probably noninfectious after the first week of jaundice, but prolonged viral excretion—for up to 6 months—has been reported in children.*
   C. *Transmission of HAV is by the fecal–oral route with the virus transmitted from person to person between household contacts, sex partners, or by contaminated food or water.*
   D. There is no chronic, long-term infection, nor is there crossover to other types of hepatitis.
   E. There is immunity to HAV after infection.
   F. History of direct exposure.
   G. History of eating contaminated shellfish or drinking contaminated water.
   H. Children are generally asymptomatic.
   I. Onset is abrupt with adults and older children.
   J. Prodromal phase: fever, anorexia, nausea and vomiting, malaise, abdominal pain, headache, enlarged or tender liver.
   K. Icteric phase (5 to 7 days after initial symptoms): sclera and skin are jaundiced, urine is darkened, stools are light-colored.
IV. **Initial Management**
   A. Refer students with symptoms to parent or caregiver for medical care.
   B. HAV is a reportable disease in all states.

C. Use good hand-washing techniques after toileting and before and after eating or preparing food.

D. Treatment and management of HAV infection is supportive.

E. Dispose of feces in a sanitary manner. Infants and young children can shed the virus for longer periods.

F. Determine what health education is needed in the school and community. Support family and stay in close contact.

G. Refer close contacts to their HCP or Public Health Department (PHD) for information regarding immunoglobulin.

H. Inform and educate all school staff who may be at risk (e.g., special health services staff, custodians, bus transportation personnel) of any necessary cleaning or precautions.

I. Review and implement Occupational Safety and Health Administration (OSHA) regulations.

V. Exclusion/Readmission

A. Exclude student from school.

B. Student may return after a minimum of 1 week after onset of jaundice or as directed by PHD.

VI. Additional Information

A. Transmitted by drinking water or using ice contaminated with HAV; eating raw or partially cooked shellfish harvested from waters containing raw sewage; and eating vegetables, fruits, or other uncooked contaminated foods. Diaper changing tables, when not cleaned or cared for properly, may facilitate the spread of hepatitis A infections, because *HAV can survive on an object or surface for months.*

B. The Advisory Committee on Immunization Practices (ACIP) recommends routine childhood immunization against hepatitis A in those states with rates of the disease that are twice the national average or greater. Consult local or state health department for current recommendations. The vaccine dosages and schedules vary according to student's age and the type of vaccine. Advise families to check with their HCP.

C. Hand washing is the most important measure for prevention and control. Young children are more likely to have poor hand-washing habits, so education is an important service provided by the school nurse.

D. Maintain strict OSHA protocols. Heating foods to 185° F for 1 minute or washing surfaces with a 1:10 solution of household bleach can inactivate HAV (this solution is caustic, so be careful: wear gloves and avoid direct contact with skin and eyes).

E. Immunoglobulin injections should be given as soon as possible and no later than 2 weeks after exposure. Staff and children in day care centers or schools that care for children in diapers should receive injections, if there is more than one case a month. In addition, all members of households whose diapered children attend the center or school should get injections when the disease exists among three or more families. If the infected person is directly involved in handling foods that will not be cooked, or in handling cooked foods before they are eaten, then other kitchen employees—and possibly even those served—should be given an IG injection. Local or state public health departments should be contacted for current recommendations.

WEB SITES

Medline Plus: Hepatitis
http://www.nlm.nih.gov/medlineplus/hepatitis.html
Immunization Action Coalition
http://www.immunize.org/hepa/index.htm

IMPETIGO

I. Definition
A. Impetigo is a highly contagious skin disease characterized by pustular eruptions. It is seen primarily in infants and children.

II. Etiology
A. Impetigo is caused primarily by *Staphylococcus aureus;* group A beta-hemolytic streptococcus, alone or in combination with *S. aureus*, is also associated with the infection.

III. Signs, Symptoms, and History
A. *Incubation period is 2 to 5 days.*
B. *Period of communicability lasts until lesions are dry.*
C. *Transmission is by direct contact.*
D. Lesions are most commonly found on the face and extremities.
E. Secondary infection to insect bites, abrasions, chickenpox, scabies, burns, and any break in the skin.
F. Rapid progression from macules to vesicles to pustules (see color plates, Primary and Secondary Skin Lesions).
G. Pustules rupture, producing an oozing, sticky, honey-colored crust (see color plate 5).
H. Pruritus.

IV. Initial Management
A. Ensure good hand-washing technique. Wash area with soap and water, cover with clean dressing if exposure to others is possible, but leave open to air if not.
B. Call parent or caregiver.
C. Clean toys and items the child uses (see Box 3-2).

V. Exclusion/Readmission
A. Exclusion depends on student's age and ability to practice good personal hygiene.
B. Day care students are excluded until 24 hours after treatment has been initiated.
C. Without medical treatment, student cannot return to school until lesions are dry.

VI. Additional Information
A. Medical treatment is with antibiotic of choice applied locally or systemically. Topical baciguent (Bacitracin) and mupirocin (Bactroban) are used, and cephalexin (Keflex), cloxacillin (Cloxapen), dicloxacillin (Dynapen), and erythromycin (E-mycin) are used systemically.

Topical treatment is used for isolated lesions; if no improvement shows within 3 days, oral medication is prescribed. Oral medication is used for widespread lesions when deeper tissue is involved and with constitutional symptoms.
  B. Complications are rare. One complication is acute glomerulonephritis, which is often accompanied by a headache, elevated blood pressure, and dark brown urine. Other complications include osteoarthritis, septicemia, septic arthritis, and pneumonia.

WEB SITES

Kids Health for Parents: Impetigo
    http://www.kidshealth.org/parent/infections/bacterial_viral/impetigo.html
eMedicine.com: Impetigo
    http://www.emedicine.com/emerg/topic283.htm

KAWASAKI DISEASE

I. Definition
  A. Kawasaki disease is an acute febrile vasculitis that affects the arterioles, venules, and capillaries. It is seen mainly in infants and children, about 80% of whom are under age 5, and it is the leading cause of acquired heart disease in children in the United States and Japan. It is also known as *mucocutaneous lymph node syndrome (MCLS).*
II. Etiology
  A. The cause of Kawasaki disease is not known. It is more prevalent in Asian children, seen more in males than females, and is rare in children over 8 years of age, but it can affect older children and adolescents.
III. Signs, Symptoms, and History
  A. Acute phase: lasts up to 10 days.
      1. Significant irritability and mood change.
      2. Fever of 101° F (38.5° C). Can spike to 104° F or higher.
      3. Reddened oral cavity; strawberry tongue.
      4. Reddened conjunctiva with no discharge.
      5. Edema of hands and feet with reddening of palms and soles.
      6. Erythematous, nonpruritic rash.
      7. Dry and red lips with fissuring (cracking).
      8. Swelling of cervical lymph nodes.
      9. Tachycardia and gallop rhythm.
  B. Subacute phase: around tenth to twenty-fifth day.
      1. Peeling of fingers and toes.
      2. Fever subsides.
      3. Rash desquamates (skin cells shed).
      4. Temporary arthritis and arthralgia (joint pain).
      5. Temporary hearing loss.
      6. Abdominal pain, enlarged gall bladder.
      7. Possible cardiac complications such as arrhythmias, aneurysms or thromboses, congestive heart failure, pericardial effusion, and mitral valve insufficiency with resulting heart murmur. Of these, the most *serious health threat is an aneurysm, and there is a risk of sudden death.*

C. Convalescent phase: 25 to 60 days.
 1. All signs of illness have disappeared.
 2. Preceding coronary complications may also occur during this phase.

IV. Initial Management
 A. Isolate feverish students from other children.
 B. Notify parent or caregiver for referral to primary HCP.

V. Exclusion/Readmission
 A. Exclude student as you would any student with elevated temperature.
 B. Readmit student on HCP's release.
 C. Consult with HCP upon student's return regarding level of activity, medications, and signs of complications.

VI. Additional Information
 A. Illness is self-limiting, but treatment of intravenous immunoglobulin (IVIG) and high dose of aspirin is given as soon as possible after diagnosis; when aspirin is given, children should avoid exposure to flu or chicken pox due to the risk of Reye syndrome. Aspirin treatment helps to diminish the risk of coronary aneurysm or disease. Recovery is generally complete for those without coronary disease, and prognosis with coronary disease depends on severity.

WEB SITES

Kawasaki Disease Foundation
 http://www.kdfoundation.org
Lucile Packard Children's Hospital: Kawasaki Disease
 http://www.lpch.org/DiseaseHealthInfo/HealthLibrary/cardiac/kawasaki.html

MEASLES (RUBEOLA)

I. Definition
 A. Measles is a contagious childhood disease marked by fever and skin eruption. It is a vaccine-preventable disease.

II. Etiology
 A. The measles virus causes measles, and one attack almost invariably conters immunity, although second occurrences have been recorded.

III. Signs, Symptoms, and History
 A. *Incubation period is 7 to 18 days.*
 B. *Period of communicability lasts at least 7 days beyond the onset of the first symptoms.*
 C. *Transmission is via respiratory droplets and by contact with articles freshly contaminated by nose, throat, mouth, and eye secretions.*
 D. Prodromal phase: 4 to 5 days.
 1. Fever, malaise, runny nose, cough, conjunctivitis.
 2. Koplik spots—small, irregular, red spots with minute grayish-white centers on buccal mucosa—usually disappear 1 or 2 days after onset of rash.
 E. Rash: 3 to 4 days later.
 1. Abrupt rise in temperature as rash appears.

2. Fine, reddish brown eruptions begin on face, hairline, behind ears, and gradually spreads downward.
3. Rash is more severe in earlier sites and less intense in later sites.
4. About 2 days after rash appears, symptoms begin to subside.
5. Complications include otitis media, pneumonia, laryngotracheo-bronchitis and obstructive laryngitis, encephalitis, permanent disability, and death.

IV. Initial Management

A. Treatment is symptomatic and supportive.
B. Call parent or caregiver to pick up the child and provide infectious disease information.
C. Ensure proper hand-washing techniques among school personnel.
D. Dispose of soiled tissues appropriately.
E. Isolate student from other students.
F. Maintain a list of students lacking measles vaccination.
G. Following school and county or state guidelines, notify the parents or caregivers of the infected student and those of any students not previously immunized.
H. Notify and follow local health department regulations regarding reporting of disease.
I. Observe all students closely for possible additional cases.
J. Those with severe measles have low vitamin A levels. A one-time dose of 100,000 units of vitamin A for children 6 to 12 months of age and 200,000 units for children 1 year of age or older may be prescribed. The dose is repeated the following day and 1 month later if ophthalmologic evidence of vitamin A deficiency exists.

V. Exclusion/Readmission

A. Exclude student from school immediately.
B. Student may return to school a minimum of 4 days after rash appears; parents should check with their HCP.

VI. Additional Information

A. Measles vaccine is administered as part of the measles, mumps, and rubella (MMR) series to children, starting at 12 to 15 months and again at 4 to 6 years of age and 11 to 18 years (see Appendix B, Immunizations).
B. Contraindications for MMR include immunocompromised individuals, febrile individuals, pregnant women, and recipients of recent blood products or IG, in which case the vaccine should be postponed for 3 months.
C. Immunoglobulin (IG, 0.25 ml/kg) may be given to a susceptible, exposed individual within 5 days for prevention of disease, but if given after 5 days, it will reduce severity of illness. HIV-infected children, regardless of vaccination status, should be given IG if measles exposure has occurred.

WEB SITE

Kids Health for Parents: Measles (Rubeola)
   http://www.kidshealth.org/parent/infections/lung/measles.html

INFECTIOUS MONONUCLEOSIS

I. **Definition**
   A. Infectious mononucleosis, also referred to as the *kissing disease,* is an acute, self-limiting viral disease that can occur at any age but is most commonly seen in adolescents and young adults. The infection is characterized by increased mononuclear leukocytes in the blood.

II. **Etiology**
   A. Mononucleosis is usually caused by the Epstein-Barr virus (EBV) and can occur in both sporadic and epidemic forms. EBV can be shed in oral secretions up to 6 months after acute infection and intermittently throughout life.
   B. Infrequently, cytomegalovirus, HIV, *Toxoplasma gondii,* and human herpesvirus type 6 can cause the infection.

III. **Signs, Symptoms, and History**
   A. *Incubation period is 4 to 6 weeks but may be shorter in young children.*
   B. *Period of communicability may last for months in pharyngeal excretions, making asymptomatic carriers common (15%).*
   C. *Transmission is generally by direct, intimate contact with infected saliva and rarely by blood transfusions or bone marrow transplantation. Repeated and prolonged contact with infected oral secretions is thought to be required, making the contact unknown.*
   D. Generally a mild illness and difficult to recognize in children but overt illness in adolescents and young adults. Usually mild but can be serious with complications.
   E. Symptoms vary in type, duration, and severity.
   F. Acute symptoms typically disappear within 2 to 4 weeks; some students require restricted activity for 2 to 3 months because of continued fatigue, malaise, or enlarged spleen.
   G. Prolonged fever with generalized lymphadenopathy and splenomegaly.
   H. Malaise, fatigue, and persistent, low-grade headache.
   I. Epistaxis and severe sore throat, frequently exudative or accompanied by palatine petechiae.
   J. Discrete maculopapular skin rash may occur, particularly over trunk. Occurs more often in young children, whereas older children may have abdominal pain.
   K. Jaundice from hepatic involvement.
   L. Can be confused with many conditions, including those characterized by neurological and cardiac symptoms.

IV. **Initial Management**
   A. Notify parent or caregiver to pick up student. Discuss symptoms and referral to HCP for diagnostic laboratory tests, especially if abdominal pain or sore throat cause difficulties drinking, eating, or breathing.
   B. Dispose of, or properly disinfect, all articles that may have been soiled with saliva or nasal secretions.
   C. Determine the type of information needed to educate the infected person, their family, and contacts.
   D. Avoid administering live vaccines until several months after recovery.

E. Treatment is usually symptomatic.

F. On student's readmission to school, discuss with student and staff the necessity for good hand washing and proper disposal of articles contaminated with saliva or nasal secretions.

G. Allow time for students to express feelings and concerns regarding the illness or the limitations on sports and social activities, and provide a safe place for students to vent their anger and frustration about activity limitations when they return to school.

H. Student may need additional rest and regulation of activities according to tolerance.

V. Exclusion/Readmission

A. Exclude student from school.

B. Student may return after acute symptoms have disappeared.

C. Discuss with parent/HCP any restriction on activities and any recommendations regarding rest or reduced school days.

VI. Additional Information

A. Clinical manifestations, positive heterophil agglutination test, an increase in atypical leukocytes in a peripheral blood smear, spot test (monospot), and heterophil antibody test are tools for diagnosis.

B. Acyclovir and corticosteroids decrease oropharyngeal shedding and viral replication, but they do not change the severity or duration of symptoms or the clinical outcome. The level of individual tolerance and symptoms dictates regulation of activities. Severe manifestations are often treated more aggressively.

WEB SITES

Mayo Clinic
http://www.mayoclinic.com/health/mononucleosis/DS00352
TeensHealth
http://www.kidshealth.org/teen/infections/common/mononucleosis.html

MUMPS (INFECTIOUS PAROTITIS)

I. Definition

A. Mumps is an acute, contagious, febrile disease marked by inflammation of the salivary glands. It was widespread worldwide but occurs less frequently as a result of the 1967 introduction of the MMR vaccine.

II. Etiology

A. The cause of mumps is a ribonucleic acid (RNA) virus of the genus *Paramyxovirus.*

III. Signs, Symptoms, and History

A. *Incubation period is 16 to 18 days.*

B. *Period of communicability is approximately 6 days before and 9 days after salivary gland swelling has appeared.*

C. *Transmission is by direct contact, airborne droplets, saliva, and possibly by urine from an infected person.*

D. Prodromal: first 24 hours.
  1. Low-grade fever, headache, malaise, and loss of appetite.
  2. Earache aggravated by chewing.
E. Third day:
  1. Swelling—either unilateral or bilateral—of one or more salivary glands, usually parotid, accompanied by pain and tenderness.

IV. Initial Management
A. Call parent or caregiver to pick up the child and discuss concerns of infectious disease.
B. Treatment is symptomatic and supportive.
C. Follow appropriate separation practice from other students.
D. Ensure good hand-washing techniques by school personnel.
E. Disposal of soiled tissues properly.
F. Review immunization records of all students for mumps vaccination.
G. Notify student's parents and parents of any unimmunized students; follow school, county, or state guidelines.
H. Notify and follow local health department regulations regarding reporting of disease.
I. Be aware of other students with symptoms and refer for care.

V. Exclusion/Readmission
A. Isolate and exclude student from school.
B. Student may return to school a maximum of 9 days after start of swelling.

VI. Additional Information
A. Mumps vaccine is administered as part of the MMR series to children, starting at 12 to 15 months, then again at 4 to 6 years, or at 11 to 12 years (see Appendix B, Immunizations).
B. Complications of mumps disease include sensorineural deafness, epididymitis/orchitis, myocarditis, postinfectious encephalitis, arthritis, hepatitis, and mastitis. Around one half of the males with mumps have atrophy of the testicles; the condition is generally unilateral, so sterility rarely occurs. Pregnant women should contact their primary care provider, since exposure to the virus in the first trimester of pregnancy may increase the likelihood of spontaneous abortion.

WEB SITE

Centers for Disease Control and Prevention: Childhood Diseases
  http://www.cdc.gov/ncidod/diseases/children/diseases.htm

OTITIS MEDIA

I. Definition
A. Otitis media (OM) is an inflammation of the middle ear and the most common cause of conductive hearing loss in children. It can be described as acute otitis media (AOM) with or without effusion, chronic otitis media with effusion (see "Additional Information"), OM with or without cholesteatoma, and atelectasis of the tympanic membrane/middle ear/mastoid. If it lasts 6 weeks or more, it is considered to be *chronic otitis media*.

II. Etiology

    A. *S. pneumoniae* or *H. influenzae* are major causes. Frequently, OM is associated with allergic rhinitis or hypertrophy of the adenoids. Secondhand smoke is a significant factor in the incidence of OM.

III. Signs, Symptoms, and History

    A. Most commonly a result of eustachian tube dysfunction and does not require antibiotics.

    B. Concurrent upper respiratory or pharyngeal infection.

    C. Pain, fever, malaise, irritability, and lethargy.

    D. Anorexia, nausea, vomiting, diarrhea, and headache occur less often.

    E. Enlarged postauricular and cervical lymph glands.

    F. Infant may become irritable, pull at ears, and roll head from side to side.

    G. Middle ear fluid may be serous (thin), mucoid (thick), purulent (pus-filled), or a combination.

    H. Otoscopic exam reveals bright red, bulging tympanic membrane with no visible landmarks or light reflex; indicates effusion.

    I. Impedance testing shows negative pressure and low compliance.

    J. Foul smell may result from eardrum rupture.

    K. Feeling of fullness in ear; popping sensation with swallowing.

    L. Fever or severe pain often absent with OM; child may seem well.

    M. Babies who are put to bed with a bottle are more likely to have increased incidence of OM.

IV. Initial Management

    A. Call parents and discuss referral of care to HCP.

    B. Treat discomfort and fever.

    C. Monitor impedance and hearing acuity testing.

    D. Discuss hearing acuity variance with speech therapist for ongoing monitoring.

    E. If pressure-equalizing (PE) tubes are placed, use precautions for water play to avoid middle ear infections. Provide impedance testing to monitor patency of tubes.

    F. Symptoms of conductive hearing loss (see Chapter 2, Vision and Hearing).

V. Exclusion/Readmission

    A. Does not apply.

VI. Additional Information

    A. Otitis media effusion (OME) is fluid in the middle ear associated with a viral upper respiratory infection, or it can be a precursor to otitis media, or it can occur after OM. It is treated with decongestants and monitoring but not antibiotics. If the condition continues, PE tubes may be inserted. Educate parents and staff that inappropriate use of antibiotics contributes to antibiotic-resistant bacteria.

WEB SITES

American Speech-Language-Hearing Association: Questions and Answers about Otitis Media, Hearing, and Language Development
http://www.kidsource.com/ASHA/otitis.html

National Institute on Deafness and Other Communication Disorders
http://www.nidcd.nih.gov/health/hearing/otitism.asp

PEDICULOSIS CAPITIS (HEAD LICE)

I. Definition

A. This condition is an infestation of lice in the scalp and facial hair. Three types of human lice are *head, body,* and *pubic.* They all have similar life cycles. However, head and pubic lice spend their life cycles on the skin of the human host, whereas body lice live in clothing, coming to the skin only to feed. Head lice generally cannot live longer than 24 hours without access to a human host; however, nits— the eggs—may survive up to a week. The female louse lays 3 to 5 eggs per day, which take 7 to 10 days to hatch and another 7 to 10 days to mature and lay eggs. Lice do not jump, fly, or live on animals.

II. Etiology

A. The louse *Pediculus humanus capitis* is the cause of the infestation.

III. Signs, Symptoms, and History

A. Itching of scalp or back of neck.

B. Presence of live lice found on the scalp.

C. Presence of nits on hair shaft.
   1. Observed on hair shaft close to head; difficult to remove with fingernails.
   2. Nits resemble dandruff, but dandruff can be easily removed from hair shaft, whereas lice nits cannot.
   3. Lice nits are small, grayish white, tear-shaped, and hatch in 1 week.
   4. Nits a half inch or more from the scalp are nearly always hatched and do not generally indicate active infestation.

D. Reddened areas around scalp, behind ears, and behind neck.

IV. Initial Management

A. Be aware of school and district policies and standards.

B. Practice good hand-washing techniques.

C. Refer to parent for treatment of head lice.

D. Examine siblings of those identified as having head lice.

E. Advise parents to consult HCP for prescription or purchase of over-the-counter medication and follow instructions on product (see Box 3-3).

F. All individuals living in the household should be inspected and *only treated* if infested. Encourage parents to notify relatives and other contacts of infestation.

G. Advise family to wash all bedding, linens, combs, brushes, and headgear in hot soapy water.

H. Seal contaminated objects that cannot be laundered or dry cleaned in a plastic bag for a week.

I. Educate family and school faculty that the transmittal of lice can occur by sharing hats, combs, and so on.

J. Spend time with student to allow for expression of feelings, because psychological impact is stressful.

K. Educate public regarding prevention, transmission, detection, and treatment.

V. Exclusion/Readmission

A. Exclude student from school until the hair has been properly treated.

CHAPTER 3

Acute Conditions

Box 3-3   *Instructions for Pediculicide Products*

1. Infected household members must be treated at the same time. Uninfected family members should be checked every 2 or 3 days.
2. DO NOT shampoo with combination shampoo and conditioner or apply cream rinse prior to product application. For extra-long hair, two bottles of product may be needed.
3. Apply permethrin-based or synthetic molecule products, such as Nix and Elimite creams, to freshly shampooed, towel-dried hair. Hair must be partially dry for product to be effective. Permethrin continues to kill newly hatched nits for several days (CDC, 2005).
4. Apply pyrethrin-based shampoos or natural products—such as RID, Clear, Pronto, A-200, and various generic products—to dry hair. These shampoos kill live lice but do not affect the nits (CDC, 2005).
5. Remove all clothing from the waist up prior to treatment. Have infected person put on all clean clothing after treatment (CDC, 2005).
6. Entire scalp and hair close to scalp should be saturated.
7. Application is more effective when a few drops are placed over various parts of the head, rather than putting a large amount in the middle and spreading out from there.
8. Leave all treatments in hair for the time period indicated by product instructions to avoid scalp irritation. Do not cover with a shower cap.
9. Begin nit comb-out process at the nape of the neck, around the ears, and work upward. Several combs are available: metal combs are more effective than plastic, but flea combs used on cats and dogs are also effective (CDC, 2005).
10. DO NOT shampoo for at least 1 to 2 days after treatment.
11. Apply second application in 7 to 10 days as recommended to kill any newly hatched lice.

B. Recheck on return to school and evaluate the student in 7 to 10 days to determine if nit reinfection has occurred, which may require a second treatment for newly hatched eggs.
C. School nursing organization policies differ on nit-free guidelines. Refer to your district or school policy, check the National Association of School Nurses (www.nasn.org), and your state school nurse organization for specific policies and guidelines. Some chronic infestations require more stringent management than a one-time infestation. The potential for epidemic spread is minimal, although epidemics may occur in day care centers, which requires discreet and stringent management.

WEB SITES

National Pediculosis Association
   http://www.headlice.org
Centers for Disease Control and Prevention, Division of Parasitic Diseases
   http://www.cdc.gov/ncidod/dpd/index.htm
   http://www.cdc.gov/ncidod/dpd/parasites/headlice/factsht_head_lice.htm

PINWORMS (ENTEROBIASIS)

I. Definition

A. *Pinworms,* which cause *enterobiasis,* are white, threadlike parasites that live in the large intestine and are found in and about the rectal area. They are the most common helminthic infection in the United States. Infections are more frequent in preschool and younger school-age children and in crowded living conditions.

II. Etiology

A. The cause is a parasitic infection with *Enterobius vermicularis.*

III. Signs, Symptoms, and History

A. *Incubation period starts when eggs are inhaled or ingested (see "Additional Information" for life cycle).*

B. *Period of communicability is the entire time the eggs exist in the environment.*

C. *Transmission is either directly by the transfer of infective eggs by hand from the anus to the mouth or indirectly through articles contaminated with eggs. The eggs can survive up to 2 weeks, without a human host, on objects such as bed linen, underwear, food, shared toys, bath items, doorknobs, and toilet seats.*

D. May be asymptomatic.

E. Perianal itching and scratching, especially at night.

F. Vaginal and anal irritation because of scratching.

G. Migration of worms to vagina or urethra may cause infection.

H. Sleeplessness, irritability, restlessness, distractibility, and short attention span found in young children.

IV. Initial Management

A. Call parents immediately and discuss assessment using a flashlight to observe the area 2 to 4 hours after child is asleep or the tape test (see "Additional Information").

B. Inform parents that bed linens, hand towels, and clothing should be machine washed using hot water and dried using a high heat setting.

C. Notify teaching staff and provide education.
   1. Follow standard hygienic procedures.
   2. Wash hands after toileting and before eating or preparing food.
   3. Provide adequate toilet and hand-washing facilities.
   4. Discourage habits of nail biting and scratching bare perianal area.
   5. Clean contaminated areas and routinely disinfect.
   6. Remove sources of infection by treating known cases.

V. Exclusion/Readmission

A. Exclude young child from school until 24 hours after treatment has been initiated.

VI. Additional Information

A. After the eggs are inhaled or ingested, they hatch in the upper intestine, mature in 2 to 8 weeks, and migrate to the cecum. Females mate and migrate outside the anus, where they lay up to 17,000 eggs. The movement of worms on the skin and mucous membranes causes intense itching. The eggs adhere to many surfaces because of their adhesiveness and durability. While

CHAPTER 3

Acute Conditions

scratching or during toileting, eggs can easily be deposited on hands or under fingernails, which can create reinfestation of young children in preschool care.
B. Treatments include mebendazole (Vermox), albendazole (Albenza), and pyrantel pamoate (Antiminth). Mebendazole is not recommended for children under 2 years of age, and only pyrantel pamoate can be taken by a pregnant woman. Reinfection is common, and in some cases, entire families require treatment.

WEB SITES

Centers for Disease Control and Prevention: Pinworm Infection Fact Sheet
http://www.cdc.gov/ncidod/dpd/parasites/pinworm/factsht_pinworm.htm
FamilyDoctor.org: Pinworms and Your Child (also available in Spanish)
http://www.familydoctor.org/handouts/139.html

POISON IVY, OAK, AND SUMAC DERMATITIS

I. **Definition**
   A. Contact with dry or succulent segments of poison ivy, oak, or sumac can induce a potentially serious dermatitis. Poison ivy is common east of the Rockies; poison oak is generally found west of the Rockies; and poison sumac is usually found in standing water in peat bogs in the Northeast and Midwest and swampy areas in parts of the Southeast. However, the plants can be found in all states except Hawaii and Alaska.

II. **Etiology**
   A. The dermatitis is caused by the oily substance urushiol, which transverses the roots, stems, leaves, and fruit of the plant. It can also result from contact with smoke, burning leaves, contaminated clothing, tools, or the fur of a cat or dog.

III. **Signs, Symptoms, and History**
   A. Rash may begin within 12 to 24 hours after exposure.
   B. Redness, itching, and swelling.
   C. Multiple vesicles and blisterlike lesions that appear in linear streaks (see color plates, Primary and Secondary Skin Lesions).
   D. Lesions usually rupture, followed by oozing of serum and subsequent crusting.
   E. Blisters become crusted and heal in about 10 days.

IV. **Initial Management**
   A. With known exposure, flush with cold running water immediately to neutralize the oil that has not bonded to skin; leave clothes on and rinse skin and clothing, and clean well under fingernails.
   B. Use of mild soap may be helpful; harsh soap removes protective skin oil.
   C. Avoid hard scrubbing that may further irritate skin.
   D. Remove clothing carefully and launder in hot water and detergent.
   E. Wash camping and sporting equipment and other objects that may have been in contact with the urushiol oil, because it can remain active on objects for many months.

F. Treatment is symptomatic.

G. Before blisters form, apply topical corticosteroid to relieve or prevent inflammation. Oral corticosteroids may be needed for severe reactions, and sedatives such as diphenhydramine (Benadryl) are useful for itching and to promote sleep. Encourage student not to scratch, since this may cause secondary infections.

H. Blistering phase can be soothed by cool baking soda bath (use up to 1 cup baking soda per tub); Aveeno baths, calamine lotion, and Burow's solution compresses may also be used to quell the itching.

V. Exclusion/Readmission

A. Student may remain in school as long as itching does not interfere with student's ability to function in the classroom. The rash is not contagious, but if the oil is transferred, it can cause a reaction.

VI. Additional Information

A. Prevention is best accomplished by teaching staff and students to recognize the plants and avoid them. Urushiol is in the roots and the stems of the plant, so contact can occur even when there are no leaves. Tecnu, an OTC skin wash, can be used to remove urushiol oil after exposure.

B. Those who are known to be allergic can secure a protective cream, such as Stokoguard, for exposed skin.

WEB SITES

American Academy of Dermatology
http://www.aad.org/pamphlets/PoisonIvy.html
Poison Ivy Organization
http://www.poison-ivy.org

UPPER RESPIRATORY TRACT INFECTION (COMMON COLD)

I. Definition

A. The common cold is an acute infection of the upper respiratory tract, nose, and pharynx, usually lasting 5 to 7 days. Upper respiratory infections (URI) are the most commonly occurring infectious disease in the United States, and they account for the highest number of absences from school and visits to the doctor. Colds occur more frequently in fall and winter.

II. Etiology

A. URIs are known to be caused by more than 200 viruses, and rhinoviruses account for more than a third of these URIs. Respiratory syncytial virus (RSV) is seen in infants.

III. Signs, Symptoms, and History

A. *Incubation period is 2 to 5 days and can be up to 8 days.*

B. *Transmission is directly from contaminated large or small particle droplets or indirectly from contaminated secretions on hands or objects.*

C. Symptoms depend on age, living environment, and preexisting health concerns.

D. Infection rate appears to be higher in the toddler and preschool-age child. Infants younger than 3 months have a lower infection rate, and those over age 5 have URIs less frequently.
E. Disease is self-limiting and can last up to 10 days.
F. General malaise.
G. Fever appears abruptly in ages 3 months to 3 years and is associated with irritability, restlessness, and decreased activity and appetite.
H. Nasopharyngitis, which is more severe in infants and younger children.
I. Older children may experience dry and irritated nasal passages and pharynx, followed by chilly sensations, muscular aches and pains, sneezing, nasal discharge, and unproductive cough.
J. Nasal inflammation can lead to obstruction and open-mouth breathing, making sleeping and feeding laborious.
K. Nasal discharge.
L. Red and watery eyes.

IV. Initial Management
A. Management is symptomatic.
B. Emphasize good general hygiene, such as use of individual utensils and drinking glasses, proper disposal of tissues, and proper hand washing.
C. Notify parent or caregiver.
D. Determine temperature, vital signs, and behaviors.
E. Note consistency and color of nasal discharge. *Decongestants* may be prescribed for children 2 years and older to decrease swollen nasal openings to make sleeping and breathing easier. FDA advises not giving cold medicines to children under 2 years of age. FDA is investigating the efficacy and safety of OTC cold remedies for children 2 through 11 years of age (FDA, 2008).
F. If cough is present, note frequency and whether it is productive. When cough is dry and hacking, cough suppressants may be prescribed for older children. AAP recommends not giving OTC cough or cold medicines to children ages 6 and under. Research demonstrates that buckwheat honey can diminish a nighttime cough. *Do not use* honey for children under age 1 because it may cause botulism. Recommended dose of honey is ½ tsp for 2- to 5-year-olds, 1 tsp for 6- to 11-year-olds, and 2 tsp for ages 12 and older (Penn State, 2008).
G. Antihistamines may be used to dry secretions, but they may cause drowsiness or excitability, so they may offer few benefits.
H. Do not give aspirin because of its association with Reye syndrome, and antibiotics must not be used for viral infection. Educate caregivers to check for ingredients to avoid overdose, because many OTC products and prescribed medications have the same active ingredients.

V. Exclusion/Readmission
A. It is difficult to exclude from school every child who has a simple cold, and decisions regarding dismissal depend on individual circumstances, including student's age, personal hygiene, classroom setting, and developmental level. URIs are contagious before and after symptoms are present, so excluding student does little to

reduce chance of spread. Student may be dismissed from school for any of the following reasons:
1. Purulent or discolored nasal discharge, especially in very young children.
2. Temperature of 101° F or above.
3. Student feels too ill or uncomfortable to adequately function in classroom setting.
4. Student can return to school when temperature-free for 24 hours, nasal drainage is clear, is well enough to participate in class, and ceases to be threat to well-being of others.

WEB SITE

Kids Health for Parents: Common Cold
    http://www.kidshealth.org/parent/infections/common/cold.html

RINGWORM OF THE BODY (TINEA CORPORIS)

I. **Definition**
    A. Ringworm of the body is a shallow fungal infection of the skin, hair, and nails. Ringworm is generally, but not always, ring-shaped.
II. **Etiology**
    A. Ringworm is caused by *Trichophyton tonsurans, Microsporum canis,* and *Epidermophyton* fungi.
III. **Signs, Symptoms, and History**
    A. Rash begins as small, red, colorless, or depigmented circle that progressively becomes larger.
    B. Circular border is elevated and perhaps scaly and dry or moist and crusted.
    C. Center of circle starts to heal as area becomes larger.
    D. Mild pruritus, pain, and scaling.
    E. Close contact with infected humans or animals, such as dogs, cats, or pet mice.
    F. Usually seen on arms, face, and neck but may occur elsewhere on body.
    G. Most common cause of alopecia.
IV. **Initial Management**
    A. Cover area; exclude younger student from school, but an older student may return to class.
    B. Use good hand-washing techniques.
    C. Clean toys or other items contaminated by infected younger student.
    D. Over-the-counter antifungal ointments are available for most conditions. *Tinea capitis,* ringworm of the scalp, must be treated by oral administration of griseofulvin.
V. **Exclusion/Readmission**
    A. Depends on the age and developmental level of student. If student is very young or disabled and lesion cannot be covered, exclude student from school until treatment has started.
    B. After treatment, recheck in 1 to 2 weeks for improvement; if no improvement, refer student back to HCP.

CHAPTER 3

Acute Conditions

WEB SITE

American Academy of Family Physicians
    http://www.familydoctor.org/handouts/316.html

ROSEOLA INFANTUM (EXANTHEM SUBITUM)

I. Definition
  A. Roseola is an acute illness of children younger than 4; it commonly occurs around 1 year of age. The incidence is highest in the spring.
II. Etiology
  A. The cause of roseola is human herpesvirus type 6 (HHV-6).
III. Signs, Symptoms, and History
  A. *Incubation period is approximately 5 to 15 days.*
  B. *Period of communicability is unclear.*
  C. *Transmission seems to be salivary contact with parents, caregivers, and siblings. The virus has also been found in the saliva of healthy adults.*
  D. Illness is self-limiting.
  E. Sudden fever as high as 104° to 106° F (40° to 41.1° C) lasting 3 to 5 days; temperature drops with appearance of rash.
  F. Discrete, rose-pink, maculopapular rash, initially on trunk; spreads to face, neck, and extremities; fades on pressure; nonpruritic; and lasts from 1 to 2 days.
  G. Cervical/postauricular lymphadenopathy.
  H. Reddened pharynx, coryza, cough, lethargy.
  I. Complications are rare but include encephalitis, febrile seizures, and mononucleosis-like illness.
IV. Initial Management
  A. Treatment is supportive and symptomatic.
  B. Isolate child from other children.
  C. Treat fever (refer to fever discussion).
  D. If prone to febrile seizure, discuss precautions with parents and caregivers.
V. Exclusion/Readmission
  A. Exclude student from school.
  B. Student may return to school when fever and rash have gone.

WEB SITE

eMedicine: Pediatrics, Roseola Infantum
    http://www.emedicine.com/emerg/topic400.htm

RUBELLA (GERMAN MEASLES)

I. Definition
  A. Rubella is a mild infectious childhood disease that was widespread but is now infrequent because of the availability of the measles, mumps, and rubella (MMR) vaccine. The greatest danger of rubella is its effect on a fetus.
II. Etiology
  A. The cause is an RNA virus of the genus *Rubivirus*.

Dermatologic Conditions and Skin Lesions

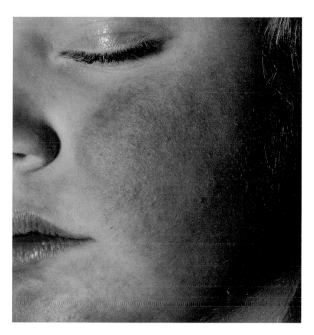

PLATE 1 Erythema infectiosum (fifth disease). Facial erythema "slapped cheek." Red plaque covers cheek and spares nasolabial fold and circumoral region. *(From Habif T: Clinical Dermatology: A Color Guide to Diagnosis and Therapy, ed 4. Philadelphia, 2004, Mosby.)*

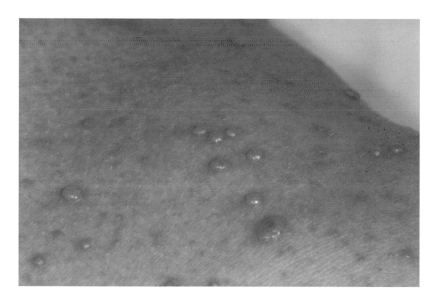

PLATE 2 Varicella (chickenpox). Note vesicular lesions. *(From Lemmi FO, Lemmi CAE: Physical assessment findings CD-ROM, Philadelphia, 2000, WB Saunders.)*

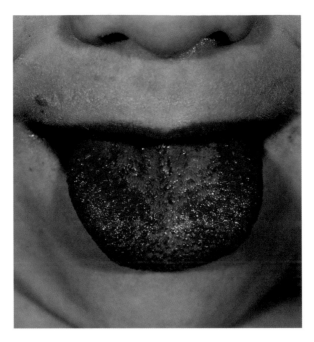

PLATE 3 Portions of the white coat remain in the center, but the remainder of the tongue is red with engorged papillae ("strawberry tongue"). *(From Habif T: Clinical Dermatology: A Color Guide to Diagnosis and Therapy, ed 4. Philadelphia, 2004, Mosby.)*

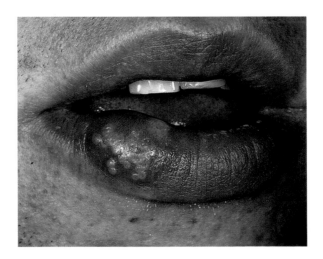

PLATE 4 Herpes. A small group of vesicles on an erythematous base are the primary lesion. *(From Habif T: Clinical Dermatology: A Color Guide to Diagnosis and Therapy, ed 4. Philadelphia, 2004, Mosby.)*

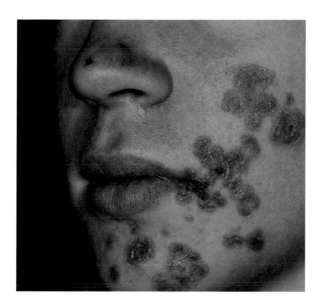

PLATE 5 Impetigo. A thick, honey-yellow adherent crust covers the entire eroded surface. *(From Habif T: Clinical Dermatology: A Color Guide to Diagnosis and Therapy, ed 4. Philadelphia, 2004, Mosby.)*

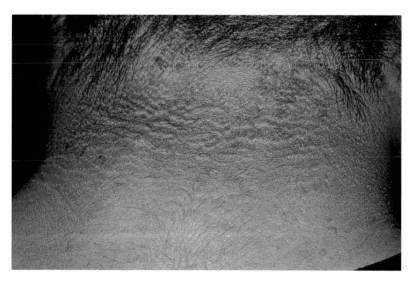

PLATE 6 Brownish-colored warty hyperkeratosis on the nape of the neck, in a patient with acanthosis nigricans and insulin resistance. *(From White GM, Cox NH: Diseases of the Skin: A Color Atlas and Text, ed 2. Philadelphia, 2006, Mosby.)*

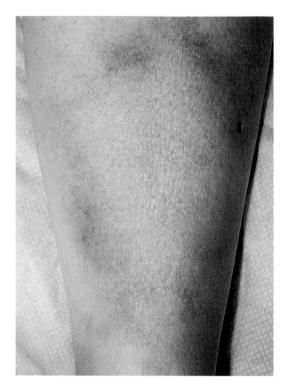

PLATE 7 Erythema migrans (early stage Lyme disease). Broad oval area of erythema has slowly migrated from the central area. *(From Habif T:* Clinical Dermatology: A Color Guide to Diagnosis and Therapy, *ed 4. Philadelphia, 2004, Mosby.)*

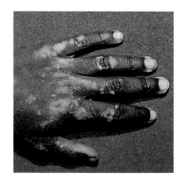

PLATE 8 Vitiligo. *(From Weston WL, Lane AT, Morelli JG:* Color Textbook of Pediatric Dermatology, *ed 2. St. Louis, 1996, Mosby.)*

PRIMARY SKIN LESIONS

Macule: A flat, circumscribed area that is a change in the color of the skin; less than 1 cm in diameter

Examples: Freckles, flat moles, rubella, rubeola, scarlet fever, photoallergic or phototoxic drug eruptions

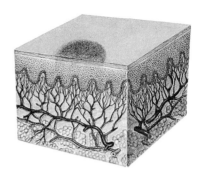

Papule: An elevated, firm, circumscribed area; less than 1 cm in diameter

Examples: Warts, elevated moles, pigmented nevi, scabies, closed comedone, skin tags

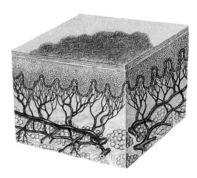

Patch: A flat, nonpalpable, irregular-shaped macule greater than 1 cm in diameter

Examples: Vitiligo, port-wine stains, Mongolian spots, café au lait patch

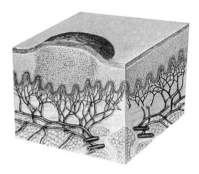

Plaque: Elevated, firm, and rough lesion with flat top surface greater than 1 cm in diameter

Examples: Psoriasis, seborrheic and actinic keratoses

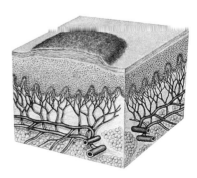

Wheal: Elevated, irregular-shaped area of cutaneous edema; solid, transient, variable diameter

Examples: Insect bites, uticaria, allergic reaction

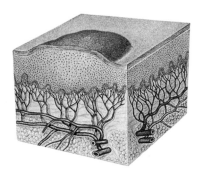

Nodule: Elevated, firm, circumscribed lesion; deeper in dermis than a papule; 1 to 2 cm in diameter

Examples: Erythema nodosum, lipomas, warts, neurofibromatosis

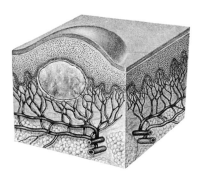

Cyst: Elevated, circumscribed, encapsulated lesion; in dermis or subcutaneous layer; filled with liquid or semi-solid material

Examples: Sebaceous cyst, cystic acne

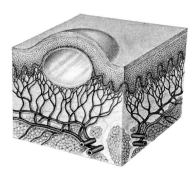

Vesicle: Elevated, circumscribed, superficial, not into dermis; filled with serous fluid; less than 1 cm in diameter

Examples: Varicella (chicken pox), herpes zoster (shingles), herpes simplex, blister, impetigo, scabies

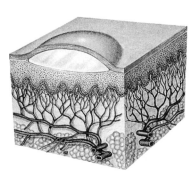

Bulla: Vesicle greater than 1 cm in diameter

Examples: Blister, pemphigus vulgaris

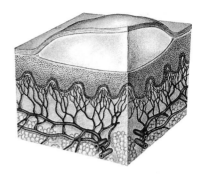

Pustule: Elevated, superficial lesion; similar to a vesicle but filled with purulent fluid

Examples: Impetigo, acne, varicella, herpes simplex, scabies

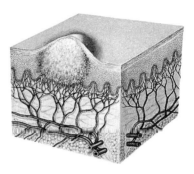

SECONDARY SKIN LESIONS

Scale: Heaped-up, keratinized cells; flaky skin; irregular; thick or thin; dry or oily; variation in size

Examples: Flaking of skin with seborrheic dermatitis following scarlet fever, or flaking of skin following a drug reaction; dry skin

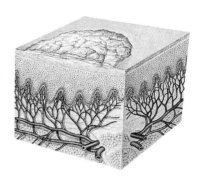

Crust: Dried serum, blood, or purulent exudates; slightly elevated; size varies; brown, red, black, tan, or straw-colored

Examples: Scab on abrasion, eczema, tinea capitis, impetigo

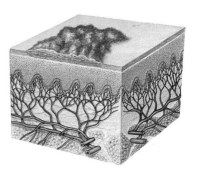

Fissure: Linear crack or break from the epidermis to the dermis; may be moist or dry

Examples: Athlete's foot, cracks at the corner of the mouth

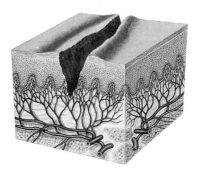

Excoriation: Loss of epidermis; linear hollowed-out, crusted area

Examples: Abrasion or scratch, scabies

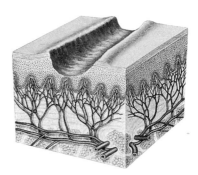

Lichenification: Rough, thickened epidermis secondary to persistent rubbing, itching, or skin irritation; often involves flexor surface of extremity

Examples: Chronic dermatitis

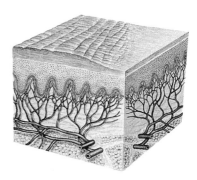

Modified from Seidel HM, Ball JW, Dains JE, Benedict GW: Mosby's Guide to Physical Examination, *ed 6. St. Louis, 2007, Mosby.*

III. Signs, Symptoms, and History

A. *Incubation period is 14 to 21 days.*

B. *Period of communicability is from 7 days before rash appears to at least 5 days after the rash appears. Immunization prevents the disease.*

C. *Transmission is by direct contact with nasopharyngeal secretions or urine from infected individual.*

D. Prodromal stage is 1 to 5 days; subsides 1 day after rash has appeared.

E. Low-grade fever, headache, malaise, anorexia, mild conjunctivitis, nasal discharge, cough, pharyngitis, and swelling of lymph nodes behind ears.

F. A distinct, faint pink rash appears first on face and rapidly spreads downward. Disappears in same order as it began; usually gone by third day, hence name *3-day measles*. Sometimes resembles measles or scarlet fever.

G. Complications are rare but include arthritis, encephalitis, and purpura.

IV. Initial Management

A. Treatment is supportive and symptomatic.

B. Follow appropriate isolation practice from other students.

C. Encourage good hand-washing techniques and hygienic procedures by school personnel.

D. Dispose of soiled tissues properly.

E. Review immunization records of all students.

F. Notify the student's parents and caregivers and those of any student not immunized, following school and county health guidelines.

G. Notify and follow local health department regulations; rubella is a reportable disease.

H. Become aware of other students, staff, or family members with symptoms, and refer for care as needed.

I. Refer any pregnant woman exposed to rubella to her HCP. In early pregnancy, rubella may cause congenital rubella syndrome, which is a serious, multisystem disease that may result in heart damage, blindness, deafness, mental retardation, miscarriage or stillbirth.

V. Exclusion/Readmission

A. Immediately isolate and exclude student from school.

B. In infant and day care centers, any child under 12 months who has not been vaccinated against rubella should be excluded from the center until immunized or until 3 weeks after the onset of rash in the last case.

C. Student may return to school a minimum of 6 days after rash has appeared.

WEB SITE

Kids Health for Parents: Infections
http://www.kidshealth.org/parent/infections

SCABIES

I. Definition

A. Scabies is a highly pruritic, communicable infection of the skin.

II. Etiology

A. Scabies is caused by the itch mite *Sarcoptes scabiei*. The pregnant female mite burrows beneath the stratum corneum layer of the epidermis and deposits her eggs and fecal material. These burrows are minute, linear, grayish-brown, threadlike lesions that are a distinctive sign; the mite may be seen at the end of the lesion, appearing as a black dot.

III. Signs, Symptoms, and History

A. *Incubation period is 2 to 6 weeks for new infestation. In a person who has had scabies previously, symptoms appear within a few days.*

B. *Period of communicability is while mite is alive. The mite cannot live over 48 to 72 hours away from a host.*

C. *Transmission is by prolonged, direct contact with infected individuals or indirect contact of infected garments or linens.*

D. Intense itching, more severe at night.

E. Raised grayish-white, linear burrows, papules, or vesicles.

F. Child under 2 years, largest eruption usually found on feet and ankles.

G. Child over 2 years, largest eruption usually found on hands and wrist.

H. Skin eruptions are commonly found in the webbing of the fingers; the skin folds of the wrist, elbow, or knee; the penis; the breast or shoulder blades; the axillary folds; and the abdomen, buttocks, and groin.

I. Pustules present, with secondary infection from scratching (see color plates, Primary and Secondary Skin Lesions).

J. Exposure to scabies at home or school.

K. Mites found on animals cannot establish infestation on humans.

IV. Initial Management

A. The decision to isolate a student will depend on the age of the child, the developmental level, and the location of the lesions.

B. Use good hand-washing techniques.

C. Instruct parents to treat all family members and to wash all bed linens, towels, underwear, and so forth, in hot water (140° F).

D. Treatment with permethrin 5% (Elimite) is generally safe and requires one application. Instructions for treatment must be followed (see Box 3-4). Several lotions and treatments are available.

V. Exclusion/Readmission

A. Exclude student from school until 24 hours after treatment has been completed.

WEB SITES

Centers for Disease Control and Prevention: Scabies Fact Sheet
http://www.cdc.gov/ncidod/dpd/parasites/scabies/factsht_scabies.htm
McKinley Health Center
http://www.mckinley.uiuc.edu/Handouts/scabies.html

SCARLET FEVER

I. Definition

A. Scarlet fever is an acute, systemic, contagious childhood disease that usually occurs in spring or late winter. It is also called *scarlatina*.

| Box 3-4 | *Instructions for Scabies Treatment* |

1. Infested household members must be treated at the same time, as well as anyone who has had close, prolonged, personal contact with an infested person (CDC, 2005).
2. Treatment is most easily applied at bedtime.
3. Bathe or shower and dry skin completely.
4. Trim nails and use a brush to apply product under fingernails.
5. Apply lotion from the neck down to the soles of the feet; massage into all surfaces, including skin folds.
6. If lotion gets into eyes, immediately flush with water.
7. Leave on overnight, 8 to 14 hours, following pharmaceutical instructions.
8. Remove product during a warm bath, shower, or shampooing of hair.
9. Stinging may occur, which may be normal for some individuals.
10. Change and either wash or dry-clean all clothing, linens, and towels used and dry them in a hot dryer.
11. No new burrows or rashes should be seen 1 to 2 days after treatment. Second treatment may be necessary in 7 to 10 days (CDC, 2005).
12. Itching may continue for 2 to 3 weeks.
13. Always check medication instructions for changes.

II. Etiology
  A. The cause is group A beta-hemolytic streptococci (GABHS), generally following streptococcal pharyngitis.
III. Signs, Symptoms, and History
  A. *Incubation period ranges from 1 to 3 days.*
  B. *Period of communicability is during incubation period, and active phase of illness is approximately 10 to 21 days but may persist for months.*
  C. *Transmission is by direct contact with an infected person, by droplet spread, by indirect contact with contaminated articles, or by ingestion of contaminated food (e.g., milk, milk products, deviled eggs).*
  D. Complications are otitis media, rheumatic fever, glomerulonephritis, peritonsillar abscess, sinusitis, carditis, and polyarthritis.
  E. Prodromal phase: 1 to 2 days.
    1. Abrupt fever from 102° to 104° F (38.8° to 40° C); increased pulse that is out of proportion to fever, headache, pharyngitis, chills, and malaise.
    2. Abdominal pain may occur.
  F. Exanthem on skin.
    1. Rash appears 12 to 48 hours after onset of pharyngitis; red, punctiform (pinpoint) lesions with fine papules that blanch under pressure appear on trunk and extremities.
    2. Increased redness in Pastia's lines, found in inguinal, antecubital, or other skin folds; skin feels rough or like sandpaper; rash persists for about 1 week. Desquamation occurs on fingers and toes, occasionally on palms of hands and on soles of feet. May be complete by 3 weeks, but may take longer.
  G. Exanthem in mouth.
    1. Red pharynx and uvula; tonsils are enlarged, red, edematous, and covered with gray-white exudate.

CHAPTER 3

Acute Conditions

2. Tongue is swollen, red, and has a white coating from which red papillae project for 1 to 2 days (white strawberry tongue); white sloughs off, displaying prominent papillae and palate, which persist with erythematous, punctate lesions (red strawberry tongue) by 4 to 5 days (see color plate 3).

IV. Initial Management

A. Isolate child from other students.

B. Use good hand-washing technique.

C. Implement supportive measures.

D. Call parent and refer for evaluation by HCP. Diagnosis should be reported back to school, so other children can be observed.

E. Treatment of choice is penicillin, or erythromycin for penicillin-sensitive children; fever usually subsides 24 hours after initiation of therapy.

V. Exclusion/Readmission

A. Exclude student from school.

B. Students may return to school 24 hours after antibiotic therapy has been initiated and when they have been fever-free for 24 hours.

WEB SITE

Kids Health for Parents
http://www.kidshealth.org/parent/infections/bacterial_viral/scarlet_fever.html

---

SHIGELLOSIS (ACUTE DIARRHEA)

I. Definition

A. Shigellosis is a dysentery-like acute diarrhea involving the large and distal small colon. It can be a serious disease, particularly in children younger than 2 years of age, and it can be epidemic in day care centers and institutions.

II. Etiology

A. Shigellosis is caused by *Shigella dysenteriae;* there are four subgenera of bacilli. The pathogen stimulates loss of fluids and electrolytes, and peak incidence is in late summer.

III. Signs, Symptoms, and History

A. *Incubation period is 1 to 3 days, but may range from 12 to 96 hours.*

B. *Period of communicability is during acute infection and until bacteria are no longer present in feces, usually 4 weeks after illness.*

C. *Transmission is by direct or indirect fecal–oral transmission of a symptomatic individual or by infected food or water.*

D. Onset is variable but generally abrupt.

E. Fever up to 104° F (40° C) with nausea, vomiting, and sometimes toxemia.

F. Watery diarrhea with mucus and pus 12 to 48 hours after onset.

G. Convulsions associated with fever in young children.

H. Stools preceded by abdominal cramps, tenesmus, and straining.

I. Headache, nuchal rigidity, delirium.

J. Complications: severe dehydration and collapse.

K. Usually self-limiting, lasting several days to weeks; average is 4 to 10 days.

IV. Initial Management

A. Use good handwashing techniques (e.g., after diapering, toileting, and fecal accidents).

B. Call parent(s) and advise going to HCP.

C. Discontinue formula, milk, and solids.

D. Provide clear liquids.

E. Treat fever.

F. Treatment is with antibiotics.

G. Educate school staff, caregivers, and parents about outbreaks caused by contaminated water or food that can occur in youth activity groups, such as sports teams, or on field trips or overnight trips.

H. Shigellosis is a reportable disease in the United States.

V. Exclusion/Readmission

A. Depends on age of child and physical involvement.

B. Exclude from school until diarrhea has stopped and local health department recommendations have been met. Readmission requires two negative stool cultures.

WEB SITE

Centers for Disease Control and Prevention: Shigellosis
    http://www.cdc.gov/nczvcd/dfbmd/disease_listing/shigellosis_gi.html

STREPTOCOCCAL PHARYNGITIS (STREP THROAT)

I. Definition

A. Streptococcal sore throat is an inflammation of the upper airway. The infection is not serious, but the complications—acute rheumatic fever (ARF) and acute glomerulonephritis—are.

II. Etiology

A. The cause is group A beta-hemolytic streptococci (GABHS).

III. Signs, Symptoms, and History

A. *Incubation period is 1 to 3 days.*

B. *If untreated, period of communicability is 10 to 21 days, and the organism can exist for weeks or months. With adequate antibiotic therapy, the illness may be over in 24 hours.*

C. *Transmission is person-to-person contact with infectious respiratory secretions and rarely by contaminated objects.*

D. Sudden onset of fever and acute onset of pharyngitis.

E. Acute pharyngitis is often viral, so a throat culture is necessary.

F. Headache, fever, nausea, and abdominal pain.

G. Pharynx and tonsils may be inflamed or covered with exudate; foul breath.

H. Tender anterior cervical lymph nodes.

I. Pain is mild to severe and makes swallowing difficult.

J. Clinical symptoms subside in 3 to 5 days unless complications occur.

1. Acute glomerulonephritis can occur in about 10 days.
2. Rheumatic fever can occur in about 19 days.
3. Rheumatic heart disease and Sydenham's chorea, also called *Saint Vitus Dance*, may occur several months later.

IV. Initial Management

A. Isolate individual from others and call parents or caregivers.
B. Use good hand-washing technique.
C. Control fever elevation with cooling measures (see Fever).
D. Advise parents to obtain a throat culture for their child to rule out GABHS. Office, clinic, and OTC test kits are available for identification; but even if test results are negative, a confirmatory throat culture is recommended.
E. Treatment is oral antibiotics for approximately 10 days.
F. Advise parents to ensure the child to take all the prescribed medication, which is crucial to eliminate the organism that can cause rheumatic fever.
G. Remind students and parents to discard toothbrush and replace it after 24 hours of antibiotic treatment when there is a positive throat culture for GABHS.
H. Share information with other parents and staff, since GABHS can be epidemic in day care and school sites.

V. Exclusion/Readmission

A. Call parents to pick student up from school.
B. Readmit student after 24 hours of antibiotic treatment, if there is no fever for the preceding 24 hours, and when no symptoms are present that interfere with school activity.

WEB SITE

American Academy of Family Physicians
   http://www.familydoctor.org/handouts/670.html

STY (HORDEOLUM)

I. Definition

A. A sty is a localized inflammation of the sebaceous gland near the eyelashes and is generally on the lower eyelid.

II. Etiology

A. The most common cause is *S. aureus*.

III. Signs, Symptoms, and History

A. Localized edema and redness.
B. Tenderness or pain.
C. Often comes to a head and resembles a pimple in 2 to 3 days.
D. Two types of sty: in an *internal sty*, the abscess is large and may be observed through the skin or conjunctival surface; an *external sty* is smaller, superficial, usually seen at the lid margin, and involves the gland.
E. Usually unilateral.
F. Visual acuity not affected.

IV. Initial Management

A. Ask student or call parents to inquire if they are aware of the problem and if treatment has been initiated.

B. Ensure good hand-washing technique by school staff to prevent spread of organism.

C. Instruct students not to rub or touch their eyes or attempt to squeeze the sty, because doing so may spread the infection.

D. Frequent warm compresses 2 to 3 times a day may bring a sty to a head.

E. Discuss with student and parents that if spontaneous rupture does not occur, and the sty is large and edematous, it may need surgical incision and drainage.

F. Topical antibiotics can be prescribed.

G. If no result from medication, refer to primary care practitioner for systemic antibiotic.

H. When untreated, cellulitis of the lid or orbit may develop, which requires systemic antibiotics.

V. Exclusion/Readmission

A. Depends on student's age, level of functioning, and personal habits.

B. Excluded student may return after treatment has been initiated.

WEB SITE

Intelihealth
    http://www.intelihealth.com/IH/ihtIH/WSIHW000/9339/10151.html

TAPEWORM

A tapeworm has a small head, or scolex, and up to 4000 proglottids, or segments. It has a characteristic ribbonlike shape and can be up to 30 ft long. Although infestation is not particularly common in the United States, it is frequent in other parts of the world. Because of the large number of visitors and immigrants entering the United States daily, health personnel are seeing more people with infections. The four types of tapeworm are *beef*, *pork*, *fish*, and *dwarf* (see Table 3-2).

BEEF, PORK, FISH, AND DWARF TAPEWORMS

I. Definition

A. A parasitic infestation of the intestinal tract.

II. Initial Management

A. Refer suspected cases to parent or caregiver for referral to HCP for diagnosis and treatment.

B. Use good hand-washing technique.

III. Exclusion/Readmission

A. Exclude student from school until treatment can be verified.

WEB SITE

U.S. Department of Agriculture, Food Safety Inspection Service
    http://www.fsis.usda.gov/Fact_Sheets/Parasites_and_Foodborne_Illness/index.asp

Acute Conditions   CHAPTER 3

Table 3-2 *Etiology, Symptoms, Treatment, and Prevention of Tapeworm Infestation*

Tapeworm	Etiology	Signs, Symptoms, History	Treatment	Prevention
Beef				
Adult worm is 15-30 ft long	Cestode *Taenia saginata* Transmission only by raw or poorly cooked infected beef.	Usually asymptomatic; epigastric pain, diarrhea, weight loss. Active proglottid may be felt crawling in anus, visible in stool.	Praziquantel (Biltricide), 20 mg/kg per day in four divided doses for 1 day. Niclosamide (Yomesan, Niclocide) is also effective.	Thoroughly cook beef. Freeze below temperature of −5° C (23° F) for more than 4 days. Adequate toilet facilities and meat inspection help to control.
Pork				
Adult worm is 8-10 ft long	Cestode *Taenia solium* Transmitted directly through ingestion of egg-infested food or water, directly from contaminated feces to oral cavity.	Usually asymptomatic; heavy larval infestations may cause muscle pains, weakness, fever. If CNS involved, meningoencephalitis or seizures. Eggs near anus or in stool.	Same as beef.	Thoroughly cook pork. Same as beef prevention.

Fish				
Adult worm is 15-30 ft long	Cestode *Diphyllobothrium latum* Transmitted directly through ingestion of egg-infested fish or water; directly from contaminated feces to oral cavity.	Usually asymptomatic; mild GI symptoms. Eggs or segments of the worm in stool.	Praziquantel (Biltricide) or niclosamide (Niclocide) are drugs of choice.	Thoroughly cook all fresh fish; freeze at −18° C (0° F) for 24 hr. All fish and shellfish for raw or semiraw consumption should be blast frozen to −35° C or −31° F or below for 15 hr.
Dwarf				
Children more susceptible	Cestode *Hymenolepis nana* Transmitted directly through ingestion of egg-infested food or water; directly from contaminated feces to oral cavity; ingestion of larvae-carrying insects.	May be asymptomatic; diarrhea, abdominal discomfort, dizziness, lethargy in children. Eggs in stool.	Same as beef.	Elimination of rodents from home environment. Protect food and water from contamination. Education regarding hygienic practices and personal hygiene.

TESTICULAR TORSION

I. Definition
   A. Testicular (spermatic cord) torsion (TT) is an acute loss of blood supply to the testis, which causes ensuing ischemic injury and possible tissue death of the testicle.

II. Etiology
   A. May follow trauma but most often occurs without known cause. Peak incidence is 12 to 18 years of age, but may occur at any age. The left testicle is more likely to be involved because of a longer spermatic cord.

III. Signs, Symptoms, and History
   A. Sudden onset of abdominal or testicular pain that is excruciating and unremitting.
   B. Frequently occurs during sleep.
   C. Scrotum may be edematous, reddened, and warm to the touch.
   D. Often bilateral.
   E. Minimal elevation of the testis increases the pain.
   F. Earlier episodes of transitory pain are reported in about half of all cases.
   G. Absence of blood flow to the testis for 4 to 6 hours may cause loss of spermatogenesis.
   H. Complications of untreated TT include testicular atrophy, abscess, and loss of testis or decreased fertility.

IV. Initial Management
   A. *This is urgent.*
   B. Contact parents regarding prompt evaluation by physician.
   C. Begin treatment within 6 hours from onset of pain to avoid loss of the testis.
   D. May be reduced manually if pain has been present for less than 4 to 6 hours, but usually requires surgical exploration and detorsion to prevent recurrence and to preserve fertility.
   E. Rule out infection, tumor, trauma, hydrocele, kidney stone, and hernia.

V. Exclusion/Readmission
   A. Does not apply.

WEB SITE

eMedicine: Testicular Torsion
   http://www.emedicine.com/emerg/topic573.htm

URINARY TRACT INFECTION

I. Definition
   A. Urinary tract infection (UTI) is a clinical condition that involves primarily the growth of bacteria within the urinary tract, which is normally sterile. May involve the *lower urinary tract,* the urethra and bladder; the *upper urinary tract,* which comprises the ureters, renal pelvis, renal calyces, and renal parenchyma; or both. There are three classifications of UTI: *asymptomatic bacteriuria, cystitis,* and *pyelonephritis.*

B. Not including structural anomalies, most often occurs in children between 2 and 6 years of age. At age 1 year and younger, the incidence is higher in males, and it occurs more frequently in uncircumcised boys. Beyond age 1, it is more common in females (Kliegman, et al, 2006). Box 3-5 provides information on how to prevent urinary tract infections.

II. Etiology

A. The most common cause of UTI is bacteria. The most prominent bacterial organism is *Escherichia coli,* followed by *Klebsiella, Proteus,* and then *Pseudomonas, S. aureus, Haemophilus,* and coagulase-negative *Staphylococcus.* Viral infections, especially adenovirus, are a cause for cystitis.

B. Increased incidence of bacteriuria in the female is due, in part, to the short urethra, about ¾ in (2 cm), in young females and 1½ in (4 cm) in mature women. The length of the male urethra, 8 in (20 cm) accounts for inhibition of entry and growth of pathogens. In the uncircumcised male, bacterial pathogens ascend the urethra from the flora beneath the prepuce.

III. Signs, Symptoms, and History

A. Unrecognized symptoms, referred to as *asymptomatic bacteriuria,* occur most frequently in girls. Note day or nighttime incontinence or perineal discomfort and a positive urine culture; usually a benign infection, except during pregnancy, when it can result in more severe symptoms if not treated.

B. *Cystitis* is an inflammation of the bladder and ureters; there is no fever or renal injury.

C. *Pyelonephritis* is an infection involving the upper urinary tract and renal parenchyma.

D. Manifestations depend on age. In newborns and those under age 2:
   1. Poor feeding; failure to thrive; vomiting, diarrhea, and abdominal distention; and jaundice, which may indicate pyelonephritis.
   2. Fever, hypothermia, or sepsis.
   3. Altered voiding pattern, strong-smelling urine, irritability, squirming, or persistent diaper rash.

E. In preschool and those over age 2:
   1. Fever.
   2. Increased frequency of urination, dysuria, or urgency.
   3. Lower abdominal pain or costovertebral tenderness.
   4. Pyelonephritis indications: high fever with chills, severe abdominal or flank pain, malaise, vomiting, and diarrhea.

Box 3-5   *Preventive Education for Urinary Tract Infections*

1. Discuss diet high in animal protein to avoid alkaline urine.
2. Encourage generous fluid intake.
3. Teach proper perianal hygiene: wipe from front to back.
4. Teach avoidance of holding urine.
5. Avoid wearing tight panties.
6. Use cotton underwear instead of synthetic underwear.
7. Avoid use of bubble baths if susceptible to UTIs.
8. Educate sexually active teenagers to void after intercourse.

F. In adolescents (classic signs):
   1. Lower tract infection: frequency and urgency, dysuria (pain and burning), enuresis; fever is often absent.
   2. Upper tract infection: fever and chills, flank pain, lower abdominal pain, costovertebral tenderness; lower tract symptoms occur a few days later.
   3. May develop UTI after first time intercourse.

IV. **Initial Management**
   A. Discuss with parents the clinical manifestations and need for diagnostic evaluation; stress the need for follow-up.
   B. Treat the fever, following school guidelines and procedures.
   C. If enuretic, assure student it is only a symptom of the infection.
   D. For infants and toddlers, check diaper every half hour to determine signs of discomfort, straining, intermittent starting or stopping, dripping of small amounts, frequency, and odor.
   E. Educate children and parents about prevention and treatment of infection.
   F. Rule out sexual abuse, especially with young children.
   G. Treatment.
      1. Midstream urine culture for identification.
      2. Mild symptoms: treatment is delayed until culture results are available, then nitrofurantoin or amoxicillin may be prescribed.
      3. Severe symptoms: culture is obtained and treatment begins immediately, and therapy with trimethoprim-sulfamethoxazole may be suggested.
      4. Increase fluids; unsweetened cranberry juice or cranberry tablets prevent bacteria binding to the host cell in urinary tract membranes.
      5. Acute febrile infections that suggest pyelonephritis are treated with a broad-spectrum antibiotic for 14 days.
      6. Hospitalization for acute symptoms of pyelonephritis with parenteral antibiotics.
      7. Single antibiotic dose or 3-day treatment for adolescent girls can be considered for uncomplicated UTI.
      8. When child is younger than 5, and the UTI is complicated, radiological evaluation of kidneys and bladder may be done to rule out renal scarring.
      9. If untreated, child is at risk for pyelonephritis.

V. **Exclusion/Readmission**
   A. Does not apply.

WEB SITE

National Kidney and Urologic Diseases Information Clearinghouse
   http://kidney.niddk.nih.gov/kudiseases/pubs/utichildren/index.htm#points

VARICELLA-ZOSTER VIRUS (CHICKENPOX)

I. **Definition**
   A. Chickenpox is a highly contagious, self-limiting disease marked by an eruption on the skin and mucous membranes. The initial infection

results in a lifelong dormant infection of the sensory ganglion nerve cells. Reactivation of this latency condition is the cause of herpes zoster (HZ) or shingles. There is a vaccine for prevention of Varicella (See Appendix B, Immunizations).

II. Etiology
A. Varicella-zoster virus (VZV) is a human herpes virus. It is the cause of primary, latent, and recurrent infections. Epidemics are most frequent in winter and spring.

III. Signs, Symptoms, and History
A. *Incubation period is 10 to 21 days.*
B. *Period of communicability usually begins 1 to 2 days before the rash appears, and it lasts until all lesions are scabbed—about 5 to 6 days after the appearance of the rash.*
C. *Transmission is by contact with secretions from the respiratory tract of infected persons and, to a lesser degree, through the discharge from skin lesions and scabs until these are dry.*
D. Generally a mild illness in childhood.
E. In immunocompromised children and adolescents, there can be increased morbidity and mortality.
F. Predisposes individual to GABHS and *S. aureus* infections.
G. Prodromal stage:
   1. Slight fever.
   2. Malaise.
   3. Anorexia.
   4. Headache.
   5. Mild abdominal pain.
H. Rash.
   1. First appears on back and chest, spreading outward to face and extremities, but sparse on distal limbs. May be limited to a few lesions.
   2. Continues to make its appearance for 3 to 7 days.
   3. Begins as a flat red macule that rapidly progresses to lesions resembling itchy insect bites.
   4. These lesions develop into blisters filled with an amber fluid.
   5. Blisterlike eruptions are in crops; after they rupture, crusts form.
   6. All stages present in varying degrees at one time: macules, papules, vesicles, and scabs (see color plate 2 and color plates, Primary and Secondary Skin Lesions).

IV. Initial Management
A. Isolate student.
B. Maintain good hand-washing technique.
C. Keep infected student isolated from immunosuppressed individuals and those with eczema, malignancies, and human immunodeficiency syndrome or acquired immunodeficiency syndrome (HIV/AIDS), because such individuals are at high risk for greater complications.
D. Disease can be prevented by immunization with a live-attenuated VZV vaccine (See Appendix B, Immunizations).
E. If high-risk students are exposed, varicella zoster immunoglobulin (VZIG) given within 72 hours may alter the course of the disease.

V. Exclusion/Readmission
   A. Exclude student from school.
   B. Student may return to school a minimum of 7 days after onset of rash; all vesicles (blisters) must have crusted.
VI. Additional Information
   A. Gestational chickenpox can cause a severe reaction in a pregnant woman and a rare but identifiable syndrome in the fetus. The infection can be life threatening to the fetus.

WEB SITE

Centers for Disease Control and Prevention: Varicella
   http://www.cdc.gov/vaccines/vpd-vac/varicella/default.htm

GENERAL WEB SITES FOR CHAPTER 3

American Academy of Dermatology
   http://www.aad.org/public
American Academy of Pediatrics: Children's Health Topics
   http://www.aap.org/topics.html
Centers for Disease Control and Prevention, Division of Parasitic Diseases
   http://www.cdc.gov/ncidod/dpd/index.htm
Infectious Disease Information: Childhood Diseases
   http://www.cdc.gov/ncidod/diseases/children/diseases.htm
Children's Hospital Boston
   http://www.childrenshospital.org
Kids Health
   http://www.kidshealth.org
MedlinePlus Health Information
   http://www.nlm.nih.gov/medlineplus
Merck Manual of Diagnosis and Therapy
   http://www.merck.com/pubs
National Foundation for Infectious Diseases
   http://www.nfid.org
National Immunization Program
   http://www.cdc.gov/vaccines
University of Iowa, Department of Dermatology
   http://tray.dermatology.uiowa.edu

BIBLIOGRAPHY

American Academy of Dermatology: *What is eczema?* (available online): www.skincarephysicians.com/eczemanet/whatis.html#who. Accessed Sep 1, 2006.
American Academy of Otolaryngology: *Head and neck surgery: children and secondhand smoke* (available online): www.entnet.org/healthinfo/tobacco/secondhand_smoke.cfm. Accessed Sep 9, 2006.
American Academy of Pediatrics: School health. In Pickering LK, ed: *Red book: 2006 report of the Committee on Infectious Diseases,* Elk Grove Village, Ill, 2006.
American Ophthalmology Association: *Optometric clinical guideline: care of the patient with conjunctivitis,* (available online): www.aoa.org/documents/CPG-11.pdf. Accessed Aug 2, 2006.

American Ophthalmology Association: *Preferred practice patterns: Blepharitis* Available online: http://www.aao.org/aao/education/library/ppp/upload/Blepharitis_.pdf Accessed Aug 1, 2006.

Burns CE: *Pocket reference for pediatric primary care,* Philadelphia, 2000, WB Saunders.

Centers for Disease Control and Prevention: *Epidemiology and Prevention of Vaccine Preventable Diseases,* Atkinson W, Hamborsky J, McIntyre L, Wolfe S, editors. Washington, DC, 2006, Public Health Foundation.

Childers K: Health problems of toddlers and preschoolers. In Hockenberry M, Wilson D, Winkelstein ML, eds: *Wong's essentials of pediatric nursing,* St Louis, 2005, WB Saunders.

Heyman DL: *Control of communicable diseases manual,* Washington, DC, 2004, American Public Health Association.

Hockenberry MJ, Wilson D, Winkelstein ML: *Wong's essentials of pediatric nursing,* St Louis, 2006, Mosby.

Jenson HB, Baltimore RS: Infectious diseases. In Kliegman RM, ed: *Nelson essentials of pediatrics,* Philadelphia, 2006, WB Saunders.

Kliegman RM: *Nelson essentials of pediatrics,* Philadelphia, 2006, WB Saunders.

Lucile Packard Children's Hospital: *Fever, Stanford* (available online): www.lpch.org/HealthLibrary/ParentCareTopics/FeverInfectionsCrying/Fever.html. Accessed Sep 19, 2006.

Lynch DM: Cranberry for prevention of urinary tract infection, *Am Fam Physician* 70 (11): 2175-7, 2004 (available online): www.aafp.org/afp/20041201/2175.html. Accessed Sep 19, 2006.

Mosby's Dictionary of Medicine, Nursing and Health. St. Louis, 2006.

Nettina SM: *Lippincott manual of nursing practice handbook,* Philadelphia, 2006, Lippincott Williams & Wilkins.

Osborn LM: *Pediatrics,* Phildelphia, 2004, Mosby.

Penn State Social Science Research Institute: *Honey proves better option for coughs than OTCs,* 2007. Available online: http://www.ssri.psu.edu/news/120307.htm. Accessed March 18, 2008.

Proctor SE: *To see or not to see: Screening the vision of children in school,* Castle Rock, Colo, 2005, National Assoc of School Nurses.

Robertson J, Shilkofski N: *The Harriet Lane handbook,* St Louis, 2005, Mosby.

Skidmore-Roth L: *Mosby's nursing drug reference,* Philadelphia, 2007, Mosby.

U.S. Food and Drug Administration (FDA): Public Health Advisory: *Nonprescription cough and cold medicine use in children,* January 2008. Available online: http://www.fda.gov/cde/drug/advisory/cough_cold_2008.htm. Accessed March 18, 2008.

Chronic Conditions

Chapter Outline

*T*he school-age population with chronic illness is increasing and will continue to increase as medical technology saves and extends the lives of affected students daily. The physical, emotional, intellectual, and social impact of chronic illness on children is immense, and nurses and educators contribute greatly to the goal of enabling each individual to achieve maximum potential in all areas of functioning.

This chapter provides comprehensive, concise information on 31 chronic conditions found in the school-age child that require nursing assessment and management. Each chronic condition is described in the same format to enhance usability and ease of reading for the nurse. The complexity of the chronic condition and the need for the school nurse to be aware of current and pertinent knowledge dictate the information included in this chapter.

As the nurse reads the individual chronic conditions in this chapter, a picture of the great number of health concerns and emergencies each condition could produce will emerge. There is no question as to the importance of nursing care to the physical well-being and safety of each student with a chronic illness. The school nurse is in a position to facilitate a networking and learning environment between school staff and community health care providers (HCPs) that will bridge the gap in understanding the unique school health care and support provided during the school day to students and their families.

Individualized Health Care Plans (IHCPs) and Individualized Emergency Care Plans (IECPs) are now a part of the student's school records. Subsections included with each condition will assist in developing these plans.

The Effects on Individual section provides some insight into the stress and uncertainty that may accompany each condition. Recognition of the psychological effects of long-term illness on both child and family will better equip the nurse to help students and their families cope and adjust to the many difficulties of living with a chronic illness. The nurse can have a positive influence on attitudes among staff and families by emphasizing the child's strengths rather than focusing on deficits.

CHAPTER 4

Chronic Conditions

AMBIGUOUS GENITALIA

I. Definition

A. Normal sexual differentiation occurs in utero with external and internal genitalia consistent with the sex chromosome of either 46 XX (female) or 46 XY (male). Embryos have the potential to develop as either males or females, and differentiation into one sex or the other (i.e., the development of testes or ovaries) occurs during the seventh or eighth week of gestation. Errors in embryonic sex determination and differentiation result in diverse degrees of intermediate sex, a condition known as *hermaphroditism* or *intersexuality*. The condition in which the chromosomal sex is different from the phenotype sex is often referred to as *intersex* or *disorders of sex development (DSD)*.

B. *Hermaphroditism* suggests a discrepancy between the morphology of the gonads, ovaries/testes, and the appearance of the external genitalia.

C. *True hermaphroditism* presents itself with both ovarian and testicular tissue as separate organs or combined in the same organ, or ovotestis; this is an extremely rare condition (Kliegman et al, 2006). *Female pseudohermaphrodites* have ovaries, and *male pseudohermaphrodites* have testes; both have ambiguous genitalia.

D. Disorders of sex development are classified by the histological appearance of the gonads but include situations in which the chromosomal and phenotype sex are different.

E. The terms *hermaphrodite* and *sex reversal* are stigmatizing and not anatomically correct. The American Academy of Pediatrics has proposed changes in terminology, from *male pseuodohermaphrodite* to *46 XY DSD:* from *female pseudohermaphrodite* to *46 XX DSD;* and from *true hermaphrodite* to *ovotesticular DSD* (Lee et al, 2006).

II. Etiology

A. May be caused by atypical differentiation of primitive gonads and differentiation and development of internal duct systems and external genitalia. Alterations in these processes may result in a defect of embryogenesis, abnormalities of chromosomal complement, and biochemical abnormalities that include androgen insensitivity, defective sex hormonal synthesis in a male, placental transfer of masculinizing agents in a female, or congenital adrenal hyperplasia (CAH), also called *adrenogenital syndrome.*

   1. CAH is the most common cause of ambiguous genitalia.

B. *Female pseudohermaphroditism* usually occurs when the female fetus is exposed to excessive androgens, and *male pseudohermaphroditism* usually occurs from androgen insensitivity. True hermaphroditism is not completely understood. (See "Additional Information" for other ambiguous sex conditions.)

III. Characteristics

A. *True hermaphroditism.*

   1. Has both an ovary and a testis or an ovotestis, which are usually nonfunctional.

B. Other.

   1. The phenotype may be female or male; however, the external genitalia are ambiguous.

   2. Gender assignment may not be the same as genetic or gonadal sex.

IV. Health Concerns/Emergencies

A. An electrolyte imbalance such as CAH can be life threatening if unidentified and untreated at birth.

B. Gender assignment, when doubt exists, can be psychologically distressing to the family and the growing child and may continue throughout life.

C. May need hormones or assistive medications at particular times of life.

D. May have lifelong emotional difficulties.

E. May need long-term management.

V. Effects on Individual

A. Will need to make decisions about sexual identity, a developmental process that lasts through childhood, adolescence, and into adulthood.

B. Emotional/Psychological.

   1. May have feelings of guilt and shame, as may parents.

   2. May not have been told about their gender assignment secondary to ambiguous genitalia.

      3. Cannot understand development of sexual body parts and may have feelings of inadequacy, shame, or inferiority.

      4. May not identify with the gender selection that has been made.

      5. Consider delaying surgery until child is old enough to participate in decision.

  C. Social/Familial.

      1. Often not accepted by one or both parents.

      2. May face criticism, comments, and judgments because of sexual differences.

      3. May lack or not identify with parent role model.

VI. Management/Treatment

  A. Listen to and support student.

  B. Be supportive, understanding, honest, and encouraging with parents. Encourage openness with their child; secrecy compounds the problem.

  C. Teach staff who work with the student about the condition in honest and supportive ways.

  D. Be alert for mental health issues and any need for counseling.

  E. Consider referral to peer support for both child and parents.

  F. Be aware of medication and any side effects.

  G. Monitor anthropometry.

  H. At birth, four conditions that produce ambiguous genitalia require prompt and accurate assessment: (1) female pseudohermaphroditism, (2) male pseudohermaphroditism, (3) true hermaphroditism, and (4) mixed gonadal dysgenesis.

      1. Gender determination may take days or weeks; tests may include history, physical examination, chromosomal analysis, endoscopy, ultrasonography, radiographic contrast tests, biochemical tests, and laparotomy or gonad biopsy.

      2. Consideration of gender assignment should include both anatomical findings and genetic sex determinations.

      3. Surgery may or may not be performed, but preliminary sex assignment should be made shortly after birth. Child may later decide to change sex assignment.

  I. Treatment is centered on the cause and degree of ambiguity.

      1. *Hermaphroditism* and mixed gonadal dysgenesis: choose an appropriate gender, maximize potential for adult sexual function, and decrease psychosocial difficulties. After gender decision, surgical intervention is usually undertaken, and hormonal replacements are given at puberty.

      2. Defective testosterone biosynthesis of male infant: testosterone injections in adolescence and adulthood to initiate puberty and sustain adult masculinization.

      3. Controversy exists regarding treatment and surgery before the child's participation in the decision.

      4. Studies have not shown any increased rates of social ostracization or psychological illness as a result of delaying surgery until the child is older.

VII. Additional Information

  A. The Intersex Society of North America (ISNA) supports a paradigm for the management of disorders of sex development. They are a resource for those seeking help by offering positive advocacy, policy advice, and caring support for individuals and families dealing with DSDs.

B. *Female pseudohermaphroditism:* These individuals have chromatin-positive nuclei and a 46 XX chromosome constitution. This anomaly occurs when the female fetus is exposed to excessive androgens that affect the external genitalia, resulting in clitoral enlargement and labial fusion. Ovarian abnormalities do not exist, but the most common cause of this condition is increased production of androgens, which produces masculinization of the external genitalia. This varies from enlargement of the clitoris to almost masculine genitalia.

1. The most common cause of this condition is CAH. Androgenic agents administered during pregnancy may cause similar anomalies to the external genitalia. This condition may also result from benign adrenal adenoma, ovarian tumors, and the treatment for threatened abortions.

2. Untreated CAH results in early sexual maturation with development of facial, axillary, and pubic hair; acne; early sexual maturation; deepening of the voice; and a noticeable increase in musculature toward an adult male physique. The females do not develop breasts and are amenorrheic and infertile. The male testes remain small, and spermatogenesis does not occur.

C. *Male pseudohermaphroditism:* These individuals have chromatin negative nuclei and a 46 XY chromosome constitution. External and internal genitalia vary according to degree of development of the external genitalia and internal female organs. These anomalies are caused by defects in testicular differentiation, inadequate production of testicular hormones, or defects in androgen action.

D. *Androgen insensitivity syndrome* (testicular feminization): This syndrome follows X-linked recessive inheritance. In individuals with this condition, 1 in 20,000, appear as normal females despite the presence of testes and a 46 XY chromosome constitution. External genitalia are female, the vagina generally ends blindly, and the uterus and uterine tubes are absent or rudimentary. Normal development of breasts and female characteristics occurs during puberty; however, pubic hair is scant or absent, and menstruation does not take place. Psychosexual orientation is usually completely female, and medically, socially, and legally, these are women.

1. Testes are generally in the abdomen or inguinal canals but can descend into the labia majora. These individuals are not considered ambiguous because of normal external genitalia, even though embryologically, these females represent an extreme form of male pseudohermaphroditism.

E. *Hypospadias:* Hypospadias occurs in one of every 300 male infants. With this condition, the external urethral orifice is on the ventral surface of the glans of the penis or on the ventral surface of the shaft of the penis. The penis is generally underdeveloped and curved ventrally, known as *chordee*. There are four types of hypospadias, but glandular and penile types make up 80% of cases.

1. This condition is the result of inadequate production of androgens by the fetal testes, inadequate receptor sites for the hormones, or

both. In perineal hypospadias, the labioscrotal folds fail to fuse, and the external urethral orifice is found between the unfused halves of the scrotum. Because in this severe type of hypospadias the external genitalia are ambiguous, those individuals with perineal hypospadias and cryptorchidism (undescended testes) are occasionally diagnosed as male pseudohermaphrodites.

F. *Epispadias:* This condition occurs in about one of every 30,000 male infants. The urethra opening is on the dorsal surface of the penis.

G. *Micropenis:* The penis is almost hidden, since it is so small. This abnormality results from a hormonal deficiency of the fetal testes and is often associated with hypopituitarism. A number of uterine and vaginal anomalies result from arrests of development of the uterovaginal primordium during the eighth week of gestation.

H. *Double uterus:* This results from a lack of fusion of the inferior parts and can be associated with a double or a single vagina. Occasionally the uterus appears normal externally but is divided internally by a thin septum. When only the superior portion of the body of the uterus is involved, the condition is called *bicornuate uterus.* When one duct has retarded growth and it does not fuse with the other one, a bicornuate uterus with a rudimentary horn develops.

I. *Absence of vagina and uterus:* This condition occurs in one of every 4000 female births. It results from failure of the sinovaginal bulbs to develop and form the vaginal plate. If the vagina is absent, then the uterus is generally absent, since the developing uterus induces the formation of the vaginal plate.

J. *Vaginal atresia blockage:* This vaginal condition occurs as a result of failure of canalization of the vaginal plate. Failure of the inferior end to perforate results in an anomaly known as *imperforate hymen.*

WEB SITE

Intersex Society of North America
http://www.isna.org

IRON DEFICIENCY ANEMIA

I. Definition

A. In iron deficiency anemia, the blood is deficient in erythrocytes (red blood cells [RBCs]) and hemoglobin (oxygen-carrying pigment in RBCs). This is the most common type of nutritional anemia in all age groups.

II. Etiology

A. Factors causing anemia are:

1. Inadequate iron stores at birth from prematurity, low birth weight, severe maternal iron deficiency, and fetal or maternal blood loss.

2. Insufficient daily iron intake during rapid growth in children 3 months to 6 years old, during adolescent years combined with poor eating habits, and during adolescent pregnancy.

3. Excessive milk intake (milk is extremely low in iron) delays or reduces the addition of solid food to the infant's diet; may also cause an infant to be chubby although nutritionally deficient.

CHAPTER 4

Chronic Conditions

4. Iron loss from acute or chronic hemorrhage (e.g. heavy menstrual flow) or parasitic infection.
5. Impaired absorption of iron from chronic diarrhea or gastrointestinal (GI) disturbances.
6. In children older than 2, anemia may be due to blood loss rather than poor nutrition.
7. Inability to form hemoglobin due to lack of vitamin B_{12} and folic acid.
8. Lead poisoning.

III. Characteristics

A. Obscure and insidious symptoms; severity directly related to length of nutritional deficiency.
B. Condition characterized by microcytes (small) and hypochromic (pale) erythrocytes.
C. Fatigue and shortness of breath occur from reduced hemoglobin levels, which decrease oxygenation of tissues.
D. Early symptoms are:
  1. Pale skin and pale mucous membranes.
  2. Decreased activity and apathy.
  3. Prone to infection.
  4. May be asymptomatic and not diagnosed until routine physical examination.
E. Late symptoms are:
  1. Easy fatigue, irritability, and anorexia.
  2. Headaches, dizziness.
  3. Slow nail growth; brittle nails.
  4. Poor muscle tone.
  5. Soft systolic precordial murmur.
  6. Enlarged spleen.
  7. Pica, usually ice.
  8. Psychological disturbances (e.g., hyperactivity, decreased attention span).

IV. Health Concerns/Emergencies

A. Iron preparations may cause GI upset, nausea, anorexia, diarrhea, and constipation.
B. Liquid iron temporarily stains teeth; straw or medicine dropper placed at back of throat may be used for administration. Brushing teeth after dosage may lessen discoloration.
C. Black or dark green stools when iron preparation is given; absence of discolored stools may indicate medication is not being administered or compliance is poor.
D. Individuals with iron deficiency absorb lead more easily and are at higher risk for lead poisoning.

V. Effects on Individual

A. May have difficulty in academic performance because of low energy level, frequent headaches, and dizziness.
B. Difficulty with sports participation because of poor muscle development and easy fatigue.
C. Frequently absent from school because of recurrent infections.
D. Fatigue may limit student's participation in play and social activities.
E. Cognitive and psychomotor development may be affected.

VI. Management/Treatment

A. Avoid giving medication with meals; giving juices with vitamin C enhances absorption. Coffee, tea, bran foods, milk, and antacids impede absorption of iron. If iron supplements cause vomiting and diarrhea, give them with meals.

B. Avoid giving solid food at or near breast feedings, because it interferes with bioavailability of the small amount of iron in human milk.

C. Achieve normal hemoglobin level by replenishing depleted iron stores.

D. Diagnosis of underlying conditions (e.g., bleeding ulcer).

E. Assist family in meal planning; provide list of foods high in iron; educate family regarding disease, medication, and dietary compliance.

VII. Additional Information

A. Iron medication is highly toxic and must be kept out of the reach of children. If it is in the classroom, keep it locked in a drawer or cabinet. Usual dosage is 3 to 5 mg/kg of elemental iron per day. Commonly prescribed ferrous iron is more readily absorbed than ferric iron.

B. In cultures where tea is a common beverage, advise giving iron with another beverage, since tea forms an insoluble complex with iron. Some herbal tea may have a negative effect on the absorption of iron.

C. There are various nutritional recommendations: Give infants iron-fortified formula. Give foods containing iron. The best sources are fish, poultry, and meat, especially organ meat; soybeans; dried legumes; dry enriched cereals; and whole grain breads. Other sources are egg yolks; dark green, leafy vegetables; dried fruits, apricots, peaches, prunes, and raisins; nuts and peanut butter; and molasses.

D. Vitamin C helps the body absorb iron. A deficiency of vitamins B_6, B_{12}, and E can contribute to anemia. Preparing foods in iron skillets increases the iron content.

WEB SITE

Iron Disorders Institute
http://www.irondisorders.org

SICKLE CELL ANEMIA

I. Definition

A. Sickle cell disease (SCD) is the term used to describe a number of diseases called *hemoglobinopathies,* of which sickle cell anemia is the most common. It is a severe, chronic, incurable, anemia characterized by sickle-shaped red blood cells, and it results in acute and chronic organ damage. RBCs with sickle-cell hemoglobin (Hb S) change and become crescent-shaped with the following conditions: low oxygen tension, dehydration, and acidosis.

II. Etiology

A. Sickle cell anemia is inherited by an autosomal recessive pattern. The abnormality occurs in the globin portion of the hemoglobin. The hemoglobins (Hb) are identified by letters. Hb A denotes *normal adult hemoglobin,* Hb AS refers to *sickle cell trait* (carrier state of one normal hemoglobin gene and one sickle hemoglobin gene), and Hb SS designates *sickle cell anemia.* Those with SCD have parents who both have the trait. It is one of the most common genetic disorders affecting persons of African descent. The gene is also found in ethnic groups from sections of Turkey, the Middle East, India, the Mediterranean, and the Caribbean. Those with Hb AS demonstrate a mutation with the ability to resist malarial parasites.

   B. In the United States, 8% of African-Americans are carriers of the sickle cell trait, and 1 in 500 manifests the disease (NIH, 2005).
   C. Most states now perform newborn screening for sickle cell anemia with Hb electrophoresis (Robertson and Shilkofski, 2005).

III. Characteristics
   A. Around 5 or 6 months of age, other clinical manifestations may be observed.
   B. Dactylitis occurs; it is characterized by painful, nonpitting edema of hands and feet and is often accompanied by a fever as high as 103° F (39.4° C); it most frequently occurs from 6 months to 4 years of age.
   C. Enlarged spleen in early childhood because of its function in removing sickle cells from circulation; functional activity is generally lost during first few years of life.
   D. From approximately 6 to 8 years, spleen decreases in size from repeated infarcts and is replaced by fibrous mass.
   E. Splenic sequestration crisis, a sudden pooling of blood in the spleen, generally occurs between 4 months and 3 years of age.
   F. Bacterial infections from functional asplenia are a major cause of death in all age groups. Infective organisms: *Haemophilus influenzae, Streptococcus pneumoniae,* and *Neisseria meningitis.*
   G. Aplastic anemia crisis, which is caused by a decrease in RBC production secondary to an infection.
   H. Painful vasoocclusive crisis, in which sickle cells obstruct blood vessels: causes occlusion, ischemia, and possible necrosis, and can potentially affect every organ. In older children, there is pain and tenderness in bones, back, and joints of extremities from infarctions.
   I. Central nervous system (CNS) infarction or stroke may appear at any age and can cause paralysis or death.
   J. In middle childhood, a zinc deficiency may contribute to underweight and delayed puberty.
   K. Older children may have cardiomegaly, symptomatic gallstone formation, and damage of the liver, pancreas, and heart from the increased iron absorption.
   L. Skeletal problems include osteoporosis, skeletal deformities, and osteomyelitis.
   M. Other possible clinical manifestations are growth retardation, underweight, delayed sexual maturation, frontal protuberance, retinopathy, sensorineural hearing loss, priapism (abnormal, constant, painful penile erection), urinary retention, leg ulcers, and renal complications.

IV. Health Concerns/Emergencies
   A. Young children with fever, nonproductive cough, pain, or respiratory distress may have acute chest syndrome (ACS), a life-threatening

pulmonary complication. ACS is the second most common condition requiring hospitalization.

B. Aphasia, seizures, visual disturbances, headache, or any other neurologic symptoms may indicate cerebral insult.

C. Hematuria, enuresis, and dilute urine indicate kidney ischemia.

D. Spleen sequestration often follows an acute febrile illness, requiring immediate hospitalization. It is one of the most life-threatening complications and is responsible for the highest incidence of death in the young child; symptoms of fever, headache, and nausea may be present.

E. Eleven percent of children have strokes that can lead to lifelong disabilities. The highest risk is between 2 and 5 years of age.

F. Routine blood transfusions seem to decrease the risk for a stroke, based on research using brain ultrasound data. Transfusions pose another risk by increasing iron in the body, which can damage the heart and other vital organs, unless steps are taken to reduce iron levels.

V. Effects on Individual

A. The toddler may interpret pain as punishment.

B. Misses school frequently; grades, along with motivation, may drop. Pain may interfere with concentration.

C. Child may not want to spend the night at a friend's house, because bed wetting is common in some children with sickle cell anemia. Using Depends or similar diapering product may be a solution if done in privacy.

D. May be teased because of short stature.

E. Tires easily.

F. Teenager often matures later than peers, making physical appearance a concern.

G. Disfigurement, jaundice, surgical scars, and dental deformities may cause embarrassment.

H. With good treatment and supportive counseling, individual can lead a full and productive life.

I. Life expectancy is increasing with new and innovative treatments.

VI. Management/Treatment

A. Treatment is symptomatic and supportive; there is no cure.

B. Febrile infants with SCD should be seen immediately because of risk of bacterial and subsequent secondary infection.

C. Daily antibiotic (penicillin) treatment beginning at 2 months and continuing to age 5 or 6 can reduce serious infections by about 85%.

D. Review for or vaccinate with H. influenzae type B (HIB) vaccine at age 2 months to protect against life-threatening bacterial infections. Other vaccinations that prevent respiratory complications are advised (National Institutes of Health [NIH], 2002).

E. Encourage fluid intake because of need to maintain hemodilution; dehydration increases the sickling process; 150 ml/kg/day (Nettina, 2006).

F. Discuss extreme necessity of wearing medical alert identification.

G. Routine visual screening up to age 10 and annual retinal examination for sickle retinopathy thereafter. Referral to ophthalmologist in the event of any eye trauma.

CHAPTER 4

Chronic Conditions

H. Routine audiological assessments, because individual is at high risk for sensorineural hearing loss in the high-frequency range due to reduced circulation in the inner ear (vasoocclusive episodes).

I. Scoliosis screening should be done according to individual's delayed maturational level.

J. Educate teachers and other school staff regarding basic concerns during school day, field trips, sports, and other physical activities; have water available for hydration; avoid temperature extremes, stress, overexertion, and fatigue.

K. Be aware of symptoms that require urgent medical care: fever, shortness of breath, chest pain, progressive fatigue, atypical headache, abrupt visual changes, sudden loss of sensation or weakness, unrelieved pain, priapism, and abdominal distention.

L. Do not use ice on any injury; the extreme temperature change can cause localized sickling.

M. Discourage adolescent smoking, which increases vasoconstriction.

VII. Additional Information

A. Prenatal diagnosis for known carriers of hemoglobinopathies is available by chorionic villi sampling (CVS) during the first trimester. Amniocentesis can be done in the second trimester. A simple hemoglobin electrophoresis test can determine if someone is a carrier of the sickle cell trait.

B. If both parents possess the trait, there is a 25% chance that a child will have Hb S. There is also a 25% chance that the child will have neither the trait nor the disease, and there is a 50% chance that the child will have the trait, like both the parents, but not the disease.

C. The drug hydroxyurea reduces the number of pain crises in about 50% of severely affected adults and is also being used in children (NIH, 2002). Bone marrow transplant has been successful in some severely affected children, whereas about 5% to 8% with severe hemoglobin disorders die. Hematopoietic stem cell transplantation has been successful in curing many children. Gene therapy approaches continue to be researched.

D. Vasoocclusive episodes are caused by sickling that is precipitated by a variety of factors (e.g., weather changes, stress, menstruation). A physiological process causes the accompanying pain and is associated with a psychosocial component based on the individual's tolerance and reaction to pain and family beliefs and interpretations.

WEB SITES

American Sickle Cell Anemia Association
http://www.ascaa.org
Sickle Cell Disease Association of America (SCDAA)
http://www.sicklecelldisease.org

JUVENILE ARTHRITIS

I. Definition

A. Juvenile arthritis (JA) is an inflammatory disease of children. There are three main forms of the disease: (1) monoarticular (involving one joint) or pauciarticular (involving four or fewer joints), (2) polyarticular (involving five or more joints), and (3) Still's disease (systemic onset). JA diagnosis is given when onset is before age 16, and duration lasts longer than 6 weeks without other known cause. The term juvenile arthritis is becoming popular to distinguish more clearly between JA and adult rheumatoid arthritis. JA was previously known as Juvenile Rheumatoid Arthritis (JRA) but JRA applies to a small percentage of children. The newer, broader term is Juvenile Idiopathic Arthritis (JIA).

II. Etiology

A. The cause of JA is unknown; present theories include infections, autoimmunity, and genetic predisposition. Approximately 1 in 1000 children has JA (Haftel, 2006).

III. Characteristics

A. General characteristics:
   1. Two peak ages of onset: 1 to 3 years and 8 to 12 years
   2. More prevalent in girls.
   3. Probable duration of disease, degree of disability, and eventual functional ability are based on onset, type, extent of joint involvement, and extent of systemic involvement. Long-term prognosis is good; about 75% enter long remissions without significant impairment.
   4. Early in the disease process, a child may exhibit irritability, fatigue, poor appetite, poor weight gain, growth delay, early morning joint stiffness, and walking with knees flexed to protect inflamed joints and avoid pain.
   5. Most common handicapping complications are hip disease or loss of vision because of iridocyclitis (inflammation of iris and ciliary body).

B. Three types of JA:
   1. *Monoarticular and pauciarticular arthritis:*
      a. Involves approximately 50% of children with JA.
      b. Mildest form and best prognosis regarding long term joint disability.
      c. Involves four or fewer joints.
      d. May be accompanied by mild rash, low-grade fever, and other systemic involvement.
      e. Commonly seen in ankle, wrist, hip, cervical spine, and proximal interphalangeal joints, but knee joint is most commonly involved.
      f. May not complain of pain; however, can be listless and have difficulty getting up in the morning.
      g. Chronic iridocyclitis is a common serious systemic complication that may precede arthritis by several years and is usually asymptomatic. Also called *uveitis* and *iritis*.
   2. *Polyarticular arthritis:*
      a. Occurs in approximately 40% of children with JA.
      b. Similar to adult variety.
      c. Seen at any age, but there is a peak in early childhood and again in adolescence with a positive rheumatoid factor.
      d. May exhibit low-grade fever, listlessness, and anorexia.
      e. Multiple joint involvement, and the form most likely to cause deformity.

CHAPTER 4

Chronic Conditions

    f. Joint symptoms may occur abruptly, with several joints swollen and painful.

    g. Involvement of joints is usually symmetrical.

    h. High incidence of involvement of temporomandibular joint (TMJ), causing a receding chin; also involves hips, wrist carpal bones, and cervical spine.

    i. Finger and toe joints become inflamed, swollen, and develop spindlelike shape.

    j. Ankylosis, immobility, and fixation of joints or cervical spine.

    k. Can cause growth retardation.

    l. Likely to persist into adulthood.

  3. *Systemic-onset juvenile arthritis:*

    a. Occurs in about 10% of children with JA.

    b. Onset usually before age 5; at highest risk for long-term disability.

    c. Temperature spikes once or twice daily and subsides without treatment.

    d. Salmon-colored macular rash frequently comes and goes with fever or may be brought on by hot shower or trauma; appears over trunk or extremities and is nonpruritic.

    e. Joint symptoms generally do not appear for several weeks or months and at first are only subjective; warmth, swelling, and tenderness may be observed later.

    f. Other symptoms are:

      (1) Splenomegaly (70%) and hepatic enlargement.

      (2) Lymphadenopathy.

      (3) Pericarditis and pleuritis.

      (4) Elevated white blood count is common.

IV. Health Concerns/Emergencies

  A. School staff should be aware that a student with JA may have pain or discomfort.

  B. Work with staff to accommodate student's inability to be punctual because of morning stiffness and pain; allow rest time at school, and have extra sets of text books available, because heavy loads can increase pain. May need shortened day to decrease fatigue.

  C. Promote independence in activities of daily living whenever possible, and make adaptive devices available (e.g., railing in bathrooms, elevated commodes).

  D. Monitor weight; decreased physical activity may lead to excessive weight gain, causing increased strain on inflamed joints of lower extremities; may be secondary to decreased physical activity. Weight loss can indicate arthritis of TMJ, which causes pain while chewing, malnutrition, poor disease management, and anorexia.

  E. Discuss interactions of oral contraceptives with medications, effects of arthritis medications on fetal development, and delayed sexual maturation.

  F. Encourage good oral hygiene.

V. Effects on Individual

  A. Pain and physical limitations may interfere with daily activities and self-care and may contribute to weight gain.

B. Academic performance can suffer from frequent absences from school or inability to concentrate because of discomfort.
C. There may be social isolation from inability to participate in many activities with peers or failure of peers to accept the child who is "different."
D. May be irritable and demanding and feel angry and resentful.
E. May be embarrassed because of deformities.
F. May be anxious and concerned regarding the future and career options.
G. May constantly depend on others if limitations prevent the child from doing even simple tasks, such as turning on a faucet, opening a door, or cutting meat.
H. Difficulty in maneuvering steps can make the use of public transportation difficult.
I. Susceptible to increased dental caries secondary to painful TMJ and poor oral hygiene because of limited use of upper extremities.

VI. Management/Treatment
A. At risk for chronic iridocyclitis, also called *uveitis* or *iritis*. Presence of positive antinuclear antibody (ANA) indicates child—girls especially—at high risk for chronic uveitis, which is the primary treatable cause of blindness in children (Haftel, 2006). Sometimes asymptomatic, but can be detected by a special slit-lamp examination. Need annual ophthalmologic exam.
B. Three major management goals:
   1. Prevent deformities.
   2. Preserve joint function.
   3. Relieve symptoms without iatrogenic complications.
C. Consult with physical therapist regarding classroom activities, exercises, and positioning that might help preserve function and prevent deformities.
D. Occupational therapists provide information and design therapy for fine motor movements, ADLs, and when TMJ is involved.
E. Periods of rest may be necessary to avoid excessive fatigue.
F. Splints, braces, and casts are used to immobilize the joints in a neutral position and prevent contractures. Passive, active, and resistive exercises are a daily routine to maintain range of motion and muscle strength. Swimming is an excellent activity.
G. Unconventional therapies introduced by family may interfere with prescribed medical treatment, such as dietary regimens and supplements.
H. Use of surgery is limited but may be performed to relieve pain, correct deformities, or restore range of motion (e.g., soft tissue releases, tendon lengthening, and joint replacements).
I. Medication:
   1. Make provisions for prescribed medication to be administered while student is at school.
   2. The primary drugs for alleviating pain and inhibiting inflammation are nonsteroidal antiinflammatory drugs (NSAIDs), which include naproxen (Naprosyn), tolmetin (Tolectin), indomethacin (Indocin), and ibuprofen (Advil or Motrin). May take up to 8 to 12 weeks to observe improvement. Most common side effect for

CHAPTER 4

Chronic Conditions

this group of medications is GI irritation, which may be avoided if NSAIDs are taken with food. Other side effects that may interfere with school include dizziness, headache, and drowsiness.

3. Second-line drugs include disease modifying antiinflammatory drugs (DMARDS), which include gold compound (Solganal), penicillamina (DePen), and hydroxychloroquine (Plaquenil). These are added to the medication schedule when NSAIDs are not effective.

4. Corticosteroids are very strong antiinflammatory drugs used when life-threatening events occur (e.g., pericarditis), when systemic disease does not respond to NSAIDs, and for iridocyclitis.

5. Cytotoxic drugs are prescribed for severe debilitating disease and those not responding to NSAIDs or DMARDS. These are antineoplastics or immunosuppressants, such as cyclophosphamide (Cytoxan) and azathioprine (Imuran).

6. Salicylates are seldom used, since frequent, large doses may have adverse effects that include bleeding, acute gastritis, hyperventilation (from acidosis), drowsiness, tinnitus, and Reye syndrome.

VII. Additional Information

A. The arthritic process (Figure 4-1) begins with inflammation of the synovial membrane (synovitis) and joint capsule, which increases

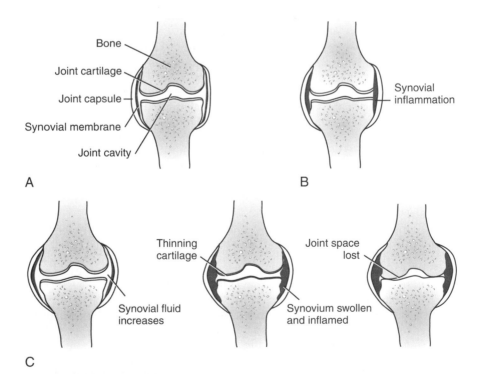

FIGURE 4-1 Juvenile arthritic process. **A,** Normal synovial joint. **B,** Early-stage synovitis. **C,** Chronic synovitis leading to joint destruction.

fluid in the joint (joint effusion), making it feel swollen and boggy. Chronic synovitis may lead to erosion of joint structure and loss of joint space. Immobilization of the joints (ankylosis), bone deformity, and subluxation (partial dislocation) occur over time. These inflammation processes can extend to other systems, causing pericarditis, pneumonia, uveitis, or organomegaly.

B. JA may last as little as several months to a year or may go away indefinitely. Most children have exacerbations and remissions for many years, but the exacerbations tend to diminish over time.

C. Remission is defined as being symptom-free for 6 months after stopping medication. Inflammation has a unique effect on the growing child. Severe arthritis can slow growth (e.g., knee inflammation may inhibit growth compared with an uninflamed knee). May resume normal growth patterns when arthritis is in remission. If the premature epiphyseal fusion has not occurred, the normal height curve will resume within 2 to 3 years.

WEB SITES

Arthritis Foundation
    http://www.arthritis.org
American College of Rheumatology
    http://www.rheumatology.org

ASTHMA

I. Definition
A. Asthma is a chronic inflammatory disorder of the airways characterized by airflow obstruction, which is usually reversible either spontaneously or by treatment, and bronchial hyperresponsiveness to a variety of stimuli.

II. Etiology
A. The inherited tendency to develop an immunoglobulin E (IgE) mediated response to allergens, known as *atopy,* is the strongest predisposing factor for developing asthma. Environmental causes include viruses, allergens, or anything that irritates and impacts the respiratory tract. Respiratory syncytial virus (RSV) is one of the viral infections, and exposure early in life can increase the risk of developing asthma. The allergic triggers are generally those carried in the air, such as plant pollens, molds, animal dander, and dust mites. In some instances, no allergic process can be detected. Secondhand smoke, an irritant, can trigger asthma attacks and increase severity of an episode. It is more of a concern in younger children due to their rapid breathing rate. Asthma is a complex disorder in which biochemical, immunological, endocrine, infectious, and psychological factors are involved to varying degrees in different people.

B. In the United States in 2005, 6.5 million children under the age of 18 had asthma, suggesting around 9% of children were affected (CDC, 2006a). Asthma is the number one cause of school absenteeism and is responsible for 12.8 million days of school missed in

2003. It is the most prevalent cause of chronic illness and a leading cause of pediatric hospital admissions (Hall and DeFrances, 2003).

C. Asthma is more common in African-Americans. At a ratio of 2:1, it is more common in boys until adolescence. After puberty prevalence is higher in girls. Childhood asthma is not usually outgrown. Adolescents or young adults may experience relief, but symptoms usually return later.

III. Characteristics

A. Diagnosis generally occurs between 3 and 8 years of age, and many have symptoms during the first year of life; however, approximately 80% of children with asthma develop symptoms before age 5 (Bloom, Dey, and Freeman, 2006).

B. Diagnosis is based on individual's health history; family history of asthma, allergy, rhinitis, or sinusitis; spirometry and challenge tests (e.g., histamine, methacholine, cold air); as well as response to appropriate therapy.

C. Diagnostic symptoms include:
1. Cough, more common at night.
2. Cough with exercise, laughing, or crying; wheezing may not be present.
3. Wheeze with prolonged expiratory phase.
4. Shortness of breath.
5. Chest tightness.
6. Symptoms worsen with precipitating factors, especially viral respiratory infections.

D. Precipitating factors:
1. Plant pollens, molds, dust mites, cockroach droppings, animal dander or secretory products, and air pollutants, especially secondhand smoke.
2. Viral respiratory infections and weather changes (e.g., excessively cold, wet, or humid conditions).
3. Physical exercise or strong emotional expressions (e.g., fear, frustration, or hard laughing or crying).
4. Medications (e.g., aspirin, NSAIDs, β-blockers, eye drops); sensitivity increases with age and severity of asthma; aspirin is in many over-the-counter (OTC) medications, including Pepto-Bismol; these drugs may precipitate a severe or fatal exacerbation in a small percentage of people.
5. Foods, additives, and preservatives.
6. Endocrine changes (e.g., menses, pregnancy, thyroid disorders).

E. Prodromal signs:
1. Cough is usually the first sign.
2. Wheezing, shortness of breath, and increasing respiratory difficulty.
3. Tightness in chest, irritability, restlessness, and anxiety.

F. Exacerbations are caused by edema or inflammation in the bronchial wall and constriction of the small and large airways in the lungs, which results from bronchial smooth muscle spasm and excessive production of mucus.

G. Children younger than age 5 may experience more airway obstruction than do older children, perhaps because they have smaller airways.

H. Often associated with gastroesophageal reflux disease (GERD).
I. Most children with asthma have allergies in the form of rhinitis or atopic dermatitis (Liu, Spahn and Leung, 2004).
J. *Mild intermittent* asthma is treated with a bronchodilator as needed and does not require daily medication. A child who usually meets the criteria for mild intermittent asthma may have exacerbations during a cold that increase the requirement for rescue medication. The illness may actually require a daily medication for a short period because of the possibility of damage and the ongoing repair process associated with chronic inflammation that could lead to permanent airway damage, called *remodeling,* which is not responsive to treatment.
K. *Mild, moderate,* and *severe persistent asthma* are treated with daily preventive and acute inflammation treatments. Use of inhaled corticosteroids is frequently the recommended treatment (see Box 4-1).

Box 4-1	*Classifications of Asthma*

Individuals at any level can experience mild, moderate, or severe exacerbations.

Mild Intermittent Asthma
1. Symptoms no more than twice a week.
2. Responds to bronchodilator treatment.
3. Does not require daily medication for control.
4. Exacerbations brief, from a few hours to a few days; may vary in intensity.
5. Asymptomatic and normal peak expiratory flow rate (PEFR) between exacerbations.
6. Little interruption of school attendance.
7. Nighttime symptoms no more than twice a month.
8. PEFR no less than 80% of predicted value; PEFR less than 20% variability.

Mild Persistent Asthma
1. Symptoms more than twice a week but less than once a day.
2. Exacerbations may affect level of activity.
3. Nighttime symptoms more than twice a month but less than once a week.
4. PEFR no less than 80% of predicted value; PEFR variability 20% to 30%.

Moderate Persistent Asthma
1. Daily symptoms.
2. Daily treatment with inhaled short-acting β_2-agonist.
3. School attendance and exercise tolerance affected.
4. Exacerbations at least twice a week and may last for days.
5. Nighttime symptoms more than once a week.
6. Coughing and wheezing disrupt normal activities and make it difficult to sleep.
7. PEFR 60% to 80% predicted; PEFR variability greater than 30%.

Severe Persistent Asthma
1. Continual symptoms.
2. Frequent exacerbations.
3. Limited physical activity.
4. Frequent nighttime symptoms, disrupting sleep.
5. Occasional hospitalization may be needed to bring symptoms under control.
6. PEFR 60% predicted or less; PEFR variability greater than 30%.

Modified from the National Asthma Education and Prevention Program: *Expert panel report 2: guidelines for the diagnosis and management of asthma* (NIH Pub No 97-4051), Bethesda, Md, 1997, National Heart, Lung, and Blood Institute.

IV. Health Concerns/Emergencies
A. *Status asthmaticus,* a long lasting or severe asthma episode that does not respond to treatment, can lead to respiratory failure and death.
B. Acute, prolonged asthmatic attack may result in reduced oxygenation. Symptoms of status asthmaticus include restlessness, increased anxiety, and heavy sweating.
C. Silent chest may indicate severe spasm or obstruction with no movement of air and therefore no breath sounds; this condition requires immediate emergency treatment.
D. Emergency symptoms:
1. Difficulty walking or talking (e.g., unable to speak in complete sentences, using phrases or single words).
2. Hunched over (tripod position to allow expansion of diaphragm), struggling to breathe.
3. Sternal or intercostal retractions.
4. Perioral or nail bed cyanosis are both extremely serious signs that indicate impending respiratory arrest.
5. Treat according to individual's emergency (rescue) plan.

V. Effects on Individual
A. The longer the asthma attack, the greater the anxiety.
B. May feel isolated, and academic studies may suffer because of school absenteeism.
C. May be self-conscious about need for medication or monitoring, and may avoid going to health office for assessment or treatment. Some students may carry their own medications.
D. May use asthma as an excuse to avoid activities.
E. May experience delay in puberty and growth because of disease and corticosteroid use; maximal height usually possible through appropriate disease management.
F. May be negatively affected by the impact this chronic illness has on family routines, economic resources, activities, and dynamics.
G. Increasing control of the treatment plan and self-management by the student, especially in adolescence, improves compliance, diminishes exacerbation, and promotes self-empowerment.

VI. Management/Treatment
A. Individualized Health Care Plan (IHCP).
1. Perform initial health assessment (see Box 4-2).
2. Develop IHCP in consultation with parents and HCP; student should have written plans for both school and home care.
a. Prescriptions for daily, rescue, and prn medications signed by parent and HCP.
b. Peak expiratory flow rate (PEFR) monitoring instructions.
c. Emergency contacts and plan.
d. Guidelines for activities.
e. Factors that increase asthma symptoms.
f. Back-up inhaler at school for students who carry rescue inhalers.
B. 504 Accommodation Plan
1. Student may need 504 plan developed to attain success in school (see Special Education, Chapter 9).

| Box 4-2 | *Sample Questions for the Initial Assessment of Asthma* |

A "yes" answer to any question* suggests that an asthma condition is likely.

In the past 12 months:

1. Have you had a sudden severe episode or recurrent episodes of coughing, wheezing (high-pitched whistling sounds when breathing out), or shortness of breath?
2. Have you had colds that "go to the chest" or take more than 10 days to get over?
3. Have you had coughing, wheezing, or shortness of breath during a particular season or time of the year?
4. Have you had coughing, wheezing, or shortness of breath in certain places or when exposed to certain things (e.g., animals, tobacco smoke, perfumes)?
5. Have you used any medications to help you breathe better? How often?
6. Are your symptoms relieved when the medications are used?

In the past 4 weeks, have you had coughing, wheezing, or shortness of breath:

1. At night that has awakened you?
2. In the early morning?
3. After running, moderate exercise, or other physical activity?

From the National Asthma Education and Prevention Program: *Expert panel report 2: guidelines for the diagnosis and management of asthma* (NIH Pub No 97-4051), Bethesda, Md, 1997, National Heart, Lung, and Blood Institute.
*These are suggested questions for student interviews.

NOTE: Most states have laws allowing students to carry medication for asthma and anaphylaxis. Self-administration of medication is allowed when determined appropriate by school nurse, parent, and HCP, and management procedures are in place when necessary. Be knowledgeable about the Nurse Practice Act and state and school district policies and guidelines. The National Association of School Nurses (NASN) has a position statement on asthma.

    C. Prevention of exercise-induced bronchospasm (EIB).

        1. Do breathing exercises and physical training to strengthen respiratory muscles, improve breathing patterns, prevent overinflation, improve cough for clearing the airway, and provide physical and mental relaxation.

        2. Take preventive medication before exercise as prescribed.

        3. Use combination of two to three drugs if a single medication is ineffective.

        4. Do warm-up exercises.

        5. Use a scarf, muffler, or cold-weather mask to warm and humidify air as needed.

        6. Pace exercise.

        7. Maintain adequate hydration by taking in adequate fluids.

    D. Monitoring.

        1. Use a daily check-off list of factors: respiratory status, medications used, PEFR, adherence to treatment plan, inhaler technique, amount of prn medications needed, side effects of medications, and sleep disturbances. Provide verification of effective protocol or need for change and monitor growth, especially when on long-term inhaled steroids. Avoid obesity; kids usually experience catch-up growth. (see Table 4-1 and Table 4-2).

CHAPTER 4

Chronic Conditions

Table 4-1   Key Points Regarding Asthma Management Medications

Medication Category	Indications/Actions Per Drug Category	*Potential Side Effects Per Drug Category	Comments Per Drug Category
Corticosteroids (Inhaled) *Beclomethasone* (Beclovent, QVAR, Vanceril) *Budesonide* (Pulmicort) *Flunisolide* (AeroBid) *Fluticasone* (Flovent) *Mometasone furonte* (Asmanex Twisthaler) *Triamcinolone* (Azmacort) *Fluticasone with salmeterol* (Advair) Dosing varies by product and delivery device; usually given bid.	**Indications:** Long-term prevention of symptoms; suppression, control, reversal of inflammation. Decrease need for oral corticosteroid. **Actions:** Antiinflammatory, reduce airway hyperresponsiveness. Inhibit late-phase allergic reaction. Improve PEFR. Prevent exacerbations. May prevent airway remodeling.	Upper respiratory infections, hoarseness, dry mouth, oral thrush. In high doses, systemic effects may occur (e.g., osteoporosis, growth suppression, adrenal suppression, skin thinning, easy bruising). Compare risks of uncontrolled asthma against adverse affects of drugs; potential but small risk of adverse events is well balanced by drug efficacy.	Spacer or holding chamber devices: rinsing mouth or gargling after inhalation decreases oral side effects and systemic absorption. Preparations are not entirely equivalent on puff or µg basis; new delivery systems may be even more efficient. Inhaled corticosteroids are most potent antiinflammatory drugs presently available. *FDA Warning:* Advair Diskus (salmeterol component) may increase risk of asthma-related deaths.
Corticosteroids (Systemic) *Methylprednisolone* (Medrol, Duralone, Methpred) *Prednisolone* (A-Delta-Cortef, Prelone, Pediapred) *Prednisone* (Orasone, Meticorten, Deltasone)	**Indications:** Short term "burst" (3-10 days) for prompt control. To gain prompt control of inadequately controlled, persistent asthma.	**Short-term use:** depression, mood swings, hypertension, diarrhea, nausea, abdominal distension, blurred vision, skin rash, headache, flushing, sweating, mood changes, increased appetite, fluid retention, hypertension, peptic ulcer, delayed wound healing.	Give at lowest effective dose. Give with food or milk to reduce GI symptoms. Consideration should be given to conditions that could be exacerbated by systemic corticosteroids (e.g., herpes virus infections, varicella, tuberculosis). Avoid live attenuated vaccinations while on steroids.

Alternate-day A.M. dosing produces least toxicity when needed for long-term therapy. If daily dosing is needed, 3 P.M. is more efficacious than A.M. dose

Long-term use: in severe persistent asthma to suppress, control, and reverse inflammation.
Actions: Antiinflammatory; reduce airway hyperresponsiveness.
Inhibit late-phase allergic reaction.
Improve PEFR.
Prevent exacerbation.
May prevent airway remodeling.

Long-term use: acne, osteoporosis, growth suppression, Cushing syndrome, cataracts, hypothalamic-pituitary-adrenal suppression, hypertension, diabetes, muscle wasting, impaired immune function (rarely)

Long term use: carry emergency ID as steroid user.
Do not discontinue abruptly.
Avoid OTC products with alcohol or salicylates.

Mast Cell Stabilizers:
Cromolyn (Intal)
Nedocromil (Tilade)
Usual dosing is qid; nedocromil has been effective on bid schedule.

Indications: Long-term prevention of symptoms; may modify inflammation.
Use before exercise or exposure to known allergen.
Severe perennial bronchial asthma.
Actions: Antiinflammatory; inhibits early and late-phase reaction to allergens; inhibits acute response to exercise, cold dry air, and sulfur dioxide.

May have coughing with DPIs; using MDI or nebulizer may prevent cough.
Occasionally unpleasant taste.

Therapeutic response to cromolyn and nedocromil often occurs within 2 wk, but 4-6 wk period may be needed to measure maximum benefits.
MDI cromolyn (1 mg/puff) may be inadequate, may need nebulizer delivery (20 mg/amp).
Clinical response is less predictable than response to inhaled corticosteroids.
Safety is primary advantage.

Continued

Chronic Conditions

CHAPTER 4

Table 4-1 *Key Points Regarding Asthma Management Medications—cont'd*

Medication Category	Indications/Actions Per Drug Category	*Potential Side Effects Per Drug Category	Comments Per Drug Category
Long-Acting β₂-Agonists Inhaled: *Salmeterol* (Serevent Diskus) *Formoterol* (Foradil Aerolizer) Usual dosing: bid 12 hr apart.	**Indications:** Long-term prevention of symptoms, especially nocturnal; used as adjunct to antiinflammatory therapy. Prevention of EIB: Inhaled, use 15 min before exercise. Not to be used to treat acute symptoms or exacerbations. **Actions:** Bronchodilation, relaxes smooth muscles; effects last at least 12 hr.	Tachycardia, skeletal muscle tremors, anxiety, headache, hypokalemia, nausea, and vomiting. May have diminished bronchoprotective effect within 1 wk of chronic therapy, and clinical studies have demonstrated development of tolerance. Inhaled long-acting β₂-agonists are longer acting and have fewer side effects than the tablets.	Correct use of inhaler is essential. FDA warning: Foradil Aeolizer and Serevent Diskus may increase risk of severe asthma episodes and possible death. Inhaled meds: rinse mouth after using inhaled cortico teroids. Should not be used in place of antiinflammatory therapy. Remind not to stop antiinflammatory therapy even though symptoms may improve significantly. Not for acute symptoms or exacerbations. Avoid excessive use of caffeine in colas, chocolate, coffee, and tea. Keep canister at room temperature; cold decreases potency.
Methylxanthines *Theophylline* (Slo-Bid, Theo-Dur, Theolair, Uniphyl) Usual dosing is 2-4 times/day at 6-12 hr intervals.	**Indications:** Long-term control and prevention of symptoms, especially at night. Used when not responding to inhaled medications. **Actions:** Bronchodilation, smooth muscle relaxation.	Effects at therapeutic dose include insomnia, increase of hyperactivity in some children, gastric upset, aggravation of ulcer or reflux. Dose-related acute toxicities include tachycardia, dysrhythmias, nausea and vomiting, irritability, seizures, CNS stimulation, headaches, hematemesis, hyperglycemia, hypokalemia.	Routine serum concentration monitoring essential because of significant toxicities, narrow therapeutic range, and individual differences in metabolic clearance. Maintain serum concentration between 5 and 15 μg/mL. Not generally recommended for exacerbations. Take with 8 oz water. Avoid taking with food. Ephedrine in OTC products or medications will increase stimulation.

Oral Leukotriene Modifiers

Montelukast (Singulair)
Usual dosing: 1 tablet or granule packet in evening.

Zileuton (Zyflo Filmtab)
Usual dosing: 1 tablet qid.

Zafirlukast (Accolate)
Usual dosing: 1 tablet bid.

Indications: Long-term control and prevention of symptoms in mild persistent asthma for age 12 and above.

Actions: Inhibits the enzyme responsible for producing inflammatory leukotriene products, which induce bronchoconstrictor response, enhance vascular permeability, and stimulate mucus secretion. Mildly anti-inflammatory.

Headache, nausea, diarrhea
Increased risk of URI when used with inhaled corticosteroids.
Zileuton: Elevation of liver enzymes; limited reports of reversible hepatitis and hyperbilirubinemia.

Singulair: May take with food.
Accolate: Take one hour before meals or 2 hours after meals.
Do not crush or break tablets.
Coadministration with warfarin increases PT; monitor PT.

* Potential side effects are typical for the medication category; please consult the PDR or other reference for specific profile of each medication. *DPI*, Dry powder inhalation; *MDI*, metered dose inhaler; *PT*, prothrombin time; *URI*, upper respiratory infection; *PEFR*, peak expiratory flow rate; *EIB*, exercise-induced bronchospasm; *bid*, twice a day.

Chronic Conditions

CHAPTER 4

Table 4-2 *Key Points for Asthma Rescue Medications*

Medication Category	Indications/Actions Per Drug Category	*Potential Side Effects Per Drug Category	Comments Per Drug Category
Short-Acting Inhaled β₂-Agonists *Albuterol* (Proventil, Ventolin, Airet, AccuNeb) *Terbutaline* (Bricanyl, Brethine) *Levalbuterol* (Xopenex) *Pibuterol* (Maxair) Usual dosing for EIB: 1-2 puffs before exercise; for symptoms: 2 puffs tid or qid as needed.	**Indications:** Acts within 30 min, relief of acute symptoms. Preventive treatment for EIB. **Actions:** *Bronchodilation,* relax bronchial smooth muscle, increase vital capacity, decrease airway resistance. Increasing use or lack of expected effect indicates inadequate asthma control. Use of more than one canister/mo may indicate overreliance on this drug.	Tachycardia, tremors, hypokalemia, headache, hyperglycemia, nausea, nervousness, weakness, insomnia, increased BP. Inhaled route generally causes few systemic adverse effects. More than two canisters/mo poses risk of adverse side effects.	Drugs of choice for acute bronchospasm; faster and more effective than systemic route. Regularly scheduled daily use not recommended; does not provide better control than prn. *Isoproterenol* (Isuprel), *metaproterenol* (Alupent), *isoetharine* (Bronkosol), and *epinephrine* (Adrenalin) are not recommended
Anticholinergics *Ipratropium* (Atrovent) Usual dosing: MDI 1-2 puffs qid; nebulizer 1-unit dose qid. Combination of *albuterol* and *anticholenergic* (DuoNeb, Combivent)	**Indications:** Relief of acute bronchospasm (see Comments). **Actions:** *Bronchodilation,* competitive inhibition of muscarinic cholinergic receptors; may decrease mucus gland secretion.	Dry mouth and decreased respiratory secretions, increased wheezing in some individuals, blurred vision if sprayed in eyes. Does not have atropine's side effects. Combination treatments: Side effects same as for the individual drugs.	Reverses only cholinergically mediated bronchospasm; does *not* block EIB; does *not* modify reaction to antigen. May provide additive effect to β₂-agonist but has slower onset of action. Alternative for those with intolerance for β₂-agonists.

* Potential side effects are typical for the medication category; please consult the PDR or other reference for specific profile of each medication.
BP, Blood pressure; *MDI,* metered dose inhaler; *prn,* as required; *qid,* four times a day; *tid,* three times a day.

    2. Screen for glaucoma or cataracts when on daily high-dose systemic corticosteroids; otherwise, routine vision screening is acceptable.

E. General.

    1. Controlled breathing, including pursed lips with expiration, may calm a student in respiratory distress, but it does not improve lung function.

    2. Annual influenza vaccine is recommended.

    3. Avoid cough suppressants, which mask symptoms.

    4. Consider allergen immunotherapy when individual is sensitive, unable to avoid allergens, medications are not controlling symptoms, and reactions are noted most of the year.

F. Training: Educate teachers, coaches, bus drivers, and other school staff regarding:

    1. Basic facts about asthma.

    2. Awareness of animal allergies; do not allow those animals in classroom.

    3. Signs and symptoms of respiratory distress.

    4. Treatment of acute asthmatic episode and correct use of devices (e.g., metered-dose and dry-powder inhalers, nebulizers, space holding chambers).

    5. Medications for use before exercise or exposure to known irritants.

    6. Ways to minimize exposure to triggers and techniques to prevent EIB (e.g., warm-up period).

    7. Individual's treatment plan with all phone numbers.

    8. When to call parents, HCP, or 911.

VII. Additional Information

A. Pregnancy poses risks for the asthmatic, and good asthma control is needed to avoid perinatal mortality, premature delivery, and low birth weight. Most of the medications used for asthma pose little risk to the fetus. Pregnant women generally use Sudafed and antitussives, which are typically not problemlematic during pregnancy.

B. Physical activity is generally not limited; there are Olympic medalists who are asthmatics, including 40 gold medal winners. EIB is associated with hyperventilation of cold, dry air. Thus running, ice skating, and cross-country skiing are difficult, but swimming is an excellent exercise, because it builds up lung capacity without compromising the airway.

    1. EIB is caused by pulmonary loss of water and heat when hyperventilation occurs in air that is drier and cooler than the air in the lungs. EIB may be the only symptom of asthma for some students, but the condition should be evaluated to make certain symptoms are under control as much as possible. Symptoms of EIB usually occur during or a few minutes after vigorous exercise; they are generally at their worst 5 to 10 minutes after stopping exercise, and should resolve within a half hour.

C. School environment can aggravate or trigger asthmatic symptoms because of poor air quality, unregulated temperature, pesticide use, animals in the classroom, and excessive humidity or mold. Environment can be evaluated and improved with tools such as the IAQ

Tools for Schools Kit, which is free through the Environmental Protection Agency (EPA): phone 866-837-3721 to order.

D. Peak Expiratory Flow Rate (PEFR).

1. Peak flow monitoring provides:
   a. Means of determining effectiveness of treatment plan.
   b. Early detection of progression in the disease, so changes can be instituted.
   c. Means of identifying triggers.
   d. Method of determining need for emergency care (National Heart, Lung, and Blood Institute [NHLBI], 2007).

2. Personal best PEFR is the highest PEFR obtained over a 2 to 3 week period, when asthma is in control. Baseline reading should be taken 2 to 4 times a day: on awakening, between noon and 2 p.m., and before and after taking a short-acting β_2-agonist, if prescribed. This becomes the reference point for individualized care. Charts for PEFR are available based on height and age; however, estimated normal lung function varies among racial and ethnic groups. Results cannot be applied to all populations, and the individual's personal best PEFR value is the preferred method for monitoring asthma (NHLBI, 1997). The same brand of peak-flow monitor should be used consistently, since various brands can give widely differing values. PEFR measurements depend on the effort and procedure used, so encouragement and frequent review of correct technique is important.

3. Ongoing PEFR is usually taken in the morning soon after waking, before treatments, 5 to 15 minutes after inhaled treatments, and with increased respiratory symptoms (see Table 4-3).

NOTE: Individualized plan indicating rates and actions should be written by the HCP.

Table 4-3   *Peak Flow Interpretation System*

Zone	Peak Expiratory Flow Rate (PEFR): Personal Best or Predicted for Age	Action/Recommendation
Green—All clear	80% or better More than ____L/min	Full activity; may use medication before exercise or exposure to allergens; routine management plan.
Yellow—Caution needed	50%-80% Between ____L/min and ____L/min	May be having acute exacerbation, asthma not well controlled; follow plan supplied by PCP and call if student does not improve.
Red—Medical alert	50% or less Less than ____L/min	Implement rescue plan immediately and call PCP if PEFR does not move to yellow or green zone after rescue medication; prepare for transport as needed.

PCP, Primary care provider.

WEB SITES

National Asthma Education and Prevention Program
http://www.nhlbi.nih.gov/about/naepp
National Heart, Lung, and Blood Institute Information Center
http://www.nhlbi.nih.gov
Allergy and Asthma Network Mothers of Asthmatics
http://www.aanma.org
American Academy of Allergy, Asthma, and Immunology
http://www.aaaai.org
American Lung Association
http://www.lungusa.org
Asthma and Allergy Foundation of America
http://www.aafa.org
U.S. Environmental Protection Agency: Indoor Air Quality
http://www.epa.gov/iaq

CEREBRAL PALSY

I. Definition
   A. Cerebral palsy (CP) is the term used to designate a number of non-progressive disorders of the central nervous system (CNS); it is primarily characterized by impaired muscular control and aberrant movement and posture. The four classifications are *spastic, dyskinetic, ataxic,* and *mixed.*

II. Etiology
   A. CP can be attributed to prenatal, perinatal, and postnatal factors. The three most significant risk factors are low birthweight, intrauterine infection, and multiple births. (Odding, Roebroeck, and Stam, 2006). About 2 to 3 in 1000 live-born children have CP.
      1. *Prenatal* factors include malfunctioning placenta, intrauterine infection, teratogens, Rh incompatibility, maternal metabolic disorder, brain malformations, and genetic disorders (rare). CP occurs most commonly in the prenatal period.
      2. *Perinatal* factors include premature birth, birth trauma, anoxia, low birth weight, metabolic or electrolyte disturbance, and hyperbilirubinemia.
      3. *Postnatal* factors include trauma to the head, infections of the brain (such as meningitis and toxins), cerebral hemorrhage or embolus, anoxia, and tumors of the brain. In most cases the cause is unknown.
   B. The neuromuscular dysfunction is directly associated with the area of the brain injured and the stage of development reached when the injury occurred.

III. Characteristics
   A. Spastic CP:
      1. Most common type, representing 70% to 80% of all cases.
      2. Limb muscle contracts strongly with stretching or sudden attempted movement.
      3. Disorder of the adductor muscles or hip, legs crossed, scissoring.
      4. Fixed contractures common.

5. Muscle may continue to contract and relax repetitively (clonus).
6. In involved limbs, deep tendon reflexes are increased (e.g., ankle and knee jerk).
7. With growth, spastic muscle becomes shorter, and pelvis, spine, and limb deformities are common.
8. Poor control of posture and balance.
9. Abnormal postures at rest or with change of position.
10. Risk for hip subluxation and dislocation.
11. Impaired fine and gross motor skills.
12. Spastic CP is classified by limb involvement.
    a. *Monoplegia:* one limb involved.
    b. *Hemiplegia:* only upper and lower limbs of one side involved; 25% develop homonymous hemianopsia (sees straight ahead but not to the affected side). Most common type of spastic CP.
    c. *Paraplegia:* lower limbs affected.
    d. *Diplegia:* both upper and lower limbs involved, but lower limbs are more severely affected.
    e. *Triplegia:* usually one upper limb and both lower limbs affected.
    f. *Quadriplegia:* also known as *tetraplegia;* all four limbs involved and musculature around trunk, mouth, tongue, and pharynx may be involved, affecting speech, chewing, and swallowing; emotions are more labile with inappropriate laughing and crying.
    g. *Double hemiplegia:* both sides of body involved, but upper extremities more involved than lower.
B. Dyskinetic (athetoid) CP:
    1. Involuntary movements are aggravated by stress.
    2. Two subtypes: *athetoid* and *dystonic.*
       a. *Athetoid* movements are common (slow writhing movements or chorea movements [jerky and rapid]) of extremities, neck, trunk, facial muscles, and tongue.
       b. *Dystonic* movements are slow, twisting movements of trunk and extremities, resulting in an abnormal position.
    3. Voluntary movements contorted.
    4. Movements and rigidity disappear during sleep.
    5. All extremities are generally involved.
    6. Drooling and dysarthria, poor speech articulation.
    7. Muscles not spastic.
    8. Deformities rare.
    9. Impaired swallowing.
    10. Motor manifestations exacerbated by emotional stress.
    11. Frequently has high-frequency hearing loss or deafness.
C. Ataxic CP:
    1. Walks with wide-based gait, weaving trunk, arms out.
    2. Unable to turn rapidly, falls frequently.
    3. Unable to perform rapid, coordinated movements well.
    4. Hypotonia during infancy and decreased tendon reflexes.
    5. Tone ranges from ataxic to hypotonic to atonic.

D. Mixed CP:
    1. Combination of athetosis and spasticity.
    2. Generally quadriplegic.
E. Other associated characteristics:
    1. Mental retardation.
    2. Seizures present in 20% to 40%, particularly in spastic type.
    3. Attention-deficit disorder.
    4. Low visual acuity in nearly 75%, strabismus present in about 50%; hearing impairments in about 10%.
    5. Tactile perception impaired.
    6. Speech impairment in up to 80% of CP cases.
    7. Visual-motor and perceptual problems.
    8. Gastrointestinal and feeding difficulties in 50%.

IV. **Health Concerns/Emergencies**
    A. At high risk for injury, possibility of falls because of gross motor impairment, spasticity, and seizures.
    B. At risk for status epilepticus or uncontrolled seizures.
    C. Choking, aspiration, or feeding problems because of uncoordinated chewing, sucking, and swallowing.
    D. Susceptible to latex allergies (see Chapter 9, Special Education).

V. **Effects on Individual**
    A. Depend on age, extent of involvement, and degree of mental disability (See Table 4-4).
    B. Simple daily tasks can be monumental or impossible (e.g., self-feeding, dressing, toileting, turning on television, answering telephone).
    C. Student may have normal intelligence but be unable to communicate thoughts and needs verbally.
    D. Those who can verbalize may encounter impatience or ridicule because of slow and inarticulate speech.
    E. Delayed social development.
    F. May have to face numerous surgeries to correct contractures and to provide mobility.
    G. Often must depend on peers for assistance at school, and thereby left vulnerable to thoughtlessness and rejection.
    H. Social and recreational outlets and career opportunities may be limited, but application of new technology is expanding choices in many areas.
    I. Low feelings of self-worth emerges with more awareness of being different from peers and siblings, and guilt may be felt for the numerous problems the family must face in daily management.
    J. Behavior problems frequently develop because of rejection by others.
    K. Constant stress from meeting with the numerous professionals involved in therapy: orthopedist, physical therapist, occupational therapist, speech therapist, neurologist, psychologist or psychiatrist, and so on.

VI. **Management/Treatment**
    A. Hearing loss and vision impairment—usually refractive errors, such as farsightedness and strabismus—must be ruled out and referred for correction if indicated.

Table 4-4	*Educational Issues Resulting from Brain Insult*		
Class	Type	Brain Involvement	Educational Issues
Spastic	Diplegia, quadriplegia, hemiplegia	Motor cortex and pyramidal tract	Cognitive: 70% are within normal IQ range. Retardation varies from mild with learning disabilities to profound.
Dyskinesis	Athetoid, dystonic	Basal ganglia or extrapyramidal tracts	Motor skills: Both fine and gross affected, which interferes with handwriting, drawing, computer, and cutting skills, almost all classroom skills. Often nonambulatory or walks with unsteady gait.
Ataxic	Range of tone and coordination; ataxic-hypotonic-atonic	Cerebellum	Speech and language: Weak if any perioral tone, which affects articulation. Often nonverbal. May benefit from augmentative communication device.
Mixed	Combinations of spastic and dyskinesia	Various areas in brain	Sensory integration: Impaired or limited vision, hearing, and tactile methods of learning. Dysfunctional figure ground differentiation, eyehand coordination. Visual motor and perceptual problems. Behavioral and affective: ADHD, hyperactive, impulsivity, noncompliant and moody at times, cries.

B. Monitor medication and possible side effects:
   1. Some persons with athetosis have benefited from diazepam (Valium) to control tension and excessive movement.
   2. Dantrolene (Dantrium) reduces spasticity in the muscles, but it may affect liver function. Botulinum toxin-A (Botox) injections and baclofen (Lioresal) are also used to reduce spasticity and prevent permanent contractures. Baclofen given as a continuous infusion may help with ambulation.

3. Barbiturates (e.g., phenobarbital), which generally sedate, may excite individuals with brain damage. The stimulant dextroamphetamine is sometimes used to calm individuals with brain damage.

4. Anticonvulsants are administered to those with seizure involvement.

C. Caries, malocclusion, and bruxism (grinding of teeth) are common; refer for dental care when necessary.

D. Eating and feeding difficulties are prevalent because of poor perioral muscle tone and coordination. This problem, along with high caloric expenditure from spasticity and tremors, creates a calorie deficit. Evaluate, including monitoring anthropometry, and provide lists and techniques to caregivers for increasing calories in diet at home and at school. Some students benefit from special eating utensils; severe, unresolved problems may require gastrostomy tube placement.

E. Urinary retention and bladder control difficulties are common, as well as the inability to sense urination urge or bladder fullness. A number of medications are available.

F. High risk for pulmonary infection secondary to abnormal muscle tone, inactivity, contractures, and scoliosis. Infections last longer because of ineffective cough and inability to blow nose.

G. At increased risk for latex allergies. It is prudent to minimize contact with latex products.

H. Prevent breakdown of skin by encouraging staff to frequently change position of severely disabled and periodically check braces and other appliances for possible rubbing, pressure points, and necrosis.

I. Awareness of safety needs:
1. Helmet to prevent head injury.
2. Wheelchair in good working order.
3. Provide proper support when sitting balance is inadequate.
4. Rails and other means of support should be available, particularly in toilet facilities.
5. Evaluate usability and safety of school routine and pathways via wheelchair.
6. Emergency evacuation plans should be in place.

J. Know physical and occupational therapy goals to determine nursing role.

K. It may be necessary to coordinate care provided by a number of professionals and community agencies while working with the parents. Assist parents when appropriate for respite services, meeting other parents with the same needs, finding support groups; include siblings.

L. Develop IHCP or IECP as needed. Prepare nurse assessment report for individualized education program (IEP) and participate in IEP meeting as appropriate. Nurse may be case manager for severely involved students.

VII. Additional Information

A. Common terminology associated with bracing (orthotics):
1. Ankle–foot orthosis (AFO). The metal AFO has an adjustable ankle joint; the plastic AFO keeps the foot in a fixed position.

CHAPTER 4

Chronic Conditions

2. Knee–ankle–foot orthosis (KAFO) is also made of metal and plastic. The metal brace can be adjusted and lengthened for growth more easily than the plastic one.
3. Hip–knee–ankle–foot orthosis (HKAFO) is a pelvic band that fits around the waist and is attached to a long leg brace.

WEB SITES

American Academy for Cerebral Palsy and Developmental Medicine
   http://www.aacpdm.org/home.html
American Association on Intellectual and Developmental Disabilities
   http://www.aamr.org
Best Buddies
   http://www.bestbuddies.org
United Cerebral Palsy
   http://www.ucp.org

CLEFT LIP AND/OR PALATE

I. Definition
A. A cleft of the lip results from an incomplete fusion of the medial nasal and maxillary processes. A cleft of the palate occurs because of failure of the palatal shelves to fuse. These anomalies occur during the fifth to twelfth weeks of gestation. The malformation may involve only the lip, the palate, or both the lip and palate. The severity of the defect depends on the timing of the insult on fetal development; the lip and palate develop and fuse at different times during fetal life.
B. In an incomplete unilateral cleft of the lip, only the vermilion border on either side of the lip is involved. In a complete unilateral cleft, either side of the lip is involved and extends into the nasal septum. In complete bilateral clefts, both sides of the lips are involved.
C. A unilateral complete cleft of the lip and palate extends through either side of the premaxilla alveolar arch and the lips. No fusion occurs in the premaxilla and maxilla or the bones of the hard palate and nasal septum. A bilateral complete cleft of the lip and palate extends through both sides of the premaxilla, alveolar arch, and the lips. Neither side of the premaxilla, maxilla, or palatal bones fuses together. Clefts of the palate only involve either a cleft of the soft palate or clefts of both the hard and soft palate. Figure 4-2 illustrates the variations of cleft lip and palate.

II. Etiology
A. When numerous factors cause clefts, the term *multifactorial inheritance* is used to indicate a combination of chromosomal, genetic, teratogenic, and environmental factors. Over 300 syndromes exist that include clefts as a characteristic. Some syndromes are identified as chromosomal abnormalities, mutant genes, or teratogens (e.g. drugs or alcohol). Environmental factors often associated with clefts are maternal vitamin deficiencies, such as in folic acid; maternal smoking; and x-ray exposure during the first trimester of pregnancy.

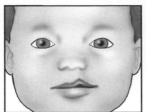
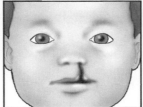
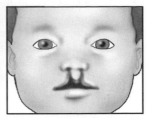

| Unilateral incomplete cleft lip | Unilateral complete cleft lip | Bilateral complete cleft lip |

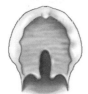

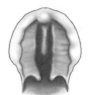

| Soft palate involvement only | Unilateral complete cleft palate | Bilateral complete cleft palate |

FIGURE 4-2 Cleft lip and palate.

CHAPTER 4   Chronic Conditions

    1. Each year, one out of every 700 infants is born with a cleft lip and/ or palate (Bishop, 2006). It is the fourth most common birth defect in the United States and appears more frequently in Asians and certain Native American tribes. It occurs less frequently in the African-American population and affects boys more often than girls.

III. Characteristics

  A. Usually observed at birth:
    1. Notch in vermilion border of lip.
    2. Complete bilateral or unilateral separation of lip.
    3. Bilateral or unilateral opening in the roof of the mouth.
    4. Bifid uvula is associated with a submucous cleft.
  B. Submucous clefts of the palate are not usually observed at birth but become apparent when feeding or speech problems occur (e.g., nasal sounding).
  C. Normal developmental patterns of feeding, speech, and language are disrupted.

IV. Health Concerns/Emergencies

  A. Presence or severity of medical problem depends on degree of involvement.
  B. Feeding difficulties with the newborn or infant pose an immediate problem, because malformation may cause an inefficient suck, resulting in prolonged feeding time, poor weight gain, or weight loss.
  C. Recurrent otitis media and eustachian tube infections are common.
  D. Braces and dental prosthetics increase probability of tooth decay and gum disease; regular visits to a pedodontist are necessary.
  E. Displacement of maxillary arches and malposition of teeth require intervention with orthodontia.

F. Frequently, congenital anomalies that require additional care and medical intervention are present.

V. Effects on Individual

A. Child becomes frustrated because others cannot understand their speech.
B. Facial disfigurement may cause difficulty with parent relationships and, later in life, peer groups.
C. May develop hearing loss, causing more delays in speech and language.
D. Low self-esteem because of obvious deformity.
E. Fears and trauma related to surgery and possible separation from parents.

VI. Management/Treatment

A. Initial concern for infant is provision of adequate nutrition and prevention of aspiration and infection:
  1. Feed in upright position.
  2. Cleft palate nipples and plastic palatal coverings are available.
  3. Use specialized nipple as needed, staying with one nipple for at least 24 hours.
  4. If unable to adapt to a nipple, infant may be gavage-fed or fed with a medicine dropper.
B. Follow-up with periodic, complete hearing evaluations.
C. Coordinate health plan with parents and cleft lip/palate clinical team.
D. Orthodontic repairs occur in stages until about age 18.

VII. Additional Information

A. Cleft lip surgical closure is generally done when child is 2 to 3 months old. Before surgery, an infant should weigh at least 10 lbs and be free of respiratory, oral, or systemic infections. Z-plasty is the common surgery performed and minimizes notching of the lip caused by retraction of scar tissue. The surgery enhances the child's appearance and enables intake of food in a normal manner.
  1. Additional repair or revision may be needed, depending on severity of cleft lip. If the nose is involved and rhinoplasty is necessary, corrective surgery is generally delayed until adolescence, when growth has stopped.
B. Cleft palate surgical repair timing varies and should be individualized. Time of repair depends on size, shape, and degree of child's cleft palate; in a healthy child, surgery can be done before 1 year of age to unite the segmented cleft, provide pleasant and intelligible speech, and prevent injury to growing maxilla.
  1. Improved techniques are lowering the age of repair to as early as 1 month. Prosthetic devices may be necessary when cleft palate interferes with dentition.
C. After palatal surgery, the nurse should frequently examine the oral cavity and report fistulas or tissue collapse to the surgeon. When not a health hazard, enlarged tonsils and adenoids create extra tissue mass that may aid in velopharyngeal function.
D. Secondary complications of cleft lip and palate include speech and language, hearing, and dental concerns. Speech and language delays occur in more than half of the affected children. Both receptive and

expressive language are affected; absent teeth may cause an interdental lisp, and there may be voice problems.

E. Hearing is affected by the eustachian tube dysfunction. Cleft palate exposes the eustachian tube to foods and liquids, causing a predisposition to inflammation. Upper respiratory disease also increases the incidence of middle ear and eustachian tube infections. This results in middle ear pathology, which may cause a bilateral conductive hearing loss. Dental involvement may necessitate the need for regular dental visits, preferably with a pedodontist, or it may require orthodontics or prosthodontics.

F. A child with cleft lip or palate should be evaluated by a dysmorphologist for any associated syndromes and to provide genetic consulting for the parents. The interdisciplinary management team involves at least seven people, and many more specialists are involved in the correction of the birth defect.

1. The *pediatrician* prescribes routine health care.
2. The *otolaryngologist* follows up middle ear pathology and eustachian tube dysfunction.
3. The *audiologist* diagnoses hearing impairment.
4. The *orthodontist* handles dental occlusion prevention and correction.
5. The *prosthodontist* constructs an appliance for absent teeth and or reconstructs the opening between the oral and nasal cavities.
6. The *speech and language pathologist* oversees and remediates speech and language development.
7. The *surgeon* repairs the cleft.

WEB SITES

Wide Smiles, Cleft Palate and Lip Resource
    http://www.widesmiles.org
Operation Smile
    http://www.operationsmile.org

CYSTIC FIBROSIS

I. Definition
A. Cystic fibrosis (CF) is an autosomal recessive disorder that affects multiple systems. Viscous mucus obstructs all, or nearly all, ducts of the exocrine glands. This obstruction is responsible for the clinical manifestations.

II. Etiology
A. The condition is genetically transmitted, and both parents must be carriers of the gene. The CF gene is found on the long arm of chromosome 7 and is associated with production of the cystic fibrosis transmembrane conductance regulator (CFTR) protein. This defect results in abnormal electrolyte and fluid transport across cell membranes. The incidence is 1 in 3200 Caucasians in the United States, with progressively lower incidence in Hispanics (1:8000), African-Americans (1:15,000), and Asians (1:31,000) (Marshall and Debley, 2006). The recessive gene is carried in 1 out of 28 Caucasians. It is

one of the most common genetic disorders. Prenatal testing is available and has a 90% sensitivity for detecting the CF gene. Most states have routine newborn screening for CF.

III. Characteristics

A. Pulmonary involvement:
   1. Dry or productive cough, which may be paroxysmal.
   2. Hemoptysis not uncommon over age 10.
   3. Rapid, wheezing respirations.
   4. Shortness of breath (SOB) with increased activity, progressing to chronic SOB.
   5. Chronic sinusitis, nasal polyps.
   6. Repeated episodes of bronchopneumonia, bronchitis, bronchiectasis.
   7. Cyanosis.
   8. Clubbing of fingers and toes.
   9. Barrel chest.

B. Gastrointestinal system:
   1. Malabsorption.
   2. Gastroesophageal reflux disease (GERD).
   3. Meconium ileus (intestinal obstruction caused by failure to pass meconium) occurs in 7% to 10% who have the disease.
   4. Distal intestinal obstruction syndrome (DIOS) is partial or complete obstruction that may occur at any age but is more common in adolescence and young adulthood.
   5. Fibrosing colonopathy, prestricture state, or true stricture of the colon associated with excessive doses of pancreatic enzymes; greater than 6000 lipase units/kg per meal in children under age 12.
   6. Pancreatic involvement, which prohibits production of digestive enzymes and may lead to diabetes.
   7. Pancreatic insufficiency, as manifested in slow growth; failure to thrive; decreased muscle mass; voracious appetite but poor weight gain; protuberant abdomen; and frequent loose, foul-smelling, oily, floating stools.
   8. Prolapse of rectum is common in infancy and childhood.
   9. Anemia secondary to vitamin E or iron deficiencies.
   10. Frequent bruising as a result of vitamin K deficiency.

C. Hepatobiliary system:
   1. Prolonged neonatal jaundice.
   2. Biliary cirrhosis.
   3. Portal hypertension.
   4. Cholelithiasis.

D. Reproductive system:
   1. Delayed puberty.
   2. Sterility in 98% of males from maldevelopment or obstruction of epididymis, vas deferens, and seminal vesicles.
   3. Females may be less fertile because of abnormal cervical mucus.
   4. Inguinal hernia, hydrocele, and undescended testes more common.

E. Integumentary abnormalities:
   1. Elevated concentrations of sodium and chloride in the sweat.

2. Abnormal salt loss and dehydration secondary to electrolyte imbalance.
3. Hyponatremic metabolic alkalosis.
4. Heat stroke.

IV. Health Concerns/Emergencies
A. Constipation and pain may indicate bowel obstruction.
B. Prolapse of rectum can occur secondary to bowel obstruction.
C. Anemia from impaired absorption of fats, which causes deficiency of fat-soluble vitamins A, D, K, and E.
D. Pulmonary obstruction or infection:
   1. Fatigue.
   2. Irritability.
   3. Decreased appetite and exercise tolerance.
   4. Increased cough (especially at night) or sputum production.
   5. Rales, wheezes, or increased respirations.
   6. Inability to gain weight; weight loss.
   7. Intermittent low-grade fever.
E. Excessive dosage of enzyme preparations may cause:
   1. Constipation.
   2. Frequent loose, green stools.
   3. Abdominal pain.
F. Enzymes should not remain on lips or skin, because they can break down tissue.
G. Salt loss caused by weather, vomiting, fever, or heavy exercise. Symptoms include:
   1. Weakness.
   2. Lethargy.
   3. Irritability.

V. Effects on Individual
A. Demands long-term medical management.
B. Hospitalizations may be dreaded or feared.
C. Dependency on parents for care.
D. Uncertain future may cause depression.
E. May feel different and excluded from peers because of physical limitations, medical complications, and frequent hospitalizations.
F. May experience guilt feelings because of the disruption the illness has caused the family.
G. Puberty delayed in most young people with CF.
H. Activities have to be built around treatment, diet, and medication.
I. May be subject to ridicule from peers because of retarded growth or delayed puberty.

VI. Management/Treatment
A. Monitor height and weight.
B. Coordinate school health management with clinical management team.
C. Be aware of prescribed medications and side effects.
D. Discuss using school bell sound as a reminder to do deep breathing and coughing.
E. Encourage fluids to keep lung secretions thin.
F. Do not restrict salt, especially during hot weather.

CHAPTER 4

Chronic Conditions

    G. Salt tablets may be necessary to prevent salt loss for active child.

    H. Recognize signs of respiratory distress, and intervene before respiratory failure develops.

    I. Perform chest physiotherapy (CPT) before meals when prescribed.

    J. Give digestive enzymes at beginning of each meal and snack to facilitate absorption of fats and proteins.

    K. High-protein, high-calorie, and high-carbohydrate diet; high-fat foods not tolerated.

    L. Minimize exposure to those who have respiratory tract infections.

    M. Encourage participation in activities of interest, because activity increases movement of mucus from airways.

    N. Encourage use of horn blowing instrument in the school band.

    O. Encourage peer counseling with another student who has a chronic illness.

VII. Additional Information

    A. Suspect CF in any infant who fails to thrive even with adequate intake of food. The sweat chloride test remains the best diagnostic measure.

    B. Multiple medications are used: antibiotics (some aerosolized) for pulmonary disease exacerbations, corticosteroids for airway inflammation and severe bronchospasm, mucus-thinning drugs, and enzymes for pancreatic insufficiency.

    C. There are two devices on the market to help maintain a patent airway:

        1. The Vest airway clearance system (Advanced Respiratory, St. Paul, Minnesota) helps loosen mucus by high-frequency chest wall oscillation.

        2. The Flutter mucus clearance mechanism (Scandipharm, Birmingham, Alabama) helps to remove mucus in 5 to 15 minutes by blowing into the handheld device.

    D. Annual screening for diabetes is standard in CF clinics; type 2 diabetes is found in 9% of children and 26% of adolescents with CF. Onset is gradual and related to impaired pancreatic function; treatment is difficult due to the complex medical and nutritional problems of CF (Alemzadeh and Wyatt, 2004).

    E. Advanced lung disease may be treated with lung or heart/lung transplant. New treatments now in clinical trials include gene therapy and CFTR protein repair. Life expectancy is now into the thirties and forties.

WEB SITE

Cystic Fibrosis Foundation
    http://www.cff.org

CYTOMEGALOVIRUS

I. Definition

    A. Cytomegalovirus (CMV) is a common viral infection that is found throughout the world but seldom causes clinical illness in healthy children or adults. CMV is of particular significance to pregnant women, however. It is the most common of the intrauterine infections and can result in severe mental retardation, neurological damage, and death to the fetus or newborn.

II. Etiology

A. CMV is a member of the herpes virus group *Herpesviridae*. CMV is congenital or acquired and is transmitted by exposure to infected body fluids and sexual contact. Congenital CMV is a common cause of serious disability. About 1 in 150 children are born with congenital CMV and 1 in 750 children are born with or develop permanent disabilities due to CMV. The exact mechanism of CMV transmission and the incubation period is unknown. It affects between 50% and 80% of adults by 40 years of age in the United States (CDC, 2006b). Risk of transmission through casual contact is very small.

III. Characteristics

A. Congenitally acquired, asymptomatic CMV:
   1. Of congenitally infected infants, 85% to 90% have a *silent infection* and are asymptomatic at birth (CDC, 2006b). Asymptomatic infections are still a major cause of deafness, retardation, and blindness, and late manifestations occasionally appear in early childhood.
      a. Progressive auditory damage (deafness) in about 10%.
      b. Learning disabilities.
      c. Neuromuscular disturbances.
   2. These children excrete virus through their urine, tears, saliva, or other bodily excretions or secretions.

B. Congenitally acquired, symptomatic CMV:
   1. Also called *cytomegalovirus inclusion disease (CID)*.
   2. Degree of involvement is thought to be related to gestational age of fetus at time of maternal infection.
   3. Newborns with CID exhibit some of the following abnormalities:
      a. Low birth weight.
      b. Petechia.
      c. Jaundice.
      d. Microcephaly.
      e. Obstructive hydrocephaly.
      f. Hepatosplenomegaly.
      g. Chorioretinitis, cataracts.
      h. Heart disease.
      i. Encephalitis.
      j. Intracranial calcifications.
      k. Anemia.
   4. Later manifestations include:
      a. Progressive hearing loss.
      b. Visual impairment.
      c. Mental retardation.
      d. Motor disabilities.
   5. Death may occur in utero; neonatal death rate is high in severely infected infants.
   6. Severely involved children excrete virus through their urine, tears, saliva, and other bodily excretions or secretions until 4 to 8 years of age.

CHAPTER 4

Chronic Conditions

NOTE: Only a very small percentage of children born with congenital CMV suffer devastating effects of classic CID.

    C. Connatal CMV, acquired during or shortly after birth:
       1. Almost always asymptomatic.
       2. A very small percentage of children who do exhibit symptoms may have any of the following conditions:
         a. Failure to thrive.
         b. Hepatosplenomegaly.
         c. Chronic gastroenteritis.
         d. Hemolytic anemia.
         e. Hepatitis.
    D. Those who acquire the virus in childhood or as adults:
       1. Usually asymptomatic.
       2. Mononucleosis-like symptoms can occur in immunocompromised children and adults:
         a. Fever.
         b. Lymphadenopathy.
         c. Splenomegaly.
         d. Hepatitis.
       3. Reactivation or reinfection may also produce same mononucleosis-like symptoms in susceptible persons.
       4. Both asymptomatic people and those with symptoms excrete CMV through their urine, saliva, and other bodily secretions or excretions.
         a. Infected children may have prolonged periods of intermittent excretion of CMV.
         b. Infected adults may also intermittently shed virus, but it is a negligible means of transmission.
    E. Immunosuppressed or immunodeficient individuals (e.g., patients with leukemia or human immunodeficiency virus [HIV], those on steroids) exposed to CMV suffer serious morbidity and mortality, and they also excrete virus through their urine, saliva, and other bodily secretions or excretions.
       1. Such individuals are susceptible to:
         a. Disseminated infection.
         b. Pneumonia.
         c. Retinitis.
         d. Hepatitis.
       2. Suffer serious morbidity and mortality.
       3. Excrete virus through their urine, saliva, and other bodily secretions or excretions.
       4. Combination antiviral treatment has greatly reduced CMV in persons with HIV.

IV. Health Concerns/Emergencies
    A. Vary according to extent of involvement.
    B. Of known congenitally infected infants who are asymptomatic at birth, 5% to 20% will exhibit late manifestations of infection; these children need to be monitored for:
       1. Hearing loss. CMV is one of the leading causes of sensorineural hearing loss.

2. Visual impairment.
3. Neuromuscular disturbance.
4. Poor intellectual performance.
5. Learning disabilities.

C. Immunocompromised individuals are more susceptible to severe clinical manifestations and should be protected from exposure to CMV; this is a reminder that universal precautions should be practiced in all situations.

V. Effects on Individual

A. Congenital asymptomatic infants—who later exhibit lower intelligence quotient (IQ) levels, motor deficits, learning disabilities, and hearing loss—will require close clinical assessments and follow-up for special education services.

B. CID infants may die shortly after birth or be profoundly damaged, requiring lifelong care.

C. Children with mental retardation will require special education services.

D. Uninformed teaching staff and other professionals working with CMV-infected infants and children may be frightened of the condition and its effects. This emotion can detract from their relationships with the children and negatively impact the children's welfare and development.

VI. Management/Treatment

A. Varies according to extent of involvement.

B. Treatment is symptom specific.

C. Severely involved students will have an IEP, which covers all necessary nursing services, identifies involved personnel, and outlines procedures performed at school.

D. Educate and practice universal precautions and follow individual state, county, or school district policy manuals.

E. Students should receive information about the epidemiology, transmission routes, and hygienic procedures for CMV.

F. Pregnant women should be counseled concerning the risk of acquiring CMV infection and the disease's possible effects on the fetus; women may want to be tested for CMV antibodies; refer to HCP.

G. Transfer to another position requiring less contact with infants and very young children should be considered.

VII. Additional Information

A. CMV is transmitted transplacentally (intrauterine); connately (during or shortly after birth); through the breast milk of an infected mother; by close or intimate contact with individuals excreting CMV through their urine, saliva, tears, and other bodily secretions or excretions; through blood transfusions; or through transplanted organs.

B. Regarding the period of communicability:

1. Infants and young children excrete the virus through their urine (viruria) often up to 4 years and, in the more severely involved, up to 8 years after birth. Excretion is generally intermittent.

2. Infected adults seem to excrete the virus for shorter periods of time and intermittently.

3. At present, it has not been determined how many negative urine specimens should be tested to be reasonably confident that the infant is no longer excreting CMV.
4. Infection rates vary with socioeconomic levels of the population and are higher in developing countries.

C. Prevention of CMV involves using universal precautions. Treatment is symptomatic. Drug therapy for infants is being evaluated, and vaccines are in the research and development stage. Evidence indicates that maternal antibody does reduce the severity of infection but does not protect the fetus from infection. Diagnosis of a maternal primary infection during pregnancy is difficult; blood tests can be performed, but isolation of CMV from the genital tract does not indicate whether the infection is primary. It is currently impossible to determine if the fetus has been affected when maternal primary CMV has been documented. The National Center for Infectious Diseases does not presently recommend routine serologic testing for CMV antibodies but suggests testing based on case-by-case evaluation.

D. Recommendations concerning infants and children include:
1. Not excluding normal infants from nursing when the mother is a known excretor of CMV.
2. Because CMV can be transmitted by breast milk, the risks and benefits for its use need to be evaluated before it is given to immunosuppressed or premature infants.
3. Universal precautions should be practiced, and appropriate procedures for contaminated secretions should be exercised. For those women working with infants and high-risk children, and those working in hospitals and other institutions, there is concern regarding acquiring CMV. Hospital nurses appear to run a lower risk of contracting primary CMV infection from hospitalized infants and children than do community home workers, perhaps because of the short contact and the controlled environment. Research is lacking regarding the risk of community workers in contact with the disease (e.g., school nurses, teachers, and others who work directly with children with CMV). Applying universal precautions in schools should provide the needed protection.

E. In immunosuppressed or immunodeficient individuals, CMV infections are a major cause of morbidity and mortality. Risk factors and the type of infection that predispose these individuals to CMV infections are not as well defined as those for the previous groups. Immunodeficient individuals include HIV and cancer patients, organ transplant recipients, hemodialysis patients, and those receiving systemic corticosteroids and immunosuppressive drugs. Posttransfusion CMV infection occurs and can be especially threatening to immunocompromised patients, infants, those receiving immunosuppressive therapy, and pregnant women.

WEB SITE

CDC National Center for Infectious Diseases, CMV
http://www.cdc.gov/cmv

DIABETES MELLITUS: TYPE 1 AND TYPE 2

DIABETES MELLITUS: TYPE 1

I. Definition

    A. Both types of diabetes mellitus are metabolic diseases caused by a deficiency in the production or action of the hormone insulin, which converts sugar, starches, and other food into energy. Insulin is usually produced by specialized cells in the islets of Langerhans in the pancreas. Each type of diabetes (see Table 4-5) has its own etiology, clinical course, and treatment management.

        1. Type 1 diabetes was previously known as *insulin-dependent diabetes mellitus*.

        2. Type 2 diabetes was previously referred to as *non-insulin-dependent diabetes mellitus;* it is covered later in this section.

Table 4-5	*Comparing Types of Diabetes*	
Characteristics	**Type 1**	**Type 2**
Type of onset	Rapid	Insidious
Age at onset	Under 20 years of age	Previously adults, now often in puberty
Sex ratio	Males slightly more than females	Females more than males
Percentage of diabetics	5%-10%	85%-90%
Family history	5% have first or second degree relatives with type 1 diabetes	74%-100% have first or second degree relatives with type 2 diabetes
Ethnicity	Primarily Caucasian	More prevalent in Native Americans, Hispanics, African-Americans
Weight at onset	Typically normal or underweight	85% are overweight
Diagnosis on routine physical	Infrequent	Frequent
Ketoacidosis	35%-40 % have keto-acidosis	33% have ketonuria and 5%-25% have mild ketoacidosis
Acanthosis nigricans	Rare	60%-90%
Dyslipidemia	Less frequent	Frequent
Hypertension	Less frequent	Common
Polyuria, polydypsia, weight loss	Frequent	Less frequent
Vaginal infections	Rare	Frequent
Chronic complications	More than 80%	Variable
Insulin	Always	20%-30%
Oral medications	Ineffective	Often effective
Diet and exercise	Ineffective	Often effective
Prevention	No known method	Lifestyle changes; medication (metformin)

(Adapted from Cerasuolo, 2007 and Kaufman, 2005).

II. Etiology

A. In type 1 diabetes, the body produces insufficient insulin, or the insulin produced is ineffective, resulting from a predetermined genetic susceptibility or from environmental factors that influence an autoimmune response. Particular viruses and toxins, as well as seasonal influences, have been linked as causative factors. Changes in the body induced by obesity, pregnancy, illicit drugs, or the use of certain medications may also trigger the onset of different diabetic types.

B. Diabetes is the most common metabolic disease of childhood and adolescence; approximately 1 in 523 persons younger than 20 years had diabetes in 2006 (CDC, 2007). Peak incidence is about 7 to 15 years, but may present at any age (Alemzadeh and Wyatt, 2004). Approximately one in every 400 to 600 children and adolescents has type 1 diabetes (CDC, 2005b).

Brain Findings

Studies on animals have demonstrated that neurons die as a result of hyperglycemia. Insulin-like growth factor 1 (IGF-1) and some antioxidant agents were found to prevent this cell death or dysfunction. Other animal studies demonstrated that uncontrolled periods of hyperglycemia damage the hippocampus, which is important for memory function. Controlling blood glucose levels and having an islet cell transplant were both found to protect against such damage.

III. Characteristics

A. Usually seen in children but can occur at any age.

B. Symptoms generally manifest around preschool or school age; however, it has been diagnosed in infants as young as 6 months.

C. Rapid onset.

D. Presenting symptoms:
1. Polyphagia (excessive eating).
2. Polydipsia (excessive drinking).
3. Polyuria (excessive urination).
4. Fatigue and weakness, sometimes extreme.
5. Irritability.
6. Extreme hunger.
7. Sudden weight loss, sometimes striking.
8. Nausea and vomiting (acute symptoms).

E. Other manifestations:
1. Dry skin.
2. Skin infections that heal slowly.
3. Blurred vision.
4. Constipation from dehydration.
5. Children most likely underweight and adolescents overweight.
6. Monilial vaginitis in adolescent girls.
7. Enuresis in previously toilet-trained child.
8. Lethargy.
9. Fruity breath odor.

      10. Abdominal pain.
      11. Rarely, diabetic coma is the first sign.
IV. Health Concerns/Emergencies
    A. Chronic complications:
      1. Vascular and nervous system damage, hypertension, and amputations.
      2. Neuropathy.
      3. Retinopathy and cataracts.
      4. Renal disease.
      5. Cardiovascular disease.
      6. Peridontal disease.
      7. Short stature and underweight.
    B. Acute complications (see Box 4-3 and Box 4-4).
NOTE: Must check Nurse Practice Act, state, and school district policies and guidelines for administration of treatment and medication before storing medication or administering it to students. Emergency treatment is also discussed in Chapter 12.
V. Effects on Individual
    A. Poor self-image as a result of being "different."
    B. Altered mood and mental alertness.
    C. Doubles the risk for depression, which increases risk for hyperglycemia and other complications.
    D. Parental relationships may be strained from having parent who does too much or too little.
    E. May feel insulin injections are form of punishment.

Box 4-3	*Hyperglycemia (Excess Blood Glucose) Ketoacidosis*

Characteristics	**Action**
1. Less common than insulin reaction.	If uncertain whether individual is hyperglycemic or hypoglycemic, the following will not do harm if person is hyperglycemic but will alleviate hypoglycemia:
2. Slow onset.	
3. Precipitating events:	
a. Undiagnosed diabetes.	
b. Too little or no insulin.	1. Check student's emergency care plan (ECP).
c. Infection, illness, or injury.	
d. Emotional stress.	2. Give conscious person sugar-containing drink; if no response, activate emergency medical services (EMS) and call parent(s).
e. Nonadherence to diet.	
4. Symptoms:	
a. Gradual drowsiness.	3. If unconscious, activate EMS and call parent(s).
b. Increased thirst and urination.	
c. Flushed skin.	4. To differentiate between the two, the nurse or designee should check blood glucose level and ketones.
d. Nausea, vomiting.	
e. Anorexia.	
f. Weakness, abdominal pains, generalized aches.	5. If no ketones present, exercise moderately and give extra insulin per ECP.
g. Fruity or wine breath.	
h. Rapid pulse.	
i. Hyperventilation or tachypnea.	
j. If untreated, eventual stupor or unconsciousness.	

Box 4-4 | *Hypoglycemia (Low Blood Glucose)*

Characteristics
1. Rapid onset.
2. Usually occurs before mealtime and at peak effective time of insulin.
3. Precipitating events:
   a. Too much insulin.
   b. Delayed or missed meal.
   c. Excessive exercise without adequate food.

Mild Reaction
1. Behavioral problems, temper tantrums, irritable, "not themselves."
2. Hunger.
3. Increased pulse and respiratory rate.
4. Hyperactivity.
5. Weakness.
6. Pallor.
7. In children, first sign may be behavioral problems.

Action
1. Provide immediate source of food, milk, fruit juice, glucose tablets, gel, or icing (milk is good because it provides lactose, protein, and fat); can follow with starch or carbohydrate snack.
2. Do not use diet drinks and do not give insulin.
3. Check blood glucose level.

Moderate Reaction
1. Cerebral function affected.
2. Confusion and disorientation.
3. Poor coordination.

4. Increased irritability.
5. Blood glucose severely lowered.
6. Sweating.
7. Extreme nervousness, tremors.
8. Headache, abdominal pains.
9. Nausea and vomiting.
10. Blood pressure lowered.
11. Pulse rate increased.

Action
1. Check blood glucose level, if indicated provide 10 to 15 g simple carbohydrates, 3 tsp sugar in water, orange juice (3 to 6 oz), apple juice, or grape juice, or treat as prescribed (e.g., glucose tablets, gel, or icing).
2. Repeat in 10 to 15 min if no response.
3. Follow with larger carbohydrate protein snack, or if mealtime, allow student to eat lunch.
4. Provide rest, but do not leave unattended.
5. Do not give insulin.

Severe Reaction
1. Tachycardia.
2. Loss of consciousness.
3. Seizure activity.
4. Deep coma.
5. Decreased reflexes.

Action
1. Activate EMS, notify parent(s).
2. Administer glucagon as prescribed, intramuscularly or subcutaneously.

   F. Can be healthier than peers when following recommended diet and medical regimen and remaining alert to symptoms of illness and fatigue.
   G. Unable to participate in certain sports, which may be due primarily to parental concerns.
   H. Must check feet every day and be vigilant in looking for signs of bruising, infection, or other trauma to prevent secondary complications.
   I. Very little or no limitations on career or lifestyle when practicing proper self-care.
   J. Unable to enlist in armed forces.
VI. Management/Treatment
   A. School nurse responsibilities:
      1. Coordinate school plans with parents and HCP.

2. Develop IHCP for care of student that includes emergency action plan.
3. Develop and participate in student 504 Accommodation Plan; may use IHCP if accommodation plans are complete (see Chapter 9, Special Education).
4. Provide appropriate diabetic care and supervise health paraprofessional or designated trained adult.
5. Have trained back-up personnel available at all times.
6. Identify location of testing and insulin administration; follow district policy for safe disposal of equipment and supplies.
7. Make classroom adaptations to avoid penalizing students who require diabetic care.
8. Check availability of glucose supply and snack foods.
9. Educate teachers and staff regarding disease and emergency procedures; include computer, music, and physical education teachers, coaches, playground supervisors, bus drivers, and cafeteria workers.
10. Advise parents regarding field trips; make arrangements as needed.
11. Be aware of Nurse Practice Act and state and district educational mandates, since they vary regarding who can be taught and who can administer glucose or insulin injections.
12. Post generic emergency procedures for easy access and visibility.

B. Encourage need for personal medical identification alert.
C. Monitor anthropometry (height and weight). Any rapid changes in weight gain or loss may be in reaction to medications or poor control.
D. Assess teeth integrity and check for skin lesions.
E. Stress need for annual eye examination with funduscopic (red reflex) examination and cardiac and kidney function screenings.
F. Review vaccinations for annual influenza shot; needs at least a one-time pneumococcal vaccination.
G. Monitor carbohydrate intake and ensure consistent day-to-day eating; meals and snacks should be eaten within 1 hour of scheduled time; avoid excessive protein.
H. Be aware of drug interactions; many OTC medications contain glucose, alcohol, or glucose-neurogenic substances.
I. Encourage exercise, which improves glucose utilization, and give frequent praise to overcome negative feelings and inadequacies that arise regarding reporting of and treatment for negative glucose results.
J. Encourage involvement in sports, but be aware that hypoglycemic reactions can occur up to 12 hours after participating in an athletic event.
K. Be alert to classroom learning or behavioral difficulties; both hypoglycemia or hyperglycemia can affect learning.
L. Understand that inappropriate behavior can be misinterpreted as acting out (e.g., belligerent, defiant) but may be due to hypoglycemia; blood-level testing should be monitored before disciplinary action or discussion.

M. Adolescent-specific issues:
   1. Monitor closely for candidiasis; adolescents are prone to infection.
   2. Susceptible to hyperglycemia during menstruation.
   3. Eating disorders, such as bulimia and anorexia nervosa, can complicate diabetic management; adolescent may manipulate or withhold insulin to control body size.
   4. Pregnancy creates risks five times greater than for an adolescent without diabetes; use low-dose estrogen contraceptive because of complications with high doses of estrogen.
   5. Adolescent should be aware of blood glucose levels before driving.
   6. Push for independence and feelings of omnipotence and exceptionality promote greater risk-taking behaviors, which make diabetic control difficult.
N. Alcohol and drug use: Alcohol consumption inhibits the release of glycogen from the liver, causing hypoglycemia; the diabetic may be confused regarding the effects of alcohol and may self-treat with additional insulin rather than a sugary or food snack. In a party environment, a hypoglycemic state and intoxication could be confused. Cigarettes and stimulants can accelerate the complications of diabetes.
O. Insulin administration technology:
   1. *Insulin pens:* A cartridge of insulin is fitted into a penlike device. A special needle tip fits onto the end of the pen, and the dosage is dialed before giving. When the end of the pen is cocked and pressed, insulin is delivered. The needle is changed at every use. Cartridges hold 150 and 300 units. A variety of insulin pens are available. Some are completely disposable, whereas others have single dose or multidose cartridges. The insulin cartridges may or may not need refrigeration; check manufacturer's recommendations. Administration of insulin is faster and needles are sharper, because they do not go through a vial first. Children can become independent at an earlier age with this method.
   2. *Insulin pumps:* These provide a continuous subcutaneous infusion of insulin and are a bit larger than a credit card. Age for beginning use is about 10 years but is dependent on developmental level, motivation, and supportive network. The pump is computer programmed to deliver insulin from a syringe to a catheter to a needle placed in the subcutaneous tissues in the abdomen or thigh. The pump is worn on the belt or in a shoulder holster; the needle and catheter should be changed every 48 hours. After eating, a bolus can be given to cover food consumed. A pump can accurately deliver insulin in 0.1 unit increments.
      a. Advantages include consistent blood glucose level; reduced number of injections; improved control, flexibility, and convenience—child can sleep late without worrying about early morning hyperglycemia.
      b. Disadvantage is that if disconnected, individual can go into diabetic ketoacidosis (DKA); provide back-up insulin pen at school, during sports, and for bathing and intimate moments.

VII. Additional Information

A. Insulin effects vary with each preparation and from person to person, by injection site, activity, and physical or emotional well-being. Effects may vary in an individual from day to day. Absorption is faster and most reliable in the abdomen, followed by the arms and legs (see Table 4-6).

B. Injection sites include upper arms, thighs, buttocks, and abdomen. Sites are rotated to various areas of the body, with approximately four to five injections given in each area. Each injection is spaced about 1 in (2.5 cm) from the previous injection (see Figure 4-3).

C. *Lipodystrophy* is a complication of insulin administration. It is a localized manifestation of disordered fat metabolism and takes the form of hypertrophy or atrophy, which is prevented by systematically rotating insulin injection sites, administering insulin at room temperature, and pinching up the skin before injection to ensure that the insulin goes between the fat and muscle tissue.

1. *Hypertrophy* is a mass of fibrous scar tissue that can cause malabsorption of insulin.

2. *Atrophy* appears as dimpling and pitting of the skin and underlying tissue.

D. Future trends for insulin management:

1. *Inhaled insulin* technology converts large or small molecules into a fine-particle aerosol and delivers the insulin deep into the lungs, where it is rapidly absorbed. Advantage is more rapid peak insulin concentration than some injected insulins. Inhaled insulin is

Table 4-6	*Types of Insulin*			
Insulin		**Onset**	**Peak**	**Duration**
Rapid acting:		15-30 min	30-90 min	3-4 hr
aspart (Novalog)				
lispro (Humalog)				
Short acting:		30-60 min	2-3 hr	3-6 hr
regular (Novalin R,)				
(Velosulin for insulin pump)				
Intermediate acting:				
isophane suspension (NPH)		2-4 hr	6-10 hr	10-16 hr
zinc suspension (Lente)		3-4 hr	6-12 hr	12-18 hr
Long acting				
ultralente (Novolin U)		6-10 hr	10-16 hr	18-20 hr
glargine (Lantus)		5 hr	No peak	≥ 24 hr
detemir (Levemir)		1-2 hr	6-8 hr	Up to 24 hr
Mixtures				
NPH and regular (70/30)		30-60 min	2-4 hr	10-16 hr
NPH and insulin mixtures				
50/50		30-60 min	2-5 hr	10-16 hr

NPH, Neutral protamine Hagedorn (insulin).
Adapted from Skidmore-Roth L, editor: *2007 Mosby's Nursing Drug Reference*, 20th ed, 2007, St Louis, Mosby Elsevier.

Chronic Conditions

CHAPTER 4

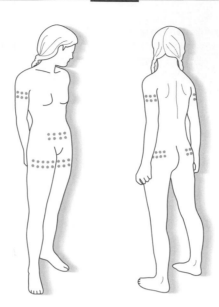

FIGURE 4-3 Rotation sites for insulin injection.

used before mealtimes, and peak values are attained within 5 to 60 minutes. In type 2 diabetes, inhaled insulin may be used alone or with oral preparations. Inhaled insulin will probably not eliminate the need for injectable insulin.

a. Advantages: rapid delivery and peak value without injection.

b. Disadvantage: partial loss of drug in the device, in the environment, or in the oral cavity.

c. Exubera was the first inhaled insulin approved by the FDA in 2006.

2. *Temporary glucose sensors:* Continuous blood glucose monitoring systems are used on a temporary basis to record frequent blood glucose levels throughout the day and night.

a. The GlucoWatch Biographer is worn like a watch. A transdermal pad is next to the skin on the wrist, which induces sweating, displaying the blood glucose level on the face of what looks like a watch.

b. The Continuous Glucose Monitoring System (CGMS) is used by the HCP to obtain frequent readings to assess the patient's condition. It is inserted under the skin in the abdomen and records 288 readings in 3 days.

c. Several other devices are being researched, all of which determine blood glucose level by measuring the concentration in the interstitial fluid, the clear fluid under the skin. These devices provide continuous blood glucose monitoring and have alarms to alert for hypoglycemia or hyperglycemia.

3. New treatments for diabetes include islet and pancreas transplantation, which have been successful in some adults but are not recommended in children or adolescents. Cell-based therapy,

gene therapy, and drug therapy to advance beta-cell growth are being researched as possible cures for diabetes (see Box 4-5).

DIABETES MELLITUS: TYPE 2

I. Definition and Etiology

A. Previously referred to as *non–insulin-dependent diabetes mellitus,* type 2 diabetes is most often found in adults. This disorder is increasing in the adolescent population secondary to obesity and a sedentary life style. Type 2 diabetes includes those with insulin resistance, a pancreatic disease resulting in decreased insulin secretion; hormonal changes; genetic predisposition; impaired glucose tolerance; gestational diabetes mellitus; or adverse effects of drugs. Of the diagnosed diabetic children and adolescents, 8% to 45% are type 2 (Kaufman, 2005).

B. Contributing to the increase in child and adolescent diabetes is a combination of environmental and genetic factors. Environmental factors are poor diet, weight gain, physical inactivity, and a family history of diabetes. Type 2 diabetes is more common in Native Americans, African-Americans, and Hispanic/Latino Americans. Symptoms include obesity with little or no weight loss, mild or no polyuria, polydipsia, glycosuria without ketonuria, and acanthosis nigricans (60% to 90%; see color plate 6). Nurses should counsel staff, high-risk students, and others regarding development of type 2 diabetes and prevention strategies.

C. Can often be controlled or prevented by managing weight, blood pressure, and blood lipid levels through exercise and diet, but may require oral medication if not successful. Some will require insulin, especially when first diagnosed. Some medications for children have been approved by the FDA; metformin (Glucophage) is often used, which decreases hepatic glucose production and increases sensitivity to insulin.

WEB SITES

American Diabetes Association
http://www.diabetes.org
Centers for Disease Control and Prevention: Diabetes Public Health Resource
http://www.cdc.gov/diabetes
Juvenile Diabetes Research Foundation International
http://www.jdrf.org
National Diabetes Education Program
http://www.ndep.nih.gov
National Institute of Diabetes and Digestive and Kidney Diseases
http://www.niddk.nih.gov

Box 4-5	*Current Diabetic Research Focus*

- Islet cell or pancreatic transplantation
- Cell therapy and beta cell development
- Laser technology
- Genetic research

CHAPTER 4   Chronic Conditions

DOWN SYNDROME

I. Definition

A. Down syndrome is a genetic disorder in which proper cell division does not occur. It is the most common chromosomal abnormality that causes mild to moderate mental retardation and medical problems. It is sometimes erroneously called *mongolism.*

II. Etiology

A. Normally, an individual has 46 chromosomes in each cell body, 23 from each parent. The 46 chromosomes are in pairs of 23 and are numbered 1 to 23. An individual with Down syndrome almost always has 47 chromosomes in each cell, 23 from one parent and 24 from the other parent; the extra genetic material is responsible for the syndrome's characteristics. There are three types of Down syndrome: *trisomy 21 (nondisjunction), mosaic,* and *translocation.*

B. Down syndrome affects approximately 1 in 800 live births in the United States (Levy and Marion, 2006). The chances for an error in chromosome division increases with maternal age; at age 25 the incidence is 1:1250, but at age 40 it is 1:100 (NIH, 2007). However, the majority of affected infants are born to women under age 35. This may be explained by prenatal detection being more common for women over 35 and the birth rate being higher in younger woman.

C. Approximately 95% of children with Down syndrome display *trisomy 21,* which is caused by failure of the cells to divide properly during meiosis. There is an extra chromosome with the twenty-first pair of the numbered chromosome, making three in that group. The normal egg has 23 chromosomes, and when combined with a normal sperm, it has 46 chromosomes. When a meiotic nondisjunction event occurs, it results in 47 chromosomes. This type is more common in boys and is not inherited.

D. In *mosaic Down syndrome* there is a combination; some cells have the normal number of chromosomes, and other cells have an extra chromosome 21. The individual will have the normal number of chromosomes (46) in some cells but will have 47 chromosomes in other cells. The error in cell division occurs spontaneously after normal division has begun, and the range of involvement depends on the number of cells with the additional chromosome 21. This type is nonhereditary and is the cause of 2% to 3% of the observed Down syndrome children.

E. *Translocation Down syndrome* occurs during meiosis and is caused by a defect in chromosomal structure rather than an error in cell division. The twenty-first chromosome attaches or translocates to another chromosome 21, generally the fourteenth. This form of Down syndrome results in features of Down syndrome and may be inherited from a parent carrier. It occurs more frequently in children of younger parents and occurs more often in girls. With the translocation type, the chances of having a second child with Down syndrome is 10% if the carrier is the mother and 2% if the carrier is the father.

III. Characteristics

A. No individual with Down syndrome has all the physical characteristics or same degree of mental retardation, which may range from low-average intelligence to severe mental retardation.

B. Trisomy 21 and translocation Down syndrome present the same physical characteristics.

C. Individuals with mosaic trisomy 21 may have less noticeable physical features and higher intelligence than the other two types, because they have a number of normal cells.

D. Physical characteristics:

1. Head:
   a. Head is generally small and round with flattened occiput.
   b. Brachycephaly.
   c. Separated sagittal suture and enlarged anterior fontanel.
   d. Sparse hair.
   e. Hypoplasia of midfacial bones with small, flattened nose.
   f. Undersized maxilla, short palate, and narrowed nasopharynx.
   g. Susceptible to obstructive sleep apnea; large, protruding tongue observed at birth.
   h. Chronic rhinitis.
   i. Teeth erupt late, some may never erupt.
   j. Voice somewhat husky; has delayed speech and poor articulation.

2. Eyes/vision:
   a. Brushfield's spots (no clinical significance); hypoplasia of the iris.
   b. Eyes tend to slant upward (98%) and are almond shaped with epicanthal folds, narrow palpebral fissures, and increased incidence of glaucoma.
   c. Blepharitis and blocked tear ducts.
   d. Strabismus, pseudostrabismus, nystagmus, cataracts, astigmatism and refractive errors.

3. Ears/hearing:
   a. Small, low-set ears with folded helix (margin of external ear).
   b. Narrow canals with cerumen impaction common.
   c. Susceptible to middle-ear fluid and ear infections.
   d. Conductive, sensorineural, or mixed hearing loss.

4. Musculoskeletal:
   a. Moro reflex absent in newborn.
   b. Hypotonia common in newborn but improves with age.
   c. Short, broad neck with loose skin at nape.
   d. Little fingers are curved inward; small, short, and broad hands, digits, and feet; clinodactyly.
   e. Palms have single transverse crease called a *simian line.*
   f. Wide space between first and second toes; deep vertical crease on sole that runs between these two toes.
   g. Shorter than average.
   h. Atlantoaxial instability (AAI), which is an increased distance between cervical vertebrae 1 and 2 that may predispose the individual to C1–C2 dislocation or other injury (Levy and Marion, 2006).

       i. Hyperflexibility or an extreme ability to extend joints.

       j. Patellar dislocation; hip subluxation.

   5. Sexual:

      a. Male sex organs poorly developed.

      b. Females often have enlarged labia majora and clitoris and small breasts; pelvic bone is wide, flattened, and smaller.

      c. In boys, sperm count is decreased and they are sterile; in girls, menarche usually occurs in normal age range; recorded incidence of pregnancy is low; offspring have high risk of some abnormality.

   6. Structural manifestations:

      a. Congenital heart defects (40%) especially septal defects (Levy and Marion, 2006).

      b. Tracheoesophageal fistula; esophageal atresia.

      c. Renal agenesis.

      d. Duodenal atresia or obstruction.

   7. Other characteristics:

      a. Prone to respiratory infections.

      b. Thyroid dysfunction (20%); celiac disease; gastrointestinal tract anomalies.

      c. Increased incidence of autoimmune disorders.

      d. Increased risk of developing acute leukemia.

      e. Failure to thrive common in infancy; obesity may occur in adolescence.

IV. Health Concerns/Emergencies

   A. Children with congenital heart defects require close observation and care:

      1. Watch for respiratory distress, cyanosis, failure to thrive, or signs of congestive heart failure.

      2. Children on digitalis may need their pulse rate monitored daily.

      3. When necessary, obtain instructions from physician for any restrictions on activity.

      4. Cardiac defects may be asymptomatic, especially atrioventricular defects. Monitor closely for fatigue and failure to thrive, which may be subtle indicators.

   B. Tendency toward frequent otitis media and middle-ear fluid necessitates frequent otological examinations and audiological and impedance audiometry screenings, along with referrals as necessary.

   C. Hearing loss is common, and hearing aids may be necessary; 70% to 80% have hearing deficits, and risk persists through adulthood.

   D. Upper respiratory tract infections may easily progress to involvement of bronchi and lungs.

   E. Susceptible to obstructive sleep apnea.

   F. Chronic constipation is common; consider Hirschsprung's disease.

V. Effects on Individual

   A. Hearing loss caused by frequent otitis media will affect language acquisition, emotional and social development, and educational progress.

   B. Surgical intervention for cardiac anomalies can be a frightening experience.

   C. May be isolated from others because of parents' fears of social rejection.

D. In adolescence, the person's desire for independence may not be fulfilled, since parents may view the individual as a child.

E. Parents may deny the individual's sexual maturation, which can cause inappropriate behavior and additional social isolation.

F. Predisposition to premature aging; more susceptible to diseases associated with older adults.

G. Self-image and self-worth can be affected if relationship between the parents, caregiver, and child is not positive.

VI. Management/Treatment

A. Monitor hearing every 6 months until age 3 and annually thereafter.

B. Evaluate vision by 6 months of age and annually thereafter.

C. Monitor height and weight using Down syndrome charts and body mass index (BMI; see Appendix B).

D. Periodic otoscopic examination for children who tend to develop cerumen impaction.

E. Mucus may have to be cleared from nose with bulb syringe because small, depressed nasal passages impede drainage.

F. Myringotomy tubes may be placed; take precautions to ensure that fluid does not enter into middle ear by using earplugs during showering, swimming, or water play.

G. Testing of thyroid function annually. Risk of hypothyroidism increases with age.

H. Radiographic screening for AAI is recommended between 3 and 5 years of age and before participation in sports, physically active exercise, or surgical procedures. Avoid activities involving strain or stress on the neck (e.g., somersaults) until AAI is ruled out.

I. Celiac disease screening between 2 and 3 years of age. Treatment is gluten-free diet.

J. Cardiology evaluation in adolescence for possible valvular disease.

VII. Additional Information

A. For *prenatal diagnosis* there are several screening methods and diagnostic tests. The American College of Obstetricians and Gynecologists recommend first-trimester screening for all pregnant women. The use of nuchal translucency (NT), an ultrasound exam that measures the thickness at the back of the neck of the fetus, and a blood test are an effective screening tool in the general population. Women with an increased risk of having a baby with Down syndrome should be offered further counseling and diagnostic testing. Amniocentesis is frequently recommended for women aged 35 or older at about 12 to 20 weeks gestation. Chorionic villus sampling (CVS) is done between 8 and 12 weeks of pregnancy. Percutaneous umbilical blood sampling (PUBS) is performed during the eighteenth to twenty-second weeks of pregnancy. All of these tests are associated with the risk of miscarriage. Complete genetic counseling should be obtained along with a discussion of family history relative to the benefits and risks of pursuing diagnostic procedures (NIH, 2007).

B. *Postnatal diagnosis:* during the physical examination, the examiner notes signs commonly associated with the syndrome, extent of muscle hypotonia, any congenital defects, and adjustment of the infant to extrauterine life. Chromosome analysis confirms diagnosis.

C. Developmental screening should begin as soon as possible and is necessary for planning and implementing special programs. The child with Down syndrome needs an early intervention program best suited to their individual needs with emphasis on language and speech development and large and small muscle stimulation.

D. Development is frequently close to normal during the first 6 months of the child's life, causing parents to question the diagnosis. Affected individuals can vary widely in intellectual functioning; the majority are moderately retarded, whereas others may be borderline or severely retarded. A child with mosaic Down syndrome can have higher intellectual ability, because there are some normal cells as well as some misdivided cells.

E. Approximately 10% of individuals with Down syndrome have AAI, which is generally asymptomatic (Levy and Marion, 2006). When symptomatic, there is risk of cord compression. Symptoms include deteriorating ambulatory skills, changes in bowel or bladder function, weakness in any of the extremities, limited neck movement, neck pain or weakness, changes in neck posturing, and neurological signs (e.g., hypertonicity, clonus of the ankles, hyperreflexia, extensor responses). Surgery may be required.

F. Increased incidence of autoimmune thyroid disease; symptoms may be subtle; mood changes, depression, abnormal menstrual cycles, and worsening of dry skin.

G. Alternative and complementary medicines are sought by some parents and may include nutritional supplements or megavitamins, cell therapy, growth hormone, acupuncture, homeopathy, chiropractic manipulation, patterning, or surgery for relief of midfacial hypoplasia for cosmetic reasons and for facilitated communication.

H. Life expectancy has increased from 25 years in 1983 to 49 years in 1997 (Yang, Rasmussen, and Friedman, 2002).

WEB SITES

Down Syndrome: Health Issues
    http://www.ds-health.com
National Association for Down Syndrome
    http://www.nads.org
National Down Syndrome Society
    http://www.ndss.org

EATING DISORDERS

I. Definition

A. *Anorexia nervosa:* Restriction of food intake as weight falls below minimal normal body weight for age and height due to a fear of fatness and a compulsion to be thin (see Box 4-6).

B. *Bulimia nervosa:* Patterns of binge eating exist while individual continues to manifest concern with body weight and shape. Overeating and the fear of gaining weight are followed with purging by forced vomiting, fasting, laxative or diuretic use, or excessive exercise (see Box 4-7).

Box 4-6   *DSM-IV Criteria: Anorexia Nervosa*

1. Refusal to maintain body weight at or above a minimally normal weight for age and height (i.e., weight loss leading to maintenance of body weight < 85% of that expected); or failure to make expected weight gain during period of growth, leading to body weight < 85% of that expected.
2. Intense fear of gaining weight or becoming fat, even though underweight.
3. Disturbance in the way in which one's body weight or shape is experienced, undue influence of body weight or shape on self-evaluation, or denial of the seriousness of the current low body weight.
4. In postmenarchal females, amenorrhea (i.e., the absence of at least three consecutive menstrual cycles).

From American Psychiatric Association: *Diagnostic and statistical manual of mental disorders,* ed 4, text revision, Washington, DC, 2000, American Psychiatric Association.

Box 4-7   *DSM-IV Criteria: Bulimia Nervosa*

1. Recurrent episodes of binge eating, characterized by both of the following: (a) eating an unusually large amount of food in a discrete period (within 2 hours) and (b) a sense of lack of control over eating during the episode.
2. Recurrent inappropriate compensatory behavior to prevent weight gain (e.g., self-induced vomiting; misuse of laxatives, diuretics, enemas, or other medications; fasting; excessive exercise).
3. Binge eating and compensatory behaviors both occur on average twice a week for 3 months.
4. Self-evaluation is unduly influenced by body shape and weight.
5. The disturbance does not occur exclusively during episodes of anorexia nervosa.

From American Psychiatric Association: *Diagnostic and statistical manual of mental disorders,* ed 4, text revision, Washington, DC, 2000, American Psychiatric Association.

1. Prevalence in the United States for teenage girls is approximately 1.5% for anorexia and 1% to 3% for bulimia. Prevalence for both anorexia and bulimia among boys is about one-tenth that of girls (APA, 2000). Between 10% to 25% of female adolescents have some disorganized eating habits characterized by binge eating or purging.
2. Anorexia and bulimia in boys occurs most frequently when competing in sports with weight limitations, such as wrestling.
3. Age of onset for anorexia is bimodal; it peaks at ages 13 to 14 and 17 to 18 years; childhood onset is reported between ages 7 to 11 years. Onset of bulimia appears to occur during middle to late adolescence.
4. Eating disorders affect all socioeconomic and racial-ethnic groups.

II. Etiology

A. May involve biological, nutritional, psychological, and sociocultural factors. There is a disturbance in the way the shape or weight of the body is perceived.

1. Eating disorders tend to run in families. Anorexia and bulimia are three times more common in relatives of eating-disordered individuals than in the general U.S. population.

B. Risk factors include dieting, obesity, family history of eating disorders, groups placing value on thinness (e.g., models, ballet dancers, figure skaters, gymnasts). Certain personal characteristics also create an increased risk; these include low self-esteem, rigidity, compliance, dependency, competitiveness, impulsiveness, perfectionism, difficulty with boundaries, and self-regulation.
  1. Comorbidity with psychiatric disorders is common and includes depression; with anorexia, social phobic, simple phobic, and obsessive-compulsive disorders are often seen; with bulimia, anxiety disorders and substance abuse.
C. American culture and other Western societies emphasize thinness, with role models observed on television and in movies, newspapers, and magazines, as well as in families. During adolescence, girls are more conscious of their bodies and are more prone to diets and restrictive food intake.

Brain Findings

Both disorders have abnormalities in the noradrenergic, dopamine, and serotonin systems of the brain that normalize with weight gain. This finding may explain why serotonin reuptake inhibitors are beneficial.

III. Characteristics
A. Trigger factors include sexual abuse, traumatic loss, chronic dieting, family difficulties, peer pressure, sensitivity to teasing about body size and shape, and demands on performance from family and school staff.
B. Feeling a lack of control over eating.
C. Low frustration tolerance, poor self-esteem, suppressed anger, rebellion, hostility, and depression.
D. Binge eating–purging cycles or not purging with rigorous dieting, fasting, or rigorous exercise.
E. Anorexics are usually model children, obsessive-compulsive, high achievers who deny illness; they usually are not sexually active.
F. Bulimics often act out, are impulsive, lose self-control, fluctuate in school performance; they are aware of their illness, and they may be sexually active (see Table 4-7).

IV. Health Concerns/Emergencies
A. Death related to cardiac arrhythmia, hypokalemia, suicide.
B. Osteoporosis.
C. Alcohol and drug abuse or addictions.
D. Growth retardation.
E. Dehydration.
F. Gynecological difficulties associated with prolonged amenorrhea.

V. Effects on Individual
A. Fatigue, weakness, and poor wound healing.
B. Cold hands or feet and thinning hair.
C. Bloated stomach.
D. Headaches.
E. Dental problems include damage to enamel and decay secondary to vomiting.

Table 4-7	*Associated Symptoms of Eating Disorders*	
Body System	**Anorexia Nervosa**	**Bulimia Nervosa**
General concerns	Excessively underweight Irritability, dizziness, syncope, confusion, sleep difficulties Lethargy, hyperactivity Hypothermia Amenorrhea, malnutrition Decreased growth parameters	Usually normal weight, or ranges from obese to extremely underweight Weakness, fatigue Irregular menses
Sensory system	Decreased concentration, drowsy, irritable, confused	—
Vital signs	Decreased temperature, pulse, blood pressure, and respiration	—
Dermatological	Hair dry, brittle, dull or hair loss, lanugo on body Skin dry, rough, yellowish or grayish, cracked	Ulcerations, scars/calluses on back of hand Skin dry, cracked, rough; sores on mucous membranes in mouth and around fingernails Face edema, broken blood vessels
Extremities	Peripheral edema of feet/ hands	Edema of feet and sometimes hands
Oral	—	Enamel erosion or discoloration of teeth, dental caries, parotid gland hypertrophy
Cardiovascular	Bradycardia, hypertension	Arrhythmia
Genitourinary	Thin, dry, pale, atrophic vaginal mucosa	—
Gastrointestinal	Decreased bowel sounds, constipation	Abdominal distension, epigastric tenderness, GER, diarrhea, or constipation
Musculoskeletal	Decrease in bone mass (osteopenia), fractures	—
Neuromuscular	Muscle wasting/weakness Decreased deep tendon reflexes and decreased mass and definition, weakness	Muscle wasting/weakness with chronic use of ipecac

GER, Gastroesophageal reflux.
Individuals with both disorders can exhibit signs and symptoms of both diseases.

CHAPTER 4

Chronic Conditions

    F. Guilt, depression, and anxiety regarding binge-eating behavior.
    G. Teasing, personal rejection by family or peers, and social stigma.
    H. Family stress.
VI. Management/Treatment
    A. Detailed history needs to be taken with student and must include:
       1. Weight and dietary intake.

2. Issues around being fat or thin.
3. Perception of body image.
4. Diet methods used.
5. Exercise regimen.
6. History of binging and purging.
7. Symptoms or diagnosis of psychiatric disorders.
8. Abuse of drugs or alcohol.

B. Management and treatment depend on the history, stage of illness, diagnosis of one or both eating disorders, presence of affective disorder or substance abuse, level of family support, and other indicators for referral and treatment. Many schools have nurses, counselors, or other individuals who are trained to work with the student population for at-school supplemental counseling.

C. Referrals for physical examination, clinical assessment, nutritional counseling, individual and group psychotherapy, and family therapy. May require hospitalization for stabilization of electrolyte imbalance and nutrient intake, supplements, and medications that may include antidepressants, metoclopramide, estrogen, progesterone, and minerals such as calcium, phosphate, zinc, potassium, iron.

D. Support students with empathetic listening, and express your acceptance of them. Focus discussion on body movement, performance, health, and nutrition rather than on what the body looks like. Express the respect you have for the student's ability to make wise choices.

E. Promote prevention by discussion in classrooms on healthy eating and the necessity of exercise suitable for individual students. Enlist support of coaches in promotion of healthy lifestyles with less emphasis on weight.

WEB SITES

National Eating Disorders Association
  http://www.nationaleatingdisorders.org
Girl Power
  http://www.girlpower.gov/girlarea/bodywise/eatingdisorders
Harris Center Massachusetts General Hospital
  http://www.harriscentermgh.org
National Association of Anorexia Nervosa and Associated Disorders (ANAD)
  http://www.anad.org

ENCOPRESIS (CHRONIC CONSTIPATION/RETENTION)

I. Definition

A. Encopresis is involuntary fecal soiling by a child beyond the usual age for toilet training. *Primary encopresis* is when a child has never achieved bowel control, and *secondary encopresis* occurs after bowel control has been established. The two subtypes of encopresis are with or without constipation and overflow incontinence. Organic pathology or illness is not present.

II. Etiology

A. Encopresis is believed to be psychogenic and/or physiological. It is associated with chronic constipation, fecal impaction, and overflow incontinence in about three fourths of cases and may progress to an enlarged colon. One cause may be the conscious or unconscious manipulation of the environment. Another cause is *chronic diarrhea* or *irritable bowel syndrome* in which the child is incontinent as an apparent reaction to stress or emotional upset.

    1. Before age 4, chronic constipation occurs equally in boys and girls. In school-age children, encopresis affects approximately 1% to 3% of children and is three to six times more common in boys (Christopherson and Friman, 2004).

III. Characteristics

  A. More prevalent in males; often unreported because of family embarrassment.

  B. Often precipitated by upsetting or stressful event.

  C. Retention of stool continues for days or weeks.

  D. Frequent refusal to defecate in the toilet.

  E. Often defecates in supine or standing position.

  F. Abdominal pain.

  G. Palpable abdominal fecal mass.

  H. Poor appetite and lethargy.

   I. Most accidents take place during the day.

  J. Frequent presence of fecal odor.

  K. Retentive posturing.

  L. Organic factors have been explored and ruled out.

  M. History of straining, constipation, and intervention with laxatives and enemas.

IV. Health Concerns/Emergencies

  A. Organic factors need to be ruled out.

  B. Chronic megacolon from constipation.

  C. Anorexia.

  D. Lesions or perianal dermatitis may cause child to withhold stool.

  E. Fever and headache.

  F. Superficial fissures with bleeding may develop because of passage of large stool.

  G. Urinary tract infections and disease from obstruction of urinary tract are serious complications of chronic fecal retention; however, this rarely occurs.

  H. Ulceration with significant rectal hemorrhage is a possible complication of constipation but uncommon.

V. Effects on Individual

  A. Irritable and avoids play.

  B. Embarrassed by soiling and fecal odor.

  C. Attempts to deny the problem exists.

  D. Abdominal discomfort and pain.

  E. Passage of a gigantic stool causes physical discomfort and fear.

  F. Detects disapproval of parents and peers; may affect self-esteem.

  G. Recipient of parental anger because of repeatedly clogged toilets and soiled clothing.

  H. May not want to attend school because of social difficulties that soiling may cause.

VI. Management/Treatment

  A. Listen to student to evaluate need for medical referral or psychological counseling.

  B. Contact with parents and home visit when possible to lend support and educate regarding relationship between toileting and nutritional management.
  C. Enemas, suppositories, or laxatives may be prescribed to clean out the colon with continued use of laxatives or stool softeners until bowel habits are established.
  D. Mineral oil may be used as a gentle laxative; however, nurse should educate parents regarding its use. Mineral oil retards absorption of fat-soluble vitamins; thus it should be administered 1 to 2 hours after meals or at bedtime.
  E. Use behavioral techniques (e.g., stickers on a chart or simple rewards) or biofeedback to teach child how to correctly use abdominal, pelvic, and sphincter muscles for toileting.

VII. Additional Information
  A. Referral to a psychologist or psychiatrist may be the only means toward improvement. The nurse may be able to alleviate parental anxiety by explaining that the following common fears have little or no scientific basis:
   1. The colon ruptures if it accumulates too much stool.
   2. Retained waste substances will cause a toxic state; headache is directly caused by retention.
   3. A dilated rectosigmoid impedes defecation.
   4. The temporary anorexia preceding massive evacuation causes nutritional damage.

ENURESIS

I. Definition
  A. Enuresis is persistence of intentional or involuntary urination in the bed or clothing by a child beyond the age of being toilet trained. Primary enuresis is when control was never established, and secondary enuresis is present when child has been continent for at least 1 year. Nocturnal enuresis is voiding only at night, whereas diurnal enuresis is voiding while awake.
   1. Diagnosis is made when frequency of enuresis is twice a week for at least 3 consecutive months, or there is significant clinical distress or impairment in important functional areas of the child's life because of the incontinence.

II. Etiology
  A. Enuresis may be caused by an organic disorder, an emotional disturbance, or developmental delay. Organic causes include structural disorder of the urinary tract, neurological deficits, infection, diabetes, spastic bladder, epilepsy, sickle cell anemia, food allergies, or chronic renal failure. Emotional disturbances also account for only a relatively small percentage of the problem. In most situations, the etiology is unknown.
  B. There is a genetic predisposition for enuresis; approximately 75% of children with enuresis have a first degree relative with the disorder. Enuresis prevalence at age 5 years is 5% to 10%, at age 10 it is 3% to 5%, and it falls to 1% for individuals over age 15 (American Psychiatric Association, 2000).

III. Characteristics
  A. More common in boys than in girls.
  B. Family history of enuresis.
  C. Child may sleep more soundly than other children.
  D. Child has smaller functional bladder capacity.
  E. May have an abnormal level of antidiuretic hormone (ADH).
  F. Most cases spontaneously resolve by adolescence (Gahagan, 2006).

IV. Health Concerns/Emergencies
  A. Organic cause needs to be ruled out.
  B. Be aware of dosage and drug side effects, since antidepressants are most popular form of treatment, and children are more sensitive than adults to medication.
  C. Be alert to punitive techniques of control that may be used in the home.

V. Effects on Individual
  A. Suffers disapproval of parents and ridicule of peers, and self-esteem may be affected.
  B. May experience side effects of medications.
  C. If diurnal wetting occurs, the child may resist going to school because of embarrassment.

VI. Management/Treatment
  A. Management depends on an understanding of underlying causative factors: physical, psychosocial, or both.
  B. Physical examination will determine whether organic or inorganic cause and lead to recommendations for treatment.
  C. History and a chart indicating date, time of incidents, and estimated volume may be helpful in diagnosis.
  D. Screening for emotional or behavioral problems can be done using Achenbach Child Behavior Checklist or Behavioral Assessment System for Children (see Appendix A).
  E. Types of treatment and control:
    1. Bladder training.
    2. Withholding or restricting fluids after the evening meal.
    3. Waking child during night to void.
    4. Psychotherapy, hypnotherapy, and behavioral techniques.
    5. Conditioning devices: bell and pad—wire pad is attached to a bell, buzzer, or occasionally a light; when urine touches the pad, buzzer is activated, waking child to go to the bathroom; child then resets equipment and goes back to bed. Initial success rate of 70% with relapse rate of 10% (Gahagan, 2006).
  F. Medications used include antidiuretics, tricyclic antidepressants, and anticholinergics.
  G. Desmopressin (DDAVP) is a fast-acting antidiuretic administered at bedtime that may be useful for overnights and other special occasions, but the relapse rate is high when medication is discontinued.
  H. Imipramine (Tofranil) is an antidepressant given to control enuresis; dosage should not exceed 2.5 mg/kg given daily, 1 hour before bedtime. Side effects are potentially serious and overdose may be fatal (cardiac arrhythmia). Relapse rate is 90% when medication is discontinued (Gahagan, 2006).

I. Anticholinergic drugs, such as oxybutynin (Ditropan) or hyoscyamine (Levsinex), reduce or stop bladder contractions and increase bladder capacity. Anticholinergics may be helpful for children who have daytime wetting due to bladder contractions or small bladder capacity.

J. If on medication, be aware of side effects.

K. Be supportive and educate the child, family, and school staff regarding this phenomenon.

VII. Additional Information

A. A child is considered enuretic if daytime wetting occurs beyond the chronological or mental age of 5 (APA 2000). Most clinicians diagnose nocturnal enuresis if the child has a problem at age 4 or 5, but others say 6 or 7 or older.

WEB SITE

National Kidney Foundation
http://www.kidney.org/patients/bedwet.cfm

FETAL ALCOHOL SYNDROME AND EFFECTS

I. Definition

A. *Fetal alcohol syndrome (FAS)* is used to describe a pattern of physical and mental birth defects. It is defined by three criteria: a characteristic pattern of facial abnormalities, growth retardation, and brain damage. Maternal alcohol use during pregnancy may or may not be established.

B. The term *alcohol-related neurodevelopmental disorder (ARND)* is used when signs of brain damage appear after fetal alcohol exposure without other indications of FAS. Those affected may have some or no facial anomalies and may exhibit difficulties in mental development and behavioral difficulties that impact learning and long-term development. The symptoms often are not apparent until in a school setting, and they vary in severity. Also referred to as *fetal alcohol effects (FAE)* and *alcohol-related birth defects (ARBD)*. Fetal Alcohol Spectrum Disorder (FASD) is an umbrella term that includes the whole range of effects.

II. Etiology

A. The syndrome is found in children whose mothers consumed alcohol during pregnancy. Alcohol is a teratogen that interferes with the ability of the fetus to receive adequate oxygen and nourishment for normal brain and body structural cell development. Prenatal alcohol exposure is the known leading preventable cause of mental retardation in the United States. Prevalence of FAS is 1 to 2 per 1000 live births (Jones, 2006). The wider spectrum of children affected by fetal alcohol exposure is thought to be ten times that of FAS (Ridgeway and Clarren, 2005).

Brain Findings

Magnetic resonance imaging (MRI) studies demonstrate reduced overall brain size and structural or functional changes in the brain, which are reflected in behavioral and cognitive impairments in those with FAS.

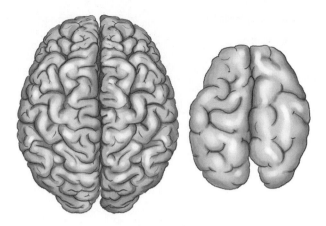

FIGURE 4-4 **A,** Normal brain. **B,** fetal alcohol brain.

Decreased size of the cerebellum is noted, which is associated with balance, coordination, gait, and cognition. The changes noted in the basal ganglia can impair spatial memory and set-shifting (state rigidity) in animals and are known to impair cognitive processes in humans. The corpus callosum, which is a major communication link between the right and left hemispheres of the brain, is either absent or development is impaired (National Institute on Alcohol Abuse and Alcoholism, 2000; see Figure 4-4).

III. Characteristics
    A. Facial (see Figure 4-5).
        1. Microcephaly.
        2. Short palpebral fissures, microphthalmia, hypertelorism, and ptosis.
        3. Epicanthal folds.
        4. Flattened midface.
        5. Low-set or poorly formed ears.
        6. Low nasal bridge; short, upturned nose.
        7. Hypoplastic philtrum.
        8. Smooth and thin upper lip.
        9. Small mouth with high-arched palate.
       10. Micrognathia or prognathia in adolescence.
       11. Some facial features may diminish in adolescence.
    B. Growth retardation.
        1. Birth head (BH) size average 33 cm (normal full-term BH average 35 cm).
        2. Birth weight (BW) average 6 lb (normal full-term BW average 7 lb, 8 oz).
        3. Growth deficiencies usually continue postnatally.
    C. Neurological.
        1. Microcephaly, defined as decreased head size and growth.
        2. Mental retardation; average IQ is 65, but ranges from 20 to 120.
        3. Motor retardation and poor coordination of body, hands, and fingers.

Chronic Conditions

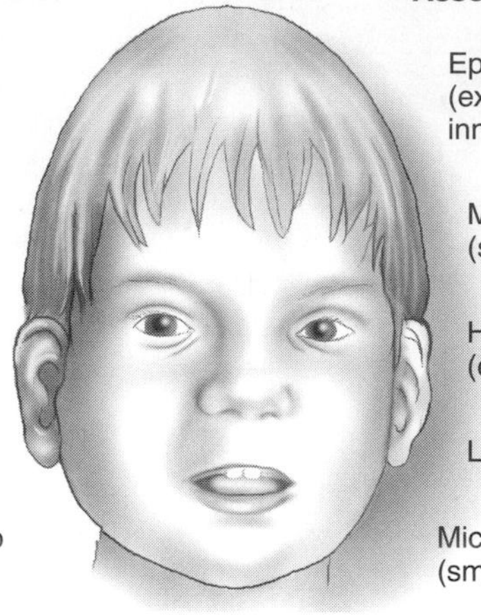

Discriminating features

Microcephaly
(small head circumference)

Low nasal bridge

Flat midface

Short palpebral fissures
(small eye openings)

Hypoplastic philtrum
(absent or
underdeveloped groove)

Thin upper lip

Associated features

Epicanthal fold
(extra skin fold at
inner angle of eye)

Micropthalmia
(small eyes)

Hypertelorism
(eyes wide set)

Low set ears

Micrognathia
(small jaw/chin)

FIGURE 4-5 Fetal alcohol syndrome features.

    4. Hypotonia.
    5. Hyperactivity.
    6. Hearing disorder.
  D. Other.
    1. Cardiac defects, including ventricular septal defect (VSD) or atrial septal defect (ASD).
    2. Kidney abnormalities: hydronephrosis, horseshoe kidneys.
    3. Urinary defects.
    4. Increased risk of hearing loss, eighth nerve deafness, and ear infections. Ears and kidneys form during the same time in utero, stressing the importance of diagnostic procedures of kidneys when ear anomalies are found.
    5. Small teeth with enamel hypoplasia, malocclusion.
    6. Myopia (nearsighted).
  E. FAS and ARND cognitive and behavioral impairments.
    1. Attention: able to focus and maintain attention but display difficulty in shifting attention from one task to another; set shifting (transitioning).
    2. Executive functioning: perseveration, distractibility, and impulsivity contribute to attention and learning problems.
    3. Verbal learning: language and memory difficulties; may have difficulty learning words (encoding, which is an initial stage of memory formation), but once a task is learned, they can recall the information.
    4. Visuospatial learning: demonstrate poor performance on tasks that involve learning spatial relationship of objects.
    5. Reaction time: affected school-age children often exhibit slower, less-efficient processing of information.

IV. Health Concerns/Emergencies
   A. Severity of health problems varies according to extent of involvement.
   B. Birth anomalies may be present that require additional care and medical intervention.
   C. Ethanol effects transferred through breast milk can produce motor delays in the baby and decrease prolactin hormone secretion, which is essential to maintain adequate lactation.
   D. Birth parents may be alcoholic, and child is at risk for neglect and physical and emotional abuse.
   E. Lifelong health and learning disabilities may exist.

V. Effects on Individual
   A. Frequently in out-of-home placement; some have multiple placements, which can impair bonding and attachment, impact educational achievement, and interfere with peer relationships.
   B. Often petite and short, which can be especially detrimental for boys.
   C. May have feelings of academic inadequacies because of learning problems.
   D. May have poor school performance, even with normal IQ.
   E. May be self-conscious because of facial features.
   F. Often oversensitive to the environment, light, sound, touch, and in need of sensory integration.
   G. At risk for becoming alcoholic.
   H. When adopted or in a consistent placement at an early age, prognosis may improve.

VI. Management/Treatment
   A. Early identification is imperative for intervention to be most effective.
   B. Provide prompts and cues to facilitate transitioning.
   C. Monitor anthropometry.
   D. Monitor dental health, encourage good oral hygiene and frequent check-ups, and pursue fluoride sealant.
   E. Encourage fluids, and be alert for signs of possible urinary tract infection.
   F. Needs referral for special resources when having difficulty in academic achievement.
   G. Contact receiving school nurse when student changes schools due to parental transfer or multiple home placements to update health and educational concerns, provide smooth and consistent transition, and avoid gaps in services.

VII. Additional Information
   A. The embryonic period, the first 2 to 8 weeks of gestation, is a time of great vulnerability to teratogenic effects of alcohol as evidenced by the structural symptoms of FAS. There are data that cessation of drinking in the third trimester, which is also a critical stage for brain development, can improve fetal outcome and minimize prenatal growth retardation. Some studies suggest binge drinking can be more dangerous to the fetus than drinking smaller amounts more frequently.

WEB SITES

National Institute on Alcohol Abuse and Alcoholism (NIAAA)
    http://www.niaaa.nih.gov
National Organization on Fetal Alcohol Syndrome
    http://www.nofas.org

FRAGILE X SYNDROME

I. Definition
A. Fragile X syndrome (FXS) is the most common inherited disorder in males, and it can cause mental impairment. Down syndrome is more common but is not usually inherited. A spectrum of cognitive involvement ranges from normal to subtle learning disabilities to severe mental retardation. Disabilities are found in three major areas: *cognitive, physical,* and *behavioral.*

II. Etiology
A. The incidence of FXS in males is 1 in 4000, and in females it is 1 in 6000. One in 246 females and 1 in 1000 to 1 in 2000 males is a carrier (CDC, 2001; Hagerman, 2005).
B. FXS is caused by a mutation of the X chromosome. The name is derived from the fragile site or break in the X gene, the fragile X mental retardation 1 gene (FMR-1). Males have one X and one Y chromosome, and females have two X chromosomes. An end section of the X chromosome normally contains between 6 and 50 repetitions of the genetic code CGG. When a code breakdown occurs, the repetitions of CGG can increase. An increase of 50 to 200 CGG repeats, called a *permutation,* causes few symptoms; but an increase of over 200 CGG repeats, called a *full mutation,* results in FXS.
C. Cognitive, physical, and behavioral problems are presumed to be caused by the lack of normal FMR-1 protein (FMR-P) production from the dysfunctional FMR-1 gene. This absence of adequate protein produces changes in brain structure; thus, changes in neurotransmitter systems can be improved by medication. Executive function deficits are common (e.g., lacking in attention, organizational skills).

III. Characteristics
A. Male.
   1. Boys are more severely affected than girls.
   2. Long, narrow face noted after puberty and large, cupped or prominent ears.
   3. Subtle features: prominent jaw and forehead, long palpebral fissures.
   4. Enlarged testicles, generally postpuberty.
   5. Connective tissue disorder manifestations: mitral valve prolapse; high, arched palate; hyperextensible finger joints; flat feet; and hypotonia.
   6. Most boys have IQ levels in mild-to-moderate range of mental retardation; a small percentage are severely to profoundly retarded.

7. Difficulty with mathematics, abstract reasoning, and attention.
8. Delayed onset of speech and language.
9. Majority of boys, especially younger boys, appear to have normal physical characteristics but can exhibit perseverative behaviors and speech and language difficulties.
10. ADHD or hyperactivity, impulsivity.
11. Psychosocial deficits: anxiety, withdrawal, and depression.
12. Poor eye contact, fascination with spinning objects.
13. Hand biting or hand flapping.
14. Some symptoms seem similar to autistic children.

B. Female.
1. Long, narrow face.
2. Prominent forehead, ears, and jaw; high-arched palate.
3. Hyperextensible finger joints, flat feet.
4. Generally higher cognition than boys; about 30% will have a normal IQ, others will have moderate to severe mental retardation.
5. Difficulty with mathematics, speech, and language.
6. Learning disabilities, poor attention, and low organizational skills.
7. Poor eye contact, shyness, and social or emotional disturbances.
8. Perseveration in behaviors and speech.
9. Anxiety, depression, impulsive behavior, and ADHD

IV. Health Concerns/Emergencies

A. Health concerns depend on the state and level of involvement of the syndrome.
B. Visual concerns, such as strabismus (esotropia/exotropia), may be present and may interfere with learning and physical activity. Occasional deficits: nystagmus, myopia, ptosis, hyperopia, astigmatism.
C. Recurrent otitis media, which may be caused by an unusual angle or collapsibility of the eustachian tube, can lead to a conductive hearing loss that may interfere with speech and language development.
D. Detection of a murmur or click indicates cardiac involvement, such as mitral valve prolapse, which requires a referral for cardiac evaluation.
E. High-arched palate, which can be associated with dental malocclusion.
F. Hypotonia, scoliosis, or flat feet (*pes planus*) require adequate assessment and referral.
G. Seizures that may be complex, partial, or generalized, create a need for a school health emergency plan. Medications may be required during the school day.
H. Autistic-like behaviors and sensory integration difficulties may create safety issues at school and home and may decrease social opportunities with peers.
I. Infants are often diagnosed with failure to thrive.
J. Obesity can be the result of obsessive–compulsive behaviors, such as food cravings, as well as hypothalamic dysfunction or sensory integration issues (e.g., difficulties with food textures and consistencies). A school plan for exercise and diet should be in place: provide support for the parents and counseling for the individual and family.
K. Masturbation and forms of self-stimulating behavior can be problematic for the adolescent and will require individual or family

CHAPTER 4

Chronic Conditions

counseling. Fertility is normal. Sex education needs to be provided based on the individual's level of development.

L. Anxiety in social encounters or shy and withdrawn behavior may create abnormal social situations that require intervention.

M. Hypersensitive to touch; tactile defensiveness and environmental overstimulation caused by sensory integration issues can cause delay in early development and later can produce a variety of behaviors, including temper outbursts, aggression, and emotional instability.

V. Effects on Individual

A. Depends on level of involvement.

B. Developmental delays and vision and hearing issues impact academic learning.

C. Difficulties around eating, toileting, and inappropriate personal behaviors play an important role in making and keeping friends.

D. May be teased because of physical appearance or behaviors and left out of recreational and social activities.

E. Lack of confidence and self-esteem.

F. Side effects from medication.

G. Unable to screen out noises, lights, or confusion in the environment because of sensory integration issues.

H. Visual learner more than auditory learner due to auditory processing problems.

I. Sibling can have the same disorder.

VI. Management/Treatment

A. Genetic counseling, including all family members.

B. Complete school assessment, including nurse assessment for special educational needs and services as indicated.

C. Assessment of hyperactivity and appropriate treatment, including counseling or medication.

D. Assessment of behavioral problems, aggression, anxiety, and mood instability to determine appropriate treatment with medication, counseling, or both.

   1. Carbamazepine (Tegretol) has been useful for those with mood disorders.

   2. Obsessive thinking, compulsive behavior, aggression, and anxiety may be helped by fluoxetine (Prozac), sertraline (Zoloft), paroxetine (Paxil) fluvoxamine (Luvox), cetalopram (Celexa), and all selective serotonin reuptake inhibitors (SSRIs).

   3. Psychological and behavioral therapy may be an important intervention for child and family.

E. Medications for hyperactivity and poor attention span include methylphenidate (Ritalin), pemoline (Cylert), and dextroamphetamine (Dexedrine). These medications work by stimulating both the dopamine and the norepinephrine neurotransmitter systems, which improves attention, hyperactivity, inhibition, and visual motor coordination. Clonidine (Catapres) is better for calming hyperactivity and minimizing tics but does not work as well as stimulants for attention and concentration difficulties. Clonidine has also been used successfully with children as young as 3 yrs. It works by lowering overall norepinephrine levels and can be used together with stimulants.

Although controversial, folic acid has been used with prepubertal boys with improvements noted in attention, activity level, coping skills, and unusual mannerisms.
   F. School treatment often includes speech and language therapy, occupational therapy, sensory integration, physical therapy, and special education.
VII. Additional Information
   A. FXS occurs in all racial and ethnic groups and the majority of families are unaware of its presence. Individuals with undiagnosed mental retardation or autism should have a fragile X DNA test performed. Those with learning disabilities (LD) who exhibit several of the known characteristics should have the X (FMR-1) DNA test done; testing must include the carrier, grandparent, and all siblings of the proband (Parker, Zuckerman, and Augustyn, 2005). Any carriers, especially men over 50, are at risk for the Fragile X-Associated Tremor/Ataxia syndrome. If gait instability or tremors are observed, they should immediately consult with a neurologist.
   B. A diagnosis can be made prenatally by chorionic villus sampling (CVS) as early as 10 weeks and an amniocentesis between 16 and 20 weeks gestation. Testing is reserved for women who are shown to be a carrier of a fragile X mutation. Prior to prenatal screening, the couple should meet with a genetic counselor to discuss prenatal diagnostic methods and their risks and benefits. However, a negative result for any of the intrauterine testing does not entirely rule out the syndrome.
   C. *Affected* refers to those with FXS and mental retardation. *Permutation* refers to those with fewer CGG repeats and immediate alteration who are usually unaffected. *Full mutation* refers to those with FMR-1 repeats in the 200 and above range; boys will have FXS, and about 50% of girls will have intellectual and cognitive deficits and some level of LD. Girls with normal IQs may also have LD. *Mosaic* refers to those with variability in the number of working genes, showing a mosaic status and a range of symptoms less severe.

WEB SITES

Conquer Fragile X
   http://www.conquerfragilex.org
The Fragile X Research Foundation
   http://www.fraxa.org
The National Fragile X Foundation
   http://www.fragilex.org

HEMOPHILIA A, B, AND C

I. Definition
   A. Hemophilia is a common hereditary disorder characterized by prolonged bleeding episodes that are either spontaneous or traumatically induced. There are three types of hemophilia: *A (classic)*, *B (Christmas disease)*, and *C (Rosenthal syndrome)*. Most hemophiliacs

are type A; type B is the second most prevalent form. Hemophilia C is rare and is a milder disease. Another common bleeding disorder is von Willebrand disease.

II. Etiology

A. Each type of hemophilia is caused by a deficiency or abnormal functioning of specific clotting factors: factor VIII in type A, factor IX in type B, and factor XI in type C. Bleeding problems are related to the plasma level of activity of the affected factor, classified as *mild, moderate*, and *severe hemophilia*. Types A and B are transmitted to the male by a carrier female, X-linked recessive gene. Type C is inherited as an autosomal dominant trait and affects both males and females. Hemophilia also occurs by spontaneous genetic mutation and about one third of children affected have no prior family history. Hemophilia A occurs in approximately 1:5000 males; Hemophilia B occurs in about 1:25,000 males. Von Willebrand disease is an autosomal dominant bleeding disorder found in 1% of the population (Scott, 2006). This disease has several subtypes each requiring different therapy (see "Additional Information").

III. Characteristics

A. *Mild hemophilia* (factor activity greater than 5%):
   1. May go undiagnosed until surgery or major trauma.
   2. First indication may be prolonged bleeding after a dental extraction.
   3. Spontaneous bleeding does not occur.
B. *Moderate hemophilia* (factor activity 1% to 5%):
   1. Seldom bleeds spontaneously.
   2. Victims may suffer joint and muscle bleeds several times a year after moderate injury.
   3. Additional factor replacements are necessary to stop bleeding after surgery or major injury.
C. *Severe hemophilia* (factor activity 1% or less):
   1. Major category of hemophiliacs (60%).
   2. Usually diagnosed by 12 to 18 months of age, some identified at birth.
   3. Spontaneous bleeding or bleeding with minor injury.
   4. Joints and muscles are most common bleeding sites (hemarthrosis).
   5. Additional factor replacements are needed after surgery.
D. Bleeding is not harder or faster, just prolonged, and delayed bleeding is common.
E. Bleeding can occur anywhere in the body, internally or externally; the ankle is the most common joint bleed as the toddler learns to ambulate; hemarthroses of the elbows and knees are the most debilitating bleeds for the older child and adolescent.
F. Signs of bleeding episode:
   1. Reported tingling or other sensation.
   2. Limb held in an abnormal position.
   3. Obvious signs of discomfort or pain.
   4. Area of bleeding warm, swollen, firm, and tender on palpation.

     5. Older student aware of early symptoms of joint bleeding; fluid accumulation and major swelling in the joint space.

     6. Restriction in range of motion indicates bleeding within joint.

     7. Hemorrhage in large muscle may produce pain with movement of joint or below muscle.

     8. Discoloration of skin is *not* a good indicator of bleeding.

   G. Common cause of death (25%) is intracranial bleed, and a history of trauma is found in only half of the individuals.

   H. Subcutaneous bleeding may extend over large portion of body; site of origin is indurated, raised, and purplish-black.

   I. von Willebrand disease:

     1. Mucocutaneous bleeding (e.g., nosebleeds, bruising, gingival bleeding).

     2. Heavy menstrual flow.

     3. Posttraumatic and postsurgical bleeding.

IV. Health Concerns/Emergencies

   A. Blow to head, abdomen, or throat can be particularly dangerous, because bleeding may go unrecognized until serious complications occur.

   B. Even a suggestion of trauma to the head requires factor infusion and head scans to rule out hemorrhage.

   C. Bleeding in tongue, throat, or neck area may rapidly compromise airway; needs immediate medical attention.

   D. Ocular bleeding needs treatment and evaluation for retinal detachment.

   E. Secondary complications of joint bleeds can occur (e.g., cartilage erosion, changes in joint space, chronic arthritis, fibrosis), which can lead to a disabling condition.

V. Effects on Individual

   A. Parents may be overprotective or overpermissive.

   B. Living with chronic health problem has imposed limitations with participation in contact sports.

   C. School life disrupted because of frequent absences; may become discouraged.

   D. May feel guilt because of family's enormous financial burden for medical care and the disruption of family life. Costs may exceed insurance limits.

   E. May become disabled if joint bleeds are not treated promptly and adequately.

   F. Possibility of early death can have emotional impact.

VI. Management/Treatment

   A. Schools should have medical and emergency information up to date and plan of action in place.

   B. Coordinate treatment plan with student's health care provider and hemophilia treatment center (HTC).

   C. Encourage wearing medical alert identification.

   D. Teach parents, school personnel, care providers, and other involved persons how to control bleeding:

     1. Using gloves, apply pressure to bleeding site for 10 to 15 minutes.

     2. Elevate affected part to heart level or above.

3. Apply lightweight ice pack or cold compress.
4. Contact parents or physician as needed.
   E. Treat bleeding episodes promptly to reduce secondary complications.
   F. Do not give aspirin or products containing aspirin, because it decreases clotting time.
   G. Some antihistamines and ibuprofen can interfere with platelet action.
   H. Students may learn to self-administer factor concentrate by age 11 or 12.
   I. Factor concentrate may be kept refrigerated at school to facilitate rapid treatment in the emergency room or may be administered in school if appropriate plan is in place.
   J. Current treatments do not carry threat of infection with HIV/AIDS or hepatitis.
   K. Routine intramuscular injections, such as immunizations, should be avoided because of possible muscle hemorrhage. May be given subcutaneously. Factor concentrate usually given before injection to reduce bleeding.
   L. Use protective helmet as needed for physical activity.
   M. Encourage regular exercise to strengthen muscles, which protects joints and decreases spontaneous bleeding.
   N. Resume activity gradually after injury.
   O. Excessive body weight increases strain on affected joints.

VII. Additional Information
   A. Prenatal diagnosis may be made as early as 8 to 12 weeks by chorionic villus sampling (CVS), at 13 to 18 weeks by amniocentesis, and at 18 to 29 weeks by fetal blood sampling. Bleeding symptoms can occur in the fetus or be present at birth. Some newborns may sustain intracranial hemorrhage, and about 30% of boys will bleed during circumcision. Hepatitis B vaccine should be given during the neonatal period.
   B. Implanted venous access devices (IVAD) may be used for ease of infusion, but the frequency of line infections and clotting may outweigh the benefits.
   C. Carriers of hemophilia have lower-than-normal clotting factor, are susceptible to anemia, and may experience prolonged bleeding during menses and pregnancy. Occurs most frequently in factor IX carriers.
   D. Some children may develop an "inhibitor" or an "antibody" to the clotting factor and may need a special plan of care. This usually develops between 5 and 10 years of age and makes management more difficult.
   E. Nosebleeds are usually not serious; oral medications, such as aminocaproic acid (Amicar) and tranexamic acid (Cyclokapron) are available to decrease the bleed by maintaining the clot.
   F. Gene therapy for hemophilia is promising, because hemophilia is caused by the malfunctioning of a single gene, and just a slight increase in the clotting factor can provide substantial benefits. Human trials are in progress and are showing great potential for effective treatment. Cells have been removed from people with

hemophilia, genetically modified to produce factor VIII, and then reintroduced into the patient. Cells then begin producing factor VIII. Gene therapy does not affect the inheritance of the defective gene.

WEB SITE

National Hemophilia Foundation
http://www.hemophilia.org

HEPATITIS INFECTIONS A, B, C, D, E, AND G

I. Definition
  A. Six heterogeneous viruses are known to cause inflammation of the liver as part of their clinical manifestations and are designated hepatitis A, B, C, D, E, and G. Although similar in some ways, the infections caused by each virus differ in etiology and in some features related to epidemiology, immunology, clinical characteristics, pathology, prevention, and control (see Table 4-8).

II. Etiology
  A. Hepatotropic infections are caused by viruses identified by their respective letters. For example, hepatitis B infection is caused by the hepatitis B virus (HBV).

III. Characteristics
  A. Children often have few acute clinical symptoms.
  B. Onset is generally insidious, except for type A (see Chapter 3 for further information on HAV).
  C. Prodromal phase includes various combinations of slight or no fever; fatigue; malaise; anorexia; nausea; headache; vomiting; abdominal discomfort; myalgia (tenderness or pain in muscles); coryza (head cold); arthralgias (joint pain); rash; dark urine; and clay-colored stools approximately 1 to 5 days before jaundice.
  D. Icteric phase, usually 1 to 2 weeks after onset of initial symptoms: jaundice; enlarged and tender liver; cervical adenopathy, swelling of lymph nodes in neck, and pruritus may develop; other symptoms diminish.
  E. Chronic stage: nonspecific symptoms of lethargy, malaise, fatigue, weight loss, abdominal pain, and enlarged liver.

IV. Health Concerns/Emergencies
  A. Exposure to the virus during emergency care and clean-up during any bleeding episode is an immediate health concern.
  B. The virus can survive outside the body for 7 days and still be infectious.
  C. Chronicity and ability to transmit virus to others is an ongoing concern.
  D. Immunizations for Hepatitis A and B are the most effective means of preventing infection and are recommended by the Centers for Disease Control and Prevention (CDC) and the American Academy of Pediatrics (see Appendix C). Between 1990 and 2005, incidence of acute hepatitis B in the United States declined 78%.

Table 4-8   Hepatotropic Viruses and Clinical Data

Virus	Hepatitis A Virus	Hepatitis B Virus	Hepatitis C Virus	Hepatitis D Virus	Hepatitis E Virus	Hepatitis G Virus
Incubation	15-50 days	45-160 days	2-24 weeks	2-4 months	15-60 days	Unknown
Fecal-oral transmission	Common	No	No	No	Common	No
Percutaneous transmission	Rare	Common	Common	Common	No	Common
Sexual transmission	Rare	Common	Rare	Rare	Rare	Rare
Transplacental transmission	No	Common	Rare	No	Unknown	Rare
				Occurs as co-infection with HBV		
Chronic infection	No	Yes	Yes	Yes	No	Yes
Prophylactic	IVIG may be effective	HBIG effective	No	No	No	No
Vaccine	Yes	Yes	None	HVB vaccine prevents HDV	None	None
Rash	Rare	Common	Occasional	Similar to HBV	None	—
Jaundice	Occasional	Common	Common	Similar to HBV	Common	—
Fever	Common	Uncommon	Uncommon	Similar to HBV	Common	—
Dark urine, clay-colored stool	—	Common	—	Similar to HBV	Common	—
Joint pain	Rare	Common	Rare	Similar to HBV	—	—
Prodromal phase	Rare	Yes	Yes	Similar to HBV	—	—
Icteric phase	Yes	Yes	Yes	Similar to HBV	—	—
Mortality	Rare	Yes	Rare	Highest	Yes (pregnant women)	Rare

HBIG, Hepatitis B immunoglobulin; *IVIG*, intravenous immunoglobulin.

E. Hepatitis C is the most common cause of liver transplants. No vaccination is available.

V. **Effects on Individual**

A. Delayed or no identification of disease, because symptoms may be nonexistent, minimal, or confused with other causes of illness.

B. Feelings of guilt, shame, or the need to place blame if contracted through drug abuse or sexual activity.

C. May have difficulty concentrating in class and diminished academic performance because of fatigue, general malaise, and arthralgia.

D. Loss of weight related to nausea, vomiting, and lack of appetite.

E. Self-conscious about appearance if rash and jaundice are noticeable.

F. Fear of living with a chronic disease, cirrhosis, liver cancer, or death.

VI. **Management/Treatment**

A. Treat symptomatically.

B. Allow student to return to school after acute clinical symptoms have subsided.

C. Contact local or state health department to determine action needed for health care and education of student, family, school staff, and other contacts.

D. Refer close contacts to their primary HCP for information regarding passive immunization with IG and hepatitis B immunoglobulin (HBIG) as soon as possible, preferably within 24 hours of exposure.

E. Teach infected student procedure for control of bleeding and clean-up of any body fluids so that they can assume control of their individual bodily needs.

F. Inform school staff (e.g., direct care providers, custodians, and bus transportation personnel) of any necessary cleaning or precautions.

G. Use a 1:10 diluted solution of household bleach and water or commercial disinfectant to disinfect any contaminated surfaces or objects per CDC recommendations.

H. The Occupational Safety and Health Administration (OSHA) requires annual training on bloodborne pathogens and an exposure-control plan at each school site. See individual county or school district policy manual.

VII. **Additional Information**

A. Other viruses known to cause hepatitis include herpes simplex virus, cytomegalovirus, varicella, rubella, HIV, Epstein-Barr virus (EBV), adenoviruses, enteroviruses, arboviruses, and parvovirus B19.

WEB SITES

Centers for Disease Control and Prevention: Viral Hepatitis
http://www.cdc.gov/ncidod/diseases/hepatitis/index.htm
Hepatitis A, B, and C Prevention Programs
http://www.hepprograms.org
National Foundation for Infectious Diseases
http://www.nfid.org/info
Teenhealth: Hepatitis B
http://www.kidshealth.org/teen/infections/stds/std_hepatitis.html

CHAPTER 4

Chronic Conditions

HERPES SIMPLEX VIRUS INFECTION: TYPE 1

I. Definition
   A. One of a group of acute infections occurring as a primary infection or recurring because of reactivation of a latent virus. Herpes simplex virus type 1 (HSV-1) usually is acquired in childhood and generally involves the oral cavity, lips, and face; also called a cold sore or fever blister when on the lips. HSV types 1 and 2 can overlap, and both types can reactivate throughout life.

II. Etiology
   A. The infection is caused by human herpesvirus HSV-1, a double-stranded DNA virus. HSV-1 and HSV-2 have a significantly similar DNA structure. Eye and digital herpetic infections generally are caused by HSV-1.

III. Characteristics
   A. Incubation period is 2 to 12 days after exposure. Period of communicability for HSV-1 is unknown but appears to be about 1 week.
   B. Transmission is by infected oral secretions, by direct contact with infected genital secretions, and during both primary and recurring infections. Carriers can transmit the virus even though asymptomatic.
      1. Reactivation occurs after nonspecific internal or external disruptions to individual's system (e.g., cold, heat, stress).
      2. Infection is self-limiting.
      3. It is usually acquired before age 5.
      4. Complaints of pain, tingling, or burning in oral mucous membranes.
      5. Starts as blisters, then changes to small spots with ulcerated centers surrounded by redness.
      6. Primary infection may be found on gums, inner lips, cheeks, and tongue; reactivated infections usually involve lips and surrounding area (see color plate 4).
      7. Usually accompanied by fever, hence the term fever blister.
      8. Infection may occur in other body areas (e.g., fingers, eyes, genitals).
      9. Activated by fever, menstruation, trauma, sunlight, tension, or physical and emotional stress.

IV. Health Concerns/Emergencies
   A. HSV-1 may infect the eye and cause herpetic keratitis, which is a significant cause of blindness. The inflammation results in a sensation of something in the eye, pain, sensitivity to light, and discharge. Without prompt treatment, the eye may be scarred.
   B. HSV-1 also can cause herpetic encephalitis, which affects the orbital portion of the frontal lobe and most commonly the temporal lobe. Severe and extensive disease may occur in immunosuppressed individuals, but it occurs primarily in infants.

V. Effects on Individual
   A. Self-conscious about facial lesions and may be teased about sores.
   B. Painful lesions may interfere with eating.
   C. Risk of decreased vision or blindness if lesion is in or around the eye.

VI. Management/Treatment
   A. Initial action varies greatly, depending on student's age, site of lesion, and circumstances.

B. Proper hand-washing technique must be practiced by staff and students.
C. Use gloves when applying medicated ointment to any area.
D. Isolate infected individual from newborns and those with eczema, burns, or compromised immune systems.
E. Caution:
  1. Use sunscreen if sun is trigger factor; do not use sunscreen if lesions are present.
  2. Do not use common eating utensils when lesions are active.
F. Avoid contact sports (e.g., wrestling) when there is a possibility of direct exposure with open, active lesion; it is not transmitted through mats.
G. Acyclovir (Zovirax) might be helpful during primary infection but is not necessary during reactivation. In primary infections and with immunocompromised individuals, as well as some other individuals, medication can lessen the frequency of outbreaks and the severity of symptoms. Other medications include famciclovir (Famvir) and valacyclovir (Valtrex).
H. Isolate towels, toys, and other items from others, and thoroughly clean and disinfect the articles if infant or toddler is in early intervention program or preschool.
I. Children who have open blisters, mouth sores, or mouth toys that other children have access to should be excluded from school and cannot return until lesions are dry.
J. Each exclusion should be evaluated on an individual basis (e.g., student's age, activity level, and circumstances).

HERPES SIMPLEX VIRUS INFECTION: TYPE 2

I. **Definition**
  A. One of a group of acute infections that occurs as a primary infection or upon reactivation of a latent virus. HSV type 2 (HSV-2) infection is primarily found in the perineal and rectal area and is usually congenital or sexually acquired. HSV types 1 and 2 can overlap, and both types can reactivate throughout life.
II. **Etiology**
  A. The infection is caused by human herpesvirus 2, which is a double-stranded DNA virus. HSV-1 and HSV-2 have a significantly similar DNA structure.
III. **Characteristics**
  A. Incubation period for the primary infection is 2 to 20 days after exposure.
  B. Period of communicability is unknown but appears to be about 1 week.
  C. Transmission is by infected oral secretions, by direct contact with infected genital secretions, and during both primary and recurring infections. Carriers can transmit the virus even though asymptomatic.
  D. Reactivation occurs after nonspecific internal or external disruptions to an individual's system (e.g., cold, heat, stress).
  E. It is a self-limiting infection.

F. Primary infection begins with burning or tingling sensation.

G. Painful lesions, which erupt and develop into fluid-filled blisters that spontaneously resolve or rupture and form shallow painful ulcers that scab and heal.

H. In males, thin-walled blisters are usually located on the glans, pre-puce, and shaft of the penis or on the anus; in females, lesions are usually located on the vulva, cervix, vagina, anus, or buttocks, and edema may be present.

I. Burning sensation during urination, dysuria, and hesitancy during voiding.

J. Lymph nodes in groin area may swell and become tender.

K. Aching muscles.

L. Fever, malaise, headache, and nausea are systemic symptoms.

M. Initial infection may last 14 to 28 days.

N. Women tend to have more discomfort than men, but infection of vagina or cervix does not always cause noticeable symptoms; cervix is not sensitive to pain.

O. Activated by menstruation, heat, systemic infection, emotional stress, fatigue, and pregnancy.

IV. Health Concerns/Emergencies

A. HSV-2 complications include disseminated infection, encephalitis, pneumonia, and hepatitis.

B. Predisposes woman to cervical cancer.

C. Pregnant adolescent may transmit virus prenatally, perinatally, and postnatally, which may result in CNS damage or disseminating en-cephalitis in the infant, resulting in death; increased risk of sponta-neous abortion and premature delivery.

V. Effects on Individual

A. May have localized pain and systemic symptoms, causing school absenteeism.

B. If sexually active, may be embarrassed to tell partner about sexually transmitted disease (STD).

C. May feel disease is punishment for having sex.

D. If pregnant, individual has increased risk of premature delivery and spontaneous abortion; may affect newborn.

VI. Management/Treatment

A. Initial action varies greatly, depending on student's age, site of le-sion, and circumstances.

B. Proper hand-washing technique must be practiced by staff and stu-dents.

C. Isolate infected individual from newborns and those with eczema, burns, or compromised immune systems.

D. Use gloves when applying medicated ointment to any area.

E. Recurrent herpes can have viral shedding up to 4 to 5 days.

F. Lesion can be present for 7 to 10 days.

G. Acyclovir (Zovirax) might be helpful during primary infection but not necessary during reactivation. In primary infections and with im-munocompromised individuals, as well as some other individuals, medication can lessen the frequency of outbreaks and the severity of symptoms. Other medications include famciclovir (Famvir) and vala-cyclovir (Valtrex).

H. Younger child or developmentally delayed individual may have to be isolated.
I. Isolate towels, toys, and other items, and clean and disinfect thoroughly.
J. Exclude students who have open blisters, mouth sores, or mouth toys that other children may use. If excluded, student cannot return to school until lesions are dry.
K. Each exclusion situation must be evaluated on an individual basis (e.g., student's age, activity level, and circumstances).

WEB SITE

American Social Health Association
http://www.ashastd.org

HUMAN IMMUNODEFICIENCY VIRUS/ACQUIRED IMMUNODEFICIENCY SYNDROME

I. Definition
A. A deadly viral disease that leads to the destruction of the immune system by disabling and killing CD4+ T-cells. Children under 13 years of age with acquired immunodeficiency syndrome (AIDS) are defined as having *pediatric AIDS*. Adolescents are classified as adults.
B. There are three sequential steps of development:
  1. Stage I: A rapid viral replication occurs immediately after exposure. During this acute phase, high levels of plasma HIV ribonucleic acid (RNA) can be documented. Most people develop detectable antibodies within 2 to 6 weeks with an average of 25 days, but seroconversion may take as long as 6 months.
  2. Stage II: A continuum from initial, asymptomatic/symptomatic HIV infection to AIDS diagnosis. Includes progressive damage to the immune system. Referred to as *HIV disease* or *HIV/AIDS*. Asymptomatic HIV infection can last 10 years or more, and many individuals are unaware of their infection.
  3. Stage III: Most severe manifestation of HIV disease, as evidenced by opportunistic infections and neoplasms of various organ systems, including the brain. Final clinical stage is referred to as *AIDS*.

II. Etiology
A. HIV is a lentivirus from the subfamily of human retroviruses with two known serotypes: type 1 (HIV-1) and type 2 (HIV-2). *HIV-1* occurs in North and South America, Europe, sub-Saharan Africa and most other countries. *HIV-2* is serologically different from HIV-1. It occurs primarily in West Africa. Disease progression is slower than with HIV-1, but severe immunodeficiency can occur.
B. Approximately 900,000 individuals have been diagnosed with AIDS in the United States, including around 9300 children under the age of 13. Approximately 40,000 new cases of HIV infection occur annually in the United States (Jenson and Baltimore, 2006).

III. Characteristics
A. Three primary modes of transmission: sexual contact, exposure to blood, and perinatal transmission.

1. Sexual contact:
   a. Unprotected sexual contact is the leading cause of HIV infection in the United States. Infection can also occur during *protected* sexual contact with an infected person.
   b. Epidemiological studies support the correlation of advanced disease stage with increased likelihood of transmission to sexual partners.
   c. Semen and cervical secretions are implicated in transmission.
2. Exposure to blood:
   a. Primary exposure is through injection drug use from sharing needles or syringes.
   b. Transmission through blood transfusion or blood clotting factors is essentially eliminated. Screening of the blood supply for HIV-1 was initiated in 1985; blood testing for HIV-2 began in 1992.
3. Perinatal transmission:
   a. Vertical transmission of HIV from an infected woman to her infant can occur during gestation (in utero), at the time of delivery (intrapartum), or postpartum through breast-feeding.
   b. Administration of zidovudine (AZT) during pregnancy, labor, and to the newborn has resulted in reduction of perinatal infection rates from 25% to 2% (NIH, 2006).
B. Other modes of transmission:
   1. Casual contact: Studies have examined the risk of transmission through casual contact by evaluating more than 1000 nonsexual household contacts of both adults and children with HIV infection with no reported transmissions.
   2. Saliva, tears, and sweat: HIV has been found in low concentrations in these fluids, and transmission of HIV through tears, saliva, or sweat has never been documented. In addition, multiple studies of household contacts have found no evidence of transmission through a human bite.
   3. Pleural, cerebrospinal, synovial, peritoneal, pericardial, and amniotic fluids are potentially infectious.
C. Primary infection: Stage I.
   1. Acute retroviral syndrome occurs in 30% to 60% of individuals with primary HIV infection manifested by mononucleosis-like symptoms; fever, malaise, lymphadenopathy, pharyngitis, headache, myalgia, and sometimes maculopapular rash (Jenson and Baltimore, 2006).
   2. Symptoms may last 1 to 2 weeks.
   3. HIV testing may be negative until seroconversion (antibody creation) occurs, which can take from 2 to 8 weeks or up to 6 months. Average is 25 days.
D. Asymptomatic infection, Stage II.
   1. May be asymptomatic for 8 to 12 years and then gradually develop increasing symptoms.
   2. Persistent generalized lymphadenopathy; chronic lymph node enlargement.
   3. Oral candidiasis may exhibit as white patches on mucous membranes of the mouth or throat.

4. Oral hairy leukoplakia—painless, white, corrugated lesions— appear on lateral surface of tongue but may spread; caused by EBV.

5. Vaginal candidiasis.

6. Diarrhea (two unformed stools daily for at least 30 days).

7. Fever may be low-grade and intermittent.

8. Profound fatigue, anemia.

9. Weight loss caused by altered metabolism, poor absorption of nutrients, and decreased food intake.

10. Disease in infants and children usually progresses faster because of the immaturity of the immune system; clinical manifestations unique to this group are failure to thrive, developmental delay, recurrent bacterial infections, lymphoid interstitial pneumonitis (LIP), parotitis, and recurrent fungal infections of the diaper area.

E. Severely symptomatic, Stage III AIDS:

1. *Pneumocystis carinii* pneumonia (PCP) is the most common life-threatening infection.

2. Cryptosporidiosis, a GI disease caused by a protozoan.

3. Toxoplasmosis is a common parasitic infection and a major cause of AIDS encephalitis.

4. Esophageal candidiasis, a fungal infection.

5. Tuberculosis, CMV.

6. Histoplasmosis, fungal infection manifested as pulmonary or lymph gland infection.

7. Cryptococcosis, a yeastlike fungus; lungs are the primary site of infection, but infection may spread to meninges or CNS.

8. Kaposi's sarcoma (KS) can affect skin, mucous membranes, and internal organs.

9. Coccidioidomycosis, a pulmonary infection caused by a fungus.

10. Disseminated *Mycobacterium avium-intracellulare* complex; caused by a bacterium.

11. Lymphomas, invasive cervical cancer.

12. HIV encephalopathy; often called *AIDS dementia complex (ADC)*.

F. In adolescents with a fully developed nervous system, the neurological impact is not as pronounced, and the deficits occur at a much slower rate.

IV. Health Concerns/Emergencies

A. Adolescents, ages 13 to 19, are one of the fastest growing populations of individuals to contract HIV/AIDS; given the long incubation period, it does not manifest for 8 to 12 years after exposure.

B. Conditions and functional level vary according to opportunistic infection involved.

C. Remind staff of special precautions to prevent exposure to communicable disease. OSHA regulations and universal precautions should be in place and followed in all classrooms and throughout the school.

D. Viral infections pose significant problems.

1. Respiratory viruses may have prolonged symptoms. Most children will experience at least one episode of pneumonia. Recurrent ear and sinus infections are common.

2. Chickenpox and measles are particularly significant to the individual with AIDS. Measles may occur despite immunization and may present without the typical rash. Student should be excluded temporarily during an outbreak, 3 weeks for chickenpox, and 2 weeks for measles. Notify parents and HCP immediately if exposure occurs for administration of varicella-zoster immunoglobulin (VZIG) within 72 hours of exposure to chickenpox.

3. Live-virus vaccine immunizations are contraindicated. Most other vaccines are administered according to the American Academy of Pediatrics (AAP) or individual state guidelines. CDC recommends annual pneumococcal and influenza vaccines.

E. GI problems are common, such as chronic or recurrent diarrhea with malabsorption, abdominal pain, dysphagia (difficulty swallowing), and failure to thrive.

F. Be alert to and knowledgeable of signs and symptoms of illness, deterioration of condition, and side effects of medication.

1. Skin eruptions may appear as an allergic reaction to drugs, especially for students on sulfonamides.

2. Students with HIV/AIDS should not be in school if there are weeping lesions or skin eruptions that cannot be covered.

3. Anemia caused by chronic infection or as a drug side effect may cause the student to appear disinterested, tire easily, or require periods of rest.

G. Seizure activity is not common and usually indicates an additional pathological process, such as a tumor or opportunistic infection.

H. Elevated blood pressure may indicate renal disease.

V. Effects on Individual

A. Students may feel various degrees of anxiety regarding their condition and future.

B. May exhibit depression and social withdrawal.

C. Social contacts may be limited, and harmony with family may become disrupted.

D. May feel stress over the secretive nature of the disease, or may feel guilt over exposing others to illness.

E. Fear of pain and death may be a constant concern. HIV encephalopathy in a child infected perinatally may result in speech and language delays, cerebral palsylike motor impairment, visual and auditory short-term memory problems, attention deficits, and compromised cognitive functioning.

F. Sleep disturbances are common and may affect social, school, and family life.

G. Individual may be living with other family members with HIV infection or AIDS.

H. Frequent illness, neurological complications, medication, and treatment may negatively affect academic achievement.

VI. Management/Treatment

A. Care is supportive and depends on manifestations of virus.

B. Confidentiality is an ongoing concern; review school, county, state, and federal policy and law regarding disclosure and information on HIV status.

NOTE: In some states, the State Department of Health Services or the local health authority must notify the site principal within 3 days if a student with HIV/AIDS attends that school. They may disclose the information to the nurse, teacher, and others as needed. In other states, it is a misdemeanor to reveal the HIV status of an individual without written consent.

C. Maintain consistent communication regarding condition and recommendations of HCP.

D. Be available for dialogue and support with student and parents.

E. Maintain annual OSHA standard precautions and blood-borne pathogen inservice for all school staff, including transportation personnel and custodians.

F. Monitor pulmonary status, since majority of children with HIV disease develop lung disease.
   1. Acute onset of respiratory symptoms requires immediate evaluation, because it can progress to an emergency situation within hours.
   2. Watch for episodes of gasping, deep inhalations or sighing, and prolonged coughing, because these may indicate difficulty breathing, which may indicate respiratory distress.

G. Periodic hearing screening including impedance, since otitis media is one of the most common recurrent conditions.

H. Adequate nutrition is a concern; no special diet is needed, but a lactose-free diet may be beneficial for some.

I. Periodic dental screening is important; dental caries are a focus of infection and can become systemic. Fluoride and dental sealant may be helpful.

J. Live vaccines are generally contraindicated. Most vaccines are administered according to AAP or individual state guidelines. CDC recommends annual pneumococcal and influenza vaccines.

K. Over 20 medications are prescribed, and the most common side effects listed are nausea, vomiting, fever, rash, anorexia, diarrhea, abdominal pain, and fatigue.

L. Adolescents may resist adhering to treatment protocol out of distrust of the medical system, lack of belief in medication, avoidance of side effects, or lack of understanding of the need for medication when asymptomatic. When aware of an adolescent with HIV/AIDS, encourage medication compliance while discussing students feelings and reactions to the disease process.

M. Compliance with medications is critical, because poor adherence can result in subtherapeutic drug concentrations that promote drug-resistant infections.

N. Participation in sports should follow these general guidelines:
   1. Determined by the ability of the individual to maintain the level of activity required.
   2. All coaching staff should practice standard precautions for all participants during all sports activities, not only for sports at high risk for bleeding injuries, such as wrestling or football.
   3. If a minor injury results in a laceration or puncture wound that bleeds or an abrasion that oozes fluid or blood, participation should be limited or discontinued if the wound cannot be covered adequately to prevent any fluid contact with another participant.

CHAPTER 4

Chronic Conditions

VII. Additional Information

A. No one has been identified as infected with HIV because of contact with environmental surfaces. HIV does not survive well in the environment, and HIV is not able to reproduce outside a living host.

B. CDC recommends HIV testing for those at risk. Most people develop detectable antibodies within 3 months, with the average time being 25 days; however, it can take up to 6 months in rare cases. Therefore, CDC currently recommends testing 6 months after last exposure. In practice, most people are tested at 3 months. Enzyme immunoassay (EIA) is the most commonly used HIV antibody screening test; results are known in 1 to 2 weeks. Four rapid tests have been approved by the FDA and are being used in many settings. Results are available in 5 to 30 minutes. Rapid testing should be confirmed with another test, such as the Western blot, before a diagnosis of infection is given.

C. Medications are usually given in combinations, rather than as monotherapy, to avoid developing drug resistance observed in some children given only one drug. Medications delay progression of the disease, contribute to weight gain, diminish the effects of encephalopathy, and improve the immune system.

D. There are three classes of antiretroviral drugs:
   1. Protease inhibitors.
   2. Nucleoside reverse transcriptase inhibitors.
   3. Nonnucleoside reverse transcriptase inhibitors.

E. Combinations of drugs have been developed so that one pill can be given rather than many.

WEB SITES

AIDS Info
  http://www.aidsinfo.nih.gov
Centers for Disease Control and Prevention: HIV/AIDS
  http://www.cdc.gov/hiv
Centers for Disease Control and Prevention, National AIDS Hotline (NAH)
  800-342-2437
Positive Life
  http://www.positivelife.net

HYDROCEPHALUS

I. Definition

A. Hydrocephalus is a condition characterized by an imbalance in circulation, production, and absorption of cerebrospinal fluid (CSF) in the body, causing an abnormal increase of CSF within the intracranial cavities, leading to enlarged ventricles. The condition is often associated with myelomeningocele.

II. Etiology

A. Hydrocephalus is usually caused by an obstruction in the normal circulation of CSF. The condition may be congenital or acquired by trauma, meningitis, neoplasms, or intracranial bleeding.

B. In *nonobstructive* or *communicating hydrocephalus*, CSF passes freely between the ventricles and the subarachnoid space but is blocked from being absorbed into the subarachnoid space. The condition may result from spina bifida occulta, trauma, meningitis, or subarachnoid hemorrhage in premature infants. It may also be caused by a prenatal maternal infection, such as toxoplasmosis, cytomegalic inclusion disease, or mumps.

C. In *obstructive* or *noncommunicating hydrocephalus,* CSF is blocked from leaving ventricles and entering the subarachnoid space. This may occur from congenital defects (e.g., Arnold-Chiari malformation), tumors, trauma, or prenatal maternal infections. The most common cause of obstruction is congenital stenosis of the aqueduct of Sylvius.

III. Characteristics

A. Manifestations depend on the child's age, whether fontanels have closed and cranial sutures have fused, and the type and duration of hydrocephalus.

B. Symptoms develop slowly or very suddenly.

C. In infants, symptoms are:
   1. Abnormal increase in head size.
   2. Bulging fontanels or delayed closure.
   3. Intracranial pressure signs: listlessness, irritability, vomiting, loss of appetite, high-pitched shrill cry, change in vital signs, decreased pulse, decreased and irregular respirations, increased systolic blood pressure, coma.
   4. Motor function becomes impaired as head enlarges.
   5. Hyperactive reflexes.
   6. Spasticity of extremities.
   7. Forehead may become prominent.
   8. Scalp appears shiny, and scalp veins become prominent (transilluminated head).
   9. Increased visibility of sclera and iris (setting sun appearance).
   10. Impaired upgaze and other extraocular movements.

D. Children with closed sutures display symptoms indicative of increased intracranial pressure (ICP):
   1. Headache on awakening, which improves when sitting up or after vomiting.
   2. Papilledema.
   3. Lethargy, fatigue.
   4. Ataxia.
   5. Strabismus or pupillary changes.
   6. Separation of cranial sutures may be seen up to 10 years of age.
   7. Personality change, irritability.
   8. Decrease in academic performance.
   9. Change in vital signs similar to those seen in infants.
   10. Coma.

IV. Health Concerns/Emergencies

A. If no medical intervention, hydrocephalus causes brain damage and possible death.

B. Main health concerns center around proper function of shunt:
   1. To avoid shunt infection, whenever the child is ill or running a fever, a physician should be consulted.

CHAPTER 4

Chronic Conditions

2. Malfunction of a shunt may occur; chronic or acute symptoms include:
   a. Vomiting.
   b. Irritability.
   c. Fever.
   d. Headache.
   e. Change in behavior.
3. Holding infant in head-down position interferes with CSF flow.
4. Increased risk of head injury because of poor head control.
5. Precocious puberty, short stature, amenorrhea may occur secondary to endocrine dysfunction.
6. Incidence of migraine headaches is twice that of peers. Risk of other headaches is three times greater than that of peers.

V. Effects on Individual
A. There may be no obvious motor or educational problems.
B. Brain damage may be present, resulting in motor (60%), language, perceptual, or intellectual disabilities. Verbal IQ is usually higher than performance and full-scale IQ.
C. Memory functioning and reasoning skills may be affected.
D. Areas frequently affected are math, reading, comprehension, and writing skills.
E. Child may talk incessantly with meaningless chatter or be echolalic.
F. Visual problems are common, including strabismus, optic atrophy, and decreased acuity.
G. Hypersensitivity to noise.
H. Problems with balance and spatial awareness affect performance in PE and on the playground.
I. Low energy levels.
J. Physical and social activities can be limited by parents' overprotection.
K. Other children may laugh or make fun of individual's oversized head or ataxic gait, creating difficulties with peer relations and self-esteem.
L. Limited intellect may affect ability to adequately deal with precocious puberty.
M. Seizures may develop.

VI. Management/Treatment
A. Monitor shunt functioning and refer to parent if signs of ICP or infection are observed.
B. Measure head circumference daily until sutures are fused.
C. Be alert to signs of complications that may cause pressure on the tubing in the peritoneal cavity (e.g., constipation, pregnancy).
D. Screen vision annually.
E. Provide early developmental screening for infants and toddlers.
F. Wear helmet during activities with risk of falling (e.g., bicycling).
G. Consider restriction of high-impact contact sports (e.g., football, wrestling, ice hockey).
H. Encourage independence and taking responsibility. Emphasize optimistic prognosis.
I. Support parents and provide information as they face the fear associated with multiple procedures and surgeries involving the brain.

J. Note that medical treatment is primarily surgical: removal of obstruction, ventriculoperitoneal (VP) shunt, or ventriculoatrial (VA) shunt; rarely, medication is given to reduce production of CSF.

K. Use of serial lumbar punctures is sometimes successful in premature infants to prevent need for a shunt.

VII. Additional Information

A. Hydrocephalus can be detected in utero as early as 14 weeks. Although shunting can be done in utero, postnatal shunting is more successful.

B. With a VP shunt, a radiopaque ventricular catheter is inserted into the ventricle and connected to a one-way valve that is threaded under the skin to the abdominal cavity. This procedure enables CSF to flow out of the brain into the peritoneal cavity and be absorbed by the blood vessels surrounding those organs. In a VA shunt, the tube is inserted into the heart instead of the peritoneal cavity. This procedure is only performed if abdominal problems prevent insertion of the VP shunt. Advances in neuroendoscopy and development of techniques make this surgery less invasive and more accurate in placement of shunts.

C. Tubing is coiled in the peritoneum to allow for growth. The distal portion may need to be replaced in toddlerhood and before the adolescent growth spurt. If the shunt becomes unnecessary, it is usually left in place unless it becomes infected (see Figure 4-6).

D. Third ventriculostomy is a procedure done under general anesthesia by making a small hole in the third ventricle, which creates a natural opening for CSF to flow into the subarachnoid space. Recovery time is 1 or 2 days; occasionally, the surgery is not successful and a traditional shunt will be placed.

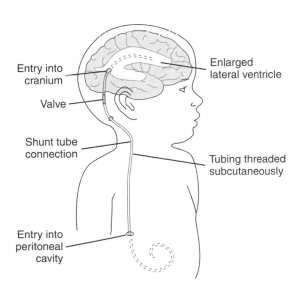

Entry into cranium

Enlarged lateral ventricle

Valve

Shunt tube connection

Tubing threaded subcutaneously

Entry into peritoneal cavity

Ventriculoperitoneal shunt

FIGURE 4-6 Ventriculoperitoneal shunt.

CHAPTER 4

Chronic Conditions

WEB SITES

Hydrocephalus Association
   http://www.hydroassoc.org
Hydrocephalus Foundation
   http://www.hydrocephalus.org

KLINEFELTER'S SYNDROME

I. Definition
   A. Klinefelter's syndrome (KS) is a genetic disorder involving the sex chromosomes.

II. Etiology
   A. Men with KS have one or more additional X chromosomes (usually only one extra X chromosome), described as 47 XXY rather than 46 XY. KS is the most common single cause of hypogonadism and infertility. It affects approximately 1 in 500 to 1 in 1000 male infants.

III. Characteristics
   A. Has an extra female chromosome and atypically high levels of female hormones.
   B. Spatial skills below the average male and may be about the same level as females.
   C. Lack of facial and body hair.
   D. Enlarged breasts, long limbs.
   E. Tendency to be taller than average and overweight.
   F. Mild elbow dysplasia.
   G. Fifth finger clinodactyly.
   H. Small penis and testes in childhood; continues into adulthood, in which length of testis is 2.5 cm or less.
   I. Inadequate testosterone production, less than one half the normal level.
   J. Usually infertile because of low sperm count; sexual dysfunction and impotence.
   K. At risk for autoimmune disorders.
   L. Wide range of IQ levels, from low to above normal, mean full-scale IQ between 85 and 90 with performance IQ higher than verbal. IQ scores are typically lower than those of siblings.
   M. Some are without noticeable learning problems in early school years, but these become more apparent as student progresses through school.
   N. Some may not speak before age 4 or 5.
   O. Problems with expressive language, auditory processing, and short-term auditory memory make reading and spelling difficult.
   P. May display immaturity, shyness, insecurity, poor judgment, and passivity.
   Q. Difficulty with peer relationships and psychosocial adjustments but no psychiatric difficulties.

IV. Health Concerns/Emergencies
   A. Risk of autoimmune disorders, such as thyroiditis, type 1 diabetes, breast cancer, and systemic lupus erythematosus (SLE).
   B. May need breast reduction because of gynecomastia (enlarged breast size).

C. If not treated with testosterone, may have increased risk for developing osteoporosis.

D. Poor gross motor coordination may affect balance and sports ability.

V. Effects on Individual

A. May feel self-conscious and embarrassed when participating in gym class or showering.

B. If lacking athletic ability, may become withdrawn and frustrated.

C. Adolescents fatigue easily.

D. The chromosomal abnormality may have an effect on the brain, producing a mild form of organic brain disorder.

E. May have gender confusion because of gynecomastia, hypogenitals, and no or decreased body and facial hair.

VI. Management/Treatment

A. May need special educational resources, especially for reading, spelling, and writing activities.

B. May need adaptation for test taking (i.e., test verbally rather than in writing).

C. May need social and emotional support.

D. Provide education and ongoing support to student, parents, and staff.

E. Testosterone injections and oral medication for delayed secondary sexual characteristics is available, but complete virilization is not usually achieved with oral replacement therapy.

VII. Additional Information

A. There are other sex chromosomal variations (SCVs) in which the cause is unclear, but there is an abnormality in the egg or sperm cell. Individuals with SCVs have 47 chromosomes rather than the normal 46, with combinations XXX, XXY, or XYY. There is a mosaic condition in which manifestations are fewer, depending on the number of cells involved.

WEB SITE

Klinefelter's Syndrome and Associates
http://www.genetic.org

LEAD POISONING

I. Definition

A. Lead poisoning (plumbism) is caused by the absorption of lead or any of its salts into the body. Once absorbed, it is distributed into three compartments: blood, bones, and soft tissue. Lead can interfere with CNS development and can cause mental impairments, such as cognitive disabilities and learning and reading difficulties. Blood lead levels ≥ 10 μg/dL (micrograms per deciliter) of whole blood are considered plumbism, but adverse effects can occur at lower levels.

B. Lead poisoning is a preventable, common, environmental and public health problem. Houses built before 1978 usually have internal and external surfaces painted with lead-based paint. Paint may chip, allowing children to eat or swallow chips or inhale lead-laden dust. Chips from lead paint have a sweet taste, which is tempting for young children to eat. Children of low-income

CHAPTER 4

Chronic Conditions

families (Medicaid-eligible) have a higher rate of lead poisoning and are the recommended target group for testing per the Centers for Disease Control (CDC) and the American Academy of Pediatrics (AAP).

II. Etiology

A. Primary sources are lead-based paints and lead-contaminated dust, soil, and water from lead-contaminated pipes. Other sources include folk remedies and traditional medicines, cosmetics, imported candy, ceramics, toys, and jewelry. Take-home exposure from occupational contact with lead, exposure to hobbies known to include lead particles, and foods, particularly spices, are also sources.

B. National Health and Nutrition Examination Survey (NHANES) from 1999 to 2000 estimated nearly 500,000 children have elevated blood levels ≥10 μg/dL (Meyer, 2003). State lead surveillance programs confirm nearly 75,000 children with blood levels ≥10 μg/dL in 2001. These statistical differences in the reporting may be due to substantial differences in methodology and reporting. However, both reports demonstrate that thousands of young children ages 1 to 5 have significantly elevated blood lead levels.

Brain Findings

Lead poisoning affects neurotransmitters and particular enzyme functions in the brain, because lead mimics and thereby inhibits the action of calcium in the human body. These actions interrupt early formation of synapses in the brain by decreasing the level of pruning, which is patterned by the response to experiences during development. Pruning is a normal process in shaping the efficiency of the brain, so such disruptions may be one of the underlying causes for learning and behavioral problems found in children with lead poisoning.

III. Characteristics

A. Often asymptomatic.

B. Central nervous system (CNS): cognitive impairment with decreased IQ; learning and reading difficulties; behavioral deficits; inattentive, hyperactive, aggressive, disorganized, antisocial behavior; decreased hearing acuity; headaches; irritability; malaise; encephalopathy; seizure, coma, and death.

C. Gastrointestinal system: abdominal pain, anorexia, vomiting, diarrhea, or constipation.

D. Hematopoietic system: Interrupts hemoglobin formation, resulting in anemia.

E. Renal system: hypertension.

F. Reproductive system: decreased sperm count and infertility, spontaneous abortion, and stillbirth; delayed puberty in girls; lead crosses the placenta and can affect the fetus; may be found in breast milk in low levels.

G. Skeletal system: affects bone growth and strength.

IV. Health Concerns/Emergencies

A. When individual is symptomatic, it is considered a medical emergency.

B. Young children are at high risk because of considerable hand-to-mouth activity, pica behavior, playing in contaminated soil, and increased GI absorption of lead.

C. Young children absorb 50% to 60% of the lead they are exposed to, whereas adults only absorb 10%.

D. Anemia: iron deficiency accelerates lead absorption.

V. **Effects on Individual**

A. Usually asymptomatic at low levels, but still can be harmful.

B. May be pale from secondary anemia.

C. Can be irritable.

D. Poor balance or clumsiness.

E. May display cognitive deficits, learning disabilities, and behavioral problems.

F. Increased rate of failure to graduate from high school and increased rate of absenteeism in senior year.

VI. **Management/Treatment**

A. Rule out blood lead levels if anemic, hyperactive, or exhibiting behavioral problems of unknown etiology.

B. Venous lead blood levels are the most accurate measurement of diagnosis. Finger-sticks are adequate for screening.

C. Radiography may indicate increased density (lead lines) of long bones.

D. Chelating agents reduce the body's burden of lead. They may be given orally, intravenously, and intramuscularly, alone or in combination with other agents. Chelation therapy may be necessary with all symptomatic exposures but cannot serve as a substitute for removing the child from the source of exposure. Notable side effects of chelation therapy include transient transaminase elevations, GI upset, headaches, hypersensitivity reactions, renal damage, transient neutropenia, and mild conjunctivitis (see Table 4-9).

E. Be alert to environmental conditions that can cause the disease, because young children may initially be asymptomatic. Such conditions

Table 4-9   *Schedule for Follow-Up Blood Lead Testing[a]*

Venous blood lead level (micrograms/dL)	Early follow-up (first 2 to 4 tests after identification)	Late follow-up (after BLL begins to decline)
10-14	3 months[b]	6 to 9 months
15-19	1 to 3 months[b]	3 to 6 months
20-24	1 to 3 months[b]	1 to 3 months
25-44	2 weeks to 1 month	1 month
>45	As soon as possible	Chelation with subsequent follow-up

[a]Seasonal variation of BLLs exists and may be more apparent in colder climates. Greater exposure in the summer months may necessitate more frequent follow-up.
[b]Some case managers or PCPs may choose to repeat blood lead tests on all new patients within a month to ensure that their BLL level is not rising more quickly than anticipated.
Source: CDC Advisory Committee on Childhood Lead Poisoning Prevention, 2005.

include children living or staying on a regular basis in a home, preschool, day care center, or caregiver's home built before 1978 with deteriorating paint.
F. Recommend routine screening at 1 and again at 2 years of age.
G. Educate parents, child care workers, and school staff about lead poisoning sources, symptoms, and complications and its learning and behavioral effects on children. Stress preventing or decreasing risk exposure (e.g., folk medications which contain lead used by various cultures, including families from China and Mexico; glazed pottery from outside the United States often contains high lead levels). Encourage proper hand washing, and promote a nutritious diet, because a malnourished child will absorb more lead; ensure adequate intake of calcium, iron, and vitamin C.
H. Notify public health officials and follow recommended guidelines.

WEB SITES

Centers for Disease Control and Prevention: Lead Poisoning Prevention Program
http://www.cdc.gov/nceh/lead/lead.htm
Alliance for Healthy Homes
http://www.afhh.org

LYME DISEASE

I. Definition
A. Lyme disease, also called *Lyme arthritis,* is a recurrent multisystemic disease named for Old Lyme, Connecticut, where the first well-known U.S. outbreak occurred in 1975. It is transmitted by a tick and may take 24 to 48 hours to transmit the bacteria. Symptoms resemble those of many other diseases, which makes diagnosis difficult. There is a direct detection test for confirmation of active disease. It is reported worldwide and in most states.
B. Ticks can harbor more than one disease-causing agent and can transfer these to their human hosts. Coinfective agents include *human granulocytic ehrlichiosis (HGE), human monocytic ehrlichiosis (HME),* and *babesiosis.*
C. Prime time for infection is in the spring, when the tick is in the nymph stage; it is about the size of a pinhead and difficult to see. In the fall, the adult stage is larger and thus the tick is easier to detect.

II. Etiology
A. The disease is caused by the spirochete, *Borrelia burgdorferi.* On the East Coast, the deer tick, *Ixodes scapularis,* transmits bacteria for Lyme disease, HGE, and HME, along with the parasite that causes babesiosis. On the West Coast, the Western black-legged deer tick, *Ixodes pacificus,* spreads Lyme disease and HGE bacteria. It is not known which tick species transmits the HME bacteria and the babesiosis parasite. Lyme disease is the most common tick-borne illness in the United States (Drew and Hewitt, 2006).

III. Signs, Symptoms, and History
A. Incubation period for B burgdorferi may be 3 to 31 days.

B. Transmission is from bacteria and parasites living on certain deer ticks.

C. Prime season for Lyme disease is April through July; for HGE, prime season is November through May; currently, season unknown for HME and babesiosis organisms.

D. The enzyme-linked immunoassay, ELISA, or the immunoflorescent assay, IFA, are blood tests used to detect Lyme disease. If questionable, they are confirmed by the Western blot.

E. First stage: early localized disease.

   1. Lyme, ehrlichiosis, and babesiosis disease.

     a. Sudden appearance of a bull's-eye rash is apparent in 1 in 2 Lyme disease cases and 1 in 5 ehrlichiosis cases. There is no rash with babesiosis. Rash is usually circular but can be oblong and hot to the touch; appears as a bruise on dark skin and red on light skin (see color plate 7).

     b. Flulike symptoms: fatigue, joint pain, muscle aches, headaches, and low-grade fever.

     c. With ehrlichiosis and babesiosis: may have nausea, vomiting, diarrhea, and appetite loss, along with flulike symptoms.

     d. With babesiosis: may have drenching sweats.

     e. Without treatment, early Lyme disease symptoms disappear within 3 to 4 weeks. Illness may return weeks or months later and manifest in late stages with debilitating symptoms, such as memory or mood disturbances and arthritis.

     f. Without treatment, ehrlichiosis symptoms disappear without long-term concerns; but some individuals develop life-threatening complications, and about 5% die.

     g. Babesiosis is usually mild, even without treatment, but severe anemia, kidney failure, and other life-threatening complications can develop and cause death.

F. Second stage: early disseminated disease.

   1. Lyme disease:

     a. Infection of the eye: retinitis, conjunctivitis, uveitis.

     b. Infection of the bone: osteomyelitis, mild arthritis.

     c. Infection of the heart: pericarditis, myocarditis, palpitations, heart pain (if inflammation of the heart muscle).

     d. Infection of the liver: hepatitis.

     e. Infection of central nervous system (CNS): meningitis, facial paralysis, drooping eyelids.

   2. Babesiosis:

     a. Malarialike illness when red blood cells are attacked.

     b. Weakened immune system.

G. Third stage: late disease.

   1. Lyme disease:

     a. May take months or years to occur.

     b. Pauciarticular: involvement of less than five joints.

     c. Arthritis, which may be recurrent with painful swollen joints, usually the knees.

     d. Late neurological concerns of deafness, chronic encephalopathy, and keratitis.

CHAPTER 4

Chronic Conditions

2. HGE.
   a. Toxic shock and death.
3. Babesiosis.
   a. Anemia and kidney failure.

IV. Initial Management

A. Remove tick as soon as possible, preferably with tweezers.
B. Pull steadily outward and away from the skin; do not twist or jerk the tick.
C. Protect fingers and hand with a tissue, paper towel, or glove.
D. Apply alcohol or disinfectant to area after tick removal.
E. Place tick in jar of alcohol and keep for identification.
F. Wash hands with soap and water.
G. Observe the site for signs of a rash for at least a month.
H. Notify parents and discuss further follow-up.
I. The disease is not treated until symptoms appear. Lyme disease and ehrlichiosis infections are treated with antibiotics. Antibiotics and medication used for malaria therapy can cure babesiosis. Antibodies remain in the system, and the individual may continue to test positive.

V. Additional Information

A. A vaccine for Lyme's disease was approved by the Food and Drug Administration (FDA) in 1988 but was withdrawn from the market in 2001.
B. See Box 4-8.

WEB SITES

Centers for Disease Control and Prevention, Lyme Disease
   http://www.cdc.gov/ncidod/dvbid/lyme/index.htm
Lyme Disease Network
   http://www.lymenet.org

Box 4-8	***Precautions to Avoid Tick Bites***

1. Cover skin with clothing.
2. Wear light-colored, long-sleeved shirts and long pants.
3. Tuck pant legs into socks and button shirts.
4. Apply tick repellents containing diethyltoluamide (DEET) to skin and clothing. Reapply every few hours, and read and follow instructions closely, because DEET can be neurotoxic. Do not apply to face, hands, or irritated skin.
5. Cover ground area with a blanket when sitting.
6. Apply medication to kill ticks on pet dogs and cats that go outside.
7. Check clothing and entire body for ticks on returning from a potentially tick-infested area, such as a grassy or woodland area. Include head and back of body.
8. Wash skin with soap and water upon returning.
9. Wash clothing and dry for at least 20 minutes.

MUSCULAR DYSTROPHY, DUCHENNE'S AND BECKER'S

I. **Definition**

    A. Muscular dystrophies (MDs) are characterized by progressive degeneration of muscle cells that are replaced by fat and fibrous tissue. They are unrelated diseases, each transmitted by a different gene, each characterized by weakness and wasting of particular groups of skeletal muscles, and each differing in expression and clinical course. Duchenne's MD is the most common type and affects 1:3500 boys (Society for Neuroscience, 2006).

II. **Etiology**

    A. Duchenne's MD *(pseudohypertrophic MD)* is inherited as an X-linked recessive trait. The X chromosome at the Xp21 locus carries the abnormal gene. The defective gene carried by the unaffected female affects all male offspring. Becker's MD is the same disease, but it follows a milder clinical course.

III. **Characteristics**

    A. Infancy: may have no symptoms or may manifest mild hypotonia and poor head control.

    B. About age 2: mild hip-girdle weakness and lordotic postures while standing may be observed.

    C. Achieves development milestones at appropriate ages.

    D. Walking on tiptoes is an early sign.

    E. Seems awkward and clumsy and has a strange way of running.

    F. By age 3, *Gowers' sign* may be observed. Child will get up from floor by "walking up" the legs with his or her hands.

    G. Has difficulty ascending stairs and rising from squatting or sitting position on floor.

    H. Age 5 to 6: Trendelenburg's gait or hip waddle appears.

    I. Weakness progresses from lower to upper limbs.

    J. Appearance of muscular enlargement due to fat replacing muscle.

    K. Progression is rapid, with all voluntary muscles ultimately involved.

    L. Calf enlargement is common because of wasting of thigh muscles *(pseudohypertrophy)*.

    M. Can be confined to a wheelchair as early as 7 years of age. Most can walk up to age 10 but with increasing difficulty. Orthotic bracing, physiotherapy, and minor surgery (Achilles tendon lengthening) can prolong ambulation up to age 12.

    N. Often overweight or obese because of limited activity or wheelchair confinement.

    O. Muscular atrophy, joint deformities, and contractures of the ankles, knees, hips, and elbows are common as disease progresses.

    P. Scoliosis can develop because of trunk's muscle weakness and can be painful.

    Q. Pharyngeal weakness can lead to nasal regurgitation of fluids, aspiration, and a nasal or airy voice quality.

    R. Cardiomyopathy is noted.

    S. Only 20% to 30% have an IQ less than 70. The majority have learning disabilities but can function in the regular classroom with help.

    T. Life expectancy is about 20 years (Society of Neuroscience, 2006).

IV. Health Concerns/Emergencies

A. Upper respiratory tract infections are frequent because of weakness of respiratory muscles and resulting decrease in vital capacity.

B. May show signs of cardiac failure, because heart muscle has weakened.

C. Osteoporosis.

V. Effects on Individual

A. Choices and activities open to student are limited.

B. Overprotective parents may also restrict activities.

C. Inappropriate behaviors may be condoned because of the parents' sympathy or guilt.

D. Health examinations and the knowledge that one is different may generate feelings of shame and doubt.

E. Social interaction with peers may be limited.

F. May have to depend on others for help at school or in social activities.

G. As the disability progresses and becomes more severe, individual must face the uncertainty of the future.

VI. Management/Treatment

A. Respiratory infections require prompt management and referral when indicated.

B. Postural drainage may be necessary because of inability to cough and accumulation of secretions.

C. Because of selective muscle involvement, contractures are common and physical therapy should be implemented. Be aware of physical therapy goals, instructions, and proper positioning. Work with physical therapist and assist family with range-of-motion exercises, stretching, or any suitable active exercises. Braces can help prevent contractures.

D. Muscles can atrophy if student must remain in bed for more than a few days (e.g., after surgery or from illness), and physical therapy or range-of-motion exercises are needed to maintain muscle strength.

E. Surgery may correct lower limb deformities and prolong ability to stand erect and walk.

F. Education of family and student regarding proper dietary intake and needs may help to prevent or treat obesity.

G. Constipation can be a problem because of limited activity; increase in fluids and use of stool softeners can help.

H. As student becomes older, fatigue increases; teaching staff and others should be aware of possible need for rest period during school day and limited energy for learning.

I. Counseling can help individuals with MD deal with body changes and prognosis.

J. Boys with Becker's MD remain ambulatory until late adolescence or young adulthood. The onset of weakness is later, and learning disabilities are not as common. Life expectancy is mid-to-late twenties; less than half of affected men are alive at age 40, and those are severely disabled (Sarnat, 2004).

VII. Additional Information

A. MD is diagnosed by signs and symptoms. Blood tests show an elevated level of creatine phosphokinase (CPK), a muscle enzyme;

electromyography (EMG), muscle biopsy, and echocardiography (ECG) may also reveal the disease.
   B. Other MDs include Emery-Dreifuss MD, myotonic MD, myotonic chondrodystrophy, myotonic congenita, limb-girdle MD, facioscapulohumeral MD, and congenital MD.

WEB SITES

Muscular Dystrophy Association
   http://www.mdausa.org
Parent Project Muscular Dystrophy
   http://www.parentdmd.org

OBESITY

   I. Definition
      A. Obesity is an increase in weight that is beyond the limitation of physical and skeletal requirements. For an adult, a body mass index (BMI) of 25 or higher is considered overweight and a BMI above 30 is considered obese. For children 2 to 20 years old, the BMI classification has a broad range of healthy weights from the fifth to the eighty-fifth percentile. The child who is at or above eighty-fifth percentile on the BMI is considered at-risk for overweight and at or above the ninety-fifth percentile is considered overweight (see Appendix B: Growth Measurements).
NOTE: BMI is a formula for determining overweight and underweight based on weight and height and is associated with body fat and health risks. For children the BMI is also age and gender specific.
   II. Etiology
      A. The results of excessive accumulation of fat in the body may occur in infancy, childhood, adolescence, or adulthood and may be caused by genetic susceptibility, hypothyroidism, overactivity of insulin secretion, hyperfunction of the adrenal cortex, hypofunction of the gonads, metabolic disorders, overeating, or inactivity. Rare mutations in the MC4-R (melanocortin receptor 4) gene account for about 4% of extreme childhood obesity and it is recommended that obese children under the age of five be screened for this gene (Farooqi et al, 2003; Vaisse, 2000).
      B. The complex neurological and peripheral systems regulate the balance between caloric intake and energy output. Intake exceeding energy output leads to imbalance and weight gain.
         1. The primary cause of overweight and obesity is life situations or habits (e.g., consumption of foods high in calories and fat, demise of home cooking and family meals, increased television viewing, decreased PE classes in schools, and reduction of physical activities).
         2. Other causes include endocrine disorders (e.g., stress-induced cortisol imbalance, hypothyroidism, insulinemia, Cushing syndrome, exogenous steroids, polycystic ovary syndrome, growth hormone deficiency, pseudohypoparathyroidism), disorders of the CNS (e.g., trauma and tumor), and dysmorphic syndromes

(e.g., Laurence–Moon–Biedel syndrome, Prader–Willi syndrome, Turner syndrome), and sleep deprivation.

C. The 2003–2004 National Health and Nutrition Examination Survey (NHANES) indicated that an estimated 17 percent of children and adolescents ages 2 to 19 years old are overweight. Overweight increased from 7.2% to 13.9% among 2- to 5-year-olds and from 11% to 19% among 6- to 11-year-olds between 1994 and 2004. Among adolescents ages 12 to 19, overweight increased from 11% to 17% during the same period (NCHS, 2004).

Brain Findings

Hunger is a basic human need, and the brain has a complex system of chemical receptors and messengers specifically for appetite, eating, and energy balance (Lasley, 2006). In 1994 Dr. Jeffrey Friedman of Rockefeller University discovered that mice lacking the hormone leptin, found in fat tissue, have lower metabolism, eat more, and grow three times the weight of normal mice. This discovery led to the identification of numerous related molecules that form signaling pathways in the hypothalamus to help regulate appetite and energy expenditure in humans. Leptin helps the brain report on the state of the body's fat stores and may have aided mammalian evolution by preventing starvation. It changes the wiring of the brain, a phenomenon known as *plasticity,* and creates new connections.

- Leptin deficient individuals lose weight when treated with leptin. Individuals who were not leptin deficient did not lose weight when treated with leptin. Further studies are needed to understand why some individuals do not respond to leptin's weight reducing effects. Doctors at the Rockefeller University Hospital are treating overweight patients who are not leptin deficient, who also subscribe to a very low calorie diet, to see the effects of leptin on weight loss (Pinto et al, 2004).

- Research on mice is providing scientific understanding of key neurotransmitters that help govern eating. Discovery of several serotonic 2c receptors provides meaningful information in regulating weight (Norris, 2000).

- Two neurons, NPY and POMC, are being studied. NPY stimulates food intake, increases weight, and reserves energy, while POMC works the opposite by curtailing eating: This happens simultaneously. It occurs as the cells connect and communicate (Pinto et al, 2004).

Leptin, found in the fat cells, has been shown to affect hunger via the hypothalamus and the mood via the hippocampus, a center of emotion and memory. Recent studies in rats show that low levels of leptin may contribute to depression, a center of emotion and memory (Lasley, 2006).

Another hormone, called *ghrelin,* is found in the brain and stomach. While leptin decreases appetite, ghrelin stimulates appetite. The hormone leptin has a slow, more long-term action, while ghrelin changes eating behaviors in moments.

III. Characteristics

A. Behaviors of eating high caloric foods containing too much fat and sugar, consuming larger portions, combined with moving about and exercising less.

B. Consuming more processed foods and simple carbohydrates with associated increased obesity and incidence of type 2 diabetes.

C. Excessive television viewing; exposure to frequent food commercials and unhealthy snacking.

D. Frequently eating fast foods.

E. Overweight children and adolescents are at risk for multiple health problems.

F. Preadolescents and adolescents may have acanthosis nigricans (darkened, thickened velvety patches on the posterior neck and in skin folds) associated with insulin resistance and increased risk of type 2 diabetes (see color plate 6).

G. Prevalence of metabolic syndrome is 30% or more in overweight adolescents (BMI ≥ninety-fifth percentile), putting them at risk for heart disease, stroke, and diabetes (Ornstein and Jacobson, 2006).

IV. Health Concerns/Emergencies

A. Obese children and teens are more likely to contract acute and chronic medical conditions, such as glucose intolerance and insulin resistance, respiratory problems (sleep apnea and asthma), orthopedic problems, early atherosclerosis, several types of cancer, gout, arthritis, and infertility (girls).

B. Obesity is the leading cause of sustained hypertension in children and adolescents.

C. Some overweight children develop a fatty liver, which is a precursor to cirrhosis, type 2 diabetes, and elevated cholesterol.

D. In diabetics, the inability to process glucose normally may cause damage to blood vessels, nerves, kidneys, and heart, which increases risk of death from heart attack, stroke, and kidney failure.

E. Obesity contributes to arthritis, back, and foot pain.

F. If stressed and made to feel ashamed, obese individuals may develop dangerous eating disorders.

G. Obesity is often associated with depression, and the two can interact and influence each other.

V. Effects on Individual

A. Negative effects on social, emotional, and physical development and self-esteem.

B. Heavy adolescents tend to be heavy adults.

C. Orthopedic difficulties, such as bowing of the tibia and a slipped femoral capital epiphysis (bone slippage at the head of the femur), can cause loss of range of motion and may manifest as knee pain.

D. More likely to experience aches and pains and impaired ability to perform daily tasks and exercise.

E. May experience educational, social, and economic disadvantages as obese adolescents and adults.

VI. Management/Treatment

A. Do a complete physical assessment.

CHAPTER 4

Chronic Conditions

B. Assess weight, height, and BMI (see Appendix B: Growth Measurements).

C. Obtain a complete history, including eating and activity patterns (e.g., television viewing, electronic games), emotional and social contributors (e.g., new in neighborhood, no friends, divorced family unit and missing one parent, depressed, having difficulty in school). Separate out possible factors to plan management strategies.

D. Be sensitive to parents feelings about overweight and develop school plan for appropriate method of communication. Success is usually related to parental involvement.

E. Consider emotional aspects of overeating; ask student to keep daily food diary and thoughts while eating (e.g., stressed over exam, fight with a friend).

F. Focus on health rather than appearance and on increased activity, not less food.

G. Form peer support groups at school by age, sex, and level of overweight.

H. Encourage student to select a "buddy" to call when tempted to overeat; do not set up a competitive situation.

I. Decrease intake of calories and fat; increase intake of high-fiber foods.

J. Avoid strict reduction of calories in younger children: weight maintenance for a period of time may be all that is necessary as they grow into their weight.

K. Advocate for increased physical activity during and after school or reinstatement of eliminated PE classes.

L. Promote walking or biking to school in groups.

M. Encourage parents to form collaborative walking groups to school rather than carpooling.

N. Advocate for healthy food choices in school cafeteria; increase fresh fruits, vegetables, and salad bars. Monitor existing school food plans.

O. Encourage selling only healthy food or nonfood products as fundraisers.

P. Support changes in products sold in vending machines at school; monitor for implementation by 2009–2010 (see "Additional Information").

VII. Additional Information

A. "Latchkey" children and those living in families who fear violence or live in an unsafe neighborhood watch an inordinate amount of television, which also contributes to decreased exercise and increased weight. The greatest amount of advertising during children's television programming is for food products, which are usually high in salt, sugar, and fat.

B. Major beverage distributors have agreed to sell only water, flavored and unflavored low-fat and fat-free milk, and unsweetened juice to elementary and middle schools. In addition to these beverages, diet sodas, diet and unsweetened teas, flavored water, and low-calorie sports drinks will be sold to high schools. Whole milk and regular soda will not be offered at any schools. Serving sizes will shrink to 8 ounces for elementary students and 10 ounces for middle schools;

Table 4-10	*List of Activities and Chores for Children*

One activity each day will burn about 1000 calories per week

Activity/chore	Amount of Time
Basketball (shooting baskets)	30 minutes
Basketball (playing a game)	15-20 minutes
Bicycling 4 miles	15 minutes
Bicycling 5 miles	30 minutes
Dancing fast (social)	30 minutes
Jumping rope	15 minutes
Pushing a stroller 1½ miles	30 minutes
Raking leaves	30 minutes
Running 1½ miles (10 minutes per mile)	15 minutes
Shoveling snow	15 minutes
Stair walking	15 minutes
Swimming laps	20 minutes
Touch football	30-45 minutes
Volleyball	45 minutes
Walking 1¾ miles (20 minutes per mile)	35 minutes
Walking 2 miles (15 minutes per mile)	30 minutes
Washing and waxing a car	45-60 minutes
Washing windows or floors	45-60 minutes
Water aerobics	30 minutes
Wheelchair basketball	20 minutes
Wheeling oneself in a wheelchair	30-40 minutes

Source: Centers for Disease Control and Prevention, Moore, 2007.

CHAPTER 4

Chronic Conditions

servings at high schools will be 12 ounces and at least 50% of non-milk beverages must be water and/or no- or low-calorie options. These guidelines were made between the major beverage companies and the Association for a Healthier Generation and are to be implemented by the 2009–2010 school year.

C. The U.S. Department of Agriculture has developed MyPyramid Plan, which provides a quick estimate of what and how much food you should eat from the different food groups by entering your age, gender, and activity level (online at http://www.mypyramid.gov).

D. Centers for Disease Control and Prevention has urged children to become more active. Even moderate activity is beneficial. (See Table 4-10.)

WEB SITES

Alliance for a Healthier Generation
   http://www.healthiergeneration.org
American Obesity Association
   http://www.obesity.org
Child Obesity Resources for Health Professionals, Educators, and Families
   http://www.childobesity.com
Centers for Disease Control and Prevention, BMI Percentile Calculator for Child and Teen
   http://www.apps.nccd.cdc.gov/dnpabmi/Calculator.aspx

Centers for Disease Control and Prevention, Table for Calculated BMI for Ages 2 to 20 Years
  http://www.cdc.gov/nccdphp/dnpa/bmi/00binaries/bmi-tables.pdf
Exercise Calorie Counter
  http://www.drgily.com/exercise-calorie-counter.php
Food Guide Pyramid
  http://www.mypyramid.gov

IDIOPATHIC SCOLIOSIS

I. Definition
A. Idiopathic scoliosis is an abnormal lateral curvature of the spine. It may or may not include deformity or rotation of the vertebrae. Idiopathic scoliosis results in a fixed rotation of the spine and is commonly observed and screened for in the school setting. It occurs more often in girls than boys, and it usually develops during periods of active growth spurts (10 to 16 years). It affects 2% to 3% of the adolescent population; the rate of mild curvature is nearly equal in boys and girls, but profound curvature is more common in girls and occurs at a ratio is 4 to 1 (King and Sarwark, 2002).
B. Of the scoliosis cases identified, 85% are considered idiopathic. The majority of these will not need treatment but should be monitored. The National Scoliosis Foundation estimates that 30,000 children with scoliosis are put into braces, and 38,000 patients undergo spinal fusion surgery.

II. Etiology
A. Because this type of scoliosis occurs without any known cause, the term *idiopathic* is used. It is a complex spinal deformity diagnosed by three main components: *balance, degree,* and *rotational component* of the curvature. Idiopathic scoliosis is the most common type and typically occurs in the growth spurts of adolescence. There may be a genetic origin, and if a family history is noted, the risk is 7 times greater (see "Additional Information" for other classifications).

III. Characteristics
A. Develops slowly.
B. Usually painless, so severe pain or chronic leg pain requires follow up.
C. Often not observed at home, because individuals dress themselves and have developed feelings of modesty.
D. Signs noted during screening procedure for scoliosis:
1. Shoulder unequally elevated.
2. Scapula prominence or elevation.
3. Prominent breast or flank area.
4. Unequal hip height and alignment.
5. Unilateral fullness of waist or extra folds.
6. Iliac crest elevation.
7. Unequal rib prominence.
8. Lumbar or thoracic prominence, or hump, when bent over; right thoracic prominence is more common.
9. Tufts of hairy patches, dimples, or café au lait spots at lower end of spine may indicate neurofibromatosis.

IV. Health Concerns/Emergencies

A. Moderate to severe curvature (> 50 degrees) involving thoracic spine reduces efficiency of heart and lungs by creating chest deformity.

B. Back pain seems to increase in adults.

C. If individual is confined to a wheelchair, neuromuscular scoliosis will prevent sitting upright without using hands to stabilize the torso; pressure sores can eventually develop from unequal pressure on buttocks.

V. Effects on Individual

A. May feel self-conscious and develop problems of low self-esteem and self-worth.

B. Bracing can be extremely uncomfortable.

C. After surgical intervention, casting or some other form of immobilization may be necessary and may limit socialization with peers and participation in school activities.

D. Must deal with reactions of others to braces, casts, or other appliances.

VI. Management/Treatment

A. Scoliosis assessment per state, county, or district requirements; usually screened at fifth or seventh grade at the latest. American Academy of Orthopedic Surgeons recommends screening girls twice, in fifth and seventh grade (ages 10 and 12 years), and screening boys once, in eighth or ninth grade (13 or 14 years).

B. *Adam's forward bend test* is given by having the student bending forward 90 degrees at the waist with feet together and knees extended. Observe symmetry of the spine from the back and the front areas. The hump is the primary marker for scoliosis and is caused by spinal rotation.

C. A scoliometer may be used to measure degree of curvature. Referrals should be made when the scoliometer shows more than 7 degrees of rotation, which corresponds to 20 degrees of deformity, or per individual school or state standards.

D. Some curvatures remain stable and require no treatment; others may increase for unknown reasons and need treatment.

E. When brace is prescribed, monitor for skin integrity.

F. Mild curvature (0 to 20 degrees).
   1. Periodic evaluation, observation, and x-rays to evaluate progression of curve.
   2. Not all curves are progressive.
   3. Mild exercise often prescribed but of questionable value.
   4. If curvature is less than 20 degrees but is secondary to another diagnosis, more aggressive treatment is initiated.

G. Moderate curvature (20 to 40 degrees).
   1. Depends on age and cause.
   2. Bracing is the usual treatment, and there are several kinds of braces: Boston brace for thoracolumbosacral orthosis (TLSO), Spine-Cor brace, and Milwaukee brace.
   3. Braces are worn day and night until skeletal maturity is attained, generally in 2 to 4 years.
   4. Braces are worn day and night to prevent progression.

H. Severe curvature (40 degrees and greater).
   1. Treatment depends on age, cause, and previous therapy.

2. Surgery considered if curvature is over 40 degrees; most likely in curves over 50 degrees. Anterior scoliosis correction by thoracoscopic surgery is less invasive, recovery is faster, and cosmetic results are better. Harrington or Dwyer instrumentation—a rod inserted along the spine to straighten it—requires a large incision, and after spinal fusion, a cast or immobilizing jacket may be required; depends on type of surgery.

VII. Additional Information

A. Scoliosis screening is controversial due to lack of research in the field that demonstrates adequate results. The American Academy of Orthopedic Surgeons (AAOS) and the Scoliosis Research Society continue to endorse scoliosis screenings in schools. However the U.S. Preventive Service Task Force recommended against routine screening in their most recent report (USPSTF, 2004).

B. Scoliosis is a deviation in normal spinal alignment that occurs in the frontal or anteroposterior plane. There are five classifications based on etiology:
   1. Idiopathic.
   2. Congenital.
   3. Neuromuscular.
   4. Syndromes.
   5. Compensatory.

C. *Idiopathic form* is divided into three forms, depending on age at onset. It is called *infantile* at birth to 3 years, *juvenile* at ages 4 to 9, and *adolescent* from age 10 to skeletal maturity.

D. *Congenital form* is caused by a vertebral anomaly that develops in utero, most likely during the third to fifth week; failure of vertebral formation, segmentation of the vertebrae, or mixed deformity (Kliegman et al, 2006).

E. *Neuromuscular scoliosis* may occur at any age and is secondary to disease and other disorders such as muscular dystrophies, cerebral palsy, syringomyelia, myelomeningocele, spinal cord tumor or trauma, and neuropathic diseases.

F. *Syndromes*: Marfan syndrome, Ehlers-Danlos syndrome, neurofibromatosis, or osteogenesis imperfecta.

G. *Compensatory* refers to such conditions as leg length inequality.

H. Other malformations of the spine include kyphosis, lordosis, and kyphoscoliosis.
   1. In *kyphosis* (roundback) an abnormally increased posterior convexity in the curvature of the thoracic spine is observed from the side. Kyphosis deformities can be congenital, structural, or postural.
   2. In *lordosis* an abnormally increased concavity in the curvature of the lumbar spine is observed from the side. It may be secondary to a disease process or trauma, or it may be idiopathic. The pain associated with severe lordosis is different than kyphosis pain.
   3. Mild kyphosis of the thoracic spine and mild lordosis of the lumbar spine may be normal, but scoliosis is never normal. *Kyphoscoliosis* is a combined abnormality of roundback and scoliosis.

I. Scoliosis screening is an opportune time to screen for acanthosis nigricans, which is a precursor of insulin resistance and type 2 diabetes (see Diabetes, page 201).

WEB SITES

National Scoliosis Foundation
    http://www.scoliosis.org
American Academy of Orthopedic Surgeons (AAOS)
    http://www.aaos.org
Scoliosis Research Society
    http://www.srs.org

SEIZURE DISORDER

I. Definition

A. A seizure is an atypical, sudden burst of excessive neuronal-electrical energy that can alter consciousness, motor activity, sensory phenomena, or behavior. A seizure disorder (epilepsy) is a condition of chronic, unprovoked, recurring seizures.

  1. Classifications of seizures:
    a. Partial seizures, simple or complex, which occur in specific areas of the brain.
    b. Generalized seizures—absence, myoclonic, clonic, tonic, tonic-clonic, atonic, and akinetic which can affect nerve cells throughout the brain. There are also unclassified seizures and hybrids.

II. Etiology

A. Seizure disorder has numerous and varied causes based on genetic and acquired factors (e.g., congenital defects, brain injury, metabolic disorders, infectious diseases, tumors, exposure to toxins). Most seizures, however, are idiopathic. Seizures are more common in children under age three but 4% to10% of all children will have at least one seizure before age 16. Almost 150,000 children will have an initial, unprovoked seizure each year, and 30,000 will go on to develop epilepsy (McAbee and Wark, 2000). Seizures continue in about 30% to 40% of children, despite regular use of medication. Onset of most epilepsy syndromes is in childhood (Donner and Snead, 2006).

Brain Findings

With seizures, nerve cells in the brain may be damaged, or difficulty may occur with the neurotransmitters, causing neuronal hyperactivity and a wide range of effects. The neurotransmitter gamma-aminobutyric acid (GABA) appears to be important in suppressing seizures, and it is suggested that a defect in the serotonin receptor may play a role in promoting seizures. Medications often act as agonists (activators) of the inhibitory transmitter GABA. Uncontrolled seizures can lead to degenerative brain alterations likely caused by excitotoxicity (a consequence of oxygen deprivation).

Juvenile myoclonic and absence seizures are heritable, and defective genes have been identified. Chromosome 22 has been implicated with absence seizures.

CHAPTER 4

Chronic Conditions

III. Characteristics
  A. Partial seizures, simple and complex:
    1. Simple, partial seizures result from local cortical discharge; symptoms depend on the area of brain involved and may be motor, sensory, somatosensory, autonomic, psychic, or a combination of all types; no loss of consciousness occurs, and individual may verbalize during the event. The seizure lasts an average of 10 to 20 seconds, and there is rarely a postictal phase.
      a. Motor: occurs in any part of the body; includes "Jacksonian march," which is an orderly sequential progression of clonic movements in foot, hand, or face as electrical impulses spread from irritable focus to indiscriminate regions of the cortex, often ending in a generalized seizure.
      b. Sensory and somatosensory: various sensations, such as visual, auditory, olfactory, gustatory (taste), and touch (e.g., paresthesias [numbness, tingling, prickling] or pain that originates in one area, such as face or extremities, and spreads to other parts of body).
      c. Autonomic: includes abdominal pain, headache, flushing of skin, rapid heart rate, perspiration, drop or rise in blood pressure, pupillary dilation, hair erection, and laughing or crying.
      d. Psychic: disturbance of higher cerebral function (e.g., dreamy states, sense of time distortion, fear, hallucinations of music or scenes).
      e. Combinations of the above types are possible.
    2. Complex partial seizures (psychomotor, temporal lobe): diffuse or focal discharges, usually unilateral or bilateral, originating in temporal or frontal lobe; seizures may be preceded by an aura, which indicates a focal onset; these seizures are the most difficult to recognize and control.
      a. Period of altered behavior in which individual is amnesic and unable to respond to environment, which can be prolonged.
      b. Consciousness is impaired during attack; children are unable to articulate feelings, or a period of impairment makes it difficult to identify seizure.
      c. Automatisms are common in infants and children (50% to 75%), including lip smacking, chewing, swallowing, picking at clothing, rubbing an object, or walking or running in a repetitive, nondirective manner.
      d. Postictal drowsiness or sleep usually follows seizure.
      e. Complex sensory phenomena may occur at the beginning of a seizure (e.g., olfactory, visual, or auditory hallucinations).
      f. Variety of motor behavior patterns may be observed during attack; sometimes it is difficult to determine whether manifestations are related to seizure activity or nonconvulsive behavioral disturbance.
      g. Average length is 1 to 2 minutes.
  B. Generalized seizures (involvement of both hemispheres):
    1. Absence (petit mal):
      a. Brief loss of consciousness or attention, 3 to 30 seconds, not associated with an aura or postictal state.

     b. Minimal or no alteration in muscle tone.

     c. May go unrecognized, since behavior is altered very little.

     d. Possibility of 20 or more attacks daily.

     e. Slight loss of muscle tone, which may cause individual to drop objects.

     f. Able to maintain postural control; person seldom falls.

     g. Frequently automatic movements (e.g., lip smacking, twitching of eyelids or face, slight hand movements).

     h. An attack is often mistaken for inattentiveness or daydreaming.

     i. Usually begins between ages of 5 to 12 years, is more common in girls, and often ceases at puberty.

2. Myoclonic:

     a. Sudden, brief contractures of a muscle or muscle group.

     b. Occurs singly or repetitively without loss of consciousness or postictal state.

     c. Usually lasts less than 3 seconds.

     d. At least five subgroupings are known: benign myoclonus of infancy, typical myoclonic epilepsy of early childhood, complex myoclonic epilepsy (Lennox–Gastaut syndrome), juvenile myoclonic epilepsy, and progressive myoclonic epilepsy.

     e. Usually begins between ages 4 and 11 and may resolve by age 18.

3. Clonic:

     a. Almost exclusively in early childhood.

     b. Begins with loss of or impaired consciousness associated with sudden decreased tone in skeletal muscles or brief generalized tonic spasm, followed by one to several minutes of bilateral jerks (often symmetrical) that may predominate in one limb.

     c. After seizure, there may be rapid recovery, prolonged confusion, or coma.

4. Tonic:

     a. Relatively rare and usually occurs between 1 and 7 years of age.

     b. Sudden increase in muscle tone produces a number of characteristic postures or stiffening.

     c. Consciousness is usually partially or completely lost.

     d. Altered consciousness after seizure is usually brief but may last several minutes.

5. Tonic-clonic (grand mal):

     a. May be associated with an aura, indicating focal origin.

     b. Eyes roll upward.

     c. Immediate loss of consciousness; falls to floor or ground.

     d. Stiffening is generalized and there is symmetric tonic contraction of entire body musculature.

     e. Arms are usually flexed; legs, head, and neck are extended.

     f. May utter peculiar, piercing cry.

     g. Tonic rigidity replaced by jerking movements as trunk and extremities undergo rhythmic contraction and relaxation.

     h. May have increased secretions and be incontinent of urine and feces.

     i. Postictally, appears to relax but may stay semiconscious and be difficult to rouse, or may waken in a few minutes but remain

CHAPTER 4

Chronic Conditions

confused for several hours; will be poorly coordinated with mildly impaired fine motor movements, and usually will sleep for several hours.

j. Occasionally lips and fingernail beds are cyanotic; condition is not unusual and should subside in a short time; if not, emergency measures may be instituted.

k. Series of seizures may occur at intervals too rapid to regain consciousness between attacks; this is known as *status epilepticus* and requires emergency intervention, because it can lead to exhaustion, respiratory failure, and death.

6. Atonic (drop attack):
   a. Loss of muscle tone.
   b. Nodding head, sudden brief dropping of head and neck, sagging at knees, and falling to the floor.
   c. Momentary or no loss of consciousness.
   d. Onset generally 2 to 5 years of age.
   e. Will get up and continue as if nothing happened.
   f. Often difficult to distinguish between atonic and akinetic seizures.

7. Akinetic:
   a. Lack of movement, muscle tone maintained.
   b. Freezes into position but does not fall.
   c. Impaired or momentary loss of consciousness.

8. Infantile spasms:
   a. Most commonly begin between 4 and 8 months of age; twice as common in boys as in girls.
   b. Classified into two groups, *cryptogenic* (unknown etiology) and *symptomatic* (associated with prenatal and postnatal risk factors). Most infants with cryptogenic spasms have a good outcome; infants with symptomatic spasms have an 80% to 90% chance of mental retardation, generally related to an underlying CNS disorder.
   c. Consist of series of sudden, brief, and symmetrical muscular contractions.
   d. Seizure may be preceded or followed by crying or giggling.
   e. Possible loss of consciousness.
   f. Flushing, pallor, or cyanosis sometimes accompanies attack.
   g. May have numerous spasms during the day.
   h. There are three types of spasms, which appear as momentary shocklike contractions of entire body: *flexor, extensor,* and *mixed.*
      (1) *Flexor* is sudden flexion of neck, arms, and legs occurring in clusters.
      (2) *Extensor* involves extension of trunk and extremities.
      (3) *Mixed* is combination of clusters of flexion and extension and is the most common.
   i. Research suggests some relationship to the sleep cycle and an underlying cause related to a particular phase of early brain development that affects neurotransmitter regulation.

IV. Health Concerns/Emergencies
A. Status epilepticus: continuous seizures or serial convulsions without return of consciousness; an emergency situation because of risk of

airway closure, aspiration, anoxia, metabolic acidosis, hypoglycemia, hyperkalemia, lactic acidosis, increased intracranial pressure, and death.

B. Noncompliance issues with medication may include discovery and experimentation with illicit drugs and alcohol during middle childhood and adolescence.

C. Parents may need help understanding the need for continuing medication even in the absence of seizures.

D. Safety concerns include falling and potential injuries. May need to wear a helmet.

E. Routine dental home care and office examinations may be difficult because of seizure activity, related disabilities, or compliance issues.

F. Chronic use of the medications ethosuximide (Zarontin) and phenytoin (Dilantin) can cause lymphoid hyperplasia, which results in gum hypertrophy or enlargement of tonsillar and adenoidal tissue, causing partial airway obstruction and snoring. Gum massage and consistent dental care may reduce gum hypertrophy.

G. Immunizations for pertussis and measles may need to be omitted or deferred for a child with seizures or a family history of seizures if the child is not neurologically stable.

H. School fire alarm systems with flashing lights or strobe lights in assembly programs may trigger seizures in predisposed individuals. Notification of health risks to school administrators is necessary.

V. Effects on Individual

A. Has to learn to live with the possibility that seizures may be lifelong.

B. Apprehensive concerning the occurrence of seizures, helplessness, care provided during an episode, and continued acceptance by peers, teachers, and others.

C. Lack of confidence and low self-esteem, because individuals see themselves as "different" from peers.

D. May be subjected to classmates' cruel remarks, or may be left out of social recreational activities.

E. Feelings of dependence (e.g., must frequently visit the physician, needs daily medication, may need to rely on a stranger's help when a seizure occurs).

F. Embarrassed when consciousness regained after a seizure, especially if incontinent.

G. Children with a seizure disorder may have a lower-than-normal IQ.

H. Temporal lobe seizures can affect language and memory functioning, and partial seizures can impair attention span.

I. There is a greater incidence of psychiatric and behavioral problems and emotional disturbances in children with seizures.

J. Side effects from medication or individual worries about the effects of prolonged use of seizure medication.

K. Difficulty obtaining a driver's license; employment opportunities may be limited.

L. Parents and school personnel can be overprotective, and child may be unnecessarily restricted from physical activity.

M. Safety at risk because of falling; may need to wear a helmet.

N. Caution while swimming; have person with lifesaving skills nearby.

VI. Management/Treatment

A. Ongoing care:
1. Treatment and management is both immediate and lifelong, involving medical, surgical, and dietary strategies and ongoing school assessments.
2. Develop IHCP or IECP for individual student, and train school staff regarding emergency procedures.
3. Special diets combined with ongoing evaluations of blood pressure, hematocrit, urinalysis, vision, hearing, and dental health; alert those on Dilantin and Zarontin regarding gum hyperplasia.
4. When student has complaints, be alert to symptoms related to medications, seizures, or diet, ruling out associations with gastroesophageal reflux (vomiting) and respiratory (apnea or breath holding), neurological (headache), and behavioral symptoms (short attention span, irritability).
5. Exercise good judgment before taking oral temperature of student with a history of seizures.
6. Emphasize need to wear medical alert identification.
7. Oxygen may be prescribed and administered at school for children with severe seizure disorders.
8. Seizure medications can be used alone or in various combinations.
   a. Be aware of medications and know their side effects (see Table 4-11).
   b. Monitor compliance; abrupt withdrawal can precipitate status epilepticus.
   c. Anticonvulsants can modify the therapeutic level of birth control medication; higher doses of birth control should be considered.
   d. Illness, fatigue, and menstrual cycle can affect seizure threshold.
   e. OTC and prescription medications may alter seizure threshold or effectiveness of anticonvulsants.
   f. Blood levels, urinalysis, and liver function tests should be determined periodically for optimum dosage levels of anticonvulsive medications.

B. Status epilepticus:
1. Requires emergency care. See Box 4-9 and Box 4-10 for guidelines for seizure management and observational notes.

NOTE: Be alert to state, county, or district guidelines for calling emergency medical services (EMS), and be aware of practitioner directives for individual students.

2. Diastat (diazepam rectal gel) may be prescribed for use in school if permitted by district policy.
   a. Specific orders must be on file. Assure student privacy during administration. Assessments of vital signs are needed every 5 to 15 minutes for 4 hours after medication is given.
   b. A second dose may be given for a single episode 4 to 12 hours after the first dose. Tolerance to Diastat may develop; should be given no more than every 5 days and not more than five times a month.

C. Other medical care:
1. A ketogenic diet is used with refractory complex myoclonic, tonic-clonic seizures, and infantile spasms.

Table 4-11   *Common Anticonvulsant Drugs*

Drug	Action and Use	Side Effects	Considerations
Corticotropin (ACTH)	Inhibitory effect on excitability of developing brain only; not used in adults. Infantile spasms Lennox–Gastaut	Increased weight or cushingoid appearance; hypertension, extreme irritability, GI distress, transient glycosuria, electrolyte disturbance. **Infections, GI bleeding, sodium retention.**	Given IM, usually a few weeks to several months.
Valproic acid (Depakene, Depakote) Usually adjunctive therapy Half-life 6-16 hr	Directly increases concentration of GABA. Absence Tonic-clonic Myoclonic Partial Akinetic Infantile spasms	GI upset, irregular menses, tremor, indigestion, weight gain, transient alopecia, sedation. **Hepatotoxicity, thrombocytopenia, polycystic ovarian disease.**	Give with food if GI upset occurs; do not crush, break, or chew enteric coated tablets; teratogenic effects. *Overdose:* somnolence, heart block, deep coma.
Phenytoin (Dilantin) Half-life 7-42 hr, average 22 hr Hydantoin class	Decreases sustained repeated firing of single neurons by blocking sodium dependent channels and decreasing calcium uptake. Tonic-clonic, partial, atonic, myoclonic, status epilepticus.	Nausea, confusion, slurred speech, irritability, nystagmus, diplopia, gum hypertrophy, hirsutism, constipation. **Hypersensitivity (rash, fever, lymphadenopathy); blood dyscrasias, osteomalacia caused by vitamin D deficiency; dizziness, ataxia, lethargy, rash.**	Abrupt withdrawal may trigger status epilepticus; pregnancy risks may outweigh benefits (fetal hydantoin syndrome). May need vitamin D supplements.

Continued

Table 4-11 **Common Anticonvulsant Drugs—cont'd**

Drug	Action and Use	Side Effects	Considerations
Felbamate (Felbatol) Adjunctive therapy Half-life 7 to 9 hr	Action unknown Partial Lennox–Gastaut Refractory severe epilepsy	Anorexia, weight loss, insomnia, nausea, vomiting; headache. **Aplastic anemia, hepatic failure.**	*PDR recommendation:* must have written informed consent of risk signed by parent(s). Not first-line anticonvulsant. Not suggested for use under age 12.
Tiagabine (Gabitril) Adjunctive therapy Half-life 7 to 9 hr	Blocks reuptake of GABA into glial and nerve cells. Partial	Ataxia, dizziness, asthenia, tremor, headache, confusion, nervousness, somnolence.	
Clonazepam (Klonopin) Benzodiazepine class Adjunctive and monotherapy Half-life 18-50 hr	Binds to specific GABA site that enhances opening frequency of chloride channel without changing duration. Absence Myoclonic Simple partial Complex partial Akinetic Infantile spasms Lennox–Gastaut	Drowsiness, ataxia. Increased salivation. **Behavioral changes (aggression, agitation, irritability), hyperactivity, cognitive dysfunction.**	Take with food. Abrupt withdrawal may result in striking restlessness, hand tremors, insomnia, status epilepticus, sweating. Psychological or physical dependence may occur. *Overdose:* somnolence, confusion, coma.
Lamotrigine (Lamictal) Adjunctive therapy for Lennox–Gastaut and monotherapy for partial therapy Half-life 12-59 hr	Inhibits voltage sensitive sodium channels, thus stabilizing neuronal membranes and regulating presynaptic transmitter release of excitatory amino acid, (e.g., glutamate). Lennox–Gastout Partial	Nausea, vomiting, dizziness, headache, ataxia, somnolence, diplopia, blurred vision. **Hypersensitivity: fever, rash, lymphadenopathy.**	Possibility of vitamin D and folic acid deficiency.

Drug	Action / Seizure Types	Side Effects	Notes
Phenobarbital (Luminal) Barbiturate class Half-life 3-23 hr	Acts on GABA receptor to increase chloride channel opening time. Tonic-clonic Partial Myoclonic	Drowsiness, hyperactivity, irritability, interferes with motor speed and concentration; mood changes. **Lethargy, learning difficulties, hepatic dysfunction, leukopenia.**	Dependence can occur with prolonged use of high dose; abrupt withdrawal may cause insomnia, tremor, delirium, status epilepticus. *Overdose:* hypothermia, severe CNS depression, severe renal impairment.
Primidone (Mysoline) Half-life 5-7 hr	Action unknown Partial Tonic-clonic	Drowsiness, dizziness, ataxia, hyperactivity, diplopia, loss of coordination. **Behavioral disturbances, GI dysfunction**	Used for age 8 and older.
Gabapentin (Neurontin) Adjunctive therapy Half-life 5-7 hr	Action unknown Partial Secondarily generalized seizures	Fatigue, dizziness, nystagmus, somnolence, ataxia, weight gain, leg edema. **Mood or behavior changes.**	Can be given with or without food.
Vigabatrin (Sabril) Adjunctive therapy Half-life 5-7 hr	Binds to specific GABA receptor, increasing GABA levels. Infantile spasms Tonic-clonic Complex partial	Appetite changes, drowsiness, sedation, abdominal pain, poor concentration. **Behavior changes, visual field constriction, psychosis.**	Not metabolized in liver like most antiseizure medications.
Carbamazepine (Tegretol) Half-life 8-20 hr	Decreases sustained repetitive firing of neurons by blocking sodium channels and decreasing calcium uptake. Tonic-clonic Simple partial Complex partial	Ataxia, drowsiness, dizziness, irritability, nausea/vomiting, visual abnormalities (spots before eyes, blurred vision, diplopia, difficulty focusing). **Rashes, movement disorders, hepatic dysfunction, bone marrow suppression, blood dyscrasias, CV disturbances.**	Take with meals to decrease GI distress. Abrupt withdrawal may precipitate status epilepticus. Erythromycin and other antibiotics increase levels, causing toxicity and increased effects.

Continued

Table 4-11 *Common Anticonvulsant Drugs—cont'd*

Drug	Action and Use	Side Effects	Considerations
Topiramate (Topamax) Half-life 21 hr Adjunctive therapy	Blocks repetitive sustained firing of neurons by inhibiting sodium channels. Tonic-clonic Partial Lennox–Gastaut	Somnolence, fatigue, diplopia, anorexia, anemia, weight loss, GI upset, headache, tremor, ataxia, renal stones, impaired cognition.	Maintain adequate hydration to prevent renal stones.
Oxcarbazepine (Trileptal) Half-life 9 hr Adjunctive therapy	May inhibit nerve impulses by limiting influx of sodium ions across cell membranes in motor cortex. Partial	Fatigue, headache, confusion, dizziness, blurred vision, diplopia, nystagmus, low sodium, GI upset, rash. May worsen seizures, rectal hemorrhage.	Give with food to decrease GI problems.
Ethosuximide (Zarontin) Half-life 60 hr	Blocks calcium channels linked with thalamocortical circulatory Absence.	GI upset, headache, drowsiness, dizziness. **Leukopenia, agranulocytosis.**	Administer with food; may aggravate tonic-clonic seizures. *Overdose:* nausea and vomiting, CNS depression.

Modified from Skidmore-Roth L: *Mosby's nursing drug reference,* St Louis, 2007, Elsevier Mosby.
NOTE: Pregnancy and breast-feeding risks are involved with many of the medications and warrant consideration for females of childbearing age.

| Box 4-9 | **Guidelines for Seizure Management** |

Protect individual during seizure and maintain airway by doing the following:

1. Make no attempt to halt seizure or restrain individual.
2. If standing or sitting in chair or wheelchair, ease down to floor immediately.
3. Do not force any object between teeth.
4. Loosen restrictive clothing.
5. Protect individual from hitting hard or sharp objects that might cause injury.
6. If salivation is excessive, turn onto side.
7. Cyanosis and cessation of breathing may occur briefly.
8. If individual appears in respiratory distress and skin is excessively blue, extend neck and gently pull on jaw. With infants, only slightly tilt head, because overextension blocks airway. If breathing does not resume, start CPR and call for medical assistance.
9. Call EMS if seizure is followed by other seizures in rapid succession, or if duration of seizure is excessive or without signs of stopping* (about 10 min for known epileptics, 5 min if no history of seizures).
10. After an episode, position individuals to lying on their side, and allow sleep until they awaken on their own.
11. Attend until the individual is conscious and oriented.

NOTE: Follow IECP or IHCP or adapt guidelines as needed.

*Epilepsy Foundation, 2008 (http://www.epilepsyfoundation.org). *CPR,* Cardiopulmonary resuscitation; *EMS,* emergency medical services; *IECP,* Individualized Emergency Care Plan; *IHCP,* Individualized Health Care Plan.

| Box 4-10 | **Observational Notes** |

During a seizure, observe and document the following information on a seizure log or health record for diagnosis and management of disorder:

1. Significant preictal events, including aura and exposure to bright lights, noise, or excitement.
2. Movements before, during, and after attack.
3. Time seizure began and length of seizure.
4. Change in color or respiratory effort, profuse perspiration.
5. Where seizure movement began (e.g., legs, arms, head).
6. Change in facial expression, eye movements, muscle tone, and automatisms.
7. Involuntary urination or defecation.
8. Note length of postictal phase, confusion, orientation to time and person, impaired speech, report of headache or muscle soreness, and changes in motor ability and sensation.

a. High in fats, low in proteins and carbohydrates, and sometimes used as treatment when control has not been achieved.
b. Burning fat instead of carbohydrates causes ketosis, but exact mechanism of action is unknown.
c. This is a strict diet with substantial risks that is initiated in the hospital to monitor metabolic and neurological changes.
d. Families may have difficulty with the precise measurement of foods, and not all children can tolerate the food restrictions. Hypoglycemia and weight loss can occur.

    e. Studies indicate a 50% to 70% reduction in seizures in about half of the patients (Jarrar and Buchhalter, 2003).

    f. Diet may be discontinued when goal is achieved.

2. Surgery is considered when seizures are uncontrolled by other methods. Regardless of the type of surgery performed, medication may still be needed for optimum control of seizures. Risks depend on type of surgery and include hemiparesis, language difficulties, and memory loss.

3. There are two major surgical techniques: resection and disconnection.

    a. Resection includes lesionectomy, lobectomy, or hemispherectomy, and it is used for infants and young children with catastrophic seizures. Lesionectomy is performed for small brain tumors or abnormalities that cause seizures. Lobectomy is conducted when focal points are limited to one lobe; small portions or the entire lobe is removed (e.g., temporal or occipital lobe). Hemispherectomy is used for seizures associated with congenital hemiplegia, chronic encephalitis, hemimegalencephaly, Sturge–Weber syndrome, and when rampant epileptic discharges extend to the normal hemisphere.

    b. Disconnection examples are corpus callosotomy and subpial transection. Corpus callosotomy is used with generalized seizures and involves partial or total removal of the corpus callosum, the white matter connecting the two hemispheres. Subpial transection entails dividing the horizontal fibers of the motor cortex while sparing the vertical fibers, thus achieving a reduction in seizures while maintaining cerebral function.

4. Vagus nerve stimulation (VNS) is considered for intractable seizures and has been demonstrated to reduce seizures by 40% to 50% in children under age 12 (Saneto et al, 2006). VNS is achieved by inserting a battery-powered device under the skin in the upper left chest with a lead attached to the vagus nerve in the lower part of the neck that provides automatic intermittent stimulation to the nerve. When seizures are preceded by an aura, the seizure activity may be aborted by passing an external magnet over the implant to initiate VNS. In young children and those with disabilities, a responsible adult can apply the magnet. Older children and adolescents with normal cognitive functioning do well with the magnet, because it can be made to appear as a bracelet, and when a seizure is sensed, the hand is simply moved across the chest area. Side effects include hoarseness, throat paresthesias, headache, and shortness of breath, which can be reduced or eliminated by adjusting the intensity of the stimulation.

VII. Additional Information

    A. Febrile seizures are the most common seizure disorder in children; associated with rapidly rising fever (102 degrees or greater), generally brief, clonic, or tonic-clonic seizures with little postictal confusion. Usually seen in children from 5 months to 5 years of age with no long-lasting effects. Etiology is unclear, but genetic predisposition is supported by strong family histories, and several gene markers have been identified. Treatment is usually limited to acute episode. Antipyretics may be used and diazepam (Valium) prescribed at the onset and for duration of a febrile illness. Prophylactic anticonvulsants are not recommended. Risk factors for developing seizure disorder are family history of epilepsy, prolonged or atypical febrile seizure, initial febrile seizure before 9 months of age, abnormal neurological examination, and delayed developmental milestones.

B. Lennox–Gastaut syndrome is refractory myoclonic and clonic seizure activity with specific electroencephalogram (EEG) patterns. It generally commences in the first year of life, and the prognosis is poor. About 75% of those affected have mental retardation and behavioral problems. Seizure control is difficult to achieve with medication alone, and a ketogenic diet may be an option (see Table 4-11).

C. Seizures can be triggered by daily events, including flashing or rotating lights, video, television's fast-moving lights (photosensitive seizures), or by high-pitched sounds. Often outgrown in adulthood.

D. Many well-known, intelligent people have had epilepsy, including Alexander the Great, Napoleon, Julius Caesar, and Vincent Van Gogh.

WEB SITE

Epilepsy Foundation
http://www.epilepsyfoundation.org

SPINA BIFIDA/MYELODYSPLASIA

I. Definition

A. Neural tube defects are anomalies of the spinal column, spinal cord, and skin that develop around the third to fourth weeks of embryonic development. There are two common forms of neural tube malformations: *spina bifida occulta* and *spina bifida cystica* (see Figure 4-7).

B. With *spina bifida occulta,* no abnormalities of the spinal cord or meninges exist. The vertebral defect is covered by skin.

C. *Spina bifida cystica* involves two major malformations. With *meningocele,* the meninges pouch out because of a defect in a vertebra of the spine, forming a saclike membrane containing cerebrospinal fluid (CSF). The area is covered by skin, and it does not involve the spinal cord. Hydrocephalus is associated with this diagnosis.

D. In *meningomyelocele* or *myelomeningocele,* the membranes, a portion of the spinal cord, and the nerves protrude through a defect in the vertebra. The sac is covered with a thin membrane, and hydrocephalus is common when the defect is in the lower vertebral area.

II. Etiology

A. The exact cause of spina bifida is unknown. There is a genetic predisposition, however, and nutritional and environmental factors play a role in the etiology. Research studies provide evidence that folic acid deficiencies are associated with neural tube defects, and an adequate intake of folic acid can reduce the incidence by 50% to 70% (Johnston and Kinsman, 2004). Particular drugs can also increase the risk for malformations, such as valproic acid.

CHAPTER 4

Chronic Conditions

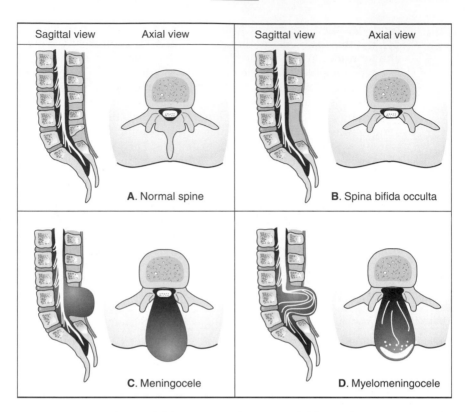

FIGURE 4-7 Forms of spina bifida. **A,** Normal. **B,** Spina bifida occulta. **C,** Meningocele. **D,** Myelomeningocele.

III. Characteristics

A. Spina bifida occulta:
1. Many individuals have no symptoms.
2. May display superficial manifestations; these signs may occur alone, together, or in combination.
   a. May be noticed as a depression or dimpling over the malformed vertebrae, which may mark the site of a dermoid sinus.
   b. Abnormal tufts of hair may be present.
   c. Telangiectasia, a small red lesion comprised of dilated capillaries.
   d. Subcutaneous lipomas (fatty tumors) are present.
3. Spinal cord and meninges are normal.
4. Defect is covered by skin and may go unnoticed, unless there are associated manifestations:
   a. Gait abnormalities become progressive.
   b. Bowel or bladder difficulties.
5. Generally occurs at L5 and S1 but may affect any area of the spinal column.

B. Spina bifida cystica:
1. Symptoms and prognosis depend on level and type of lesion, presence of hydrocephalus, or secondary complications (e.g., meningitis).

C. Meningocele:
1. Sac containing meninges and CSF protrudes through vertebral defect.
2. Cord and nerve roots generally are not involved.
3. May occur anywhere along spinal column.
4. Generally no bowel or bladder involvement.
5. Lower extremities usually not involved.
6. Hydrocephalus is associated.
7. Defects above thorax are usually meningoceles.
8. Females may have genital tract anomalies, such as vaginal septa and rectovaginal fistula.
D. Meningomyelocele:
1. Most common form of open spine defect.
2. Occurs anywhere along the neuraxis, but 75% are in the lumbo-sacral area (Johnston and Kinsman, 2004).
3. Sac contains meninges, spinal fluid, portion of spinal cord, and its nerves.
4. Leak in utero of sac or rupture after birth causes CSF drainage and makes the newborn susceptible to meningitis.
5. Surgical intervention should be within the first few days after birth, unless a CSF leakage is present.
6. Neurological, orthopedic, urological, and bowel difficulties are associated conditions.
   a. Neurological factors:
      (1) Extent of paralysis depends on location of defect.
      (2) Loss of sensation in body areas below lesions.
      (3) Hydrocephaly occurs in most children.
      (4) Hydrocephaly is usually secondary to Type II Arnold–Chiari malformation, which causes compression of cerebellar brain tissue through the foramen magnum, where the spinal cord enters the spinal column. Symptoms include feeding difficulties, choking, stridor, hoarse cry, vocal cord paralysis, apnea, and spasticity of the upper extremities.
   b. Orthopedic factors:
      (1) Dislocation of hips.
      (2) Equinovarus (clubfoot) often associated anomaly.
      (3) Scoliosis, lordosis, or kyphosis in later years.
      (4) Contractures of feet, ankles, or knees usually occur.
      (5) Prone to fractures of lower extremities.
      (6) Ambulation may or may not occur; canes and braces may be required.
   c. Urological and bowel factors:
      (1) Neurogenic bladder and bowel.
      (2) Increased susceptibility to urinary tract infections because of stasis of urine.
      (3) Poor bowel musculature or paralysis.
      (4) No bowel sensation present.

IV. Health Concerns/Emergencies
A. Medical concerns depend on state and extent of lesion and generally are associated with meningomyelocele.

    B. Loss of sensation puts individual at risk for decubiti, abrasions, and burns.

    C. If shunted for hydrocephalus, awareness of signs of increased intracranial pressure or shunt failure is necessary: irritability, restlessness, vomiting, complaints of headache, possible seizures, change in vital signs, and pupillary changes.

    D. Buttocks and areas around braces and shoes are prone to skin breakdown and must be checked frequently for rubbing and redness.

    E. Obesity can result from inactivity, inappropriate dietary management, or both.

    F. Fecal incontinence and lack of bladder control cause skin breakdown and make toilet training difficult.

    G. High risk for latex allergies.

V. Effects on Individual

    A. This condition is associated with neurodevelopmental deficits, such as visual conditions (e.g., astigmatism), memory deficits, poor organizational skills, visual-perceptual problems, impaired eye–hand coordination, and handwriting difficulties that interfere with school performance.

    B. Numerous medical appointments, surgeries, and hospitalizations take the student away from home and out of school for extended periods, interfering with academic achievement.

    C. Child may be obese from low activity level.

    D. Limitations and inconvenience are imposed by confinement to a wheelchair (e.g., certain routes may take longer to get to a class).

    E. How student is treated and viewed by parents affects his or her self-esteem and feelings of competence or incompetence (e.g., fostering independence or being overprotective).

VI. Management/Treatment

    A. Treatment and management are both immediate and lifelong.

    B. Develop IHCP or IECP to address urgent issues (e.g., VP shunt obstruction, injuries). If student is receiving special education, write nurse assessment report for IEP and attend meetings as appropriate.

    C. Monitor vision and hearing.

    D. Be alert for latex allergies (see Chapter 9).

    E. As with all children, allergy identification should be worn, such as a bracelet or necklace.

    F. Be aware of medications and their side effects.

    G. Catheterization or Credé's method may need to be taught to child or staff. Check Nurse Practice Act for guidelines related to delegation of care.

    H. Evaluate and teach designated school staff to observe periodically for skin breakdown caused by immobility, bracing, or rubbing of appliances; encourage a high-fiber diet and fluids to decrease bowel and urinary problems.

    I. Assess wheelchair for good working order and appropriate size.

    J. Evaluate usability and safety of school routine and pathways via wheelchair. Emergency evacuation plans should be in place.

    K. Be available to share and discuss health and psychosocial concerns that may interfere with friendships, family relationships, and life satisfaction with both students and parents.

L. Be knowledgeable about local resources for child and family counseling.

VII. **Additional Information**

A. Prenatal diagnosis may be possible between the sixteenth to eighteenth weeks of gestation. An elevated alpha-fetoprotein (AFP) indicates a risk, and an ultrasound of the uterus may detect an open neural tube defect.

B. Folic acid supplement, 0.4 mg daily, is recommended for all women of childbearing age. Folic acid is absolutely essential before conception and at least through the first 12 weeks of gestation, when neurulation development is complete (Johnston and Kinsman, 2004).

C. Abnormal adhesion of the spinal cord to a bony structure in the area of malformation results in a tethered cord. Manifestations include altered gait pattern, foot weakness, back pain, and problems with bowel and bladder control. These symptoms may not be seen for years, unless a child has the ability to walk or be toilet trained. Surgical intervention is based on level of involvement. May occur with both spina bifida occulta and spina bifida cystica.

D. Management of a neurogenic bladder beyond catheterization may include drug therapy with anticholinergic medication to relax the bladder and tighten the urinary sphincter; surgery, including bladder augmentation, implantation of artificial urinary sphincter, or construction of continent ileostomy for catheterization may be recommended. Reducing fluid intake in the evening may prevent nighttime incontinence.

WEB SITES

Association for Spina Bifida and Hydrocephalus
    http://www.asbah.org
March of Dimes Birth Defects Foundation
    http://www.marchofdimes.com
Spina Bifida Association
    http://www.sbaa.org

TUBERCULOSIS

I. **Definition**

A. Tuberculosis (TB) is a chronic infectious disease that primarily attacks the lungs, but it can infect any part of the body, including the kidneys, brain, joints, and spine. If not treated adequately, TB can be fatal—it is the second leading cause of death from infectious disease.

II. **Etiology**

A. TB is caused by an acid-fast bacillus, Mycobacterium tuberculosis. It is primarily transmitted by ingestion or inhalation of infected droplets. TB in the lungs and throat can be infectious, but TB in other parts of the body is generally noninfectious.

B. Children are vulnerable to the human (M. tuberculosis) bacterium and the bovine (M. bovis) bacterium. The source of M. bovis in children is unpasteurized milk or milk products.

C. In the United States, 10 to 15 million people have latent TB infection (LTBI). In 2005, about 14,000 active TB cases were reported to CDC, and the rate of TB in foreign-born people was almost nine times those born in the United States. TB has been decreasing since 1993 in the United States, but the rate of decline is waning.

III. Characteristics

A. Active TB disease is diagnosed generally when there is a positive tuberculin skin test (TST) followed by an abnormal chest x-ray, positive sputum, or extra pulmonary symptoms. Positive TST alone does not indicate active TB disease.
   1. LTBI indicates an individual who has a positive TST with a normal chest x-ray and no other physical findings of disease. They cannot spread the disease; but if LTBI is not identified and treated early, the individual can develop TB later in life.
B. Physical characteristics of active TB include malaise, fever, night sweats, anorexia, weight loss, chronic cough—which may or may not occur, but if present, progresses slowly—and aching and tightness in the chest.
C. Secondary symptoms include increased respiratory rate, anemia and pallor, diminished breath sounds and crackles, poor expansion of affected side, and dullness of percussion.

IV. Health Concerns/Emergencies

A. Young children rarely infect other children or adults, because they lack a forceful cough, and their secretions have few tubercle bacilli.
B. Children under age 4 diagnosed with TB infection are at greater risk for developing disseminated disease and need prompt and comprehensive treatment.
C. Children at or below age 5 with a positive TST are at risk for progression to disease within the first year or two after exposure.

V. Effects on Individual

A. May be asymptomatic with minor abnormalities on x-ray.
B. May have low-grade fever, malaise, lymph node enlargement.
C. Tuberculous meningitis is most commonly found in children under age 5; may exhibit low-grade fever and sudden personality change.

VI. Management/Treatment

A. The American Academy of Pediatrics and the CDC recommend targeted tuberculin skin testing for those individuals at high risk but discourage it for those at low risk for developing TB. Targeted risk categories include:
   1. Those having close contact with adults having infectious TB.
   2. Children traveling to or having visitors from countries with high TB prevalence.
   3. Children with HIV or other immunosuppressive conditions including diabetes mellitus, malnutrition, chronic renal failure, and lymphoma.
   4. Adolescents with a history of incarceration.
   5. Children exposed to high-risk individuals (e.g., homeless, HIV-infected, drug addicts, incarcerated individuals, nursing home residents, and migrant workers).

B. History of bacillus Calmette–Guerin (BCG) vaccine is not a contrain-dication for tuberculin skin testing.
C. Test all high-risk children and adolescents with the Mantoux skin test, or purified protein derivative (see Box 4-11).
D. Test school staff and volunteers as required by individual state laws and county and district guidelines.
E. Test must be read within 48 to 72 hours, interpreted, documented, and referred for treatment when indicated.
F. Perform chest x-ray and medical examination.
G. Recommended treatment for positive TST for all children.
   1. Isoniazid (INH), 10 to 20 mg per kilogram of body weight, not to exceed 300 mg per day.
   2. Daily therapy for 9 months.
   3. Directly observed therapy (DOT) is provided at the school site for consistency of therapy.
H. Medications for active disease commonly include INH, rifampin, pyrazinamide, and streptomycin.
I. Increasingly, multi–drug-resistant (MDR-TB) disease requires specific, targeted therapy.

VII. Additional Information
A. QuantiFERON-TB Gold (QFT-G) is a new blood test for TB screening. QFT-G was approved for use in 2005 for ages 17 and older. The test requires 5 cc of blood and must be processed within 12 hours. The test requires one visit, has fewer false positives, and is not affected by BCG.

Box 4-11   *Interpretation of Positive Skin Test for TB*

Definitions of positive skin tests of infants, children, and adolescents. The divisions below help to separate positive results from negative results based on specific risk factors.

Induration	Positive in child with:
Induration ≥5 mm:	Recent close contact with a person who has contagious TB; immunosuppressive disease; i.e., HIV, or on immunosuppressive drugs; Positive chest x-ray or suspected of having TB disease.
Induration ≥10 mm:	Medical conditions that place them at risk for disseminated TB; i.e.; malnutrition, diabetes, lymphoma, and being under 4 years of age. Frequent exposure to adults who are HIV-diseased, users of illicit drugs, incarcerated, homeless, residents of nursing homes, migrant farm workers.
Induration ≥15 mm:	No known risk factors and is age 4 or older.

NOTE: Induration is the elevation of the wheal, which is measured horizontally across the noted area. Redness without the hardened elevation is not a positive reaction. Record the results by mm of induration not by negative or positive reactions.

WEB SITE

Centers for Disease Control and Prevention, Division of Tuberculosis Elimination (DTBE)
http://www.cdc.gov/nchstp/tb

TURNER'S SYNDROME

I. Definition

A. Turner's syndrome (TS) is a chromosomal disorder (45 X) in which females have only one X chromosome instead of two. It is also known as XO syndrome and is called Ullrich-Turner syndrome in Europe. TS is the most common chromosomal abnormality found in the female fetus and generally (99%) are spontaneously aborted.

II. Etiology

A. TS results from complete or partial monosomy of the short arm on the X chromosome. The syndrome occurs in about 1 in 3200 live female births. Approximately 25% are mosaics (Levy and Marion, 2006).

III. Characteristics

A. Infants with TS may not be diagnosed during the newborn period due to subtle features. However, around 33% are diagnosed after birth due to congenital heart disease or physical characteristics.
   1. Symptoms recognized at birth include edema of the hands and feet, loose skinfolds at the nape of the neck (nuchal folds), epicanthal folds, low-set ears, small mandible, low birth weight, decreased length, and left-sided cardiac anomalies.
B. Another 33% of young girls are diagnosed in childhood, usually during a follow-up for short stature.
   1. Symptoms include declining growth, webbing of the neck, micrognathia (small jaw), high-arched palate, rotated or protruding ears, low hairline in back of head, or bilateral shortened ring finger.
C. Lastly, 33% are diagnosed during adolescence after they fail to develop secondary sexual characteristics (Levy and Marion, 2006).
   1. Symptoms can include pubertal delay, primary amenorrhea, and sterility. Because no ovaries exist, girls do not produce ovarian hormones.
D. Some girls have only a few features, but short stature is a cardinal characteristic.
E. Average adult height is 56 inches without treatment.
F. Hypoplastic, hyperconvex fingernails and short metacarpals or metatarsals.
G. Primary hypertension.
H. Pectus excavatum, coarctation of the aorta, and other cardiovascular abnormalities.
I. Absent kidney or renal abnormalities.
J. Hashimoto's thyroiditis (autoimmune thyroid disorder).

K. Susceptible to GI bleeding because of abnormal vascular development of the bowel.

L. Scoliosis in 10% (Rapaport, 2004).

M. Impaired vision (strabismus, amblyopia, myopia, and ptosis) and red-green color deficiency.

N. Sensorineural hearing loss.

O. Visuospatial processing, visual memory, and visuomotor integration difficulties; rarely associated with decreased IQ levels.

P. There are varying degrees of physical, emotional, and learning abilities.

IV. Health Concerns/Emergencies

A. Otitis media is more common in TS than in the general population.

B. Cardiac and kidney problems can contribute to frequent absences from school.

C. Obesity secondary to hormonal and metabolic dysfunction.

D. All of the above can affect the student's academic achievement.

V. Effects on Individual

A. Rarely fertile.

B. May grieve lack of fertility; begin discussion before adolescence.

C. Self-conscious of appearance when epicanthal folds, protruding ears, and webbed neck are prominent.

D. Susceptible to teasing and bullying due to short stature and delayed social maturity.

VI. Management/Treatment

A. Evaluate hearing and vision.

B. Assess blood pressure frequently.

C. Monitor growth using TS-specific growth chart.

D. Growth hormone treatment generally starts when student falls below the fifth percentile for normal female growth; should begin as early as age 2 for maximum benefits.

E. Initiation of estrogen replacement therapy (ERT) interrupts growth and may need to be delayed until 14 to 15 years of age; ERT typically starts at about 12 to 13 years.

F. Monitor side effects of medications given for renal, cardiac, or diabetic conditions; monitor ERT and growth hormone treatment.

G. Psychosocial support is important.

H. Encourage involvement in TS support groups for students and their families.

I. Be informative and supportive of parent or student considering plastic surgery for epicanthal folds, protruding ears, and webbed neck.

VII. Additional Information

A. Can be diagnosed prenatally by CVS or amniocentesis. Associated with polyhydramnios, oligohydramnios, unexplained anemia, or preeclampsia.

WEB SITES

The Magic Foundation (Major Aspects of Growth in Children)
   http://www.magicfoundation.org/
Turner Syndrome Support Society
   http://www.tss.org.uk

BIBLIOGRAPHY

Alemzadeh R, Wyatt DT: Diabetes mellitus in children. In Behrman RE, Kliegman RM, Jenson HB, eds: *Nelson textbook of pediatrics,* Philadelphia, 2004, Elsevier Saunders.

American Academy of Allergy, Asthma, and Immunology: *Tips to remember: childhood asthma* (article online): www.aaaai.org/patients/publicedmat/tips/childhoodasthma.stm.Accessed December 20, 2007.

American Academy of Pediatrics Committee on Environmental Health: Lead exposure in children: prevention, detection, and management, *Pediatrics* 116(4):1036-1046, 2005.

American College of Asthma, Allergy, and Immunology: *ACAAI 2007 National screening program* (available online): www.aanma.org/medicalcenter/mc_screening.htm.

American Psychiatric Association: *Diagnostic and statistical manual of mental disorders,* ed 4, text revision, Washington, DC, 2000, The American Psychiatric Association.

Anderson PM, Butcher KF: Childhood obesity: trends and potential causes, *The Future of Children* 16(1):1-46, 2006.

Ardary DA: Increasing school nurse awareness of Turner syndrome, *J Sch Nurs* 23(1):28-33, 2007.

Baer JS, Sampson PD, Barr H et al: A 21-year longitudinal analysis of the effects of prenatal alcohol exposure on young adult drinking, *Arch Gen Psych* 60:377-385, 2003.

Bertrand J, Floyd R, Weber M et al: *Fetal alcohol syndrome: Guidelines for referral and diagnosis,* Atlanta, 2004, Centers for Disease Control and Prevention (available online): www.cdc.gov/ncbddd/fas/faspub.htm.Accessed December 20, 2007.

Bishop WP: The digestive system. In Kliegman RM, Marcdante KJ, Jenson HB, Behrman RE, eds: *Nelson essentials of pediatrics,* Philadelphia, 2006, Elsevier Saunders.

Bloom B, Dey AN, Freeman G: Summary health statistics for U.S. children: national health interview survey, *Vital Health Stats* 10:231, 2005, National Center for Health Statistics (available online): www.cdc.gov/nchs/data/series/sr_10/sr10_231.pdf. Accessed December 20, 2007.

Canfield RL, Henderson CR, Cory-Slechta DA et al: Intellectual impairment in children with blood lead concentrations below 10μ per deciliter. *N Engl J Med* 348(16):1517-1526, 2003.

Centers for Disease Control and Prevention: *About CMV,* 2006b (available online): www.cdc.gov/cmv/facts.htm. Accessed March 31, 2007.

Centers for Disease Control and Prevention: Diabetes: disabling disease to double by 2050, *At a Glance,* Jan 2007a (available online): Accessed December 20, 2007.www .cdc.gov/nccdphp/publications/aag/pdf/diabetes.pdf. Accessed December 20, 2007.

Centers for Disease Control and Prevention: *Guide for primary health care providers: targeted tuberculosis testing and treatment of latent tuberculosis infection,* Atlanta, 2005a, US Dept of Health and Human Services (available online): www.cdc.gov/nchstp/tb/pubs/LTBI/pdf/TargetedLTBI05.pdf. Accessed May 5, 2006.

Centers for Disease Control and Prevention: *HIV/AIDS,* 2007b (available online): www.cdc.gov/hiv. Accessed on April 5, 2007.

Centers for Disease Control and Prevention, National Center for Health Statistics: State of childhood asthma, United States: 1980–2005, *Fact Sheet,* Dec 2006a (available online): www.cdc.gov/nchs/pressroom/06facts/asthma1980-2005.htm. Accessed March 28, 2007.

Centers for Disease Control and Prevention: *National diabetes fact sheet,* 2005b (available online): www.cdc.gov/diabetes/pubs/pdf/ndfs_2005.pdf. Accessed March 31, 2007.

Centers for Disease Control and Prevention: Trends in tuberculosis, *US 2005 Morbidity and Mortality Weekly Report* 55(11):305-338, 2006c (available online): www.cdc.gov/mmwr/preview/mmwrhtml/mm5511a3.htm. Accessed May 5, 2006.

Cerasuolo K: The child with endocrine dysfunction. In Hockenberry MJ, Wilson D, editors: *Wong's nursing care of infants and children,* St Louis, 2007, Elsevier Mosby.

Christophersen ER, Friman PC: Elimination disorders. In R Brown, ed, *Handbook of pediatric psychology in school settings,* Mahwah, NJ, 2004, Lawrence Erlbaum.

Day S, Chismark E: The cognitive and academic impact of sickle cell disease, *Journal of School Health* 22(6):330-333, 2006.

Donner EJ, Snead OC: New drugs in the treatment of epilepsy in children, *Curr Probl Pediatr Adolesc Health Care* 35(10):398-419, 2006.

Dreger AD, Chase C, Sousa A, Gruppuso PA, Frader J: Changing the nomenclature/taxonomy for intersex: a scientific and clinical rationale, *J Pediatric Endocrinol Metab* 18(8):729-33, 2005.

Drew D, Hewitt H: A qualitative approach to understanding patients' diagnosis of Lyme disease, *Public Health Nursing* 23(1):20-26, 2006.

Farooqi IS, Keogh JM, Yeo GSH: Clinical spectrum of obesity and mutations in the melanocortin 4 receptor gene, *N Engl J Med* 348(12):1085-1095, 2003.

Gahagan S: Behavioral disorders. In Kliegman RM, Marcdante KJ, Jenson HB, Behrman RE, editors: *Nelson essentials of pediatrics,* Philadelphia, 2006, Elsevier Saunders.

Haftel HM: Rheumatic diseases of childhood. In Kliegman RM, Marcdante KJ, Jenson HB, Behrman RE, editors: *Nelson essentials of pediatrics,* Philadelphia, 2006, Elsevier Saunders.

Hagerman R: Fragile X syndrome. In Parker S, Zuckerman B, Augustyn M, editors: *Developmental and behavioral pediatrics,* Philadelphia, 2005, Lippincott Williams & Wilkins.

Hagerman RJ, Hagerman PJ: *Fragile x syndrome: diagnosis, treatment, and research,* Baltimore, 2003, Johns Hopkins University Press.

Hall MJ, DeFrances CJ: 2001 National hospital discharge survey, *Vital and Health Statistics* No. 332, Hyattsville, Md, 2003, National Centers for Disease Control and Prevention (available online): www.cdc.gov/nchs/data/ad/ad332. Accessed December 20, 2007.

Hockenberry MJ, Wilson D, Winkelstein ML: *Wong's essentials of pediatric nursing,* St Louis, 2006, Elsevier Mosby.

Hodges EA: A primer on early childhood obesity and parental influence, *Pediatric Nursing* 29(3):13-22, 2003.

Howard KR: Childhood overweight: parental perceptions and readiness for change, *J Sch Nurs* 23(2):73-79, 2007.

Jarrar RG, Buchhalter JR: Therapeutics in pediatric epilepsy, part 1: the new antiepileptic drugs and the ketogenic diet, *Mayo Clin Proc* 78:359-70, 2003.

Jenson HB, Baltimore RS: Infectious diseases. In Kliegman RM, Marcdante KJ, Jenson HB, Behrman RE, editors: *Nelson essentials of pediatrics,* Philadelphia, 2006, Elsevier Saunders.

Johnston MV, Kinsman S: Congenital anomalies of the central nervous system. In Kliegman RM, Marcdante KJ, Jenson HB, Behrman RE, editors: *Nelson essentials of pediatrics, Philadelphia,* 2006, Elsevier Saunders.

Jones KL: *Recognizable patterns of human malformation,* Philadelphia, 2006, Elsevier Saunders.

Kaufman FR: Type 2 diabetes in children and youth, *Endocrinology and Metabolism Clinics* 34(3):659-76, 2005.

King EC, Saarwark JF: A look at scoliosis, *The Child's Doctor: Journal of Children's Memorial Hospital Chicago* Spring 2002 (available online):www.childsdoc.org/spring2002/lookscoliosis.asp. Accessed Oct 7, 2006.

Kliegman RM, Marcdante KJ, Jenson HB, Behrman RE, editors: *Nelson essentials of pediatrics,* Philadelphia, Elsevier Saunders.

Kwan P, Brodie MJ: Early identification of refractory epilepsy, *N Engl J Med* 342:314-319, 2000.

CHAPTER 4

Chronic Conditions

Lasley EN: Hormones play surprising roles, *Dana Foundation's Brain Work: Neuroscience Newsletter* 16(4):1-4, 2006.

Lee PA, Houk CP, Ahmed SF et al: Endorsed AAP policy statement: consensus statement on management of intersex disorders, *Pediatrics* 118 (2):e488-e500, 2006 (available online):www.aappolicy.aappublications.org/cgi/content/full/pediatrics;118/2/e488. Accessed December 20, 2007.

Levy PA, Marion RW: Human genetics and dysmorphology. In Kliegman RM, Marcdante KJ, Jenson HB, Behrman RE, editors: *Nelson essentials of pediatrics,* Philadelphia, 2006, Elsevier Saunders.

Lidsky TI, Schneider JS: Lead neurotoxicity in children: basic mechanisms and clinical correlates, *Brain* 126:5-19, 2003.

Liu AH, Spahn JD, Leung DYM: Childhood asthma. In Behrman RE, Kliegman RM, Jenson, HB, editors: *Nelson textbook of pediatrics,* Philadelphia, 2004, Elsevier Saunders.

Marshall SG, Debley JS: The respiratory system. In Kliegman RM, Marcdante KJ, Jenson HB, Behrman RE, editors: *Nelson essentials of pediatrics,* Philadelphia, 2006, Elsevier Saunders.

McAbee GN, War JE: A practical approach to uncomplicated seizures in children, *Am Fam Physician* 62 (5):1109-16, 2000.

Merkle SL, Wheeler LS, Gerald LB et al: Introduction: Learning from each other about managing asthma in schools, *J Sch Health* 76(6):202-204, 2006.

Meyer PA, Pivetz T, Dignam TA et al: Surveillance for elevated blood levels among children 1997-2001, *Morb Mortal Wkly Rep* 52 SS (10):1-21, 2003 (available online): www.cdc.gov/mm wr/preview/mmwrhtml/ss5210a1.htm. Accessed May 2, 2006.

Moore C: Chores, play can help children burn calories, *Cox News Service* (available online): www.ajc.com/health/content/shared/health/weightloss/kids_health.htm. Accessed April 12, 2007.

Murphy M, Polivka B: Parental perceptions of the schools' role in addressing childhood obesity, *J Sch Nurs* 23(1):40-52, 2007.

National Center for Health Statistics: Prevalence of overweight among children and adolescents: United States, 2003-2004 (available online):www.cdc.gov/nchs/products/pubs/pubd/hestats/overweight/overwght_child_03.htm. Accessed December 20, 2007.

National Heart, Lung, and Blood Institute, National Asthma Education and Prevention Program: *Expert panel report 2: guidelines for the diagnosis and management of asthma* (NIH Pub No 97-4051), Bethesda, Md, 1997 (available online): www.nhlbi.nih.gov/guidelines/asthma/asthgdln.htm. Accessed March 2, 2007.

National Institute on Alcohol Abuse and Alcoholism: Fetal alcohol exposure and the brain, *Alcohol Alert* 50:1-4, 2000 (available online): www.pubs.niaaa.nih.gov/publications/aa50.htm. Accessed April 4, 2007.

National Institutes of Health, Div of Blood Diseases and Resources: *The management of sickle cell disease* (NIH Pub No 02-2117), 2002 (available online): www.nhlbi.nih.gov/health/prof/blood/sickle/index.htm. Accessed March 22, 2007.

National Institutes of Health: *Down syndrome,* 2007 (available online): www.nichd.nih.gov/health/topics/Down_Syndrome.cfm. Accessed March 31, 2007.

National Institutes of Health: *Guidelines for the use of antiretroviral agents in pediatric HIV infection,* 2006 (available online): www.aidsinfo.nih.gov/contentfiles/PediatricGuidelines.pdf. Accessed April 4, 2007.

National Institutes of Health: Sickle cell anemia, *Medline Plus Encyclopedia,* 2005 (available online): www.nlm.nih.gov/medlineplus/ency/article/000527.htm. Accessed March 28, 2007.

Nettina S: *Lippincott manual of nursing practice handbook,* Philadelphia, 2006, Lippincott Williams & Williams.

Norris J: Weighing in on obesity, *UCSF Magazine* Sep:32-63, 2000.

Odding E, Roebroeck M, Stam H: The epidemiology of cerebral palsy: Incidence, impairments and risk factors, *Disability and Rehabilitation* 28(4):183-191, 2006.

Ornstein RM, Jacobson MS: Supersize teens: the metabolic syndrome, *Adolesct Med Clin* 17(3):565-587, 2006.

Pinto S, Roseberry AG, Liu H et al: Rapid rewiring of arcuate nucleus feeding circuits by leptin, *Science* 304(5667):63-64, 2004.

Rapaport R: Disorders of the gonads. In Behrman RE, Kliegman RM, Jenson HB, editors: *Nelson textbook of pediatrics,* Philadelphia, 2004, Elsevier Saunders.

Ridgeway JJ, Clarren SK: Prenatal factors affecting the newborn. In Osborn LM, DeWitt TG, First LR, Zenel JA, editors: *Pediatrics,* Philadelphia, 2005, Elsevier Mosby.

Robertson J, Shilkofski N: *The Harriet Lane handbook,* St Louis, 2005, Elsevier Mosby.

Rogers SJ, Wehner DE, Hagerman R: The behavioral phenotype in fragile X: symptoms of autism in very young children with fragile x syndrome, idiopathic autism, and other developmental disorders, *J Dev Behav Pediatr* 22(6):409-417, 2001.

Saneto RP, Sotero de Menezes MA, Ojemann JG et al: Vagus nerve stimulation for intractable seizures in children, *Pediatr Neurol* 35(5):323-326, 2006.

Sarnat HB: Neuromuscular disorders. In Behrman RE, Kliegman RM, Jenson HB, editors: *Nelson textbook of pediatrics,* Philadelphia, 2004, Elsevier Saunders.

Scott JP: Hematology. In Kliegman RM, Marcdante KJ, Jenson HB, Behrman RE, editors: *Nelson essentials of pediatrics,* Philadelphia, 2006, Elsevier Saunders.

Selekman J: *School nursing: A comprehensive text,* Philadelphia, 2006, FA Davis.

Selevan SG, Rice DC, Hogan KA, Euling SY, Pfahles-Hutchens A, Bethel J: Blood lead concentration and delayed puberty in girls, N Engl J Med 348 (16):1527-1536, 2003.

Society for Neuroscience: Muscular dystrophy. *Brain Briefings,* November 2006.

Story M, Kaphingst KM, French S: The role of schools in obesity prevention, *The Future of Children* 16 (1):109-142, 2006 (available online): www.futureofchildren.org/usr_doc/06_5562_story-school.pdf. Accessed December 20, 2007.

Sybert VP, McCauley E: Turner syndrome, *N Engl J Med* 351(12):1227-38, 2004.

Tyler C, Edman JC: Down syndrome, Turner syndrome, and Klinefelter syndrome: Primary care throughout the life span, *Prim Care Clin Office Pract* 31(3):627-648, 2004.

US Dept of Health and Human Services: *The health consequences of involuntary exposure to tobacco smoke: a report of the surgeon general,* Atlanta, Centers for Disease Control and Prevention, Coordinating for Health Promotion, National Center for Chronic Disease, Prevention and Health Promotion, Office on Smoking and Health (available online): www.surgeongeneral.gov/library/secondhandsmoke/report. Accessed April 4, 2006.

US Environmental Protection Agency: *Protect your child from lead poisoning* (available online): www.epa.gov/lead. Accessed May 20, 2006.

US Preventive Services Task Force: *Screening for idiopathic scoliosis in adolescents: recommendation statement,* Rockville, Md, 2004, Agency for Healthcare Research and Quality (available online): www.guideline.gov/summary/summary.aspx?doc_id=5302. Accessed Sep 4, 2006.

Vaisse C, Clement K, Durand E: Melanocortin-4 receptor mutations are a frequent and heterogenous cause of morbid obesity, *J Clin Invest* 106(2):253-262, 2000.

Wheeler LS, Merkle SL, Gerald LB et al: Managing asthma in schools: what have we learned? *Journal of School Health* 76 (6):201-348, 2006.

Yang Q, Rasmussen SA, Friedman JM: Mortality associated with Down's syndrome in the USA from 1983 to 1997: A population study, *Lancet* 359:1019-1025, 2002.

CHAPTER 4

Chronic Conditions

CHAPTER 5

Mental Health Disorders

Chapter Outline

Attention Deficit-Hyperactivity Disorder
Oppositional Defiant Disorder
Pervasive Developmental Disorders
    Autism
    Asperger's Syndrome
    Rett Syndrome
Pervasive Developmental Disorder–Not Otherwise Specified
School Avoidance/Refusal and School Phobia
Tics and Tourette's Disorder
Major Depressive Disorder

*T*he most prevalent mental health problems encountered in school settings are discussed in this chapter. Along with Chapter 6, Substance Abuse, these chapters provide a broad overview of the psychiatric disorders of childhood and adolescence. Mental health disorders have an impact on cognition, behavior, emotions, and social functioning. This can occur directly through neurological mechanisms affecting domains such as attention, cognitive processing, and impulse control, and it can occur indirectly through psychosocial areas such as self-esteem, motivation, emotional regulation, and peer relationships. Disabilities in any of these areas can affect the school performance and school life of a child or adolescent. Current brain research provides data regarding the areas of the brain involved and the impact these disorders may have on learning.

The phenomenon of coexisting disorders is common in all of the conditions discussed in this chapter. An illness or impairment in one domain may be associated with—or may result in—a disturbance in others, such as affective disturbances in youth with attention deficit-hyperactivity disorder (ADHD), early onset of dysthymia in children with school phobia, or anxiety disorder in oppositional defiant disorder (ODD).

Child-centered nursing interventions involve an appreciation for both the neurobiological concerns and interventions with these disorders while also noting the important role of nurturing, socialization, education, and acculturation within the educational context that need to be addressed for optimum educational outcomes. The school nurse plays an important and vital role in the assessment, educational planning, treatment management, and remediation of learning problems caused by these disorders.

ATTENTION DEFICIT-HYPERACTIVITY DISORDER

I. **Definition**
   A. Attentiondeficithyperactivity disorder (ADHD), a neurobehavioral condition, is one of the most common childhood disorders; it occurs in approximately 3% to 18% of children (CDC, 2005; Parker, 2005; Rowland, Lesesne, and Abramowitz, 2002).
      1. Boys are approximately two to three times more likely to be diagnosed with ADHD than girls (CDC, 2005), and boys are more likely to have the hyperactive-impulsive type ADHD, and girls are more frequently diagnosed with the inattentive-type ADHD (Kliegman et al, 2006; Parker, 2005).
      2. Symptoms of ADHD may persist into adolescence, and some continue into adulthood, where they may manifest as restlessness, disorganization, distractibility, job difficulties, substance abuse, accidents, or relationship problems (American Psychiatric Association [APA], 2000).
         a. There is clinical support for a *rule of thirds,* which suggests that 1 in 3 children "outgrows" the disorder, meaning they develop adequate coping capacities for it, so they no longer exhibit symptomatic states. Another child outgrows the disorder in the transition between adolescence and adulthood, and the other third continues with symptoms into adulthood (Chenven, 2006).
   B. *Diagnostic and Statistical Manual of Mental Disorders* (DSM-IV) diagnosis requires at least six symptoms of inattention and at least six symptoms of hyperactivity/impulsivity of more than 6 months' duration in two settings, and symptoms must occur before 7 years of age. Symptoms must also substantially interfere with age appropriate development and academic or job skills (see Box 5-1).
II. **Etiology**
   A. ADHD is associated with genetic factors and neuroanatomical abnormalities in the brain that are known to regulate motor and attention behaviors. Psychosocial, emotional, and environmental-exacerbating factors include coexisting mental disorders, coercive discipline, lack of consistency, exposure to media violence, parental unsociable behaviors or marital conflict, abuse, and neglect. Symptoms of hyperactivity or inattention can be secondary effects of medications (e.g., theophylline, albuterol, phenobarbital), hyperthyroidism, or lead poisoning (Kliegman et al, 2006). Prematurity and intrauterine exposure to alcohol, drugs, cigarettes, and unsafe carbon monoxide levels can contribute to ADHD.
   B. The exact cause of ADHD is unknown, but it is believed to be genetic in at least 50% of the cases based on studies of twins (Anastopoulos and Shelton, 2001) and other family members affected by the disorder (Barkley, 1998). Dopamine transporter gene DAT1, dopamine receptor genes DRD4 and DRD5 (Rosenbaum et al, 2005), and Synaptosome-associated protein 25, SNAP-25, are genes thought to be associated with ADHD (Biederman, 2005; Thapar, O'Donovan, and Owen, 2005). Research continues in this area to

Box 5-1   *DSM-IV Criteria: Attention-Deficit/Hyperactivity Disorder*

A. Either 1 or 2:
   1. Six or more of the following symptoms of inattention have persisted for at least 6 months to a degree that is maladaptive and inconsistent with developmental level:

Inattention

   a. Often does not give close attention to details or makes careless mistakes in schoolwork, work, or other activities.
   b. Often has difficulty sustaining attention in tasks or play activities.
   c. Often does not seem to listen when spoken to directly.
   d. Often does not follow through on instructions and fails to finish schoolwork, chores, or duties in the workplace (not due to oppositional behavior or failure to understand instructions).
   e. Often has difficulty organizing tasks and activities.
   f. Often avoids, dislikes, or is reluctant to engage in tasks that require sustained mental effort, such as schoolwork or homework.
   g. Often loses things necessary for tasks or activities (e.g. toys, school assignments, pencils, books, or tools).
   h. Is often easily distracted by extraneous stimuli.
   i. Is often forgetful in daily activities.

   2. Six or more of the following symptoms of hyperactivity-impulsivity have persisted for at least 6 months to a degree that is maladaptive and inconsistent with developmental level.

Hyperactivity

   a. Often fidgets with hands or feet or squirms in seat.
   b. Often gets up from seat in classroom or in other situations in which remaining in seat is expected.
   c. Often runs about or climbs excessively in situations in which it is inappropriate (in adolescents or adults, may be limited to subjective feelings of restlessness).
   d. Often has trouble playing or engaging in leisure activities quietly.
   e. Is often "on the go" or often acts as if "driven by a motor."
   f. Often talks excessively.

Impulsivity

   a. Often blurts out answers before questions have been finished.
   b. Often has trouble waiting one's turn.
   c. Often interrupts or intrudes on others (e.g. butts into conversations or games).

B. Some hyperactive-impulsive or inattentive symptoms that caused impairment were present before age 7 years.
C. Some impairment from the symptoms is present in two or more settings (e.g. at school or work and at home).
D. There must be clear evidence of significant impairment in social, academic, or occupational functioning.
E. The symptoms do not occur exclusively during the course of a pervasive developmental disorder, schizophrenia, or other psychotic disorder and are not better accounted for by another mental disorder (e.g. mood disorder, anxiety disorder, dissociative disorder, or a personality disorder).

Based on these criteria, three types of ADHD are identified:

   1. ADHD, *Combined Type*: if both criteria A1 and A2 are met for the past 6 months.
   2. ADHD, *Predominantly Inattentive Type*: if criterion A1 is met but criterion A2 is not met for the past six months.
   3. ADHD, *Predominantly Hyperactive-Impulsive Type*: if criterion A2 is met but criterion A1 is not met for the past six months.

From American Psychiatric Association: *Diagnostic and Statistical Manual of Mental Disorders,* ed 4 text revision, Washington, DC, 2000, American Psychiatric Association.

try to identify other brain neurotransmitters and receptors that may be involved.

Brain Findings

ADHD is believed to have a neurological basis. Research has found evidence of a chemical imbalance or irregularity in certain neurotransmitters, especially dopamine and norepinephrine, consistent with the genetic results described in the previous section. PET studies have demonstrated hypometabolism of glucose (Pary et al, 2002) in particular areas of the brain thought to be involved in attention. When a student is challenged with academic problems, such as math, the typical brain fires up the frontal lobe and starts working; the brain of the student with ADHD does not. With correct stimulant medication, dopaminergic activity increases in the brain, and the student is able to work on the assigned task or class problem.

National Institute of Mental Health (NIMH) brain-scan studies indicate the volume of matter in several key parts of the brain is 3% to 4% smaller in children with ADHD who have never been on medication. The areas, compared in the sample and controls, include the cerebrum, cerebellum, gray and white matter for the four major lobes, and the caudate nucleus, a part of the basal ganglia. These key parts of the brain, except for the caudate, appear to stay on a parallel developmental path during childhood and adolescence in patients and controls. This suggests that genetic and early environmental effects on brain development are unchanging and not related to medication (Castellanos, 2002). Furthermore, the decreased brain volume may be a factor in some biological processes, which can manifest as hyperactivity or impulsiveness in the educational setting (Bower, 2002).

Researchers also found a smaller volume of white matter in children with ADHD who had never been on medication compared to the control group. Another study found an enlarged hippocampus in children and adolescents with ADHD compared to the control group. This study supports the hypothesis that the pathophysiology of ADHD involves the limbic system and limbic-prefrontal circuits (Plessen et al, 2006).

III. Characteristics

A. Inattention and distractibility: difficulty in organizing, tendency to lose things, makes careless mistakes, does not understand instructions, cannot follow instructions that require mental effort.

B. Selective attention: focuses on something he or she wants or enjoys.

C. Hyperactive: squirms and fidgets in seat, climbs and moves about when inappropriate, talks excessively.

D. Impulsive: interrupts conversation, has difficulty taking turns, blurts out answers, talks or acts without thinking.

CHAPTER 5

Mental Health Disorders

E. Coexisting disorders include learning disorders, 20% to 60%; conduct disorder, 10% to 50%; oppositional defiant disorder, 30% to 60%; anxiety, 10% to 30%, tic disorders, 5% to 30%, and depression (Parker, 2005). Other disorders include obsessive-compulsive disorder (OCD), pervasive developmental disorder (PDD), and Tourette's syndrome.

F. Associated symptoms may include motor coordination difficulties, disruptive sleep, susceptibility to accidents, and poisoning.

IV. Effects on Individual

A. Difficulty maintaining friendships, social immaturity.

B. Engages in socially unacceptable behaviors.

C. Poor academic performance may result in grade retention and potential school dropout.

D. Accident prone because of impulsivity.

E. The world is confusing because of multiple sensory distractions.

F. Poor self-esteem because of the lack of success and failure to earn rewards, which result from inappropriate behavior.

G. Frequent daydreaming and excessive boredom.

H. Difficulty achieving long-term goals.

I. Strained family and peer relationships.

J. Problems with driving (e.g., impulsivity combined with poor judgment, which lead to more frequent traffic citations, especially for speeding and accidents).

K. Susceptible to drug and alcohol abuse.

V. Health Concerns and Emergencies

A. Frequent visits to nurse's office with psychosomatic complaints.

B. Poor weight gain with or without stimulant medications.

C. Higher risk for accidents.

VI. Management and Treatment

A. Rule out hearing loss or visual impairment.

B. Obtain family and social history. Address psychosocial stressors— such as parental relationship and psychopathology, chaotic living situation, and low social economic status—that may contribute to physical and behavioral symptoms, including headache, stomachache, agitation, and aggression.

C. Encourage increased caloric intake when weight gain is slow.

D. Monitor growth patterns every 6 months when medications that may suppress appetite and growth are given.

E. Various diets and nutritional supplements are advocated by family or practitioners, but research on effectiveness is inconclusive.

F. Pharmacological management is effective in 70% to 80% of children (Parker, 2005). Teens with ADHD who are treated are less likely to become involved in substance abuse than matched cohorts who did not receive treatment (Giedd, 2003; Stocker, 1999).

G. Liaison with teachers, parents, and physician regarding effectiveness and side effects of medications (See Table 5-1).

H. Count and securely lock-up prescribed medication; stimulants are subject to controlled substance rules. These medications are frequently abused by non-ADHD students.

Table 5-1   Medications for Attention Deficit-Hyperactivity Disorder

Stimulants	Action – duration	Considerations per drug category	* Potential adverse effects per drug category
Methylphenidates	*Cerebral stimulant*		
Ritalin	3-4 hours	Do not chew or crush time-released medications	Headache, anorexia, nervousness, dysphoria, sleep onset difficulties, agitation, irritability, dry mouth, increased tics and seizures, Tourette's syndrome, possibility of psychological addiction
Ritalin LA	6-8 hours	May open capsule and sprinkle over small amount of applesauce	
Focalin	5-6 hours	Hard candy or gum, sips of water may help with dry mouth	
Focalin XR	8 hours	Give at least 6 hours before bedtime or 10 hours before for extended release	
		Avoid decongestants, caffeine	
		Monitor vital signs, height, and weight every 3 months	
Concerta	9-12 hours		Concerta: Upper respiratory infection, sinusitis, vomiting, diarrhea
Methylin	3-4 hours		
Methylin ER	3-8 hours		
Metadate ER	up to 8 hours		
Metadate CD	8-12 hours		
Amphetamines	*Cerebral stimulant*		
Adderall	4-6 hours	Take 6-10 hours before bedtime	Dry mouth, diarrhea, constipation, anorexia, weight loss, rash, insomnia, hypertension, tachycardia, dizziness, restlessness, euphoria, dysphoria, depression, tics, Tourette's syndrome, angiodema
Adderall XR	9-11 hours	Avoid caffeine	
Dexedrine	4-6 hours	Risk of abuse	
Dextrostat	6-8 hours	Monitor vital signs, height and weight every 3 months	
		Report signs of excessive stimulation	Anaphylaxis (Adderall)

Continued

Mental Health Disorders   **CHAPTER 5**

Table 5-1   *Medications for Attention Deficit-Hyperactivity Disorder—cont'd*

FDA issued warning in 2006: Stimulants should not be used in children or adolescents with serious structural cardiac abnormalities, cardiopathy, or serious heart rhythm abnormalities.
Auditory hallucinations have been reported with stimulants, generally at higher dose range.

Nonstimulant options

Atomoxetine (Strattera)	Norepinephrine reuptake inhibitor First nonstimulant with FDA approval for use in children	May be taken with or without food Do not break open, capsules must be taken whole Breaking open capsule may cause eye irritation Full efficacy may take upwards of 2-3 months Monitor height and weight	Upset stomach, insomnia, palpitations, decreased appetite, growth retardation, nausea and vomiting, dizziness, and mood swings Risk of liver toxicity. ** Black box warning: Monitor for suicidal ideation

Second line option, useful when depressive component present

Bupropion (Wellbutrin) *Venlafaxine* (Effexor)	Antidepressant Antidepressant		Agitation, dry mouth, insomnia, headaches, nausea, constipation, tremor, manic episodes. May decrease seizure threshold; monitor for suicidal ideation.

See Catapres and Tofranil in Table 5-3

* Adverse effects are typical for the medication class; please consult PDR or other reference for specific profile of each medication. Note that drug interactions may need to be reviewed.
** Black box warning is the strongest warning that the FDA requires. Indicates a significant serious or life-threatening adverse effect.

I. Health intervention may include checking vital signs, observing for tics, and asking questions about medications.

J. Focus on positive behaviors, and find ways to increase child's motivation and self-esteem. Behavioral approaches are helpful when providing stability, routine, and appropriate goals.

K. Provide listening, nonjudgmental ear to parents. Be aware that some parents may also have ADHD.

L. Ensure proper supervision on playground, at special events, and during field trips.

M. Become knowledgeable regarding individual, family, and peer group therapy and behavior management; encourage multiple modalities for the child, along with individual attention; manage medication; and offer consistent and encouraging nurse–student interactions.

N. Provide information and workshop for school staff.

VII. Additional Information

A. In 1991, ADHD was recognized as a qualifying disability for special education services by Part B of the Individuals with Disabilities Education Act (IDEA) and Section 504.

B. Progressive or static neurological disease (e.g., Tourette's syndrome, absence seizures, fragile X syndrome) is ruled out before diagnosis. Treatment usually is multimodal and may include medication, behavioral modification using positive reinforcement, anger management and social skills training, and sensory integration therapy. Treatment is often complicated by coexisting disorders.

1. Less validated modalities include vision therapy, electroencephalographic (EEG) biofeedback, or neurofeedback (i.e., training the brain to increase the type of brain activity associated with sustained attention).

2. Restricted diets (e.g., Feingold) may be used. Most common diet restrictions are sugars, additives, and preservatives to eliminate possible allergens. Works best in children younger than 5 years and those with food or food additive allergies.

3. Nutritional supplements include liquid calcium and vitamin B complex to calm the nervous system or choline, which may improve memory and attention span.

4. Caution should always be used when combining nutritional and herbal supplements and pharmacotherapy. The effectiveness of over-the-counter (OTC) supplements has not been supported by research studies and may have unknown side effects in the treatment of children with ADHD.

C. ADHD can persist into adulthood. The prognosis is negatively affected by family history of ADHD; a disruptive family environment; and a comorbid condition (e.g., conduct disorders, anxiety, mood disorders). Adolescents and adults with ADHD who take stimulant medications cannot enlist in the armed services without a medical waiver, even if the medications have been discontinued; each branch has its own criteria. Career choices generally are not affected by ADHD, and many adults are successful in their chosen occupation.

WEB SITES

Attention Deficit Disorder Association (ADDA)
http://www.add.org
Children and Adults with Attention Deficit Disorder (CHADD)
http://www.chadd.org
Developmental and Behavioral Pediatrics Online
http://www.dbpeds.org
Family ADHD Resource
http://www.ADDresources.org
National Resource Center on ADHD
http://www.help4ADHD.org

OPPOSITIONAL DEFIANT DISORDER

I. Definition
A. Oppositional defiant disorder (ODD) is a negative, hostile, defiant, disobedient pattern of behavior lasting at least 6 months that includes at least four of the following symptoms: frequent loss of temper, arguments with adults, deliberate annoyance, active defiance or refusal of adult requests, a spiteful or vindictive manner, touchy and easily annoyed, angry, resentful, and blaming of others (APA, 2000). Significant impairment must also be displayed in academic, social, or occupational performance. Comorbid disorders include ADHD, anxiety disorders, mood disorders, learning disorders, language processing disorders, and substance abuse.

II. Etiology
A. Etiology is multicausal and includes biological, genetic, and environmental factors. ODD is common in families with mood disorders, serious marital discord, history of physical or sexual maltreatment of children, harsh or inconsistent discipline, or a succession of multiple caregivers. Often observed before age 8, but not later than early adolescence. More common among boys before puberty, but gender distribution is fairly equal thereafter. Prevalence rates range from 2% to 16% (APA, 2000).

B. Children with ODD may be anxious, which is often related to a learning or processing disorder that makes it difficult to function. An oppositional dynamic between the child and an adult emerges when the child with these subtle disabilities is anxious and feels the need to be in control.

C. There is evidence that genetics may be a factor, and ODD is affected by caregiver and child incompatibility.
 1. Mothers with a depressive disorder are more likely to have a child with ODD. It is also more common in families where at least one parent has a history of ODD, mood disorder, antisocial personality disorder, substance-related disorder, conduct disorder (CD), or ADHD (APA, 2000).

Brain Findings
Studies suggest the neurotransmitters dopamine, serotonin, and noradrenaline play a role in ODD with the most significant impact caused by noradrenaline (Kariyawasam et al, 2002; Comings et al, 2000).

Cortisol levels have been found to be low in children with ODD. Children taking stimulant medication for ODD have increased levels of cortisol (Kariyawasam et al, 2002; Snoek, 2004). Conclusions of the research indicate that cortisol responsivity during stress is different in these children and may manifest in how aggressive children respond to stress (McBurnett, 2002).

III. Characteristics

A. Three classic characteristics are noncompliance, exaggerated emotional response, and tendency to blame others.
B. Difficulty being comforted or soothed and high motor reactivity during early childhood.
C. Defiant, annoying, spiteful, vindictive, resentful, argumentative behaviors.
D. Stubbornness, resistance to directions, unwillingness to compromise, testing of limits, and usually unable to accept blame.
E. Oppositional behaviors tend to increase with age.
F. Symptoms same in both genders, but boys have more persistent symptoms and more confrontational behaviors.
G. Aggression is generally verbal rather than physical.
H. Behaviors usually manifest in the home or with adults the child knows well; may not be observed in the school or community.
I. Affects social functioning with peers, siblings, and parents.
J. Often comorbidities include learning problems, depressed moods, hyperactivity, and addictive behaviors.

IV. Effects on Individual

A. Affects school achievement and social success.
B. Peer rejection leads to social isolation.
C. Negative appearance to parents and teachers stigmatizes student.
D. May be precursor to conduct disorder and later antisocial personality, delinquency, and potential future criminality.
E. Risk indicator of potential school dropout.
F. Strained family relationships.

V. Health Concerns and Emergencies

A. Dependent on severity of symptoms.
B. Monitor medication, observe for hyperactivity or other symptoms.
C. Child abuse potential for parents and staff includes both verbal and physical abuse. Child may react negatively at school in response to the abuse at home.
D. Child with lower cortisol levels may not react to or fear threatening situations or aggressive actions.
E. ODD may predict later depression and suicidal ideation and attempts.

VI. Management and Treatment

A. Early identification of disruptive behaviors for intervention and support.
B. Rule out hearing loss as cause for failure to follow directions.
C. Observe for depression or other comorbid conditions.
D. Do family, home, peer, and community assessment; include situational analysis (i.e.; who or what is present when an outburst occurs and what are the precedents).

CHAPTER 5

Mental Health Disorders

    E. Set limits and be consistent during any interactions. It is important that adults do not react emotionally to child's oppositional behaviors.

    F. Setting clear limits and consequences may be difficult, because these children are affected more by the emotion of the moment and do not seem to care about the consequences.

    G. Daily privileges should be linked to the behavior that day. Over time the child begins to understand the consequences; this occurs over months not days.

    H. Reinforce socially acceptable behaviors, and provide support that may not be found in the home.

    I. Provide staff education regarding ODD and behavior management therapy.

    J. Support limits on television viewing and any media that portrays violence (e.g., games, music, movies).

    K. Encourage positive parenting, use of behavioral approach, and psychotherapy.

VII. Additional Information

    A. Conduct Disorder (CD)

        1. CD is more severe than ODD and includes persistent, repetitive behavior that ignores societal rules and can result in aggressive behaviors (bullying, threats, fighting, use of weapons, theft, arson). Behaviors may be against people, animals, and property.

        2. CD includes significant antisocial behaviors: deceitfulness, lying, thievery, truancy, and rape. These behaviors must interfere significantly with academic, social, and occupational functioning. Three of the criteria described must be present during the previous 12 months, with at least one present in the last 6 months.

        3. CD also has coexisting conditions: mood disorders, learning problems, thought disorders, anxiety, posttraumatic stress disorder, substance abuse, and ADHD. These may be diagnosed in preschool years and are not usually diagnosed after age 16 (American Psychiatric Association, 2000).

PERVASIVE DEVELOPMENTAL DISORDERS

AUTISM

I. Definition

    A. Autism is a neurodevelopmental disorder involving impairments in language, social communication, and social interactions; repetitive and stereotyped behaviors manifest in one of these areas before age 3 as defined by DSM-IV (see Box 5-2). However, the median age of diagnosis is 52 to 56 months (CDC, 2007). Table 5-2 presents early risk indicators for autism.

    B. The distinguishing behavior is a relative lack of interest in other people. Autism is the main disorder included in PDD, which are also referred to as autism spectrum disorders (ASD). This nomenclature highlights the wide range of symptomatic presentations, from severe to mild, that may occur.

Box 5-2 *DSM-IV Criteria: Autistic Disorder*

A. Total of six or more items from 1, 2, and 3, with at least two from 1 and one each from 2 and 3:
1. Qualitative impairment in social interaction, as manifested by at least two of the following:
   a. Marked impairment in the use of multiple nonverbal behaviors—such as eye-to-eye gaze, facial expression, body postures, and gestures—to regulate social interaction.
   b. Failure to develop peer relationships appropriate to developmental level.
   c. A lack of spontaneous seeking to share enjoyment, interests, or achievements with other people (e.g., by a lack of showing, bringing, or pointing out objects of interest).
   d. Lack of social emotional reciprocity.
2. Qualitative impairments in communication as manifested by at least one of the following:
   a. Delay in, or total lack of, the development of spoken language (not accompanied by an attempt to compensate through alternative modes of communication, such as gestures or mime).
   b. In individuals with adequate speech, marked impairment in the ability to initiate or sustain a conversation with others.
   c. Stereotyped and repetitive use of language or idiosyncratic language.
   d. Lack of varied, spontaneous, make-believe play or social imitative play appropriate to developmental level.
3. Restricted, repetitive, and stereotyped pattern of behavior, interests,

and activities, as manifested by at least one of the following:
   a. Encompassing preoccupation with one or more stereotyped patterns of interest that is abnormal either in intensity or focus.
   b. Apparently inflexible adherence to specific, nonfunctional routines or rituals.
   c. Stereotyped and repetitive motor mannerisms (e.g., hand or finger flapping or twisting or complex whole-body movements).
   d. Persistent preoccupation with parts of objects.
B. Delays or abnormal functioning in at least one of the following areas with onset before age 3 years:
1. Social interaction
2. Language as used in social communication
3. Symbolic or imaginative play
C. The disturbance is not better accounted for by Rett syndrome or childhood disintegrative disorder.
1. Qualitative impairment in social interaction (e.g., impairment in nonverbal behaviors, failure to develop peer relationships, lack of social or emotional reciprocity).
2. Qualitative impairments in communication (e.g., delay or lack of spoken language, inability to initiate or sustain a conversation, stereotyped and repetitive use of language, lack of varied make-believe play).
3. Restricted, repetitive, and stereotyped patterns of behavior, interests, and activities, including motor stereotypes and mannerisms.
D. The disturbance is not better accounted for by another specific pervasive developmental disorder or by schizophrenia.

From American Psychiatric Association: *Diagnostic and statistical manual of mental disorders,* ed 4 text revision, Washington, DC, 2000, American Psychiatric Association.

CHAPTER 5   Mental Health Disorders

II. Etiology

A. The etiology of this disorder is elusive; however, strong evidence exists for a genetic component, organic cause, or both. The prevalence rate of autism is reported as 1 per 150 (CDC, 2007).

1. More boys are affected than girls, generally reported to be a 4:1 ratio.
2. Autism is associated with fragile X syndrome, tuberous sclerosis, and a family history of similar disorders, depression, bipolar disorder, schizophrenia, or more subtle ASD and OCD.
3. Genes located on chromosomes 7 and 15 have been implicated as causative factors in some cases of autism. Research has also implicated gamma-aminobutyric acid (GABA) receptor genes found on chromosome 15 in some cases of autism (Rodier, 2000).
4. GABA is the major inhibitory transmitter in the brain and abnormalities of GABA transmission are associated with seizures and anxiety disorders. It is recognized that there are at least 10 or more genes involved, and that it is not the effects of a single gene but perhaps the interaction of particular genes or sets of genes that join together in certain combinations.

B. As research continues, a better understanding will emerge of how autism and related disorders occur.

Brain Findings

Results from postmortem and imaging studies have implicated many major structures of the brain in autistic disorders, including cerebellum, corpus callosum, basal ganglia, brainstem, and portions of the limbic system (see Figure 5-1). Unusually high levels of specific proteins associated with brain development have been reported in children with autism (Nelson et al, 2001), and parts of the frontal lobe are thicker than normal; this region controls decision making and planning. Other research suggests that the mirror neuronal system involved in understanding another person's actions is impaired in those with autism (Schumann and Amaral, 2006). This may result in loss of empathy and language skills, as well as the ability to learn by imitative skills. Neurons in the limbic

Table 5-2	**Early Risk Indicators for Autism**

Age	Behavior
Under age 12 mos	Little eye contact
	Lack of response to name being called.
	Seldom pointing with finger to show interest.
	Does not show object by sharing it with person.
12 mos.	No babbling.
	No gesturing, pointing, waving bye-bye.
16 mos.	No single words.
23 mos.	No two-word spontaneous phrases.
Any age	Loss of language or social skills at any age.

Cerebral cortex -
a thin layer of gray matter on the surface of the cerebral hemispheres. Two thirds of its area is deep in the fissures or folds. Responsible for the higher mental functions, general movement, perception, and behavioral reactions.

Basal ganglia -
gray masses deep in the cerebral hemisphere that serve as a connection between the cerebrum and cerebellum. Helps to regulate automatic movement.

Amygdala -
responsible for emotional responses, including aggressive behavior.

Hippocampus -
makes it possible to remember new information and recent events.

Corpus callosum -
consists primarily of closely packed bundles of fibers that connect the right and left hemisphere and allows for communication between the hemispheres.

Cerebellum -
located at the back of the brain, it fine tunes our motor activity, regulates balance, body movements, coordination, and the muscles used in speaking.

Brain stem -
located in front of the cerebellum, it serves as a relay station, passing messages between various parts of the body and the cerebral cortex. Primitive functions essential to survival (breathing and heart rate control) are located here.

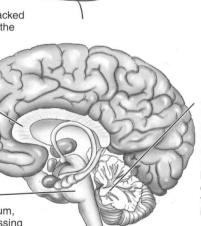

FIGURE 5-1 Major brain structures implicated in autism. *Redrawn from Strock M: Autism spectrum disorders, pervasive developmental disorders (NIH Pub No NIH-04-5511), National Institute of Mental Health, National Institute of Health, US Dept of Health and Human Services, Bethesda, Md, 2004 (available online): www.nimh.nih.gov/publicat/autism.cfm.*

CHAPTER 5

Mental Health Disorders

system where emotions are processed are plentiful but are one third fewer in number than normal.

Another biological theory is that autism may be caused by faulty wiring in the brain, or underconnectivity, that makes it inefficient (Grossberg and Seidman, 2006; National Institutes of Health, 2004). The cerebellum's ability to assist in making predictions of ensuing thoughts, emotions, and motor movements appears to be affected. Several studies have documented abnormalities in the Purkinje cells essential to the wiring of the cerebellum, including a significant decrease in their size and number (Fatemi et al, 2002; Kern, 2003). These cells inhibit the action of other neurons. Furthermore, the male autistic brain has fewer neurons in the amygdala compared to males without the disorder. Whether this occurs at birth or later as a degenerative process is unknown (Schumann and Amaral, 2006).

Data reveal a reduction of the amino acid tryptophan, a precursor to serotonin, which may interfere with serotonin synthesis. Serotonin is produced in the brain, thyroid gland, and gastrointestinal (GI) tract; and it affects mood, aggressive behavior, anxiety, memory, neural development, pain, repetitive behaviors, and sleep.

III. Characteristics
    A. Social communication.
        1. Delayed onset of intentional communication, both verbal and nonverbal (e.g., babbling, gesturing, head nods), and poor eye contact. Some children never gain useful communicative skills.
        2. Unusual language if acquired (e.g., echolalia, pronoun reversal, literal or concrete use of words, peculiar voice intonation [monotone or singsong]).
    B. Social interactions.
        1. Inability or significant difficulty in developing relationships; inability to recognize and respond to social cues; aversion to touch and cuddling; flat affect; persistent tantrums.
        2. Inability or great difficulty using facial expressions or gestures for regulation of social interactions.
    C. Restricted and repetitive behaviors and interests.
        1. Insistence on routine and sameness, narrow range of interests, bizarre attachment and inappropriate use of objects, intense preoccupation with activity or object.
        2. Motor disturbances, arm flapping, whirling, rocking, toe walking, repetitive hand and finger mannerisms, and head banging.
        3. Atypical responses to sensory stimuli (e.g., sound, pain, cold, heat).
    D. Other.
        1. Symptoms vary considerably in severity. A few children have exceptional skills in specific areas (e.g., memory, calendar calculation, solving puzzles, art, music) without lessons or practice and are called *autistic savants* (about 10%). Other high-functioning children may do well in regular classrooms with support.

2. Approximately 40% to 62% function in the mental retardation range. Females are more likely than males to have cognitive impairment (CDC, 2007).
3. Difficulty in generalizing knowledge and skills, reasoning or symbolic thinking, verbal concept formation, and integration skills.
4. Strengths in visual-spatial processing, rote learning, and memory skills.

IV. Effects on Individual

A. Negative or impaired family relationships.
B. Few if any peer relationships because of indifference, oblivious social behavior, or inability to empathize. Interactive or parallel play almost nonexistent.
C. Actions may inadvertently provoke anger in others.
D. Social isolation and ostracism, vulnerability to peer harassment and bullying.
E. Difficulty in learning because of lack of imitation and unresponsiveness to social reinforcement.
F. Difficulty transferring learning from one situation to another.
G. Autistic children may become overwhelmed by their own nervous system, resulting in heightened sensitivity to stimuli and uncontrollable repetitive actions.
H. Sleep disorders.

V. Health Concerns and Emergencies

A. Seizures occur in 25% with peak of onset in early childhood and again in adolescence.
B. Hyposensitivity or hypersensitivity to pain, noise, touch, and so forth.
C. Poor nutrition because of limited food preferences. May ingest inedible substances.
D. May express affection but indiscriminately, leading to potential child abuse.
E. Often medicated with sedatives or tranquilizers.
F. Personal safety at risk because of impulsive, disorganized motor activity and poor sense of danger.

VI. Management and Treatment

A. Rule out hearing loss.
B. Behavioral management as part of daily routine; use simple language, provide visual and verbal cues when making transitions, be mindful of child's sensory profile, especially hypersensitivity to sound or touch.
C. Monitor medications and side effects. Although there are no medications that substantially ameliorate the core disorder or disability, treatment with multiple classes of psychotropic medications is increasingly utilized to target disruptive or disturbing symptoms.
   1. Selective serotonin reuptake inhibitors (SSRIs) are often used to treat children with affective symptoms and obsessions or stereotypical behaviors. SSRI medications inhibit reuptake of serotonin, which promotes increased serotonin activity and benefits some children by improving behaviors.
   2. Ritalin and other stimulants are used for hyperactivity symptoms and are a fairly standard intervention for those diagnosed with fragile X syndrome.

3. Various vitamins are used; Vitamin B_6 with magnesium may be used to stimulate brain activity, but studies are inconclusive.
4. Sleep aids, both prescription and OTC remedies, are also used (see Table 5-3).

D. Monitor for routine illnesses, injuries, or self-abuse because of high pain threshold; youth without language skills may not be able to report pain or other distress.

E. Monitor weight.

F. Monitor nutrition and diet; vitamins and food supplements may be needed because of strong but limited food preferences. Monitor lead levels, because children with autism are known to eat inedible items, such as paint chips.
1. Tryptophan, an amino acid found to be low in some children with autism, may be provided in certain foods (e.g., beef, chicken, turkey, broccoli, brussel sprouts, eggs, fish, milk, nuts, and fennel).
2. Support parent in seeking nutritional counseling for child.

G. Diagnosis usually is made before preschool and school age years due to the impairments in communication and social interaction.

H. During the screening take a careful social and health history, a communication assessment, and psychological evaluation with tests not highly dependent on verbal abilities (see Appendix A, Assessment Tools).

I. Support parent for seeking genetic counseling for concerns about fragile X and tuberous sclerosis associated with ASD.

J. Studies do not support a link between vaccination for measles, mumps, and rubella (MMR) and autism (CDC, 2006b).

VII. Additional Information

A. Diagnoses included in the DSM-IV under PDD and ASD include autism, Asperger's syndrome, Rett syndrome, childhood disintegrative disorder, and pervasive developmental disorders not already specified (PDD-NOS).

B. Childhood Disintegrative Disorder (CDD)
1. CDD is very rare among ASDs. It is a disorder in which a child with previous normal development deteriorates in a matter of months in intellectual, language, and social functioning. It is more common among boys, and onset is after age 2 (this criteria separates the disorder from Rett syndrome) but before age 10 with normal age-related development in communication and social relationships during the first two years.
   a. For a DSM diagnosis, the child must have loss of acquired skills in at least two of the following areas: expressive/receptive language, social/adaptive behavior, bowel or bladder control, and play or motor skills. Impairment must also be evident in at least two of the following areas: social interaction, communication, or the demonstration of restricted, repetitive, and stereotyped patterns of behaviors, activities, and interests.

C. Much of the outcome data for ASD was collected before the 1980s, when fewer services were available and intervention usually was not started until the school years. Long-term outcome may improve with earlier identification and mandated services.

D. The educational focus for children with autism is to decrease unacceptable behaviors and increase social awareness and verbal communication. Important elements in the classroom include predictability and routine, assistance with transition, and family involvement. Multiple treatment approaches are used, including behavioral modification, which focuses on learning specific behaviors through repetition; teaching of more global behaviors that will affect a wide range of other behaviors (pivotal behaviors); interactive play with adults or peers; and provision of sensory integration or sensory processing therapy.

E. Examples of educational intervention techniques include Treatment and Education of Autistic and Communication-Handicapped Children (TEACCH); Floor Time/Interactive Play Therapy; Facilitated Developmentally Integrated Free Play; Applied Behavioral Analysis/Discrete Trials; Pivotal Response Training; Sensory Integration/Sensory Processing; and Picture Exchange Communication System (PECS).

Introduction to Table 5-3, Psychotropic Medications

Current scientific understanding recognizes that mental disorders are both psychosociocultural phenomena and neurobiological conditions. Clinical research documents the importance and efficacy of integrating psychosocial interventions with medication treatment for many disorders.

Following is a list of psychotropic agents prescribed to children for affective and behavioral disorders (Table 5-3). Some medications work to enhance neuropsychological functions basic to the cognitive and perceptual skills necessary for school activities; others impact mood regulatory mechanisms that affect school, home, and community functioning; still others have impact on behavioral modulation and conduct.

Many agents have multiple impacts on neuropsychological functioning and, particularly in more complex situations, multiple medications may be prescribed. Treatment efficacy and undesired side effects, both neuropsychological and physical, need to be monitored and reported. Given the proliferation of new psychotropic medications in recent decades, and given the tendency for new medications to be released with U.S. Food and Drug Administration (FDA) approval in adult patients and without extensive study in children, it is the rule rather than the exception for physicians to prescribe "off-label." (The FDA allows physicians to prescribe medications for other than approved use.) Thus careful and consistent medication monitoring is an important component of quality care.

School nurses are often at the nexus of care, given their role in monitoring, administering, and evaluating the impacts of medication on students. Their close linkage with parents, teachers, and prescribing physicians provides them with a unique opportunity to enhance both a student's academic performance and their mental health.

CHAPTER 5

Mental Health Disorders

Table 5-3   Psychotropic Medications

Off-label use: U.S. Food and Drug Administration (FDA) permits physicians to prescribe approved medications for other than intended use. Studies are not usually done on children.

Medication/Category	Off-label Clinical Indications ≤18 Years	Potential Adverse Effects*
Selective Serotonin Reuptake Inhibitors (SSRIs)		
Fluoxetine (Prozac)† *Sertraline (Zoloft)* *Fluvoxamine (Luvox)* *Citalopram (Celex)* *Escitalopram (Lexapro)* *Paroxetine (Paxil)*‡	Major depressive disorder (MDD) Obsessive-compulsive disorder (OCD) Anxiety disorders	Weight loss, weight gain, diaphoresis, dry mouth, constipation, diarrhea, nausea, vomiting, insomnia, tremors, anxiety, nervousness, mania/hypomania, hyperactivity, drowsiness, change in hepatic function; some SSRIs may alter metabolism of other drugs. Monitor for suicidal ideation.§
Serotonin-Norepinephrine Reuptake Inhibitors (SNRIs)‖		
Duloxetine (Cymbalta) *Venlafaxine (Effexor)* *Bupropion (Wellbutrin)*	MDD, OCD, anxiety disorders Effexor and Wellbutrin may be used for attention deficit-hyperactivity disorder (ADHD)	Same side effects as above (SSRIs) for all SNRIs. Effexor may raise blood pressure or produce irregular heart beat. Wellbutrin may lower seizure threshold.
Other Antidepressants		
Trazodone (Desyrel)	Sleep disorders and aggression	Sedation, dizziness, orthostatic hypotension, hypertension, blurred vision, urinary retention.
Mirtazapine (Remeron)	Sleep disorders	Sedation, dizziness.

Atypical Neuroleptics (Antipsychotics)		
Risperidone (Risperdal) *Olanapine* (Zyprexa) *Quetiapine* (Seroquel) *Ziprasidone* (Geodon) *Aripiprazole* (Abilify)	Psychotic disorders (schizophrenia, atypical psychosis, mania/hypomania, delusions, hallucinations, etc.) Behavioral disorders (agitation, aggression, impulsivity, anxiety, sleep disturbances, etc.)	Headache, dizziness, insomnia, agitation, anxiety. Sedation, weight gain, metabolic syndrome (altered lipid profile, risk of diabetes), extrapyramidal syndrome (tremor, spasms, etc.), neuro-malignant syndrome (NMS; muscle spasms, fever) tardive dyskinesia (late onset muscle dysregulation), withdrawal dyskinesia (tics and motor abnormalities with dose reduction). *Rare:* serious cardiac effects.
Anticholinergic Agents		
Benztropine (Cogentin) *Trihexyphenidyl* (Artane)	Used to counteract EPS (extrapyramidal side effects) of antipsychotic medications such as muscle spasms, parkinsonian gait, tremor, and antsy nervousness	Dry mouth, constipation, drowsiness, dizziness, headache, loss of appetite, stomach upset, vision changes, sleeplessness, trembling of the hands, decreased sweating.
Alpha 2 Agonists		
Clonidine (Catapres) *Guanfacine* (Tenex)	ADHD, tics, impulsivity, aggression	Dizziness, drowsiness, sedation, dry mouth, constipation, weight gain, weakness, bradycardia.

Continued

Mental Health Disorders **CHAPTER 5**

Table 5-3   *Psychotropic Medications—cont'd*

Mood Stabilizers	Off-label Clinical Indications ≤ 18 Years	Potential Adverse Effects*
Lithium carbonate (Lithium)	Bipolar disorder Mania MDD Aggression, labile moods, irritability	*Lithium:* Fine hand tremor, dry mouth, weight gain, thirst, nausea, kidney and thyroid changes, increased urination. *Signs of toxicity:* loss of appetite, visual impairment, tiredness, muscle weakness, tremor, unsteady gait, confusion, seizures, arrythmias, slurred speech, coma. *Drug interactions:* nonsteroidal anti-inflammatory drugs (NSAIDs), others.
Divalproex sodium (Depakote)		*Depakote:* Drowsiness, dizziness, nausea, vomiting, indigestion, diarrhea, weight loss, tremors, hair loss. *Drug interactions:* NSAIDs, others.
Lamotrigine (Lamictal)		*Lamictal:* Dizziness, somnolence, headache, double vision, blurred vision, nausea, vomiting, rash.Severe life-threatening rashes can occur. *Drug interactions:* valproic acid.
Carbamazepine (Tegretol)		*Tegretol:* Dizziness, unsteadiness, nausea, vomiting. *Serious side effects:* reduced blood cell counts, skin reactions, liver abnormalities. *Drug interactions:* theophyllin, erythromycin, birth control pills.

Oxcarbazepine (Trileptal)		*Trileptal:* Dizziness, drowsiness, fatigue, nausea, vomiting, rash, headache, trouble sleeping, acne, dry mouth, constipation. Serious side effects: double vision, change in vision, tremor, involuntary eye movements, difficulty speaking, loss of coordination, abnormal gait, dulled sense of touch, stomach pain. *Drug interactions:* birth control pills.
Tricyclic Antidepressants (TCAs)¶		
Amitriptyline (Elavil) *Desipramine* (Norpramin)	Sleep onset, anxiety	Fatigue, dizziness, blurred vision, constipation, dry mouth, orthostatic hypotension, risk of seizures, tachycardia, heart block, cardiac effects.
Imipramine (Tofranil) *Nortriptyline* (Pamelor) *Doxepin* (Sinequan) *Clomipramine* (Anafranil)	Anxiety, ADHD	Drowsiness, dizziness, confusion, dry mouth, hypoglycemia, ataxia, weakness, blurred vision, tachycardia, seizures, urinary retention, constipation, hypertension, diaphoresis, palpitations, cardiac effects.

*Adverse effects are typical for the medication class: consult *Physicians' Desk Reference* or other reference for specific profile of each medication. Note that drug interactions may need to be reviewed.

†Prozac is the only medication approved by the FDA for depression in children age 7 and older (Richardson and Katznellenbogen, 2005).

‡Paxil is not recommended by the FDA for MDD in children or adolescents as it has not been shown to be effective (FDA/Center for Drug Evaluation and Research, 2003).

§Sudden discontinuance of SSRIs may cause symptoms of withdrawal: dizziness, tiredness, tingling of the extremities, nausea, vivid dreams, irritability, poor mood, visual disturbances, and headaches.

‖SNRIs also have SSRI activity.

¶Tricyclic antidepressants are no longer recommended for MDD due to lack of effectiveness in prepubertal children. but they may be effective with adolescents (Hazell et al, 2006; Gutgeselle et al, 1999).

WEB SITES

Autism Society of America
    http://www.autism-society.org
Autism Collaboration
    http://www.autism.org
Autism Speaks
    http://www.autismspeaks.org

ASPERGER'S SYNDROME

I. Definition

   A. Asperger's syndrome is considered a form of high-functioning autism, and individuals generally display a full linguistic capability and have a normal or above normal range intellectual capacity. Deficits in social interaction are present that range from mild to moderately severe, and unusual repetitive, stereotyped patterns and behaviors are observed (see Box 5-3).

Box 5-3   *DSM-IV Criteria: Asperger's Syndrome*

A. Qualitative impairment in social interaction, as manifested by at least two of the following:
   1. Marked impairment in the use of multiple nonverbal behaviors—such as eye-to-eye gaze, facial expression, body postures, and gestures—to regulate social interaction.
   2. Failure to develop peer relationships appropriate to developmental level.
   3. A lack of spontaneous seeking to share enjoyment, interests, or achievements with other people (e.g., by a lack of showing, bringing, or pointing out objects of interest to other people).
   4. Lack of social or emotional reciprocity.
B. Restricted, repetitive, and stereotyped patterns of behavior, interests, and activities, as manifested by at least one of the following:
   1. Encompassing preoccupation with one or more stereotyped and restricted patterns of interest that is abnormal either in intensity or focus.
   2. Apparently inflexible adherence to specific, nonfunctional routines or rituals.
   3. Stereotyped and repetitive motor mannerisms (e.g., hand or finger flapping or twisting or complex, whole-body movements).
   4. Persistent preoccupation with parts of objects.
C. The disturbance causes clinically significant impairment in social, occupational, or other areas of functioning.
D. There is no clinically significant delay in language (e.g., single words used by age 2 years, communicative phrases used by age 3 years).
E. There is no clinically significant delay in cognitive development or in the development of age-appropriate self-help skills, adaptive behavior (other than in social interaction), and curiosity about the environment in childhood.
F. Criteria are not met for another specific, pervasive developmental disorder or schizophrenia.

From American Psychiatric Association: *Diagnostic and statistical manual of mental disorders,* ed 4 text revision, Washington, DC, 2000, American Psychiatric Association.

II. Etiology

A. Asperger's syndrome is believed to be hereditary; about a third of all sufferers have a close family member with the condition or a similar disability. Onset may occur later than in autism, usually after age 3; it occurs more frequently in boys (Saulnier and Volkmar, 2005).

III. Characteristics

A. Exhibits repetitive, atypical patterns and behaviors and focuses on special interests.

B. Shows interest in social relationships but often is unable to facilitate.

C. Pedantic speech, absorption in circumscribed subjects (e.g., baseball scores, weather).

D. Often verbal but tends to be egocentric in conversation, repeats words or phrases, perseveration. Unable to participate in reciprocal conversation.

E. Poor nonverbal communication and eye contact or limited understanding of facial expressions.

F. Speech is frequently repetitive and stilted with monotone, emotionless voice; vocabulary and grammar are generally very good.

G. Awkward and clumsy movements with fine and gross motor deficits.

H. No significant delays in cognitive or language development, adaptive behavior, or self-help skills.

I. May have dyslexia and difficulty with writing and math and a history of hyperlexia (i.e., reading without thought of meaning at a precocious age).

J. Depression and bipolar disorder (mood instability) occurs, and attention difficulties may be prominent.

IV. Effects on Individual

A. Socially isolated with limited friendships and vulnerability to bullying.

B. Possibility of strained family relationships.

C. Behavior problems may develop because of rejection by others.

D. Awkward motor abilities.

E. Limited interests and routines.

V. Health Concerns and Emergencies

A. Accident prone.

B. Depression and mood instability or bipolar disorder.

VI. Management and Treatment

A. Treat symptomatically and supportively. Family history is important.

B. Antidepressants, antipsychotic, stimulants, and antianxiety medications as needed.

C. Monitor medications and side effects.

D. Psychosocial intervention for depression and social skills training.

E. Occupational therapy and physical therapy as needed.

F. Facilitated and protected social intervention in class, especially on the playground.

G. May need help in acquiring social skills; can support this by allowing students to help in nurse's office, computer lab, or in some other capacity to build self-confidence and increase participation in social life at school.

H. Support parent and child interactions.

I. Be available to teach and work with staff, students, and family.

VII. Additional Information
   A. Often lead productive lives in adulthood, with independent living, a family, and job satisfaction.

WEB SITES

MAAP Services for Autism and Asperger Syndrome: The Source
   http://www.asperger.org
Online Asperger Syndrome Information and Support (OASIS)
   http://www.aspergersyndrome.org

RETT SYNDROME

I. Definition
   A. Rett syndrome is included in the pervasive developmental delay spectrum, affecting the gray matter of the brain. It is more commonly reported in girls. Affected boys generally die shortly after birth of a severe brain disorder. Although present at birth, symptoms do not manifest until 6 to 18 months of age or later. Rett syndrome is a unique neurodevelopmental disorder with severe impairment, but is similar to autism in social and language delays. Girls may live into adulthood but never regain use of their hands, and the ability to speak is rare.

II. Etiology
   A. Rett syndrome is a genetic disorder caused by mutation of a single gene, MeCP2, located on one of the two X chromosomes that determine sex. MeCP2 makes methyl cytosine-binding protein, and the mutation results in excessive amounts.
   B. Rett syndrome may be misdiagnosed as autism, cerebral palsy, or nonspecific delay. Diagnosis is based on symptoms and chromosome studies, but not all individuals have the abnormal gene. Genetic testing is available. Rett syndrome affects one in every 10,000 to 15,000 girls (NINDS, 2006).

III. Characteristics
   A. Normal development until 6 to 18 months.
   B. Purposeful hand movements replaced by repetitive hand movements—hand wringing, licking, or clapping.
   C. Loss of acquired speech.
   D. Head circumference growth decelerates from 5 to 48 mos—cerebral atrophy.
   E. Growth retardation with diminished body fat and muscle mass.
   F. Unsteady, stiff-legged gait, small feet.
   G. Disruptive sleep patterns.
   H. Irritability and agitation.
   I. Loss of interest in people and decreased interpersonal contact occur, but eye contact is maintained.
   J. Mental deficiency is severe to profound.
   K. Hypoactivity and diminished mobility with age.

IV. Effects on Individual
   A. Depends on age and extent of involvement.
   B. Activities of daily living become difficult or impossible.
   C. Behavioral problems develop because of rejection by others.
   D. Limited recreation and social outlets.

V. Health Concerns and Emergencies

A. Breathing pattern irregularities, including breath holding, hyperventilation, apnea, and air swallowing.

B. Abnormal EEG, clinical seizures.

C. Scoliosis; all are at risk for some degree of curvature.

D. Bruxism and difficulty chewing and swallowing.

E. Gastroesophageal reflux diseases (GERD), constipation, malabsorption.

F. Reduced circulation to legs and feet.

G. Instability of trunk, sometimes with limb involvement.

H. Muscle rigidity, spasticity, joint contractures.

I. At risk for injury because of motoric degeneration.

VI. Management and Treatment

A. Dependent on age, extent of involvement, and degree of disability.

B. Includes pharmacological, psychosocial, and educational interventions.

C. Monitor medication and side effects.

D. Rule out hearing loss.

E. Monitor for seizure activity.

F. Observe for breathing problems, development of contractures; monitor skin integrity on the lower extremities.

VII. Additional Information

A. Not every female with Rett syndrome displays all of the symptoms, and individual symptoms may vary in severity. Autistic-like behaviors usually disappear after preschool years. Initial deterioration is rapid, usually within a year, and then loss of skills occurs gradually up to about age 10.

WEB SITES

Rett Syndrome Research Foundation (RSRF)
   http://www.rsrf.org
International Rett Syndrome Association
   http://www.rettsyndrome.org
Rett Syndrome
   http://www.ignatz.net/unicorn.htm

PERVASIVE DEVELOPMENTAL DISORDER–NOT OTHERWISE SPECIFIED

Pervasive developmental disorder–not otherwise specified (PDD-NOS) is a diagnosis by exclusion when a child has some, but not all, of the characteristics of autism or Asperger's syndrome. Diagnosis is made when the child exhibits significant, pervasive, autistic-like impairment in communication, social, and behavioral skills, yet does not meet criteria for a specific PDD (APA, 2000).

This category is used when a severe and pervasive impairment exists in the development of reciprocal social interaction or verbal and nonverbal communication skills, or when stereotyped behavior, interests, and activities are present, but the criteria are not met for a specific PDD, schizophrenia, schizotypal personality disorder, or avoidant personality disorder. For example, this

CHAPTER 5

Mental Health Disorders

category includes *atypical autism*—presentations that do not meet the criteria for autistic disorder because of late age of onset, atypical symptomatology, or all of these (APA, 2000).

SCHOOL AVOIDANCE/REFUSAL AND SCHOOL PHOBIA

I. Definition

A. A generalized anxiety or a fixed fear associated with attending an educational facility. School avoidance/refusal generally refers to some anxiety-based absenteeism; school phobia is more specific to a fear of something related to school. School avoidance/refusal may be a developmental challenge for a preschooler leaving home for kindergarten and a social challenge for an adolescent. The terms avoidance, refusal, and phobia are sometimes used interchangeably.

B. By definition, truancy (absence from school) generally is a behavioral problem, not a phobia (see "Additional Information").

II. Etiology

A. A multitude of causes and conditions exist for these fearful or phobic behaviors. For the elementary-age child, the psychosocial issues may be separation anxiety from a caregiver, apprehension about new surroundings and strangers, or dislike of a problem person such as a peer bully or an overly harsh or strict teacher. At times the young student has an avoidant reaction to school arising from dependency on an overprotective and possessive parent. A variety of psychosocial factors may also contribute, including issues of family problems, community or school safety, or other fearful concerns.

B. School phobia is more common for students 10 years of age and older. An acute onset can be precipitated by a school-related incident. School phobia in adolescence is more likely associated with a social withdrawal syndrome, an underlying depressive disorder, or both factors. School phobia may lead to further social isolation in reaction to peer ostracism or nonconformity to peer norms.

C. Occurrence of these behaviors is approximately 5% of children in the early primary grades and 2% in junior high school. The incidence is similar in boys and girls and across socioeconomic groups (Dixon and Stein, 2006; Schmitt, 2005).

D. Delineation of the above categories or differential diagnosis depends on the severity of the problem, secondary complications, and length of absenteeism.

III. Characteristics

A. Lack of social skills, first entry to school, beginning a different school.

B. Major life change (e.g., family grief, acute or chronic medical illness, divorce, loss of peer playmate or companion).

C. Expression of shyness may be a precursor to a social phobia.

D. Conduct-disordered youths experience peer rejection.

E. Fixed learning disabilities evidenced by chronic frustration and underachievement that represent failure or avoidance.

F. Unrealistic parental standards for the student's academic and social standing, leading to feelings of inadequacy.

IV. Effects on Individual

A. Stress symptoms such as anxiety, panic states, and psychosomatic illness (e.g., nausea, vomiting, diarrhea, dizziness, headache, abdominal pain).

B. Behavioral regression to lower development.

C. Overreliance on parents or adult caregivers.

D. Diminished self-confidence and ability to take risks.

E. School absenteeism.

F. Development of perfectionist attitudes and procrastinating habits.

G. Educational underachievement.

H. Social isolation, conflicting peer relationships.

I. School dropout, employment difficulties.

V. Health Concerns and Emergencies

A. A student home alone may not receive immediate medical care for an acute health care problem or emergency (e.g., asthma attack, drug or medication overdose).

B. While at home, student may overeat, lack exercise, suffer loss of educational knowledge, and may fall behind academically; all are secondary complications leading to medical, educational, and social problems.

C. Due to chronic somatic complaints, serious physical illness may be overlooked.

VI. Management and Treatment

A. Early interruption of behaviors is critical.

B. Assess for underlying physical problems (e.g., vision, hearing, undetected or untreated physical injury or illness, fatigue related to nutritional deficiency, sleep deprivation).

C. Assess for psychosocial, emotional, and mental problems (e.g., depression, drug and alcohol abuse). School Refusal Assessment Scale measures the symptoms of school refusal and provides a basis for establishment of a treatment plan (Kearney, 2002; see Appendix A, Assessment Tools).

D. Evaluate family and home issues (e.g., Munchausen's syndrome by proxy, parental depression, parental criminal behaviors, child abuse, and lack of parental motivation).

E. Parental guidance related to dependence/independence issues.

F. Discern and differentiate stress symptoms requiring assurance and TLC versus medical-model treatment, such as rest and medication.

G. Refer for appropriate follow-up (e.g., psychosocial or emotional intervention, grief counseling, evaluation of learning disabilities, treatment with antianxiety medications).

H. Help child gain a sense of control and problem-solving skills for personal development.

I. Reprogramming of irrational fears and desensitization training.

J. Make school friendly, positive, and rewarding for student (e.g., assign duties in health office or make peer counseling referral).

K. Gradual reintegration into school can promote successful treatment.

VII. Additional Information

A. No formal DSM-IV diagnostic category exists for school phobia. However, associated diagnoses include separation anxiety disorder, adjustment disorder, social phobia, ODD, and early onset dysthymia.

B. School truancy is a choice of the student to be noncompliant with requirements to attend school, frequently without parental knowledge (e.g., willful disobedience, antisocial and delinquent behavior, conduct disorder).

C. Agoraphobia is an intense fear of a situation or of being in a place where one feels trapped and unable to get away (e.g., standing in line, riding on a bus, being in an auditorium or in a large crowd). Such situations may bring on a panic attack or extreme embarrassment, and therefore a fear of attending school can result (APA, 2000).

D. Anxiety disorders are the most common psychiatric disorders affecting children and adolescents. There are five major types; generalized anxiety disorder (GAD), obsessive-compulsive disorder (OCD), panic disorder (PD), post-traumatic stress disorder (PTSD), and social phobia, or social anxiety disorder (NIH, 2006) Anxiety is the normal reaction to stress, but when it becomes an excessive, irrational fear of everyday situations, it is a disabling disorder. Each disorder has its own set of somatic, social, and cognitive symptoms that the nurse must recognize to provide appropriate support and treatment.

WEB SITE

Anxiety Disorders Association of America
   http://www.adaa.org

TICS AND TOURETTE'S DISORDER

I. Definition

A. Tics are the most common childhood movement disorder, and various muscle groups are involved. Tics often are classified according to age of onset, duration, severity of symptoms, and by the presence of vocal and motor tics. There are other tic disorders that may last from a few weeks to more than a year. Transient, chronic, and Tic Disorder–Not Otherwise Specified (TD-NOS) are discussed in "Additional Information."

B. Tourette's syndrome, also called Tourette's disorder (TD), is the most severe disorder involving tic behaviors. It is a hereditary, neurological movement disorder, characterized by repetitive, uncontrolled tics. TD can be observed as early as 2 years of age, peak onset is 5 to 8 years; with motor tics, peak onset is 6 to 7 years. For a TD diagnosis, age of onset must be before age 18 with vocal and motor tics occurring for at least 1 year, and the child must not have been tic-free for more than 3 consecutive months (APA, 2000).

   1. Coexisting conditions are behavioral and learning disabilities including attention-deficit/hyperactivity disorder (ADHD), obsessive-compulsive disorder (OCD), depression, and anxiety.

Tics can occur sporadically, may change in character, and often are changed by the person into something that appears like a "real" thing, such as a head touch into a hair twirl, or a guttural noise into a swear word (coprolalia).

II. Etiology

A. Tics and TD can be genetic or acquired. Family history is found in more than 50% of the cases (Kliegman et al, 2006). TD occurrence is 5 to 30 out of 10,000 and is more common in boys than girls. (APA, 2000).

Brain Findings

Tics and TD are associated with abnormalities in the genes that affect the metabolism of the neurotransmitters, primarily dopamine, serotonin, and norepinephrine. These effects are thought to occur in the area of the basal ganglia, particularly the caudate nucleus (Black and Webb, 2006; NIH, 2005). The caudate nucleus is an area in the brain that is involved in the inhibition of purposeless movements, among other functions.

III. Characteristics

A. Symptoms may wax or wane over time, making diagnosis difficult.
B. Motor tics are both simple (e.g., eye twitches or blinks, grimaces, head jerks, shrugs) and complex (e.g., smelling objects; mimicking movements of another person [echopraxia], such as head shaking, repeated kicking movements, obscene hand gestures [copropraxia]). The activities may appear purposeful and coordinated but are involuntary.
C. Vocal tics include throat clearing, grunting or barking noises, outbursts of nonsensical sounds or obscene words (coprolalia, 5%), repetition of words said by others (echolalia), and repetition of one's own words (palilalia). Vocal tics may be simple (throat clearing and grunting or vocal sounds) or complex (stammering, stuttering, and swearing).
D. Rare symptoms include lip and cheek biting, head banging, and other self-abusive behaviors.
E. Tics are increased by fatigue and physical and mental stress, but in some people they manifest more when in a relaxed state.
F. Reduced or absent during sleep.
G. Tics may be suppressed for a brief period but eventually escape; they must be expressed to release tension and anxiety.
H. Tics can be exacerbated by seasonal or life changes (e.g., holidays) but tend to decrease with age.
I. Tics generally improve after puberty; some individuals are symptom-free by their twenties.
J. Associated traits include obsession, compulsion, hyperactivity, impulsivity, inattentiveness, anxiety, depression, and learning disability.
K. Treating one disorder may worsen another (e.g., stimulant for hyperactivity may increase tics).
L. Intelligence is not impaired but the individual may have learning difficulties.

IV. Effects on Individual

A. Social stigma, embarrassment and shame, self-consciousness, low self-esteem, feelings of peer rejection, social isolation.

B. If severe, symptoms can interfere with daily activities, including reading, writing, and classroom concentration.

C. Can cause physical pain and can result in deformity.

D. Side effects of medication may create resistance to medication compliance.

E. Some side effects—muscular rigidity, drooling, tremors, slow movement, and restlessness—interfere with class participation and peer acceptance.

F. Possibility of strained family relationships.

G. Some individuals with most involved symptoms can achieve outstanding social, vocational, and academic success.

V. Health Concerns and Emergencies

A. Vary according to involvement and medications.

B. Complex medication management creates possibility of negative drug interactions. Medications for one symptom can create or exacerbate other symptoms.

C. Liaison with the treating physician with parental consent to address improvement or exacerbation of symptoms is most helpful.

D. Weight gain and other health changes can occur secondary to medication.

VI. Management and Treatment

A. Take family history when appropriate and disorder is unidentified.

B. Identification of severe stressors to minimize impact whenever possible. Ask student, parents, and teachers when tics are most likely to occur and what exacerbates tics. Student may experience social and emotional effects, as may family and friends.

C. Awareness of medication side effects and contraindications. Medication is prescribed only if tics create a major educational or social impairment. May be taking medication for coexisting disorders (e.g., ADHD, OCD, depression or anxiety).

D. Monitoring of height and weight for growth retardation or excessive weight gain.

E. Classroom and staff teaching are important to develop peer and adult knowledge, understanding, and support.

F. Distinguish between student misbehavior and disorder symptoms and manage each appropriately.

G. Extended time and privacy may be needed during testing.

H. If student's movements are disruptive, nurse should consider that they are involuntary; use strategies for the moment; be calm to reduce student's stress and decrease tics.

I. Permission to leave classroom when tics are imminent; inconspicuous seating for student.

J. Cognitive behavioral therapy and habit-reversal psychotherapy may be helpful.

VII. Additional Information

A. In 2004, Tourette's disorder was recognized as a qualifying disability for special education services, other health impairment, by Part B of the Individuals with Disabilities Act (IDEA) and Section 504.

B. Transient tic disorder.
  1. Transient tics can be motor or vocal and do not last more than a year. Duration is only weeks or months, and usually they are not associated with learning or behavioral problems (APA, 2000). Tics are relatively common and are found in 1 out of 100 children. Transient tic symptoms include eye blinking, nose puckering, grimacing, and squinting. Vocalizations are less common and include humming or other mouth or throat sounds. Other bizarre behaviors may also occur (e.g., poking and pinching of the genitals, palm licking).
C. Chronic motor or vocal tic disorder.
  1. Chronic tics are motor or vocal but not both. Tics may be single or multiple and last more than a year without more than three consecutive tic-free months (APA, 2000).
D. TD-NOS.
  1. TD-NOS does not meet the criteria for a specific tic disorder, such as tics beginning after age 18 or lasting less than 4 weeks (APA, 2000).
E. Obsessive–compulsive disorder (OCD).
  1. OCD is present in 2% to 3% of children and adolescents (Obsessive Compulsive Foundation, 2006). It is a biologically based mental disorder among children who have a pattern of obsessions, worrisome thoughts or acts, compulsions, and consuming rituals. These children and adolescents are bothered with disturbing thoughts related to dirt, germs, contaminants, and ideas of harm, violence, and moral wrongdoing. These result in feelings of inadequacy, worthlessness, and self-condemnation. The repetitive rituals are performed or enacted by the child to relieve the anxiety and fears caused by the obsessions. These rituals include hand washing, cleaning, checking, counting, and confessing on a repetitive basis.
  2. OCD is more common in adolescence and can be a precursor to a diagnosis of obsessive–compulsive personality in adults, as with cyclothymia and bipolar disorder. Children, especially young children, generally do not have an awareness of the disorder. Furthermore, the association of the obsession with the compulsions in childhood OCD is less clear than for adults. Most children in elementary years are aware of their obsessive thinking and view it as "stupid," causing them embarrassment and discomfort in social situations. Younger children usually are less secretive about their compulsions and more overt in their expressions. Children express their compulsions with more irritability and moodiness than adolescents or adults. They also have more mental rituals (i.e., cognitive repetitions in their mind that are not visible to an adult or peers, such as counting exercises, reciting of phrases). Some children have vocal tics similar to Tourette's syndrome. Tics and OCD symptoms occur together in a majority of children; more than two thirds of children with OCD have tics, and 50% to 75% of children with TD have obsessive-compulsive symptoms (Swedo and Leonard, 1999).

WEB SITES

Tourette Syndrome Association
   http://www.tsa-usa.org
Tourette Syndrome Plus
   http://www.tourettesyndrome.net
The Obsessive-Compulsive Foundation
   http://www.ocfoundation.org

MAJOR DEPRESSIVE DISORDER

I. Definition
   A. Major depressive disorder (MDD) is characterized by significant in-
      termittent emotional and behavioral changes for a minimum of
      2 weeks. These may include irritability, sadness, despondency, and
      depression. There is often a marked decrease in interest and pleasure
      in most activities at home, school, and with family and peers.
      The three most typical patterns of severe mood disorders are MDD,
      dysthymia, and bipolar disorder.

II. Etiology
   A. Major depressive disorder is associated with many factors, which
      may be genetic, developmental, environmental, and biological. It is
      one of the most clearly described and thoroughly studied syndromes
      in medicine, yet unfortunately many people still see it as a weakness
      or a choice instead of an overwhelming illness.
   B. Genetic factors are associated with up to a threefold risk of MDD in
      children and may influence early onset of the disorder.
   C. Developmental changes in adolescence or their disruption—such as
      onset of puberty, establishing independence from the family unit,
      and changes in relationships and intimacy—can trigger depression.
      MDD often begins in late adolescence but can occur in the youngest
      of children.
   D. Environmental factors (stressors) occur at the time the depression
      begins and in about half of all people with depression. Trauma or
      abuse and neglect, living with a depressed parent, lack of a loving
      and nurturing parent, parental divorce or death, low social or eco-
      nomic status, and academic difficulties are just a few examples.
   E. Biological factors such as substance abuse, physical illness, and
      trauma can influence the brain and produce major symptoms by
      altering brain chemistry.

Brain Findings

The amygdala, hippocampus, and prefrontal cortex seem to play major
roles in the neural systems underlying mood. A growing body of literature
demonstrates those with mood disorders have structural changes in these
areas (Zorumski and Rubin, 2005). Perhaps most interesting is a burgeon-
ing medical literature showing how effective treatment of depression—
whether with therapy, medication, or both—is associated with improvement of right parietal lobe function to more normal levels, as seen in
functional brain imaging studies.

III. Characteristics

NOTE: Symptoms must be present for at least 2 weeks and must represent a change from previous functioning.

A. Affective.

Depressed mood most of the time, but mood can change in reaction to the environment. Mood may be much better temporarily, when the person is active (e.g., at a party), but depression returns later. Depression may be demonstrated by irritability and anger in children and in adolescents or as anxiety, melancholia, feelings of hopelessness and worthlessness, and suicidal ideation.

B. Behavioral.

1. Withdrawal, social isolation, or self-injurious behaviors may be symptoms of depression. Oppositional or defiant actions, agitation, restlessness, stealing, lying, or truancy may also be symptoms. However, it is necessary to sort out whether a person is feeling depressed because they have been caught behaving badly or because of conflicts with adults or friends, or whether a person is irritable or agitated and reactive as part of their depression. It is as important not to merely excuse bad behavior as "depression" as it is not to punish reactive anger that is in fact a part of the depression or mood disorder.

2. Many people abuse drugs or alcohol in an attempt to self-medicate, yet perhaps more often the substance abuse has brought on the mood disorder. Either way the substance abuse needs to be addressed for successful treatment.

3. Young children who are depressed may be accident prone and hyperactive, but it is important to distinguish whether the child is depressed because he or she is demoralized by preexisting ADHD, or whether a mood disturbance is creating agitation and recklessness.

4. Perhaps most important, any mention or act that implies harm to self or to others should be taken seriously and evaluated immediately by a mental health professional. Do not try to decide whether a suicidal episode is a "gesture" versus an "attempt." There is no good way to know the difference, and it is better to err on the side of caution.

C. Cognitive.

1. Significant cognitive symptoms may occur, including difficulty concentrating or thinking, inability to complete homework, indecisiveness, negative self-image, and inappropriate guilt.

D. Physical.

1. There may be loss of energy and fatigue, or there may be agitation and frenetic activity. Somatic symptoms are common, especially with people who have more difficulty talking about their lives; difficulties can include such things as frequent stomachaches and headaches. Other important neurovegatative symptoms include appetite changes with weight loss or weight gain, decreased libido, insomnia, or hypersomnia. Younger children may have encopresis or enuresis.

E. Social.

1. A loss of interest in friends, preference for time alone, school phobia, and lack of interest in after-school activities are typically

CHAPTER 5

Mental Health Disorders

seen. Missing school is considered an urgent matter, much the same as when an adult with depression is unable to work. Both are medical urgencies.

IV. Effects on Individual

A. Many adolescents with recurrent MDD will eventually develop bipolar disorder; although approximately 90% of MDD episodes remit within 18 months to 2 years after onset (Richardson and Katzenellenbogen, 2005). There is a risk of recurrence and the condition tends to be more pervasive and difficult to treat in children and adolescents than adults.

B. Frequent absences from school; decrease in school grades.

C. Becomes particularly sensitive to rejection or failure, and in any case there are often significant effects on social relationships.

D. Spends time in the nurse's office with vague somatic complaints.

E. May be suspended from school for drug or alcohol use, defiance, or aggressive behaviors.

F. Decrease in personal hygiene, increase in weight, and with long term MDD, may have poor physical health.

G. At risk for early pregnancy.

V. Health Concerns and Emergencies

A. Be aware of signs of suicide and seek help immediately. Girls attempt suicide more often, but boys are more successful (see Chapter 7, Violence).

B. Suicide is the third leading cause of death for ages 10 to 19 (CDC, 2004).

C. Lack of sleep or use of alcohol or drugs makes students vulnerable to accidents in gym, in shop classes, or while driving.

D. Drug abuse is present in 20% of adolescents with MDD (Weller et al, 2004).

VI. Management and Treatment

NOTE: Any mention or act that implies harm to self or to others should be taken seriously and evaluated immediately by a mental health professional. Contact parent and school administrator. Do not try to decide whether a suicidal episode is a "gesture" versus an attempt. There is no good way to know the difference, and it is better to err on the side of caution. Check with school district regarding school procedures.

A. Open-ended conversation to evaluate need for referral to a school mental health professional.

B. Contact parent and school administrator when indicated.

C. Take complete health and family history.

D. Screen with Beck Depression Inventory, Children's Depression Inventory, Pediatric Symptom Check List, or other appropriate tool as permitted by guardian (see Appendix A, Assessment Tools).

E. Immediate referral is imperative for any student verbalizing suicidal intentions. National hotlines: 800-784-2433 and 800-273-8255.

F. Consider referral for psychotherapy or group support services. Treatment is most effective when the family is actively involved in the process.

G. Educational team needs to strategize plan for positive reinforcement and encouraging self-worth, self-control, and optimism. Avoid "get tough" approach.

H. Monitor students for signs of increased depression or suicidal ideation, because adolescents are at increased risk of suicide. Cardiovascular monitoring required for students on Tricyclic antidepressants.

VII. Additional Information

A. Depression in Infants and Preschoolers.

1. Infants may be unresponsive to parents, irritable, crying, or consistently passive. Head banging may occur. Infants and preschoolers may have difficulties with attachment, separation, feeding, and failure to thrive. They can be nonreactive, socially withdrawn, or hyperactive and impulsive. Speech and motor skills may be delayed or regress. The child must be evaluated by a health professional familiar with depression and with developmental disorders in infants and preschoolers.

B. Adolescents and Young Adults.

1. Adults may be better able to cope with depression than adolescents, because adolescents do not have the coping skills, self-confidence, or an established identity to cope with depression and its hopelessness. Adolescents may find it difficult to seek help; they are in a stage of physical, social, and emotional change and may not recognize their symptoms as depression. Moreover, adolescents naturally avoid adults and rely on friends for support. They may ask friends to keep secrets about their suicidal feelings. Consider evaluation of adolescent mother for post-partum depression.

C. Other Types of Depression.

1. Dysthymia.

a. Dysthymia is a depressive disorder that is more difficult to recognize; it has fewer symptoms but is typically more chronic than MDD. Minimum time period for diagnosis in children and adolescents is 1 year and in adults, 2 years. In addition to a depressed mood, there may be any of the other symptoms of depression (e.g., poor appetite or overeating, loss of energy or fatigue, insomnia or hypersomnia, poor concentration, low self-esteem, difficulty making decisions, and feelings of hopelessness). At least two of the symptoms must be present for diagnosis (APA, 2000). Over time, children and adolescents accept the symptoms and feelings of depressive mood as a normal part of everyday life. This disorder colors the child's life and often impedes progress in several areas, including academic, social, and emotional growth.

b. The onset of dysthymia occurs most commonly in childhood or adolescence (Jones, 2004). It is often a precursor to affective disorders later in life, including subsequent MDD and bipolar disorder. Kovacs and colleagues (1994) found that 70% of children with dysthymia go on to develop episodes of MDD. Like MDD, antidepressants and psychotherapy are used for treatment, although efficacy of treatment is more uncertain.

2. Bipolar disorder (BPD) or manic–depressive disorder.

a. BPD and manic–depressive disorder are classically characterized by grandiosity and inflated personal worth, decreased sleep, talkativeness or rapid speech, excessive motor activity or overactivity, and distractibility alternating with periods of depression (e.g., low mood, introspection, loneliness, social withdrawal, and a generally sad affect). Mood swings cycle between severe lows and highs that generally last for many weeks or months for adults; but in children the cycles are often more rapid and more pronounced (Evans et al, 2005; Wozniak and Biederman, 2005).

b. In the past, BPD was diagnosed in adults and only rarely in children and adolescents younger than age 13. Now clinical and epidemiological research has documented an increasing prevalence of BPD in late adolescence, and some children are diagnosed as early as age 7 (Axelson et al, 2006) and many case reports exist of preschoolers with bipolar disorder. A complex etiology of BPD includes both environmental and genetic factors.

c. Comorbidity makes BPD difficult to diagnosis and manage. For children under age 12, 90% with BPD also have ADHD, and 50% to 60% of adolescents with BPD have ADHD. Other comorbid conditions include conduct disorder (40%) and anxiety (50% to 60%). Alcohol and drug abuse are common and complicate the management and treatment of BPD (Wozniak and Biederman, 2005).

D. Seasonal affective disorder (SAD).
  1. SAD is a mental health disorder which is apparently related to light exposure. Depressive symptoms occur in the fall and winter and remit in the spring, although the person may be more agitated or hypomanic in the spring.
  2. It is thought that two brain chemicals are involved in SAD: melatonin and serotonin. When days are shorter, more melatonin is produced, whereas the level of serotonin is diminished. Increased melatonin produces tiredness, and the low level of serotonin has been linked to depression. Symptoms include low energy level, hypersomnia, increased appetite, mood changes, sadness or irritability, guilt, difficulty concentrating, and loss of interest in friends and activities.
  3. Treatment includes light therapy, psychotherapy, and medication. Increased exposure to sunlight or use of a light box daily may be helpful. The light must be absorbed through the retinas to be effective, so the individual must glance occasionally at the light box. Medications are also prescribed, and current studies demonstrate that both light therapy and medication are effective (Lam, 2006). Researchers continue to pursue more data on etiology and effective treatments.

WEB SITES

Child and Adolescent Bipolar Foundation
  http://www.cabf.org
Depression and Bipolar Support Alliance
  http://www.dbsalliance.org

GENERAL MENTAL HEALTH WEB SITES

NYU Child Study Center: About Our Kids
http://www.aboutourkids.org
American Academy of Child and Adolescent Psychiatry
http://www.aacap.org
Center for Mental Health in Schools
http://www.smhp.psych.ucla.edu
Child Development Institute
http://www.cdipage.com
Federation of Families for Children's Mental Health
http://www.ffcmh.org
Healthy Minds. Healthy Lives.
http://www.healthyminds.org
National Alliance on Mental Illness: Child and Adolescent Action Center
http://www.nami.org/youth/index.html
National Institute of Mental Health
http://www.nimh.nih.gov/index.shtml
National Mental Health Information Center: Center for Mental Health Services
http://www.mentalhealth.samhsa.gov

BIBLIOGRAPHY

American Psychiatric Association: *Diagnostic and statistical manual of mental disorders, ed 4, text revision,* Washington, DC, 2000, American Psychiatric Association.
Anastopoulos A, Shelton T: *Assessing attention-hyperactivity disorder,* New York, 2001, Kluwer Academic/Plenum.
Axelson D, Birmaher B, Strober M: Phenomenology of children and adolescents with bipolar spectrum disorders, *Arch Gen Psychiatry* 63(10):1139-1148, 2006.
Barkley R: *Attention-deficit hyperactivity disorder* (available online): www.sciam.com/1998/0998issuebarkley.html. Accessed June 2006.
Biederman J: Definitions and overview of ADHD. In attention deficit hyperactivity across the life span, *Post Graduate Education Newsletter,* Massachusetts General Hospital March, 2005.
Biederman J: Pharmacotherapy of attention-deficit/hyperactivity disorder reduces risk for substance use disorder. *Pediatrics* 104(2):e20, 1999.
Birmaher B, Axelson D, Strober M: Clinical course of children and adolescents with bipolar spectrum disorders, *Arch Gen Psychiatry* 63(2):173-183, 2006.
Black KJ, Webb BS: *Tourette syndrome and other tic disorders* (available online): www.emedicine.com/NEURO/topic664.htm. Accessed March 2006.
Bower B: Attention loss: ADHD may lower volume of brain, *Science News* 162(15):227, 2002.
California Department of Developmental Services: *Autistic spectrum disorders* (available online): www.dds.ca.gov/Autism/pdf/AutismReport2003.pdf. Accessed November 2006.
Castellanos FX, Lee PP, Sharp W: Developmental trajectories of brain volume abnormalities in children and adolescents with attention-deficit/hyperactivity disorder, *JAMA* 288(14):1740-1748, 2002.
Centers for Disease Control and Prevention: *How common are autism spectrum disorders?* (available online): www.cdc.gov/ncbddd/autism/asd_common.htm. Accessed November 2006.
Centers for Disease Control and Prevention: Mental health in the United States: Prevalence of diagnosis and medication treatment for attention deficit/hyperactivity disorder: 2003, *MMWR Morb Mortal Wkly Rep* 54(34):842-847, 2005.
Centers for Disease Control and Prevention: Methods of suicide among persons aged 10 to 19 years: United States, 1992-2001, *MMWR Morb Mortal Wkly Rep* 53(22):471-474, 2004.

Centers for Disease Control and Prevention: Prevalence of autism spectrum disorders: autism and developmental disabilities monitoring network, six sites, *Surveillance Summaries,* MMWR 56 (No. SS-01):1–11, Feb 9, 2007.

Centers for Disease Control and Prevention: Prevalence of autism spectrum disorders: autism and developmental disabilities monitoring network, 14 sites, United States, 2002, *Surveillance Summaries,* MMWR 56 (No. SS-01): 12-28, Feb 9, 2007.

Centers for Disease Control and Prevention: *Research on vaccines and autism* (available online): www.cdc.gov/nip/vacsafe/concerns/autism/autism-research.htm. Accessed July 2006.

Comings DE, Gade-Andavolu R, Gonzalez N: Comparison of the role of dopamine, serotonin, and noradrenaline genes in ADHD, ODD, and conduct disorder: multivariate regression analysis of 20 genes, *Clin Genet* 57(3):178-196, 2000.

Dixon SD, Stein MT: *Encounters with children,* Philadelphia, 2006, Mosby.

Evans DL, Foa EB, Gur RE: *Treating and preventing adolescent mental health disorders,* New York, 2005, Oxford University Press.

Fatemi SH, Halt AR, Realmuto G: Purkinje cell size is reduced in cerebellum of patients with autism, *Cell Mol Neurobiol* 22(2):171-5, 2002.

Fremont WP: School refusal in children and adolescents, *American Family Physician* 68(8):1555-1560, 2003.

Ghazinddin M: Autism in mental retardation, *Current Opinion in Psychiatry* 13:481-484, 2000.

Giedd J: ADHD and substance abuse, *Medscape Psychiatry & Mental Health* 8 (1):1-2, 2003.

Gould MS: A randomized controlled trial: evaluating iatrogenic risk of youth suicide screening programs, *JAMA* 293(13):1635-1643, 2006.

Grossberg S, Seidman D: Neural dynamics of autistic behaviors: cognitive, emotional, and timing substrates, *Psychol Rev* 113(3):483-525, 2006.

Hockenberry MJ, Wilson D, Winkelstein ML: *Wong's essentials of pediatric nursing,* St Louis, 2006, Mosby.

Jones, J: Mood disorders. In Kline F, Silver L, eds: *The educator's guide to mental health issues in the classroom,* Baltimore, 2004, Paul H Brookes.

Kariyawasam SH, Zaw F, Handley SL: Reduced salivary cortisol in children with co-morbid attention-deficit/hyperactivity disorder and oppositional defiant disorder, *Neuroendocrinology Letters* 23(1): 45-48, 2002.

Kearney CA: Identifying the function of school refusal behavior: a revision of the School Refusal Assessment Scale, *Journal of Psychopathology and Behavioral Assessment* 24:235-245, 2002.

Kern JK: Purkinje cell vulnerability and autism: a possible etiological connection, *Brain Development* 25(6):377-82, 2003.

Kliegman RM, Maarcdante KJ, Jenson HB, Behrman RE: *Nelson essentials of pediatrics,* Philadelphia, 2006, WB Saunders.

Kovacs M, Akiskal HS, Gatsonis C, Parrone PL: Childhood-onset dysthymic disorder: clinical features and prospective naturalistic outcome, *Arch Gen Psychiatry* 51(5):365-374, 1994.

Lam RW, Levitt AJ, Levitan RD: The Can-SAD study: a randomized controlled trial of the effectiveness of light therapy and fluoxetine in patients with winter seasonal affective disorder, *American Journal of Psychiatry* 163(5):805-812, 2006.

McBurnett K: Low salivary cortisol and persistent aggression in boys referred for disruptive behaviors, *Arch Gen Psychiatry* 57(1):38-43, 2000.

McMahon RJ, Wells KC: Conduct problems. In EJ Mash, RA Barkley, eds: *Treatment of childhood disorders,* New York, 1998, Plenum.

National Institutes of Health: Brains of people with autism recall letters of the alphabet in brain areas dealing with shapes: finding supports theory that autism results from failure of brain areas to work together (available online): www.nih.gov/news/pr/nov2004/nichd-29.htm. Accessed July 2006.

National Institutes of Health, National Institute of Neurological Disorders and Stroke: *Tourette syndrome fact sheet* (NIH Publication No 05:2163), 2005.

National Institutes of Mental Health: *Anxiety disorders* (available online): www.nimh. nih.gov/publicat/anxiety.cfm#. Accessed November 2006.

Nelson KB, Grether JK, Croen LA: Neuropeptides and neurotrophins in neonatal blood of children with autism or mental retardation, *Ann Neurol* 49(5):597-606, 2001.

Obsessive Compulsive Disorder Foundation: *OCD in the classroom* (available online): www.ocfoundation.org/ocd.in.the.classroom.html. Accessed November 2006.

Parker S: Attention deficit hyperactivity disorder. In Parker S, Zuckerman B, Augustyn M, eds: *Developmental and behavioral pediatrics,* Philadelphia, 2005, Lippincott Williams & Wilkins.

Pary R, Lewis S, Matuschka PR: Attention-deficit/hyperactivity disorder: an update, *South Med* 95(7):743-749, 2002.

Plessen KL, Bansal R, Zhu H: Hippocampus and amygdala morphology in attention-deficit/hyperactivity disorder, *Arch Gen Psychiatry* 63 (7):795-807, 2006.

Richardson LP, Katzenellenbogen R : Childhood and adolescent depression: the role of primary care providers in diagnosis and treatment, *Curr Probl Pediatr Adolesc Health Care* (1):6-24, 2005.

Robertson J, Shilkofski N: *The Harriet Lane handbook,* St. Louis, 2005, Mosby.

Rodier PM: The early origins of autism, *Scientific American* 282(2):56-63, 2000.

Rowland AS, Lesesne CA, Abramowitz AJ: The epidemiology of attention-deficit/hyperactivity disorder (ADHD): A public health view, *Mental Retardation Developmental Disability Research Reviews* 8(3):162-170, 2002.

Saulnier CA, Volkmar FR: Asperger syndrome. In Parker S, Zuckerman B, Augustyn M, eds: *Developmental and behavioral pediatrics,* Philadelphia, 2005, Lippincott Williams & Wilkins.

Scahill L, Ort S: *Tourette syndrome and the school nurse,* Tourette Syndrome Association (Web site): www.tsa-usa.org. Accessed July 2006.

Schmitt BD: School avoidance. In Parker S, Zuckerman B, Augustyn M, eds: *Developmental and behavioral pediatrics,* Philadelphia, 2005, Lippincott Williams & Wilkins.

Schonwald A, Gonzalez-Heydrich J: Psychopharmacology. In Parker S, Zuckerman B, Augustyn M, eds: *Developmental and behavioral pediatrics,* Philadelphia, 2005, Lippincott Williams & Wilkins.

Shumann CM, Amaral DG: Stereological analysis of amygdala neuron number in autism, *Journal of Neuroscience* 26(29):7674-7679, 2006.

Skidmore-Roth L: *Mosby's nursing drug reference,* Philadelphia, 2007, Mosby.

Snoek H: Stress responsivity in children with externalizing behavioral disorders, *Development and Psychopathology* 16:389-406, 2004.

Stocker S: Medications reduce incidence of substance abuse among ADHD patients, *NIDA Notes: Research News* 14(4), 1999.

Strock M: *Autism spectrum disorders, pervasive developmental disorders* (NIH Publication No NIH-04-5511), Bethesda, Md, 2004, National Institute of Mental Health, National Institutes of Health, US Dept of Health and Human Services.

Swedo S, Leonard H: Is *this just a phase? New York,* 1999, Golden Books.

Thapar A, O'Donovan M, Owen MJ: The genetics of attention-deficit/hyperactivity disorder, *Human Molecular Genetics* 14(2):275-282, 2005.

US Public Health Service: *Report of the Surgeon General's Conference on Children's Mental Health: A National Action Agenda,* Washington, DC, 2000, Department of Health and Human Services.

Weller E, Weller R, Danielyan A: Mood disorders in adolescents. In Weiner J, Dulcan K, eds: *Textbook of child and adolescent psychiatry,* Washington, DC, 2004, American Psychiatric Publishing.

Wozniak J, Biederman J: Bipolar disorder in children. In Parker S, Zuckerman B, Augustyn M, eds: *Developmental and behavioral pediatrics,* Philadelphia, 2005, Lippincott Williams & Wilkins.

Zorumski CF, Rubin EH: *Psychopathology in the genome and neuroscience era,* Washington, DC, 2006, American Psychiatric Publishing.

CHAPTER 5

Mental Health Disorders

Clinicians are becoming increasingly aware of the staggering numbers of social and health problems created by substance abuse (SA). Much more is known about how drugs affect the brain, body, and behavior. Those who work with children and adolescents are responsible not only for understanding and teaching these facts, but also for accepting the challenge of identifying and preventing abuse. Effective intervention requires realistic, practical solutions for difficult emotions, peer affiliations, and self-defeating behaviors that can lead to SA.

SA is a major concern in our society. Not only is it prevalent among adolescents, but many more elementary-age children are now involved in substance abuse. Temporary or permanent changes in the chemistry of brain cells, associated health problems, loss of productivity, and suicide are only four of the possible devastating effects of substance abuse. The nurse can be a key person in initiating steps to remedy the problem.

The information in this chapter enables the nurse to understand the devastating effects that occur, identify at-risk students, and engage in effective interventions for drug-related health concerns and emergencies. The various categories of drugs are presented, as is the latest information on chemical interactions in the brain; but because alcohol is extensively abused, socially acceptable, and easily accessible, an entire section is devoted to it.

SA prevention programs are widespread in schools through health education and Safe and Drug-Free School programs. Although school nurses are important partners in such prevention efforts, they are crucial when individual students show symptoms of SA, or when an overdose occurs. Thus, this chapter focuses on providing basic information about drugs that are abused and defines the role of nurses in assisting individual students.

THE NEUROBIOLOGY OF REINFORCEMENT AND DRUG ADDICTION

Reinforcement is anything that increases the likelihood of a future recurrence of a given behavior. Reinforcement and drug addiction are closely linked, because they share a common brain pathway. The basic neural pathway for reinforcement involves the projection from the ventral tegmental area (VTA) of the brain to the nucleus accumbens. The VTA sends fibers along a pathway called the *medial forebrain bundle*. When neurons in the VTA increase their activity, the neurotransmitter dopamine is released onto cells in the nucleus accumbens. This activity is believed to be primarily responsible for reinforcement. Therefore, any behavior that causes a release of dopamine in the nucleus accumbens is more likely to occur in the future.

A variety of behaviors can cause a release of dopamine. Behaviors that release dopamine vary among individuals and might include eating, skydiving, jogging, weightlifting, or even reading, depending on what the individual's brain perceives as rewarding. When this happens, the individual tends to continue that particular behavior, because it is reinforced by the release of dopamine and the resulting good feeling. Many forms of drug addiction work in a similar manner. For example, cocaine, amphetamines, nicotine, and alcohol consumption all cause an increase in dopamine in the nucleus accumbens. Therefore, the behaviors that are responsible for the delivery of the drug (e.g., snorting cocaine, smoking cigarettes, drinking alcohol) are reinforced. This reinforcement can be so powerful that the individual continues to engage in these behaviors even when they become destructive. In essence, this drug addiction is not an addiction to the drug but to the behavior of administering the drug. Research indicates that the anticipation of consuming the drug can also release dopamine and that the anticipation of taking the drug is a big part of drug addiction.

UNDERSTANDING SUBSTANCE ABUSE

SA is the self-administered misuse of a chemical or toxic material to the extent that the individual's health or ability to function responsibly is adversely affected and compromised. SA may be referred to as *substance use disorder* (American Psychiatric Association [APA], 2000).

The physical, cognitive, behavioral, and emotional effects on individuals vary according to the substance used, age of the user, and body mass. Teenage substance abusers often lag behind their peers in accomplishing the adolescent tasks necessary to attain psychosocial maturity. Judgment, evaluative thinking, perception, and general function usually are impaired. Impulse control is diminished, and sleep time is interrupted. These abrupt personality and behavioral changes may threaten relationships with peers, parents or caregivers, and teachers.

Although SA is not understood completely, improved imaging technology and research continually provide new data about genetics, brain mechanisms involved, and human motivation. These data indicate that SA is the interaction among three basic factors: *the individual, the environment,* and *the substance.* Each factor contributes to the SA problem in varying degrees.

COMMON RISK FACTORS FOR SUBSTANCE ABUSE

1. Genetic predisposition
2. SA in the family of origin
3. Affective and mood disorders
4. Antisocial youth subculture affiliation
5. Inadequate coping with traumatic life experiences, including child abuse, neglect, and poverty

SYMPTOMS OF SUBSTANCE ABUSE

1. Change in choice of friends and companions
2. Change in dress, appearance, and hygienic practices
3. Change in eating or sleeping habits
4. Frequent unexplained arguments or violent actions
5. Skipping school and absenteeism
6. Failing classes and educational underachievement
7. Delinquent and runaway behavior
8. Deteriorating relationship with family
9. Severe mood swings, apathy
10. Affective disorders, depression
11. Suicide attempts
12. Legal problems

DRUG ACTIONS ON THE BRAIN

Positron emission tomography (PET), functional magnetic resonance imaging (fMRI), and single photon-emission computed tomography (SPECT) imaging scans allow scientists to view the brain and learn how drugs affect neuronal activity. Drugs are carried to the brain through the bloodstream. They stimulate a region of the brain that releases neurotransmitters, such as dopamine, in response to pleasurable experiences. Box 6-1 describes the different types of neurotramsitters and actions involved. Through various means, abused drugs increase the concentration of dopamine in cells located in the brain's pleasure and reward system in the limbic area. Many scientists believe this process is the basis of all addiction.

Two key areas in the management of the pleasure circuit are the *nucleus accumbens* and the *VTA*. The pleasure circuit is connected closely to the pathways and nuclei that manage pain, fear, anger, and gratification of hunger, thirst, and sex. Because this circuit is considered a part of the brain's control center of behavior, it also is connected to the frontal cortex and areas that assist movement. Addictive drugs produce their rewarding action by increasing dopamine in the nucleus accumbens and the VTA. Two other neurotransmitters play a role in drug abuse: *endorphins* and *norepinephrine*. The basal ganglia, which manage movement and repetitive tasks and play a role in compulsion, and the amygdala, which helps the

Box 6-1   *Neurotransmitters and Actions Involved*

Acetylcholine

The transmitter responsible for controlling all skeletal muscle activity. At the neuromuscular junction, acetylcholine is excitatory. However, it is inhibitory on the muscle fibers in the heart. This illustrates an important principle: the effect of a transmitter on a postsynaptic cell is not determined by the transmitter but by the postsynaptic receptors. In the brain, acetylcholine is strongly related to learning and memory and in controlling REM sleep.

Dopamine

Primarily inhibitory catecholamine. An important part of the brain's reward and pleasure system, causing feelings of euphoria, it has many roles. These include regulation of conscious movement and mood and management of hormonal balance and the immune system via the pituitary gland. Degeneration of dopamine-producing neurons is associated with Parkinson's disease.

Endorphins

Peptide. The broad class of endorphins that are the brain's natural morphine. The system modulates pain and pleasure and manages reactions to stress. Endorphins act not only as neurotransmitters but also as neurohormones and neuromodulators.

Gamma Aminobutyric Acid (GABA)

Inhibitory amino acid. GABA is found in the brain and other major organs and quiets the system. Because the brain is highly interconnected, any excitatory activity would quickly result in a massive chain reaction of activity without the influences of inhibitory neurons, which stabilize brain activity. Low levels of GABA combined with low levels of serotonin are associated with a tendency toward aggression and violence.

Glutamate

Principal excitatory amino acid of the brain. Involved in memory, responses to the environment, and perception of pain.

Norepinephrine, Noradrenaline

Amines. Released by the sympathetic nervous system, not subject to voluntary control. Serve as vasoconstrictors, relax the muscle walls, increase blood pressure, and dilate eyes; initiate the fight-or-flight response, anger, fear, energy, pain reduction, and mental focus. Low levels are associated with anxiety. Also present in the central nervous system, where it is involved in attention and sleep.

Serotonin (5-HT)

Primarily an inhibitory monoamine. Plays a role in the regulation of mood, control of eating, arousal, perception of pain, and sleep. Appears to be related to dreaming. Many hallucinations result from the stimulation of serotonin receptors, an effect that could be described as dreaming while awake.

---

body to respond to stress, also are believed by neuroscientists to be involved with addiction (see Figure 6-1).

Toxic substances found in illicit drugs and pharmaceuticals have mind-altering effects and can cause cell damage and death. Technology has allowed discovery of those neurotransmitters in the brain that are affected by these substances. A basic knowledge of the function of these chemical transmitters is necessary to understand the role of drugs in addiction, drug dependence, tolerance, and withdrawal.

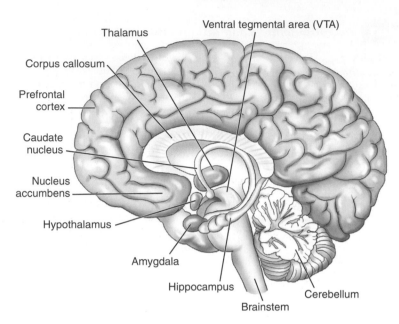

FIGURE 6-1 Brain structures involved with substance abuse.

Figure 6-2 illustrates the influence of different chemicals on brain function. All brain activity is a result of communication between neurons, which is accomplished by transmitters that are released from a neuron and change the activity of another neuron by stimulating a receptor on that neuron. Stimulation of a receptor by the transmitter requires the transmitter to have the correct chemical "shape," so that the transmitter fits neatly into the receptor. When the transmitter fits into the receptor, a process known as *binding,* it stimulates the receptor and thus allows one neuron to influence another neuron.

Some drugs block this activity. A *blocker* can bind to the receptor but is not similar enough in shape to stimulate the receptor. However, because it is bound to the receptor, the blocker prevents the neurotransmitter from attaching to the receptor and thus influences normal brain activity. Other drugs are similar enough to bind to a receptor and activate it. These activators influence normal brain activity, because they stimulate receptors in the absence of regular transmitters.

All neurotransmitters, except acetylcholine, can be classified in one of three categories: *amino acids,* chemical compounds that form the building blocks of protein; *amines,* derived from amino acids—occasionally called *neuromodulators;* and *peptides,* a chain of two or more amino acids.

Addiction is a molecular process and physiological and behavioral dependence is produced by neuronal changes. *Physical dependence* means that the body develops a dependence on the continued presence of a substance and reacts negatively when the drug is removed. This process is known as the *withdrawal syndrome. Psychological dependence* prompts a persistent desire or even undeniable compulsion to obtain and take a substance to experience

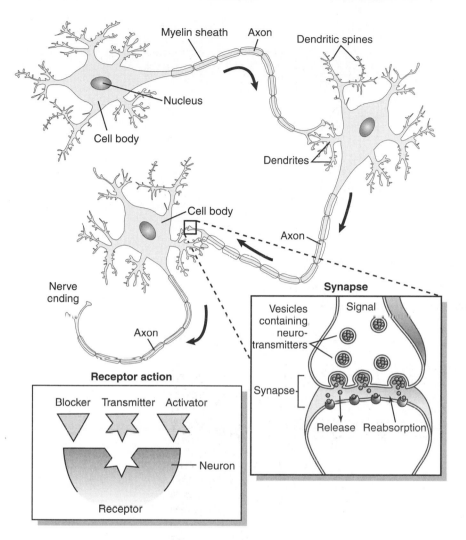

Myelin sheath Axon Dendritic spines

Nucleus

Cell body

Dendrites

Cell body

Axon

Nerve ending

Axon

Synapse

Vesicles containing neuro-transmitters

Signal

Synapse

Release Reabsorption

Receptor action

Blocker Transmitter Activator

Neuron

Receptor

Figure 6-2 Chemical influence on brain function.

satisfaction and pleasure or to avoid discomfort. The body develops resistance to the effects of a substance by requiring progressively larger doses to produce the same desired effect. This *drug tolerance* develops as the result of chronic drug abuse.

STIMULANTS

Stimulants are drugs that stimulate the central nervous system (CNS), and they can have neurotoxic effects (see Table 6-1). These drugs are used by the individual for weight control, pain control, and for alertness and feelings of calmness. Users risk a high potential for psychological dependence as tolerance develops. Commonly used stimulants are *caffeine*, found in

Table 6-1   *Drug Neurotoxic Effects*

Substance	Mental Status	Pupils	Respiratory Rate	Heart Rate	Additional Information
Stimulants	Agitation to paranoid psychosis	Mild to moderate dilation	Increased	Increased	Irritability, seizures, arrhythmias, death
Hallucinogens	Variable psychosis, coma, decreased awareness, paranoia	Mild to moderate dilation Nystagmus	Increased	Increased	Flashbacks, muscular rigidity, cardiovascular collapse
Narcotics (Opiates)	Lethargy, coma	Constricted with intoxication Dilated with anoxia or withdrawal	Decreased	Decreased	Shock, pulmonary or cerebral edema, respiratory failure
Inhalants	Disorientation, hallucinations, coma	Possible dilation Vertical and horizontal nystagmus	—	Increased Irregular heart rate	Panic, slurred speech, vomiting, cardiac arrhythmia, brain and liver damage, death
Depressants	Irritability to stupor-coma	Barbiturates: constricted Sedatives: dilated	Decreased and shallow	Decreased	Combative, violent, CNS depression, coma, psychosis
Alcohol	Drunk-like to stupor-coma	Normal or dilated	Decreased	Decreased	Slurred speech, ataxia, stupor, coma, death

NOTE: Hyperthermia may be exhibited with use of Ecstasy, PCP, and some inhalants.

coffee, tea, cocoa, and cola drinks; *nicotine,* found in cigarettes, cigars, pipe tobacco, chewing tobacco, and snuff; *amphetamines,* such as benzedrine, dextroamphetamine (Dexedrine), and dextroamphetamine with amobarbital (Dexamyl); and *cocaine,* (see Table 6-2 and Table 6-3).

I. Caffeine

A. Found in at least 60 plants, including kola nuts, tea leaves, and cacao and coffee beans. It potentiates the release of cortisol and produces effects similar to the arousal caused by stress. The effect comes by blocking the neurotransmitter adenosine, a calming chemical. In moderate amounts, caffeine appears to stimulate nerve cell activity, temporarily boosting concentration, memory, and alertness. This alertness may occur in the parts of the brain involved in arousal but not in areas managing higher-level reasoning, which seem unaffected. Too much caffeine can result in agitation, restlessness, insomnia, gastrointestinal pain or diarrhea, muscle twitching, psychomotor agitation, and tachycardia.

II. Nicotine

A. A poisonous, colorless, oily fluid with a bitter, burning taste; obtained from tobacco leaves or produced synthetically. Nicotine elevates levels of cortisol, a stress hormone. It is used in veterinary medicine as an external parasiticide and as an agricultural insecticide spray.

Table 6-2	*Stimulant Effects*

Physical and Behavioral Symptoms	Toxic Effects
General: Euphoria, exaggerated sense of well-being Increased energy and alertness Blurred vision Dizziness Talkativeness Restlessness Sleeplessness Anxiety and panic attacks Reduced appetite Insomnia Dilated pupils Increased perspiration when injected Increased blood pressure, heart rate, respiration Elevated body temperature Poor body care	Tremors Cardiac abnormalities, some fatal Seizures, some fatal Deficient immune system; malnutrition; fatal kidney, heart, and lung disorders; brain and liver damage Depression, hallucinations, violent and aggressive behaviors, panic, paranoia, formication (feelings of insects crawling on skin) Learning deficits: attention, concentration, verbal and visual memory, word production, visual motor integration Nicotine and chemicals: increased risk of miscarriages and lower–birth-weight babies, decreased sense of smell and taste; changes in DNA lead to cancer and heart and lung disease; chew and snuff can cause cancer of throat, mouth, cheek, gums, and tongue
Amphetamine: jerky, flailing, writhing movements, extreme nervousness, plus general listed symptoms	Amphetamine: can result in stroke, high fever, sudden heart failure Amphetamine/cocaine psychosis: hallucinations, delusions, paranoia

Table 6-3	*Stimulant Withdrawal Symptoms*		
Caffeine	**Nicotine**	**Amphetamines**	**Cocaine**
Headaches	Headaches	Depression	Irritability
Anxiety	Fatigue	Severe abdominal	Depression:
Dizziness	Depression	cramping or pain	exhaustion, weakness
Unusual tiredness	Anxiety	Nausea and vomiting	Poor thinking ability
Nervousness	Increased appetite	Trembling	Restless sleep
Irritability	Loss of concentration	Unusual tiredness, weakness	Decreased appetite
Depression	Loss of energy	Anxiety	Aches and pains
Nausea and vomiting	Difficulty with stress, mood control	Suicidal thoughts or actions	

B. Chemicals in cigarette smoke are toxic, and with other substances, they cause changes in deoxyribonucleic acid (DNA) that can lead to cancer, heart, and lung disease. Passive smokers, nonsmokers who inhale cigarette smoke, are exposed to the same tar and nicotine as smokers and have the same health-related concerns.

C. Smokeless forms of tobacco, such as chewing tobacco and snuff, include the same chemicals as cigarettes and have the same addictive qualities, but these also lead to an increased risk of leukoplakia (precancer) and throat and mouth cancers. Chewing tobacco can also lead to cancer of the cheek, gums, and tongue. Chewing tobacco is put between the cheek and gum, and when chewed, it releases the nicotine juices that mix with saliva. Smokeless tobacco, or snuff, is ground tobacco that can be chewed but usually is inhaled through the nose.

D. Nicotine, like other drugs, alters neuronal communication, specifically through interaction with acetylcholine receptors, either by increasing or decreasing the release or the amount of neurotransmitter. This neurotransmitter targets release of other reward-system chemicals, like dopamine, and results in feelings of pleasure, followed by feelings of increased mental alertness and acuity. The receptors targeted by nicotine become increasingly less sensitive with chronic use and habituate, a chemical basis of addiction.

E. Chronic smoking causes the brain to produce additional nicotinic receptor sites that increase nicotine craving. This biochemical demand is relieved only by more smoking. Students with attention-deficit/hyperactivity disorder (ADHD), depression, and schizophrenia are more likely to smoke, because it may be a way to self-medicate.

III. Amphetamines
A. This class of stimulants includes methamphetamine and dextroamphetamine. These drugs can be smoked, snorted, taken orally, or injected and can be made in a laboratory or at home. Chemicals similar in pharmacological qualities also are abused, such as amphetamine-like drugs used to treat ADHD (methylphenidate), narcolepsy (methylphenidate and dextroamphetamine), and over-the-counter (OTC) medications for congestion (pseudoephedrine). When taken in therapeutic dosages, these drugs are helpful and do not cause brain damage. When abused, underactivity in the temporal, parietal, and frontal areas has been noted.
B. Amphetamines have a similar but more powerful effect than cocaine on the neurotransmitters noradrenaline and dopamine by prevention of their reabsorption into neurons. Because these neurotransmitters are not deactivated by reuptake, they build up and exert a prolonged effect on their targets. This effect is seen in the continuous body movements and distractibility exhibited by the user.

IV. Cocaine
A. A natural alkaloid derived from the *Erythroxylon coca* plant grown in South America. It is used medically as a local anesthetic and appetite suppressant. Cocaine is found in different forms and can be inhaled, smoked, injected, and absorbed intraanally and intravaginally. Crack is a potent form that is smoked to produce a rapid high with intense addictive qualities.
B. The National Institute of Drug Abuse (NIDA) reports that cocaine use leads to repeated microscopic strokes that result in dead spots in the brain's circuitry (NIDA, 1998).
C. Three important neurotransmitters are disturbed with cocaine use and abuse: *norepinephrine, serotonin,* and *dopamine.* Cocaine blocks the reuptake of dopamine from the synapse. This results in dopamine remaining in the synapse for longer periods, where it can stimulate receptors to a greater extent, resulting in an extreme feeling of well-being.
D. Prenatal cocaine exposure has been documented as having subtle effects on motor skills, irritability, attention span, alertness, and intelligence quotient (IQ) level in some children. Prenatal effects are not as dramatic as previously reported, but they are significant when coupled with the environment of the child. Cocaine abuse has a financial impact related to the special education resources needed to support the children through school to succeed in their chosen endeavors.

WEB SITE

National Institute on Drug Abuse: Nicotine Addiction
   http://www.smoking.drugabuse.gov

HALLUCINOGENS

Hallucinogens are drugs that act primarily on the CNS and profoundly alter sensory perception. Individuals see images, hear sounds, and feel sensations that do not exist but seem very real. Rapid and intense emotional

CHAPTER 6

Substance Abuse

swings occur, and changes in feelings and thoughts are exaggerated and magnified. Hallucinogens are usually taken orally. Effects of these drugs vary greatly from person to person and from one episode of drug use to another episode, making "bad trips" unpredictable. Users develop psychological dependence and can develop tolerance. No withdrawal symptoms for hallucinogens have been documented, and effects can last for 12 hours. Currently no accepted medical use for these drugs exists. Commonly abused hallucinogens are *lysergic acid diethylamide (LSD)*, derived from a fungus; *psilocybin*, derived from mushrooms (found in 90 species); *mescaline*, derived from the peyote cactus; *cannabis*, the plant source of marijuana and hashish; and *methylenedioxymethamphetamine (MDMA)*, *Ecstasy*, and *methylenedioxyamphetamine (MDA*; see Table 6-4).

Hallucinogens disrupt the interaction of nerve cells and the neurotransmitter serotonin to produce their effects. Serotonin is found throughout the brain and spinal cord and is associated with the control of the regulatory, perceptual, and behavioral systems.

Dissociative drugs include *phencyclidine (PCP)* and *ketamine.* These two drugs originally were used as anesthetics, general (PCP) and veterinarian (ketamine). They affect many neurotransmitter systems, including those of norepinephrine and dopamine. They also alter or affect the distribution of the neurotransmitter glutamate, which is involved in memory, responses to the environment, and the transmission of pain signals. Dissociative drugs can interfere with glutamate signaling, leading to a sense of detachment or dissociation, hence the term *dissociative drugs,* not hallucinogens.

CHAPTER 6 Substance Abuse

Table 6-4	*Hallucinogen Effects*	
Physical and Behavioral Symptoms	**Toxic Effects**
Increased heart rate and blood pressure	Decreased awareness to touch and pain
Sleep disturbance, sweating, dizziness, tremors	Seizures
Sparse and incoherent speech	Flashbacks leading to unpredictable behaviors, accidents, panic, and suicide
Disturbances in body heat regulation, loss of appetite	
Lethargy, fatigue	Behavior similar to schizophrenic psychosis
Inability to feel pleasure	
Changes in perception, feelings, and thoughts	Catatonic syndrome: mute, lethargic, disoriented; repetitive, meaningless movements
Decreased motivation, personality change, memory impairment, sense of distance	Kidney and cardiovascular failure
Confusion, suspicion, and loss of control	
Depression, anxiety, and paranoia	
Violent behavior	

I. PCP

A. PCP can be taken orally, injected, or smoked. Long-term abusers often exhibit lack of motivation, feelings of burnout, aggressive behavior, and violence. Large doses can lead to coma and death. PCP is considered to have the most pervasive, complex effects on the brain of any of the abused drugs. When taken in excessive amounts, dextromethorphan—a drug found in some cough syrups—can produce effects like those of PCP and Ketamine.

II. Ketamine

A. Called K, special K, or vitamin K, this drug is used as a liquid applied to marijuana or tobacco items or as a white powder that is snorted. High doses can cause delirium, amnesia, impaired motor function, and occasional fatal respiratory arrest. It is one of the emerging date rape drugs. Ketamine is related to PCP and affects glutamate by blocking receptors for glutamate. Ketamine, like PCP, blocks N-methyl-D-aspartate (NMDA) receptors, which are located on the nerve cells and normally are stimulated, or activated, by glutamate. Thus, ketamine interferes with normal glutamate signal transmission.

III. Marijuana

A. Known as weed, Mary Jane, and grass (see Box 6-2 for additional slang terms), marijuana is a product of the hemp plant and includes the flowers and leaves; it contains approximately 42 chemicals and is considered a mild hallucinogen. The prime mind-altering chemical is delta-9-tetrahydrocannabinol (THC) with an average concentration of 4% to 6% THC (Drug Enforcement Administration, 2005). The amount of THC determines the strength and the effects of the plant. Different types and potencies are found in various parts of the world. Sinsemilla is a mixture of the buds and flowers of the female plant with an average concentration of 7.5% THC; some better-grade material can have up to 24% THC. Hashish, the sticky resin from the flowers of the female plant, can be even higher (Foley, 2006). Marijuana is generally rolled into a homemade cigarette called a joint, but it can be smoked in water pipes (bongs) or cigars; combined with other drugs, such as crack

CHAPTER 6

Substance Abuse

Box 6-2	*Slang and Street Terms for Marijuana*		
Airplane	Chiba Chiba	Ganja	Pot
Astroturf	Chronic	Grass	Puff
Aunt Mary	Chunky	Haircut	Reefer
Black Bart	Colombia Red	Hay	Sezz
Blow	Colombian	Herb	Sinsemilla
Blunts	Dagga	Kif	Skunk
Bobby	Dinkie Dow	Mary Jane	Smoke
Boom	Dope	MJ	Vietnamese Black
Bud	Draw	Matchbox	Weed
Cannabis	Edno	Maui Waui	Yellow Submarine
Charge	Gangster	Panama Red	Zambi

or cocaine; brewed as a tea; or mixed into foods (NIDA, 2005b). Marijuana is an example of a fat-soluble abused drug and contains up to 50% more tar and cancer-causing chemicals than cigarette smoke. Effects last longer when ingested (5 to 12 hours) than when smoked (2 to 4 hours). Users develop psychological dependency.

B. Marijuana smoking affects the brain and leads to impaired short-term memory, perception, judgment, and motor skills. It can impair the immune system and cause dysmenorrhea and lower sperm production. Marijuana affects skills required for driving a car—such as alertness, coordination, and reaction time—and the ability to concentrate for up to 24 hours after smoking. These impaired skills can make it difficult for a driver of a car to react to signals, road sounds, and judge distances.

C. Studies have shown that THC is passed to the baby in breast milk. Maternal breast milk has a higher THC concentration than THC in the maternal blood.

IV. LSD

A. Called acid and sugar, LSD is a powerful, synthetic, cheap hallucinogen. It was originally considered helpful in the treatment of mental illness. Its effects can last 8 to 12 hours. It generally is taken orally, on squares of blotter paper, sugar cubes, or pills that have absorbed the liquid drug.

B. LSD disrupts and mimics serotonin and activates areas in the temporal lobe, causing hallucinations. The most common mental symptoms are perceptual distortions and visual hallucinations. Its effects are unpredictable and range from euphoria to psychotic reactions, panic, and depression; flashbacks can occur weeks or months after use.

V. MDMA and MDA

A. MDMA (methylenedioxymethamphetamine), Ecstasy (see Box 6-3), and MDA (methylenedioxyamphetamine) are synthetic drugs that are hallucinogens when taken in high dosages; but in low dosages, they produce effects similar to those of amphetamines. MDMA is taken orally as a tablet and causes increased heart rate and blood pressure that may elevate body temperature, causing cardiovascular and kidney failure (NIDA, 2006c). Common side effects are jitteriness, jaw clenching, and anxiety. Students who have taken these drugs feel a need to grind and gnash their teeth.

B. Higher doses can cause panic and paranoid reactions and, with long-term use, exhaustion, depression, fatigue, and numbness. Long-term-use symptoms are attributed to serotonin deficiencies and long-lasting neurotoxic effects in the brain. Ecstasy is called a sensual drug rather than a sexual one, since males report decreased orgasm and

Box 6-3	*Slang and Street Terms for MDMA*		
Ecstasy	Essence	Doves	2
STC	MDM	Birds	STP
Adam	Hug Drug	5-DMA	Eve

females report sexual arousal. These drugs are often called love or hug drugs (NIDA, 2006c).

C. Ecstasy affects numerous brain neurotransmitter systems, including serotonin, dopamine, and norepinephrine. As a serotonin agonist, it causes excessive release of serotonin and then stops its reuptake; the long-term effect of use is serotonin depletion in the brain. It affects mood, sleep, pain, emotion, appetite, and other behaviors. Other possible long-term effects are residual problems with verbal and visual memory and congenital abnormalities associated with prenatal drug exposure (NIDA, 2002).

VI. GHB

A. GHB (gamma-hydroxybutyrate)—also called liquid Ecstasy, Georgia Home Boy, and G—is a CNS depressant, steroidlike substance. GHB is known to diminish inhibitions and enhance sexual experiences and has been associated with overdoses, poisonings, and date rape. It is a clear, odorless liquid that also is found in tablet or capsule form. An overdose can lead quickly to loss of consciousness, coma, and death. The purity and strength of each dose can vary greatly, making overdoses more likely.

OPIATES

Opiates are a group of toxic substances originally derived from the opium poppy; opiates include codeine, morphine, and heroin. *Synthetic opiates* also have been produced, such as methadone, meperidine (Demerol), and oxycodone with aspirin (Percodan). Opiates have pain-relieving properties, induce sleep, and are effective for diarrhea, cough, and agitation. They act primarily on the central and parasympathetic nervous system. They can be taken by injection, orally, or through smoking. Abusers develop physical and psychological dependence, and tolerance develops. Chronic users may have noticeable needle marks on their arms and legs (see Table 6-5 and Box 6-4).

Opiates are compounds that act on opiate receptors and block the reuptake of the natural neurotransmitters. Synthetic chemicals have been developed to block the opiate receptor sites, thus eliminating the high produced by these drugs in addicts. These synthetic chemicals are narcotic antagonists used to treat addiction.

I. Heroin

A. Heroin is a white powder derived from morphine. It is injected intravenously but can be smoked or taken by mouth, and it is highly addictive. Heroin is illegal in the United States and many other countries. Street names include smack, H, skag, junk, Mexican black tar, and bomb.

B. Heroin and morphine mimic natural endorphins and related pain-killing hormones. The drugs travel quickly to the brain, stimulating dopamine-containing neurons to fire and release the neurotransmitter into the nucleus accumbens. The drugs bind to the opiate receptor on the receiving terminal, sending a signal to release more dopamine.

C. Prenatal Heroin Exposure.

1. During pregnancy, heroin addiction threatens the life of the fetus and puts it at severe risk. Complications associated with prenatal heroin exposure include preterm labor and birth,

Table 6-5	Opiate Effects
Physical and Behavioral Symptoms	**Toxic Effects**
Constricted pupils, watery eyes, itching Drowsiness Early use: nausea, vomiting Slows bowel function Reduced sex, hunger, and aggressive drives Feeling of warmth and detachment Euphoria Suppression of pain and distress Clouded mental functioning Heroin: infectious diseases, HIV/AIDS, hepatitis B and C, collapsed veins, abscesses, bacterial infections, infections of heart lining and valves, arthritis and other rheumatological problems, spontaneous abortion	Slow, shallow breathing, clammy skin, sedation, seizures Overdose: respiratory depression, coma, death

Box 6-4	Withdrawal Symptoms of Opiates

- Similar to flu: aches, rhinorrhea
- Sweating, chills
- Tremors or jerks
- Anorexia
- Diarrhea, chronic nausea
- Insomnia
- Muscle and abdominal cramps
- Hypersensitivity to pain

- Restlessness, irritability
- Elevated blood pressure and pulse, increased respiration, and fever
- Severe drug craving
- Muscle spasms
- Seizures
- Coma
- Death

growth retardation, and a withdrawal syndrome after birth. The abstinence syndrome manifestations include irritability, gastrointestinal (GI) dysfunction, respiratory difficulties, tremulousness, high-pitched cry, poor feeding, increased muscle tone, and seizures. Human immunodeficiency virus (HIV) and hepatitis B are also risks related to the intravenous route of abuse. If pregnancy is known, heroin-addicted women usually are maintained on methadone during the pregnancy to reduce perinatal complications. Methadone helps to satisfy the physical cravings without the psychological high associated with heroin abuse.

II. Methadone

A. Street name Meth is used to control opiate withdrawal symptoms. It is taken orally once a day, producing a steady, unrewarding blood and brain level of the opiate. If misused and injected, it produces intense, short-term euphoria similar to that of heroin. A heroin addict receiving maintenance methadone treatment is not intoxicated or impaired because of the complete tolerance to opiate effects and the steady blood levels of the daily drug.

III. LAAM

A. LAAM (levo-alpha-acetylmethadol) is a longer-acting medication like methadone that is used in addiction treatment clinics. It is taken three times a week, thus reducing take-home abuse. When taken orally, LAAM works the same way as methadone, permitting the individual to live a more normal life by reducing cravings and preventing withdrawal symptoms.

INHALANTS

Inhalants are legal chemicals that include a variety of agents that may be inhaled to produce psychoactive effects or an intoxication similar to that of alcohol. Inhalants are sniffed or "huffed," which can cause physical and emotional problems-a one-time use can result in death. Most common abusers of these chemicals range in age from 7 to 17 years. Long-term inhalant use can cause blood chemistry disorders, fatigue, muscle fatigue, and weight loss. Deeply inhaled vapors or high concentrations of inhalants may result in disorientation, unconsciousness, or death. Users develop psychological dependency, and tolerance develops. Street names include *glue, poppers,* and *snapper* (see Box 6-5).

Inhalants can be divided into two classifications: *organic solvents* and *abusable gases.* Solvents that contain inhalant fumes include glue, quick-drying plastic cement, paint thinner, lacquer, gasoline, cleaning fluids, lighter fluid, marker pen, typewriter correction fluid, dry cleaning fluids, nail polish remover, hair spray, room deodorizers, and food products such as vegetable cooking sprays and whipped cream sprays.

Gases include nitrous oxide, amyl nitrite, and butyl nitrite. Nitrous oxide is known as "laughing gas" and is an anesthetic used for minor dental surgery. The effects of these gases are short, lasting only a few minutes, and are perceived as "safe." However, they increase the heart rate and decrease blood pressure so that the user feels light-headed and dizzy. Long or continual use can cause fainting and lead to coma. Cardiac arrhythmias caused by inhaled gases can be fatal.

A single, prolonged session of inhalant use can cause heart failure and "sudden sniffing death." Chronic use can cause long-term CNS damage, resulting in learning, movement, vision, and hearing impairments. Damage to the heart, kidneys, lungs, and liver may be permanent (see Table 6-6).

Box 6-5	Slang and Street Terms for Inhalants		
Amys	Bang	Bolt	Boppers
Bullet	Climax	Glading	Gluey
Hand Cleaner	Hardware	Hippie Crack	Kick
Locker Room	Poor Man's Pot	Poppers	Rush
Snappers	Toncho (Octane Booster)	Texas Shoe Shine	Whippets

CHAPTER 6

Substance Abuse

Table 6-6 *Symptoms and Toxic Effects of Inhalants*

Physical and Behavioral Symptoms	Toxic Effects
Solvents	
Euphoria, belligerence, dizziness	CNS system depression
Alcohol-like effects: interferes with coordination, thoughts, perceptions	Panic, disorientation, severe tissue damage, hallucinations, coma, respiratory arrest
Moderate amount: exhilaration, lessening of inhibitions	
Large amount: drowsiness, memory loss, mental confusion, physiological symptoms; slurred speech, dizziness, nausea, vomiting, tremors	
Gases	
Dizziness, light-headedness	Irregular heartbeat, fainting, coma, respiratory arrest
Increased heart rate	
Decreased blood pressure	
General	
Nausea and nosebleeds	Liver, lung, kidney impairment Irreversible brain damage Nervous system damage Chemical imbalances

Inhalants quickly enter the bloodstream and then the brain after inhalation and produce a variety of deleterious effects: reduced vision and hearing, impaired movement, lowered cognitive ability, and damage to the protective myelin sheath on the axons. This results in significant neurological impairments in movement and cognition. Solvents are fat soluble and affect the neuron membrane, which is composed of fat. Neuronal transmission is increased in low doses, whereas inhalation of large amounts inhibits neuronal transmission, causing brain dysfunction, paralysis, and death.

WEB SITES

National Inhalant Prevention Coalition
    http://www.inhalant.org
National Institute on Drug Abuse
    http://www.inhalants.drugabuse.gov

DEPRESSANTS

Depressants produce an inhibitory, constricting effect on the CNS. These drugs are used for relief of insomnia, anxiety, and pain. The three main categories are *barbiturates, nonbarbiturates,* and *tranquilizers.* Chronic users risk a high potential for both physical and psychological dependence, and tolerance develops (see Table 6-7 and Table 6-8).

Table 6-7	*Depressant Effects*

Physical and Behavioral Symptoms	Toxic Effects
Slurred speech Unsteadiness Loss of balance and falling Difficulty in thinking and faulty judgment Quarrelsome disposition Loss of inhibitions Emotional instability Drowsiness or sleep Irritability, hostility Tranquilizers: symptoms/behaviors the same but with less intensity	CNS depression, decreased respiration, decreased blood pressure Hepatic damage Respiratory arrest Unconsciousness Coma Psychosis Death

Table 6-8	*Depressant Withdrawal Symptoms*

Barbiturates	Nonbarbiturates	Tranquilizers
Restlessness, weakness	Anxiety	Anxiety
Anxiety, nervousness	Ataxia	Muscle twitching
Nose twitching, tremors	Tremors	Tremors
Abdominal cramps	Memory loss	Weakness
Headaches	Slurred speech	Abdominal and muscle
Insomnia	Perceptual distortions	cramps
Nausea and vomiting	Irritability	Seizures
Grand mal seizures	Agitation	Psychosis
Hallucinations	Delirium	Delirium
Mental exhaustion, confusion, and delirium	Insomnia Nausea and vomiting	

Commonly used barbiturates are phenobarbital (Nembutal), secobarbital (Seconal), amobarbital-secobarbital (Tuinal), and amobarbital (Amytal). Commonly used nonbarbiturates are glutethimide (Doriden), methyprylon (Notudar), ethchlorvynol (Placidyl), and methaqualone (Quaalude). Commonly used tranquilizers are diazepam (Valium), chlordiazepoxide (Librium), meprobamate (Miltown, Equanil), lorazepam (Ativan), chlorpromazine (Thorazine), alprazolam (Xanax), paroxetine (Paxil), hydroxyzine (Atarax), and oxazepam (Serax).

I. Rohypnol

A. Flunitrazepam (Rohypnol) is often implicated in sexual assaults (i.e., *rape*). It was developed as a benzodiazepine sedative to treat insomnia and as a presurgery anesthetic. It is used in 60 countries but is not approved for prescription in the United States. It is taken orally in tablet form and dissolves quickly in carbonated beverages; snorting also has been reported. It is tasteless and odorless, and its sedative and toxic effects are enhanced by alcohol. Even a small dose of Rohypnol can impair an individual for 8 to 12 hours. Profound amnesia can occur after use, so the individual may not be able to remember events experienced while under the effects of the drug. Side effects include decreased blood pressure, drowsiness, dizziness, confusion, visual disturbances, GI disturbances, and urinary retention.

CLUB DRUGS

Club drug is an ambiguous term used to describe illicit drugs used at bars, clubs, or all-night dance parties called *raves* or *trances*. They are used as mood enhancers and to increase energy for dancing. Drugs used can be stimulants, depressants, hallucinogens, or a combination of these. The common use of these drugs at a party is not perceived as risky among users; however, club drugs do cause toxic and chronic effects. For example, Ecstasy can produce hyperthermia and mask thirst, which has been reported to cause acute dehydration and death after dancing for an extended time. Six substances identified as club drugs are *Ecstasy, GHB, ketamine, Rohypnol, methamphetamine,* and *LSD.* GHB, ketamine, and Rohypnol are common date rape drugs.

WEB SITE

National Institute on Drug Abuse: Important Information and Resources on Club Drugs

http://www.clubdrugs.gov

PERFORMANCE-ENHANCING DRUGS

Ergogenic aids are performance-enhancing substances used by adolescent athletes, both boys and girls, to increase their competitive edge. These substances include steroids, dehydroepiandosterone (DHEA), androstenedione, androstenediol, creatine, human growth hormone (HGH), and dietary supplements.

ANABOLIC STEROIDS

I. Definition
A. Anabolic steroids (e.g., Deca-Durabolin, Equipoise, and Winstrol) are synthetic substances related to male androgenic hormones. These drugs promote skeletal muscle growth and androgenic effects that influence development of male sexual characteristics. Some athletes and others seeking to improve physical appearance and increase performance abuse them. These illegal uses of the drug are known to cause numerous health hazards.

II. Etiology
A. Steroids are a synthetic variant of the male sex hormone testosterone. In 2006, the prevalence of twelfth graders using steroids decreased from 2.5% (2004) to 1.8%; only 60% of twelfth graders report understanding the risk of steroid abuse. Steroid use is more prevalent among boys (NIDA, 2006a), and one out of every ten steroid users is an adolescent (Laos and Metzl, 2006).

Brain Findings

Anabolic steroids act on the limbic system, and impaired learning and memory effects from them have been demonstrated in animals. The term *roid rage* describes a sudden outburst of incredible rage. Testosterone production is controlled by neurons in the hypothalamus, which also control appetite, blood pressure, moods, and reproduction. Steroids can disrupt normal hormone functioning within the brain, causing somatic changes that include loss of scalp hair in boys and facial hair growth in girls (NIDA, 2005c).

III. Characteristics

A. Illegal in the United States, unless through prescription.
B. Used by prescription to treat delayed puberty, impotence, and body wasting in those with AIDS and other diseases.
C. Obtained illegally from clandestine laboratories, on the Internet, or by smuggling.
D. Substances sold illegally as anabolic steroids may be diluted and contaminated.
E. Used illegally by some adolescents, athletes, and competitive body builders to increase strength and body mass, reduce body fat, and improve sports performance.
F. The International Olympic Committee has numerous anabolic steroids and related compounds on its list of banned drugs.
G. Steroid abuse is higher among boys.
H. Abuse can cause trembling, fluid retention, aching joints, severe acne, hypertension, increased levels of low-density lipoprotein (LDL); lowered high-density lipoprotein (HDL) levels, jaundice, and liver tumors (see Table 6-9).
I. Withdrawal syndrome includes clinical depression, which can contribute to dependence on these drugs.
J. Steroids can be taken orally as tablets or capsules, by injection directly into muscles, or as creams, gels, or patches applied to the skin. Abusers may use more than 100 times the therapeutic dose.
K. *Stacking* is a practice in which the abuser mixes oral, injectable, or both forms of anabolic steroids to maximize the effectiveness and minimize the negative effects.
L. *Pyramiding* is a practice in which the abuser stacks compounds in cycles of 6 to 12 weeks, gradually increasing the dose, followed by slowly decreasing to none.
M. *Cycling* is a practice in which the abuser alternates cycles of 6 to 16 weeks, going from high dose to low dose and then stopping all steroids, then starting all over again later.
N. The abuser believes that stacking, pyramiding, and cycling produce larger muscles, while simultaneously helping the body to adjust between high doses of steroids.

IV. Health Concerns and Emergencies

A. In boys: hair loss, breast development, decreased testicular size, reduced or no sperm, frequent or continuing erection, impotence, sterility, difficulty or pain on urination, and prostate enlargement.

CHAPTER 6

Substance Abuse

Table 6-9   *Possible Effects of Anabolic Steroid Abuse*

Side Effects	Men	Women	General Population
Behavioral			Aggressive and combative behavior more frequent with high doses; rage, mania, delusions; mood swings; impaired judgment; depression and nervousness
Cardiovascular			Increases in LDL, decreases in HDL, heart attacks, hypertension, enlargement of left ventricle
Hormonal disruptions	Shrinking of testicles, reduced sperm count, baldness, breast enlargement, impotence	Excessive growth of body hair, male-patterned baldness, deepened voice, decreased breast size, menstrual irregularities, enlarged clitoris	
Infections			Hepatitis, HIV/AIDS, risk of other blood-borne diseases if injected
Skin diseases			Severe acne and cysts, oily scalp, jaundice
Liver diseases			Tumors and cancer
Musculoskeletal system	Tendon rupture; short stature, if taken by adolescent	Tendon rupture; short stature, if taken by adolescent	

Modified from *National Institute on Drug Abuse, Research report: steroid abuse and addiction* (NIH Pub No 06-3721); Drug Enforcement Administration (DEA): Steroid abuse in today's society, March 2004.

B. In girls: growth of facial hair, deeper voice, enlargement of the clitoris (these are irreversible symptoms), smaller breasts, and menstrual irregularities.

C. In adolescents: premature skeletal maturation, accelerated puberty, and stunted growth.

D. Muscle tissue strengthens faster than tendons increasing the risk for damage.

E. Can cause emotional instability and wide mood swings with uncontrolled anger and aggression, which can induce violent episodes.

F. Other side effects include paranoid jealousy, extreme irritability, delusions, and impaired judgment.

V. Management and Treatment

A. Know the signs and symptoms of steroid use and other sport-enhancing drugs.

B. When reviewing the sports history of students, ask if they know others who are taking steroids or performance-enhancing aids. Knowing other students who are "using" presents the dangers of peer pressure and easy access.

C. Reinforce decision of nonusers.

D. Present a balanced overall picture of both the adverse and beneficial effects of steroids and other enhancers.

E. Be aware of slang names: *arnolds, roids, juice, stackers, gym candy, pumpers,* and *weight trainers.*

F. Participate in education of coaches, trainers, school staff, and parents of adolescents; students should have the same information presented to them.

G. Encourage use of an educational course such as The Adolescent Training and Learning To Avoid Steroids (ATLAS) or Athletes Targeting Healthy Exercise and Nutritional Alternatives (ATHENA), which was designed for girls (NIDA, 2006b).

H. Be aware of government and general Web sites listed for comprehensive information.

VI. Additional Information

A. There are alternatives to anabolic steroids that adolescents are known to abuse. These substances include nonanabolic steroids, creatine, and other dietary supplements.

B. Two of the most commonly used nonanabolic steroids include androstenedione and androstenediol. These products are also called *prohormones* and were placed on the list of controlled substances, along with anabolic steroids, in the Anabolic Steroid Control Act of 2004. This act makes possession of these banned products a federal crime and provides funding for education and research relating to steroids and steroid precursors.

1. One prohormone, dehydroepiandrosterone (DHEA), was not included in the Act, because it is purported to have several health benefits, specifically antiaging properties.

2. Past studies of these products have shown no significant improvement in athletic performance, and effects of long term use is unknown. Prohormones are precursors to testosterone and estrogen. Use of androstenedione by prepubertal or pubertal

boys could bring on precocious puberty or premature closure of the epiphyseal growth plates (Laos and Metzl, 2006).

C. Creatine is a complex amino acid used to enhance anaerobic activity, and it is a popular nutritional supplement. It has been used for neuromuscular diseases and congestive heart failure. It is widely advertised in the sports media as being safe; adolescents observe many professional athletes using creatine for increased strength, weight gain, and improved performance. There are no studies of the side effects of long-term use under age 18. It is known that overloading can be harmful to the kidneys, but effects are reversible (Laos and Metzl, 2006). Short-term side effects include GI symptoms, weight gain, and muscle cramps. Creatine may be a stepping-stone to other, more harmful ergogenic aids.

D. Human growth hormone (HGH) is a polypeptide hormone used to treat children with growth failure. Athletes use HGH to increase lean body mass, build muscle, reduce recovery time between workouts, and boost overall performance. HGH is not easily detected by drug testing, and many athletes perceive it as being nontoxic. However, large amounts can lead to acromegaly, which causes enlarged extremities and facial bones, diabetes mellitus, and cardiovascular disease.

WEB SITE

National Institute on Drug Abuse: Anabolic Steroid Abuse
http://www.steroidabuse.gov

PRESCRIPTION AND OVER-THE-COUNTER DRUGS

Abuse of prescription and over-the-counter (OTC) medications by adolescents is a growing concern in the United States. The Partnership for a Drug-Free America reports that 1 in 5-about 4.5 million—adolescents have abused prescription pain medications, stimulants, and tranquilizers. The number of teens turning to prescription drugs equals that of new marijuana users. One in 10—about 2.4 million—teens have abused cough medication. Girls are more likely than boys to abuse prescription and OTC drugs.

Four out of 10 adolescents believe that prescription drugs are safer than illegal drugs. Misconceptions regarding drug use are one of the reasons for these high statistics. Teens also readily admit easy access to prescription and OTC drugs from their parents' medicine cabinet and from friends. Teens believe that medications found at home will offer a medically safe high. Pain relievers, such as Vicodin and Oxycontin, are the most commonly abused prescription drugs (Office of National Drug Control Policy, 2007; Partnership for a Drug-Free America, 2006). Teens are more prone to become dependent upon prescription medication than are young adults.

THE WIDESPREAD PROBLEM OF ALCOHOL ABUSE AND DEPENDENCY

Alcohol abuse refers to a degree of drinking that interferes with an individual's normal functioning. It is both a biological and psychosocial disease characterized by the loss of control over drinking and a dependency on alcohol. Alcohol is a CNS depressant.

The cause of alcohol abuse and dependency is now better understood. Several causative factors have been implicated: environmental influences, lifestyle choices, and genetic factors. Genetic research is focused on more than one gene. Children of alcoholics are four times more likely to become addicted to alcohol than those whose parents are not alcoholics. Approximately 50% to 60% of alcoholics have a genetic predisposition to the disease, and it is presumed that they are unable to produce adequate dopamine. The U.S. Substance Abuse and Mental Health Services Administration (SAMHSA) found in their National Survey on Drug Abuse and Health (2005) that almost 7.2 million youths between 12 and 20 years of age were binge drinkers; 2.3 million (6%) were heavy drinkers. This indicates that 1 in 5 individuals under age 20 is a binge drinker (SAMHSA, 2006).

Brain imaging techniques allow real-time visualization of the changes in the structure of the brain with chronic alcohol use. Initially, alcohol stimulates the pleasure center, which prompts repetition of the action. Alcohol eventually can turn this pleasant feeling into intense cravings and destructive behavior. Alcohol increases levels of dopamine in the nucleus accumbens, which is associated with motivation, although the exact role of this process is unknown.

Alcohol decreases neural activity through action on gamma aminobutyric acid (GABA) neurons. Drugs that block the effects on GABA neurons reduce the pleasure of drinking and, therefore, are effective in the treatment of alcoholism.

I. Health Concerns and Emergencies
  A. Alcohol abuse can lower an adolescent's resistance to infection, impair reflexes, and stunt emotional growth.
  B. An adolescent's brain appears susceptible to damage in the limbic system, prefrontal cortex, and hippocampus, which may impair personality development and sound decision making.
  C. Binge drinking damages the prefrontal cortex and associated areas more than other areas.
  D. Combined use of alcohol and another substance (polysubstance abuse) intensifies the effect of each substance and may be extremely dangerous, causing physical or mental impairment or death.
  E. Impairment of the CNS by alcohol produces changes in vision, hearing, muscular control, and judgment; these changes may lead to bodily harm (e.g., automobile accidents).
  F. The adolescent body processes alcohol differently than the adult body. Adolescents must consume more alcohol to feel its effects, and by the time they feel impairment, the blood alcohol concentration (BAC) is so high that there is a danger of alcohol poisoning.
  G. Alcohol overdose involves a great risk of suicide and death.
  H. A pregnant minor who abuses alcohol increases the chance of damage to the developing fetus (see Chapter 4, Chronic Conditions, Fetal Alcohol Syndrome).
  I. When alcohol intake interferes with an adolescent's normal dietary requirement, nutritional deficiencies can occur.
    1. Depressed appetite.
    2. Alcohol becomes a substitute for normal caloric intake.
    3. Vitamin and mineral deficiencies, particularly B vitamins (niacin and thiamin), magnesium, potassium, iron, and folic acid.

J. Possible consequences of long-term excessive use of alcohol.
1. Liver disease (cirrhosis, alcoholic hepatitis, cancer of the liver).
2. Cancer of the mouth, esophagus, or abdominal organs.
3. Peripheral neuropathy and brain damage.

II. Effects on Individual

A. A 10% difference was found in brain power between the alcohol abuser and the healthy teenager. This effect may be the difference between passing and failing a test, a class, or a grade level.
B. Frequent absenteeism and failure to complete assignments can cause academic failure, expulsion, and dropping out. In addition, career goals and opportunities become limited.
C. Alcohol abuse or dependency may prevent an adolescent's emotional growth, thereby interfering with daily functioning with significant others.
D. Alcohol-induced lack of judgment may lead to unsafe sex, unwanted pregnancy, and early marriage.
E. Arrests, loss of driver's license, and other altercations with law enforcement can affect the family and the attainment of future vocational goals.
F. Alcohol dependence causes carelessness in appearance and personal hygiene.

III. Management and Treatment

A. Some students who exhibit signs of depression, or who do not feel successful in school or friendships, experience more headaches or stomachaches, fight with parents, and generally do not feel good about themselves, may be abusing substances.
B. Students seen frequently in the nursing office often have the difficulties described above, and they may live in difficult family environments. Such students need a friendly word, smile, or compliment to promote self-esteem.
C. The formation of close bonds with students for talk time, empathic listening, and positive support may activate natural reward pathways in the brain.
D. Special education students are more at risk for SA.
E. Consider the need for peer counseling; peer counselors should receive training and be supervised by trained staff or adult.
F. Long-term dependency involves medical intervention.
1. Special diet and vitamin supplements for nutritional deficiencies.
2. Treatment of any underlying disorders caused by alcoholism.
3. Medication.
   a. Naltrexone (ReVia) is an antagonist that blocks endogenous opioids in the brain that reinforce the effects of alcohol. Naltrexone may reduce cravings and prevent relapse and has recently been approved by the FDA. Campral (acamprosate) mimics GABA and is thought to restore equilibrium between the GABA and glutamate systems. It is used for the maintenance of abstinence from alcohol.
   b. Psychotherapy and psychopharmacology are recommended as treatments of choice.

      c. Medication may be prescribed to reduce anxiety and restless-
         ness during withdrawal.

      d. Antabuse may be prescribed to discourage relapse.

  4. The symptoms of alcohol withdrawal are tremors, fever, perspira-
     tion, nausea, vomiting, anorexia, restlessness, hallucinations, and
     delirium tremens.

WEB SITES

Al-Anon and Alateen Family Group Headquarters
    http://www.al-anon.alateen.org
Alcoholics Anonymous World Service
    http://www.aa.org
National Institute on Alcohol Abuse and Alcoholism
    http://www.niaaa.nih.gov

SCHOOL NURSING ROLE IN SUBSTANCE ABUSE

I. Health Concerns and Emergencies

A. Nurses' assessment skills are necessary for prevention and intervention with students who use illicit substances. Important observation
   and assessment tasks for examination of the student in the school
   setting are listed in Table 6-10.

B. Assessment of emergencies in school settings.

  1. Assessment of substance use emergencies and action required de-
    pends on student, circumstances, and medical condition.

  2. Evaluate for need to call 911. Call if any of the following occur:

     a. Decreased or increased pulse.

     b. Decreased respiration.

     c. Hyperthermia with increased thirst and suspected use of inhal-
       ants, PCP, or Ecstasy.

     d. Extreme agitation, delirium, seizures.

     e. Any combinations of neurotoxic effects.

  3. Eliminate documented or undiagnosed medical condition (e.g.,
    diabetes). Note any prescribed medications.

  4. Identify substance whenever possible and gather information
    from teachers, other staff, peers, and parents.

  5. Notify school site administrators, parents, and site and local law
    enforcement officer as soon as possible.

  6. Follow up and coordinate with other team members (e.g., teacher,
    counselor, school social worker, psychologist).

  7. Document according to educational and health requirements.

C. School nurse interventions.

  1. Provide information for staff and parents through several meth-
    ods, including school meetings and mandated inservice sessions,
    Parent Teacher Association meetings, classroom teaching (role
    playing), newsletters, and postings in staff restrooms.

  2. Teach alcohol and drug education to students, especially pregnant
    minors.

Table 6-10   *Substance Abuse Assessment Procedures*

Nursing Assessment	Procedure	Observation or Documentation	Normal
General observations	Observation of physical, behavioral, and cognitive changes	Facial sweating, flushed or pale appearance, tense, itching, burn areas on thumb and index finger, confusion, muscle rigidity, tremors, chemical or alcohol breath, rapid or slurred speech, loss of time perception, or any of signs listed below	Normal is ability to follow simple, sequential directions; coherent Rule out disease, infectious process, or injury that can confuse observations
Pulse	Take while seated and at rest when possible. May use radial, brachial, or carotid pulse. Student may be anxious, causing increased pulse; therefore check pulse twice more at midway and at end of examination	Concern if consistently above 90 or less than 60 beats/min Physically active students may have lower heart rates	Normal pulse is 60-90 beats/min
Gaze nystagmus (horizontal)	Observe while student follows finger or pen 12-15 in from face, moving slowly from center to extreme right of nose Hold 3 sec at maximum deviation, then move slowly to left side and back to center position Rapid movement of object can result in false nystagmus	Observe for: jerky, quivering, or smooth pursuit Nystagmus at maximum deviation Angle of onset, angle at which nystagmus is noted—in degrees of 5 (e.g., 35-40-45 or none)	Normal is smooth pursuit
Gaze: nystagmus (vertical)	Assess by moving finger or pen from center of nose up, hold in position 3 sec; move down, hold 3 sec; repeat	Observe for eye bounce	Normal is smooth pursuit at all angles When positive, may indicate high blood alcohol levels

Nonconvergence of eyes	Do circular movement with finger or pen 12-15 in from face; bring stimulus slowly to bridge of nose; hold 3 sec	Observe for failure of eyes to follow stimulus, inability to cross eyes	Normally, both eyes follow stimuli to point of convergence Rule out any physical condition affecting ability to do testing
Pulse, second	Take while seated		See *Pulse*
Pupillary size	Pupil size can be seen in various settings, room light, near total darkness, or indirect/direct light Pupillary meter is available for use Size more noticeable if performed in darkened room	Observe pupillary size; note size in mm, right and left, and setting of test	Normal pupillary range is 3.0-6.5 mm, but normal adolescents may be outside this range
Pupillary reaction to light	Check reaction while checking pupil size Use penlight to evaluate pupil reaction	Note if slow, sluggish, or nonreactive and setting of test	Pupils normally constrict within 1 sec; slow or sluggish is more than 1 sec Inquire about any current medications that can influence assessment With diabetes, pupils do not dilate even in darkness Congenital anomalies can prevent dilation
Hippus	In direct light (penlight) observe for hippus (e.g., pulsating of pupil) May occur with or without stimulus	Observe for exaggerated rhythmical constriction and dilation of pupil (pulsating) under direct light	Normal is no pulsating Certain drugs produce hippus (e.g., opiate withdrawal)
Rebound dilation	Use penlight to illicit constriction of pupil Check both eyes	Observe for inability of pupil to remain constricted Positive results if pupils dilate 1 mm or more with continued direct light	Should not dilate under direct light Occurs with marijuana, certain hallucinogens

Continued

Table 6-10 *Substance Abuse Assessment Procedures—Cont'd*

Nursing Assessment	Procedure	Observation or Documentation	Normal
Romberg	Student stands erect with hands at side and feet together Tell student to wait for your instructions Cue to start, ask to tilt head slightly backward, close eyes, and hold position for 30 sec Stop task at 90 sec if not stopped earlier	Note amount of time passed when student indicates 30 sec Observe ability to maintain position	Normally holds position and can estimate 30 sec Under influence of stimulants, will call time rapidly; influence of opiates will slow call Swaying noted with alcohol use
Pulse, third	Take while seated	See *Pulse*	See *Pulse*
Ingestion-method examination	Examine nasal cavity for irritation/inflammation and debris and oral cavities for discoloration and debris Examine limbs and trunk for injection sites	Note if white coating on the tongue, blackened lips/gums or debris, irritation/inflammation in nasal passages Note track marks on skin	No evidence of substance use Rhinitis from snorting
Eyes	Observe for: droopy eyelids (e.g., upper lid touches pupil) Retracted eyelids (e.g., bug-eyed—see white sclera above iris) Swollen eyelids Reddened sclera Watering/tearing Glazed eye appearance	Note droopy, retracted, swollen eyelids Reddened sclera, tearing, or glazing	Marijuana may leave green coating or debris on tongue Rule out familial or physical conditions (e.g., ptosis or conjunctivitis)

Modified from California Department of Justice (DOJ), Sacramento, Calif, 1998, Advanced Training Center.

3. One-on-one counseling with at-risk or abusing student.
4. Referral to school SA team for possible formal SA evaluation.
5. Consider peer counseling.
6. Awareness of special school and community resources.
7. Encourage teachers, coaches, and all school staff to take time to listen to and support students, which may initiate a natural high by boosting their self-esteem; let students know someone cares about them.
8. Encourage mentoring and bonding to a positive role model, either a peer or an adult. Often a former drug user is the preferred helper.
9. Help students explore personal capabilities and determine ways to become resilient.
D. Long-term treatment and management.
1. Be aware of personal biases, prejudices, and personal value conflicts that could be a barrier to fair and humane interventions.
2. Most adolescents deny their substance use; acceptance of the problem and motivation for change is the beginning focus of treatment.
3. A continuum of services exists for adolescent substance use disorder
   a. Intervention.
   b. Rehabilitation.
   c. Maintenance.
4. Twelve-step treatment programs.
5. Treatment in an adolescent therapeutic community.
6. Family therapy.

II. Legal Requirements for School Nurses
A. Unlike child abuse, no legal requirement exists for mandatory reporting.
B. Federal and state law surrounding SA usually is interpreted by individual county or district offices of education. Nurses need a working knowledge of these policies and procedures (e.g., Education Code).
C. Local law enforcement and school administration may have memorandums of understanding.
D. Be knowledgeable regarding state Nurse Practice Act.
E. Use best practices to prevent and intervene with substance abuse patterns.
1. Opportunities can be provided in school settings for:
   a. Students to learn and practice skills necessary to promote wellness, healthy choices, ability to cope with personal struggles and adversity, and achieve academic success.
   b. Both individual and group counseling, peer counseling, and support groups for adolescents trying to achieve and maintain SA abstinence.
   c. Families to participate in educational SA workshops, support groups, and network with community agencies.
   d. Student-centered activities that attract those with various personal interests and capabilities.

CHAPTER 5

Substance Abuse

GENERAL WEB SITES

Drug Enforcement Administration: Office of Diversion Control
  http://www.deadiversion.usdoj.gov
Families Anonymous
  http://www.familiesanonymous.org
U.S. Department of Health and Human Services/SAMHSA,
National Clearinghouse for Alcohol and Drug Information (NCADI)
  http://ncadi.samhsa.gov
National Institutes of Health, National Institute on Drug Abuse (NIDA),
The Science of Drug Abuse and Addiction
  http://www.nida.nih.gov
NIDA: Drugs + HIV > Learn the Link
  http://www.hiv.drugabuse.gov
NIDA: Goes Back to School
  http://backtoschool.drugabuse.gov
NIDA: For Teens
  http://teens.drugabuse.gov
Office of Safe and Drug-Free Schools (OSDFS)
  http://www.ed.gov/about/offices/list/osdfs/index.html
Substance Abuse and Mental Health Services Administration (SAMHSA)
  http://www.samhsa.gov

BIBLIOGRAPHY

The American Psychiatric Association: *Diagnostic and statistical manual of mental disorders,* ed 4, text revision, Washington, DC, 2000, American Psychiatric Association.

Bear MF, Connors BW, Paradiso MA: *Neuroscience: exploring the brain,* Philadelphia, 2007, Lippincott Williams & Wilkins.

California Department of Justice: *The biochemistry of drugs,* Sacramento, CA, 1998, author.

Carper J: *Your miracle brain,* New York, 2000, HarperCollins.

Carter R: *Mapping the mind,* Troy, Mich, 2000, Phoenix Press.

Drug Enforcement Agency: *Chapter 7: cannabis* (available online): www.dea.gov/pubs/abuse/7-pot.htm. Accessed March 1, 2007.

Drug Enforcement Agency: *Steroid abuse in today's society: a guide for understanding steroids and related substances* (available online): www.deadiversion.usdoj.gov/pubs/brochures/steroids/professionals/index.html. Accessed Feb 25, 2007.

Foley JD: Adolescent use and misuse of marijuana, *Adolesc Med Clinics* 17(2):319-334, 2006.

Glenmullen J: *Prozac backlash: overcoming the dangers of Prozac, Zoloft, Paxil, and other antidepressants with safe, effective alternatives,* New York, 2000, Simon & Schuster.

Greene JP, Ahrendt D, Stafford EM: Adolescent abuse of other drugs, *Adolesc Med Clinics* 17(2):283-318, 2006.

Howard, PJ: *The owner's manual for the brain,* Austin, Tex, 2006, Bard Press.

Laos C, Metzl JD: Performance-enhancing drug use in young athletes, *Adolesc Med Clinics* 17(2):719-731, 2006.

Lewis KD: *Infants and children with prenatal alcohol exposure: a guide to identification and intervention,* North Branch, Minn, 1995, Sunrise Press.

Lund BC, Perry PJ: Nonsteroid performance-enhancing agents in athletic competitions: An overview for clinicians, *Medscape Pharmacotherapy* 2 (2) (available online): www.medscape.com/viewarticle/408596. Accessed Feb 28, 2007.

Mahony DL, Murphy, JM: Neonatal drug exposure: assessing a specific population and services provided by visiting nurses, *Pediatr Nurs* 25(1):27-36, 1999.

National Institute on Drug Abuse: Cocaine abuse may lead to strokes and mental deficits, *NIDA Notes* 14(3):1-3, 1998.

National Institute on Alcohol Abuse and Alcoholism: Fetal alcohol exposure and the brain, *Alcohol Alert* 50:1-4, 2000.

National Institute on Drug Abuse: *Research Report Series: Anabolic steroid abuse,* 2006b (available online): www.drugabuse.gov/ResearchReports/Steroids/anabolicsteroids5. html. Accessed April 9, 2008.

National Institute on Drug Abuse: *Drugs, brain, and behavior: the science of addiction,* (NIH Pub No 07-5605) Feb 2007a (available online): www.nida.nih.gov/scienceofaddiction/index.html. Accessed April 9, 2008.

National Institute on Drug Abuse: Ecstasy: what we know and don't know about MDMA, a scientific review, *Executive Summary,* Updated Feb 2005a (available online): www. nida.nih.gov/Meetings/MDMA/MDMAExSummary.html. Accessed Feb 28, 2007.

National Institute on Drug Abuse: High school and youth trends, *NIDA Info Facts* 2006a (available online): www.nida.nih.gov/Infofacts/HSYouthtrends.html. Accessed April 9, 2008.

National Institute on Drug Abuse: MDMA (Ecstasy) abuse, *Research Report Series* 2006c (available online): www.nida.nih.gov/ResearchReports/MDMA. Accessed April 9, 2008.

National Institute on Drug Abuse: Marijuana abuse, *Research Report Series,* July 2005b (available online): www.drugabuse.gov/PDF/RRMarijuana.pdf. Accessed Feb 21, 2007.

National Institute on Drug Abuse: *Prescription drug abuse chart,* Feb 2007b (available online): www.nida.nih.gov/DrugPages/PrescripDrugsChart.html. Accessed April 9, 2008.

National Institute on Drug Abuse: The brain's response to drugs: teacher's guide (NIDA Pub No 05-3592), Revised 2005c (available online): www.teens.drugabuse. gov/mom/teachguide/MOM TeacherGuide.pdf. Accessed April 9, 2008.

Office of National Drug Control Policy: *Teens and prescription drugs: An analysis of recent trends on the emerging drug threat* (available online): www.mediacampaign.org/teens/brochure.pdf. Accessed February 25, 2007.

Partnership for a Drug-Free America: *The partnership attitude tracking study (PATS): teens in grades 7 through 12,* 2005 (available online): www.drugfree.org/Files/Full_Teen_Report.

Schydlower M, Arredondo M: Substance abuse among adolescents, *Adolesc Med Clinics* 17 (2), Elsevier Saunders, 2006.

Substance Abuse and Mental Health Services Administration: *Results from the 2005 national survey on drug use and health: national findings,* Office of Applied Studies, NS-DUH Series H-30 (DHHS Pub No SMA 06-4194), Rockville, Md (available online): www.oas.samhsa.gov/nsduh/2k5nsduh/2k5Results.pdf. Accessed April 9, 2008.

Sylwester R: *How to explain a brain: an educator's handbook of brain terms and cognitive processes,* Thousand Oaks, 2005, Corin Press.

CHAPTER 6

Substance Abuse

CHAPTER 7

Violence

*N*urses cannot escape the consequences of violent acts toward and by the school-age population. Health problems that result from physical and emotional violence can be lifelong, and the resulting disabilities can be extensive. Violent events occur in schools, homes, and communities. This chapter focuses on *violence toward self* (including self-mutilation and suicide), *violence toward others* (sexual assault), *violence in the home* (physical, emotional, sexual abuse, and neglect), and *violence in schools* (peer harassment and bullying, physical aggression and assault, life threats and homicides, and gangs).

Self-mutilation, *violence toward self*, is a pathological yet complex behavior of youth that commonly is expressed as cutting or injury to the body for personal comfort or relief from emotional pain. Suicide is ranked as the third leading cause of death of young people (Snyder and Sickmund, 2006). Public awareness of early subtle and overt signs must be expanded, intervention services and programs require improvement, and research is needed to broaden the knowledge base and develop additional strategies for suicide prevention in all children.

Rape is a display of sexual *violence toward another person*. Three relational categories are defined within adolescent rape: *stranger, nonstranger* (date or acquaintance rape), and *incest*. All can be detrimental to the victim's health and have serious, long-lasting consequences. These categories are unique in three ways: (1) how victims process the event, which determines the prevailing cognitive and psychological behaviors; (2) how health professionals are affected by the incident, and how they sort through the salient issues; and (3) techniques and methods used for treatment. Two out of every 1000 children in the United States were confirmed victims of sexual assault in 2003 (U.S. Department of Health and Human Services [USDHHS], 2005). Sexual violence is one of the most underreported crimes.

Violence in the home is defined as physical, sexual, and emotional abuse or neglect of the child or adolescent. A child's observation of domestic violence against a sibling and elder is also considered child abuse. Often the school nurse is the first person to become aware of the incident and is the person most likely to report suspected abuse. When the nurse can identify poor relationships and stressors that place an individual or family member at high risk for child abuse, intervention strategies can be implemented.

Violence in schools occurs for students at every level of elementary and secondary education. Students experience peer conflict and aggression on a daily basis that may lead to interpersonal violence, and an increasing number of students become victims of juvenile crime. The most common types of violence in U.S. schools are peer harassment and bullying behavior. Assault and bodily injury are less common but still frequent. Between 1995 and 2001, the percentage of students who reported being victims of crime decreased from 10% to 6%. Cyberbullying is an emerging phenomenon that can create extreme social and emotional distress. It is difficult to isolate perpetrators of these aggressive behaviors, because attackers can move at great speed and may use multiple technological devices.

Gangs are peer and reference groups organized for both social and antisocial purposes, including peer violence. Gangs have been part of American culture since the colonial era, but the nature of the group has changed. The environment creates the need for violence and antisocial behavior. Participation in gangs may facilitate accomplishment of developmental tasks, even if they are also counterproductive and harmful to gang members and society. For example, the need for independence is provided by the structure and acceptance of the gang, allowing emancipation from the family. The need for intimacy may be met by peer support within the group, allowing members to redefine their gender role. Security of the gang provides the confidence to pursue intimate relationships. The gang provides acceptance, significance, and protection, allowing the cognitive and social freedom to explore various roles away from the family, thus meeting the adolescent's need for identity.

Brain Findings

Numerous studies provide data on genetic, biological, and environmental keys to aggression and violence. A biochemical link indicating an interaction between defective genes and the environment produces abnormal levels of two mood-altering neurotransmitters, serotonin and noradrenaline. Serotonin plays a key role in regulating emotions, including control of aggression, and noradrenaline organizes the brain's response to danger. Increased levels of serotonin are associated with high self-esteem and social status; low levels are associated with low self-esteem and social status, which can lead to aggression, impulsivity, and suicidal and violent behavior (Davidson, Putnam, and Larson, 2000). These two neurotransmitters

CHAPTER 7   Violence

are involved in regulating the dopamine-dependent behavioral system (Rogeness and McClure, 1996).

The orbitofrontal cortex—located in the prefrontal cortex of the brain—and interconnected structures are associated with self-regulation, social intelligence, impulse control, and attention. In violence-prone individuals, this area appears to be dysfunctional (Davidson, Putnam, and Larson, 2000). The same brain region is involved in overt expressions of aggression and also in everyday demonstrations of failed self-regulation, such as a child's temper tantrums, a teenager's driving at excessive speeds, and parents' emotional outbursts.

VIOLENCE TOWARD SELF

SELF-MUTILATION

I. Definition

A. A useful definition of *self-mutilation (SM)* that incorporates all the variables from different studies is "a direct, socially unacceptable, repeated behavior that causes minor to moderate physical injury" to oneself (Suyemoto and Kountz, 2000). Other more acceptable terms are *self-injury, self-harm, self-inflicted violence (SIV),* and *self-injurious behavior (SIB).* Such behavior is regarded as pathological, and it differs from socially acceptable bodily modifications—such as piercings or tattoos—and from indirect, risk-taking self-harm, such as driving under the influence of alcohol. Self-mutilation is not regarded as a suicide attempt, because the motivation is to inflict injury or cause suffering, not to cause death. SM is the externalization of overwhelming emotional pain. When such behavior continues, it may become chronic and debilitating.

B. SM is increasing, and a small study indicates that 13.9% of adolescents report SIB (Ross and Heath 2002). Estimates of self-mutilation in the general population range from 14 to 600 per 100,000 annually. Most researchers believe SM is underreported, because it is a secretive behavior. Rates among adolescent inpatients range from 40% to 61%. A survey of outpatient therapists showed that 47% had known a self-mutilating adolescent (Suyemoto and Kountz, 2000).

II. Etiology

A. This is not a new phenomenon: young people who self-mutilate have been studied in the medical and psychiatric community for more than 45 years. Clinicians and researchers differ on the actual diagnosis for SM, but the consensus is that the behavior can be related to the diagnosis of borderline personality disorder, which lists self-mutilating behavior as one of its criteria (American Psychiatric Association, 2000). Some authorities associate SM with eating disorders, and others document co-occurrence with dissociative identity disorder and obsessive compulsive disorder. Youths who are mentally retarded or autistic engage in SM, but these individuals are not classified in the same manner.

III. Characteristics

A. Burning, carving, cutting, hair pulling, scratching and picking of the skin, and putting objects into body openings or under the skin. Cutting is the most common form of self-mutilation. Cuts often are made by razor blades, inflicting injury to the arms, wrists, forearms, ankles, and lower legs. Other areas include the abdomen, axilla, and beneath the breasts. Girls represent the large majority of self-mutilators, and the first incident usually occurs in middle to late adolescence. Occurrence does not vary according to ethnicity, race, or class. Self-cutting usually is a secretive behavior, but scars and wounds are often visible if left uncovered. Because of shame and self-repulsion, affected individuals are socially isolated and selective in their social relationships. Substance abuse frequently is associated with self-injury. As many as three fourths of self-mutilators describe violence, abuse, and family disruptions as common in their family of origin. Bodily injury can be severe, resulting in hospitalization and the need for institutionalization as a means of protection. Some studies indicate that as many as 25% of adolescent self-mutilators have never sought medical advice regarding their self-abuse (Suyemoto and Kountz, 2000). Medication is not the treatment of choice except to treat underlying associated disorders (e.g., depression, obsessive-compulsive behavior).

B. Episodes of SM usually are less than an hour in duration and are a part of a recurring cycle in response to stress triggers that can be seen largely as unconscious, automatic processes of cognition distortion, negative feelings, and critical self-talk.

IV. Effects on Individual

A. A common theme is that self-injury helps the individual feel physical pain on the outside instead of emotional pain on the inside. Self-injury provides immediate but temporary relief from psychological pain that the individual is unable to express verbally. It is a way to externalize the intensity of the pain and turn it into an active, physical event that can be controlled. Usually the emotional incentive to mutilate is fear, hurt, anger or perceived rejection or abandonment by others, which may be precipitated by anxiety and hostility. Self-injurers have not learned how to appropriately release emotions, or they may not have been allowed to express them. Volatile and exaggerated responses can trigger events, but individuals learn to relieve overwhelming emotions through self-injury; most report feeling calm, relief, or contentment after the injury.

V. Management and Treatment

A. Depends on degree of involvement and history, such as physical or sexual abuse, chaotic family life, student alcohol or drug use, or underlying psychiatric illness. Further research in this subject is needed, and school nurses are ideally suited to perform this work.

   1. Be alert to behavioral cues, which may include low self-esteem, anxiety, anger, isolation, and inappropriate dress (e.g., wearing long sleeves and long pants in warm weather to cover up scars).

CHAPTER 7 Violence

2. Be aware of any school policies, state laws, or guidelines for reporting and management.
3. Use screening questionnaires to determine students' behaviors.
4. Understand the variance in personal triggers and usual episodes of self-mutilation among youths.
5. Develop personal care contracts.
6. Educate staff and parents—both individually and in group meetings—regarding risk factors, which include anxiety, stress, and methods used to disassociate with the overwhelming tension and impact of chaotic or negative family dynamics.
7. Conduct health classes and encourage student participation. Discuss precursors and related issues, and be a resource for parents, staff, and students.
8. Use posters, DVDs, CDs, and school nurse Web site to provide information.

B. Treatment.
1. Assess physical health and obtain detailed history of mental health.
2. Notify parents or guardians; refer to school psychologist, social worker, or mental health worker. It is important to continue dialogue with parents, but be sensitive to the fact that the student may be fearful of a parent.
3. Be aware of personal feelings about self-injury.
4. DO NOT tell the student to stop self-injury, and refrain from making judgmental comments; these can lower students' feelings of self-worth and make them more likely to self-injure.
5. Project a nonjudgmental, hopeful acceptance of the youth. Most do not want attention and hide the injury. Self-mutilators act on emotional pain and are distracted by the physical pain.
6. Provide immediate first aid and medical treatment for cuts and wounds. Make student aware of potential infection; educate and monitor the student.
7. Clarify negative emotions and identify cognitive distortions.
8. Teach alternative strategies for self-comfort and soothing (e.g., exercise, music, massage, warm bath, acupressure points).
9. Encourage students to verbalize and express emotions by modeling, and garner peer support.
10. Refer for intensive psychotherapy or group support services if appropriate.

WEB SITES

Self-Injury: You Are Not the Only One
http://www.palace.net/~llama/psych/injury.html
Self-Injury and Related Issues (SIARI)
http://www.Siari.co.uk

SUICIDE

I. Definition
A. Deliberate violence toward self or self-destruction with the intent of taking one's own life.

B. Nationwide, 16.9% of students have seriously considered suicide (Grunbaum, 2004). Suicide is the third leading cause of death among juveniles ages 15 to 19, and males outnumber females 4:1 in this age group. The suicide rate for American Indian juveniles is nearly double the white non-Hispanic rate and triple the rate for other racial and ethnic groups (Snyder and Sickmund, 2006).

II. Etiology

A. Suicide is multicausal. More than 75% of youth suicide is associated with a diagnosable mental or substance abuse disorder. Causes of childhood suicide may include escape from physical or sexual abuse, chaotic family situations, feelings of being unloved, constant criticism, depression, loss of significant relationships, humiliation, potential or actual failure in school, or intent to punish friends or family.

B. Causes of adolescent suicide—in addition to the causes listed previously—may include difficulties or lack of meaningful relationships, perfectionist expectations, serious problems with parents, sexual issues, or a fight with a close friend. In some cases, copycat suicide occurs to gain attention or to identify with a peer who has committed suicide. Suicide and attempted suicide are more prevalent in cults, homosexuals, and high-risk individuals (e.g., those who use drugs and alcohol). Teenage girls attempt suicide more frequently, whereas teenage boys have a higher rate of completed suicides. Girls more often use less violent methods of suicide (e.g., pills), and boys use guns more frequently.

III. Characteristics

A. Elementary-age student, kindergarten through sixth grade.
  1. Verbal cues: somatic complaints about headaches and stomachaches. Comments indicating loneliness, isolation, and not being loved.
  2. Behavioral cues: poor school performance, withdrawal from play and leisure interests, apathy, listlessness, erratic appetite, and sleep disturbance. Sometimes are careless and destructive toward property, both their own and others.
  3. Affective cues: feelings of sadness, irritability, lack of empathy, tend not to be carefree or engage in spontaneous laughter. Change in routine of doing chores (i.e., cleaning their room, caring for animals).

B. Adolescent student, junior and senior high school.
  1. Verbal cues: students may make subtle or obvious comments about suicide, e.g., "Will you miss me when I'm not here?" or "I won't be bothering you anymore."
  2. Behavioral cues: may stockpile pills, obtain a weapon, withdraw from activities and friends, engage in risky activities, abuse drugs or alcohol, neglect appearance and self-care, dispose of personal belongings, change sleep patterns, listen to suggestive music, suddenly receive different academic grades, change friends and relationships, engage in promiscuous sex, change appetite, or report sleep problems.

Violence

CHAPTER 7

3. Affective cues: chronic or acute depression, feelings of hopelessness and guilt, sadness, lack of empathy, boredom, decreased self-gratification.

IV. **Health Concerns/Emergencies**
   A. Physical health issues, including decreased appetite, poor sleep, and poor hygiene.
   B. Acute or recurrent depression, mood swings, or other psychiatric problems.
   C. Pattern of repeated suicide attempts.
   D. Failed suicide attempts, resulting in injury or permanent handicap.
   E. Copycat behaviors of friends or family.
   F. Mental health disorder may require suicide watch or placement in a more restrictive setting for protection.
   G. If a student takes antidepressant medication, be on the alert for suicidal ideation.

V. **Effects on Individual**
   A. Temporary or permanent handicap caused by failed suicide attempt.
   B. Emotional trauma related to repeated attempts.
   C. Depression or recurrent depression.
   D. Feelings of loss, sadness, grief, guilt, and disbelief in family, friends, and peers after failed suicide attempt.
   E. Individual may feel relief from an unsuccessful suicide attempt.

VI. **Management/Treatment**
   A. Be alert to warning signs and intervene early to prevent attempts or completion. Never ignore a warning or threat, and do not be afraid to ask: "Are you considering suicide?" "Do you have a plan?"
   B. Talk openly and directly regarding suicide.
   C. Call suicide crisis hot-line 1-800-SUICIDE (784-2433), 1-800-273-TALK (8255), when necessary.
   D. Address drug and alcohol use that contributes to depression.
   E. Support and teach students and others about stress, depression, sadness, coping with loss, and academic, social, and athletic challenges that may put the student at greater risk for suicide or attempts. This may be a component of the School Crisis Team or noncrisis intervention and prevention.
   F. Establish and support School Crisis Team with emergency guidelines and mechanism for referring at-risk students who manifest depressive behaviors, suicidal characteristics, or both.
   G. Refer for intensive counseling and treatment for underlying mental health disorders. Can utilize Columbia TeenScreen Program to screen for depression, substance abuse, and suicidal ideation (see Appendix A, Assessment Tools).
   H. Provide counseling to intervene in affective, behavioral, and self-esteem issues. Suicide attempts should always be professionally evaluated.
   I. Implement intervention centered around family support system; listen to students, show them loved ones need and respect them, set high but realistic expectations, encourage caring and nurturing, spiritual or religious involvement, and allow staff to be supportive.
   J. Counsel and refer students (friends of the victim) to a support group after the suicide and around the anniversary of the event.
   K. Acquire knowledge and skill in interviewing techniques.

VII. Additional Information

A. More people are killed by suicide than by homicide (U.S. Public Health Service, 2000). The actual rate may be higher than reported, because suicide deaths sometimes are concealed to avoid stigma, and some accidents are actually suicides. With constant media exposure to violence and homicidal behavior, youth may become desensitized to life-threatening behavior and may experience increased feelings of omnipotence or invulnerability to death. Suicide attempts may be a nonverbal cry for help. Issues related to sexual orientation and gender identity increase the risk for depression and subsequent suicide attempts and completions.

WEB SITES

ANSWER: Adolescents Never Suicide When Everyone Responds
    http://www.teenanswer.org
The American Association of Suicidology (AAS)
    http://www.suicidology.org
The American Foundation for Suicide Prevention (AFSP)
    http://www.afsp.org
Yellow Ribbon International Suicide Prevention Program
    http://www.yellowribbon.org

VIOLENCE TOWARD OTHERS

SEXUAL ASSAULT

Lisa Lewis-Javar, RN, SANE-P, FNC, and Vickie Whitson, RN, BSN, SANE-A

I. Definition

A. Sexual assault is a broad term to describe intentional sexual contact that is made without consent. It can range from kissing and fondling to penetration. Consent is a vital concept, because people cannot give consent when they are not in full command of their cognitive ability (e.g. from alcohol, drug use, or mental illness).

B. Rape is a type of sexual assault that involves penetration with both male and female victims—oral, anal, or vaginal, however slight. Most states define *penetration* as anything deeper than the labia majora, but statues may vary from state to state.

C. Family members or acquaintances commit 95% of all confirmed cases of child sexual assault. This includes members of the child's family or other persons known to or trusted by the child. Furthermore, 83% of all confirmed cases of child sexual abuse occur in the privacy of a home or residence (Snyder and Sickmund, 2006). Statistics show that 1 in 5 girls and 1 in 10 boys are sexually exploited before they reach adulthood—yet less than 35% of those child sexual assaults are reported to authorities, according to the National Center for Missing and Exploited Children. According to the Youth Internet Safety Survey II (2006) conducted by the U.S. Department of Justice, 1 in 7 children and adolescents 10 to 17 years old received unwanted sexual solicitations online (Wolak, Mitchell, and Finkelhor, 2006).

CHAPTER 7   Violence

II. Etiology

    A. Sexual assault reflects antisocial and relational problems of the perpetrator and is not something the victim provoked. It is usually an expression of power and control rather than sexuality.

Brain Findings

The hormones cortisol and corticotrophin are neurotransmitters released during stress. Repeated release of these neurotransmitters during early childhood abuse causes physical changes in brain structures that make the individual subject to increased sensitivity to minimal stress in adulthood.

    These relatively permanent brain changes caused by physical and sexual abuse of young girls can affect later life experiences, resulting in more emotional and physical difficulties, including depression, anxiety disorders, and gastrointestinal problems (Heim et al, 2000).

III. Characteristics

    A. Physical and emotional responses.

        1. Physical and emotional responses associated with sexual assault and abuse are as unique as the victims who experience them.

        2. There is no "normal" or "abnormal" response. Initially the victim's response may include shock, disbelief, shame, and self-blame.

        3. The victim's outward behavior may include a broad spectrum of emotions—anger, sobbing, crying, and inappropriate laughter—or may more often present with a quiet, calm demeanor.

        4. Common concerns after a person has been sexually assaulted include pregnancy and contraction of a sexually transmitted disease.

    B. Psychological responses.

        1. Phobias, depression, suicidal thoughts, nightmares or sleep disturbances, anxiety that manifests as chest pain, palpitation, and diaphoresis; or, individual may appear normal but may be in denial and suppressing the responses.

        2. Mistrust of the perpetrator's gender in general, mistrust of friends, or withdrawal.

        3. Reliving the event through flashbacks or intrusive thoughts.

        4. Avoidance of experiences previously enjoyed.

        5. Difficulty with memory and concentration.

        6. Avoidance of situations or place where assault occurred.

IV. Health Concerns/Emergencies

NOTE: State laws may vary regarding the time frame in which the assault must be reported, the consents needed, and the evidence required.

    A. Evidence is best gathered within 72 hours by health care professionals with special training and equipment and with scientific knowledge of DNA advances. DNA sperm has been recovered from the cervix up to 19 days post-assault with a sexual assault history of penile vaginal penetration without a condom.

    Reminder: If a student approaches you and discloses a sexual assault, remember to tell them not to shower, brush teeth, urinate, or change clothes until law enforcement can conduct a forensic interview.

    B. Victims need time to express feelings; proceed slowly. Most states have sexual advocacy organizations with twenty-four hour hotlines available. These organizations provide advocacy and emotional support to the victim even before the crime has been reported. A national hotline is available—800-656-HOPE (4673)—or contact the Rape Abuse and Incest National Network at http://www.rainn.org.

C. Advise regarding transmission of sexually transmitted diseases (STDs), including human immunodeficiency virus (HIV) and acquired immunodeficiency syndrome (AIDS). The data available regarding the transmission of HIV through a single sexual assault is limited but suggests that the rate of contraction is extremely low. Follow up with primary medical provider for HIV and hepatitis baseline testing and recommended CDC guidelines.

D. Victim may have vaginal or anal pain, tenderness, swelling, abrasions, lacerations, bruising, and bleeding. In most sexual assaults in people 12 years of age and older, there are no genital findings at least 70% of the time (Giardino, Datner, and Asher, 2003).

E. Rape trauma syndrome and post-traumatic stress disorder (PTSD) are not uncommon.

V. Effects on Individual

A. Fear of contracting HIV/AIDS or hepatitis; fear may last for years.

B. Somatic complaints often increase in frequency.

C. Individual may experience lack of trust, feelings of loss of control, and victimization.

D. Sexual assault is one of life's most devastating experiences with recurrent flashbacks and recall in long-term memory.

E. Individuals of any age who have been sexually assaulted appear to be at higher risk for depression, suicidal tendencies, self-mutilation, poor self-esteem, aggression, and inappropriate sexual behavior; these effects may manifest at any time.

F. Male sexual abuse occurs but is usually underreported, due to embarrassment and shame, and may be related to the victim's sexual orientation.

VI. Management and Treatment

A. Post-crisis support system and counseling should be in place for at least 1 year after the trauma.

B. Crisis intervention is necessary, because the victim needs time to express feelings and receive emotional support; offer techniques that increase student's sense of safety.

C. Facilitate support in the victim's social networks (e.g., school, church, community).

D. Maintain strict confidentiality and follow Family Educational Rights and Privacy Act (FERPA) and Health Insurance Portability and Accountability Act (HIPAA) guidelines.

E. When treating a sexual assault victim, a nurse must be sensitive to the individual's cultural and religious beliefs; the nurse's attitudes and emotions must not be allowed to influence their nursing role.

F. Victim assistance funds are available in most states for physical and mental health services.

G. Educate students about risky behavior, such as drug and alcohol use, that may increase the possibility of a sexual assault.

CHAPTER 7   Violence

H. Provide services to parents and family members; be concerned and sensitive to anger, guilt, blaming of the victim, and an individual's self-blame.

VII. Additional Information

A. Teach prevention in schools as early as the elementary years; discuss respect, cooperation, consideration, and other life skills necessary for healthy social relationships.

B. Use role playing, and include males and females of various ages. Most perpetrators are known to the victims. It is vital to teach the student that no one has the right to touch them inappropriately and that it is in their best interest to tell someone if that happens.

Evidentiary Sexual Assault Examination

A sexual assault nurse examiner (SANE) or sexual assault forensic nurse (SAFE), both registered nurses with specialized training and equipment, should gather evidence regarding the rape. Most metropolitan cities in the United States and Canada have SANEs or Sexual Assault Response Teams (SARTs) available; if not, the emergency room physician performs the examination.

I. Examination Procedures

A. Victim service/rape advocate is called before examination to stay with the victim through the assessment phase; she will bring a complete set of clean clothing so that personal clothing may be collected for evidence. Each step in the examination is explained before it is performed. When desired, a companion is supportive for the victim during history-taking and examination.

B. Follow state sexual assault assessment protocol for proper chain of evidence; procedures for each state may differ in requirements for the examination process.

C. An *evidentiary sexual assault examination* may include:

1. Detailed history of alleged assault, after which the examination is performed according to the victim's reported history. May include examination of genitalia, perineum, anus, rectum, and pharynx; colposcopic photographs, in which a camera is used to detect trauma of the cervix and vaginal areas, may also be used.
2. Sample collection of vaginal, anal, and oral secretions.
3. Photographs or diagrams of trauma that indicate findings, such as bruises, abrasions, lacerations, or scars.
4. Use of alternate light source to detect dried secretions on body.
5. Wet mount of vaginal secretions; slides for sperm motility.
6. Collection of foreign material.
7. Reference samples that include pubic hair, head hair, saliva, and blood are collected.
8. Pregnancy testing per hospital protocol; morning-after pill may be administered with a negative test result.
9. Treatment of acute trauma under the direction of the emergency room physician.

D. Follow discharge instructions per SART Nurse.

Acquaintance Assault

Acquaintance assault is the most common form of assault for a school age-child. Such assault may be underreported, because the victim may feel guilt and responsibility for the event. Girls usually do not consider sexual assault that occurs during a date as a reportable offense, and drugs and alcohol are frequently involved.

Several illicit drugs can be used by the perpetrator: Rohypnol, GHB (liquid Ecstasy), and ketamine. When mixed with a liquid—soda, alcohol, or water—Rohypnol dissolves instantly and is effective within 20 to 30 minutes. It is colorless, odorless, tasteless, and virtually undetectable.

WEB SITES

National Center for Missing and Exploited Children
    http://www.missingkids.com
National Sexual Violence Resource Center
    http://www.nsvrc.org
Office of Violence Against Women
    http://www.usdoj.gov/ovw
Rape, Abuse, and Incest National Network (RAINN)
    http://www.rainn.org
(800) 656-HOPE (4673) Hotline
Sexual Assault Resource Service
    http://www.sane-sart.com

VIOLENCE IN THE HOME

PHYSICAL, EMOTIONAL, AND SEXUAL ABUSE AND NEGLECT

I. Definition

    A. Child abuse is any situation in which a child suffers mistreatment or serious injury by other than accidental means. Child abuse encompasses physical, emotional, and sexual harm and neglect. The abuser can be a parent, sibling, custodian, or guardian.

    B. Types of Abuse.

        1. *Physical abuse* is any damage to the skin, bones, or internal and external organs or structures.

        2. *Emotional abuse* is a nonphysical, usually verbal, form of assault. The child does not experience the usual feelings of love, security, and worthiness.

        3. *Sexual abuse* is the use of a child for sexual gratification by an adult or a person who is significantly chronologically or developmentally older than the victim. Sexual abuse includes molestation, exploitation for prostitution, incest, or use of the child for pornographic materials.

        4. *Neglect* is a prolonged failure to provide the child with basic needs such as food, clothing, home cleanliness, safety, medical care, supervision, and education. Infants and young children are those most often neglected.

C. It is estimated that 872,000 children in the United States were determined to be victims of child abuse or neglect in 2004 (USDHHS, 2006).

II. Etiology

A. Child abuse is seldom the result of any single factor but a combination of various factors: environment, circumstances, parenting skills, coping mechanisms, and stress.

Brain Findings

Research suggests that an increase in stress hormones during childhood physical and sexual abuse produces sharper hormonal and physical responses to minor stress events in adulthood (Heim et al, 2000). Early abuse and neglect have the potential to affect brain development and functioning. During experience-dependent stages of development, where proper wiring of the brain requires appropriate stimulation, neglect or abuse can result in a lack of input that affects the development of subsequent behaviors (e.g., writing, riding a bicycle). This stimulation is analogous to failure of the visual system to establish normal connections when a child has impairment in vision, such as amblyopia or cataracts (Glaser, 2000; Perry, 2002; Post and Weiss, 1997; M. Martone [personal communication], November 10, 2006).

Early experience shapes the brain in both negative and positive ways. Whether the abuse is physical, psychological, or sexual, it affects the ability of the child's brain to cope with a turbulent world; at the same time, it may also create negative short- and long-term consequences. There is evidence that childhood maltreatment is associated with several changes in the brain, including decreased development of the left cortex and left hippocampus, diminished right–left hemisphere integration and decreased size of the corpus callosum, and abnormalities in the cerebellar vermis. The stress of chronic abuse in the young child affects specific areas of the brain and can result in hyperactivity, anxiety, sleep disturbances, conduct disorder, and learning and memory deficits (USDHHS, 2006). Early negative experiences of maltreatment resulting in brain changes may appear as mental ailments later in life and may include depression, learning difficulties, eating disorders, and PTSD. The outcomes of abuse vary by individual, because so many factors play a part: the child's age and developmental level; the type, duration, frequency, and severity of the abuse; and the relationship between the victim and abuser all play a part. The sequelae can be short-term or may last a lifetime (NCCANI, 2005). Fortunately, children's brains are more plastic than adults' brains. Early identification and aggressive intervention can minimize the negative effects of child maltreatment. Intervention in terms of removal from the home and out-of-home placement can create further traumatizing experiences for the child, thus cautions must be built into the plan. One key element to healing the child and effecting a successful therapeutic intervention is a consistent, predictable, nurturing, and caring environment at home and school (NCCANI, 2005; Perry and Marcellus, 2006).

III. Characteristics

A. Physical abuse.

1. Ecchymosis (bruises).

a. May be multiple and in various stages of healing and discoloration.

b. Often seen in places where bruising does not commonly occur as a result of normal childhood activity.

c. Marks from hands, belts, and rulers are frequently seen patterns.

2. Burns of questionable origin.

a. Recognizable by shape (e.g., iron, grill of electric heater).

b. Indication of immersion into hot water is glovelike or socklike appearance on hands and feet or doughnut-shaped scald on buttocks.

c. Burns caused by hot running water form a zebra-striped pattern on the body; creases on abdomen and folds of upper legs remain clear and occur when the child is held by the hands or legs.

d. Cigarette burns are usually multiple and found on palms and soles.

e. Rope burns are usually found around wrists or ankles.

3. Abrasions and lacerations.

a. May be found on any area of body, including mouth, lips, ears, eyes, and external genitalia.

b. Frenulum is torn from jabbing spoon into mouth during feeding.

c. Injury to oral mucosa or frontal dental ridge from poking a bottle into the child's mouth.

4. Intracranial trauma.

a. Lethargy, stupor, confusion, coma, or other signs of altered mental state.

b. Nausea, vomiting, irritability.

c. Seizures.

d. Papilledema.

e. Bulging fontanel in infant.

f. Prominent veins.

5. Damage to internal organs.

a. Shock.

b. Blood in urine or stool.

c. Increased pulse rate.

d. Abdominal pain or distention.

6. Skeletal damage, fractures.

a. Commonly skull, nose, and other facial structures involved; "spiral" fractures result from twisting of arms or legs.

b. Rib fractures.

c. Old fractures evident with x-ray films.

d. Dislocations.

7. Behavior of child.

a. Unpleasant, demanding, disobedient, and difficult to get along with.

b. Reports injury by parents.

c. Extremely aggressive or extremely withdrawn.

d. Frequently comes to school late and is often absent.

e. May linger around school after dismissal.

f. Avoids physical contact with others.

g. Wears concealing clothing (e.g., long sleeves) to hide injuries.

h. Child's explanation does not fit type or seriousness of injury.

CHAPTER 7   Violence

      i. Child appears frightened of parents or shows little or no distress at separation from parents.

      j. Eager to please or placate an angry adult to avoid injury.

      k. Indiscriminately seeks affection from any adult.

      l. Demonstrates poor self-concept.

B. Emotional abuse.

  1. Signs not as obvious as with other forms of abuse.

  2. Best indication is behavior.

      a. Apathetic, withdrawn, passive, depressed, shows lack of positive self-image.

      b. Antisocial behavior (e.g., stealing, destructiveness).

      c. Signs of emotional turmoil, such as rocking, biting, enuresis, and encopresis.

      d. Problems in school: developmental delays, excessive activity, behavior problems, school failure.

      e. Assumes inappropriate adult roles and responsibility, such as those of parent.

      f. Difficulty making friends.

      g. Fearful, prone to nightmares, anxious.

      h. Compulsively conforms to adults' instructions.

      i. Anxious when faced with new situations or people.

      j. Excessive fantasizing.

      k. Sadistic behavior.

C. Sexual abuse.

  1. Signs.

      a. Stained or bloody underwear.

      b. STD of eyes, mouth, genitalia, or anus.

      c. Lacerations, bleeding, or bruising of genitalia, anal area, mouth, or throat.

      d. Dysuria, edema, or itching in genital area.

      e. Vaginal or penile discharge.

      f. Pregnancy.

  2. Behavior of child.

      a. Informs nurse or other adult of sexual assaults.

      b. Withdrawn, preoccupied with fantasy, or may appear retarded.

      c. Infantile behavior or may act like an adult instead of a child.

      d. Poor relationships with peers.

      e. Displays early seductive behavior or knowledge of sex inappropriate for age; may engage in excessive masturbation and insertion of objects into orifices.

      f. Unwilling or hesitant to participate in physical activities.

      g. Poor academic performance, engages in delinquent acts, or runs away from home.

D. Neglect.

  1. Signs.

      a. Failure to thrive.

      b. Malnutrition.

      c. Often hungry, no breakfast, and no money for lunch.

      d. Does not receive necessary medical or dental care, immunizations, or medication.

   e. Dirty clothing or dressed unsuitably for weather.
   f. Frequently unwashed, body odor, and poor oral hygiene.
   g. Often left unattended for long periods.
   h. Child under 14 years left alone or unsupervised.
   2. Behavior of child.
      a. Constantly fatigued or sleepy.
      b. Steals food.
      c. Frequent absences from school or comes early and stays late.
      d. Few friends; seeks refuge in siblings.
      e. Uses alcohol or drugs.
      f. Engages in vandalism or sexual misconduct.
IV. Differential Diagnosis
   A. Cultural practices: traditional healing practices may be confused with physical abuse.
      1. Cupping is a Chinese practice used to treat headaches or abdominal pain; also practiced by other cultures.
      2. Coining is a Vietnamese health practice used for minor ailments; also practiced by other cultures.
      3. Native Americans have various healing rituals that may seem to delay seeking appropriate care.
      4. Homeopathic remedies are gaining wide support cross-culturally; when not effective, they can delay other care or treatment.
   B. Health conditions.
      1. Mongolian spots can be confused with bruising.
      2. Dermatological conditions have been confused with abuse, because they may resemble burns from cigarettes or scalding water (e.g., epidermolysis bullosa, bullous impetigo).
V. Health Concerns/Emergencies
   A. Long-term handicapping sequelae of physical abuse require multidisciplinary services (i.e., neurological, orthopedic, surgical, nursing, rehabilitation, and social welfare services).
   B. Subtle signs of head injury may manifest after trauma and must be monitored.
   C. Frequent colds, bronchitis, and pneumonia commonly are related to physical neglect.
   D. When immunizations have not been given because of neglect, child lacks protection from a number of serious diseases and their medical consequences.
   E. Children with poor hygiene and unsanitary living situations have frequent skin conditions (e.g., impetigo, scabies, severe diaper rash, boils); dental and periodontal problems also are common.
   F. Lacerations, punctures, and burns may become infected.
   G. STD, pregnancy, poor sphincter control, and other results of sexual abuse require immediate medical care and ongoing emotional support.
   H. *Inorganic failure to thrive* is often a consequence of neglect or inadequate parenting skills.
      1. Height and weight are under third percentile; decreased weight reflects acute malnutrition; depressed height is indicative of cumulative effects of chronic malnutrition.
      2. Unresponsiveness and withdrawal.

Violence

CHAPTER 7

   3. Little smiling.
   4. Developmental delays.
   5. Feeding difficulties.
   6. Delayed dentition.
   7. Delayed speech and social skills.
 I. *Munchausen syndrome by proxy* is a cluster of signs and symptoms in which illness in a child is simulated, faked, or produced by a caregiver, usually the mother, resulting in numerous medical appointments or procedures and frequent school absenteeism. Acute symptoms decrease or stop when separated from the caregiver. Munchausen syndrome by proxy encompasses both physical and emotional abuse. This is seen as a spectrum of medical child abuse from parental hypervigilance, fabrication, or induced illness or injury that results in unnecessary medical treatment.
 J. *Shaken baby syndrome* results from the violent shaking of a child; it causes intracranial trauma that can result in brain damage, visual impairment, or death.
 K. *Maternal deprivation syndrome* (infants) and *psychosocial dwarfism* (children) are defined as growth failure in infants and children caused by growth hormone secretory impairment. This syndrome results from living in an environment of severe emotional deprivation.
 L. Abuse of all forms causes emotional damage and frequently requires professional intervention and support of those closely associated with student.

VI. Effects on Individual
 A. Development of self-concept suffers.
 B. Difficulties in school and in making friends.
 C. Delinquency, drug abuse, alcoholism, and obesity can develop during adolescence.
 D. Lessons of violence learned in childhood frequently are used by the abused against their own children and society in general.
 E. Young child may undergo delays in cognitive, social, and motor development.
 F. As adults, the abused have difficulty maintaining relationships and choosing a good mate.
 G. Adults who have been abused as children frequently seek love and acceptance from those who are unable to meet their expectations, and as parents they have an exceptional need for love from their children.
 H. Female victims of incest have been shown to be at high risk for suicide and eating disorders.
 I. Often victims of sexual abuse, men and women, become prostitutes.
 J. Greater risk for self-mutilation and suicide attempts or completion.

VII. Management/Treatment
 A. Treatment of child's physical injuries is initial concern.
 B. Report *all* cases of suspected child abuse to child protective services. Teachers and others require education regarding the importance of early detection and mandated reporting of suspected child abuse.

    C. Damage and other long-term handicapping sequelae must be iden-
tified and services provided (e.g., schooling, rehabilitation, counseling, physical therapy).

    D. Entire family should be part of program that uses multidisciplinary
team approach in meeting both physical and psychological needs.

    E. Psychological counseling is vital for abuser and victim.

    F. Parents and victim may benefit from participation in support
groups.

    G. Many community resources are available to families; these resources
provide needed support (e.g., public health nurses, day care centers,
child abuse hotlines, volunteer organizations, mental health agencies, safe houses, or shelters).

    H. Be alert for parents who show a potential for child abuse and, when
possible, direct them to needed resources, such as parent groups,
hotlines, and counseling services.

    I. Be available and empathetic when the parent and child need some-
one who can provide practical assistance and resources.

    J. Be aware of personal feelings or bias regarding those who commit-
ted or allowed the abuse to occur.

    K. See Additional Information for preventive measures.

VIII. Additional Information

    D. Observed effects of domestic violence vary according to a student's
age.

      1. Infants through age 5 may display signs of health problems, in-
cluding loss of weight, feeding problems, and inconsolable crying.

      2. Preschoolers may appear anxious or sad, be clingy or aggressive
with peers, or regress in toilet training.

      3. Children ages 6 to 12 may be depressed, fearful, demonstrate
aggressive behavior, or have low self-esteem. May appear socially
isolated because of restricted social activity from embarrassment
of family violence.

      4. Adolescents may act out by running away from home, using
drugs and alcohol, becoming withdrawn or depressed, and
attempting suicide, often successfully. Others may assume parenting roles while caring for younger siblings and may not
attend school. Many are argumentative and verbally abusive to
parents and may have a strong fear of parental breakup and
divorce. They usually have internal conflict and ambiguous
feelings about taking sides, preferring a neutral and aloof demeanor.

    B. Statutes exist in all 50 states regarding the reporting of suspected
cases of child abuse and neglect. In all states, anyone can report a
case of suspected child abuse and neglect; however, states differ regarding who is mandated to make a report. Certain states mandate
everyone to report suspected child abuse and neglect; others mandate particular professionals to report abuse, such as, doctors,
nurses, teachers, social workers, and law enforcement officers. All
states provide the reporter with immunity from civil and criminal
liability, provided the report is made in good faith.

    C. Preventive measures.

CHAPTER 7   Violence

1. Promote prenatal classes to help the expectant mother and her partner prepare for parenting and for the changes a child will bring to their lives.
2. Develop high school parenting classes to prepare the adolescent for the physical and emotional care of a child and the enormous responsibilities of parenting.
3. Educate teachers and society in general regarding detection, prevention, and reporting of suspected child abuse.
4. Initiate parent groups, hotlines, respite services, day care centers, and other parental support systems if they are not available in the community.
5. Removal of the child from the home to prevent further abuse may be required when intervention methods have failed.
6. Involved agencies should follow up with the family after the child has returned home and should provide ongoing counseling and services as needed.
7. Refer high-risk parents for services. The high-risk parent may display any one or a combination of the following:
   a. Low self-esteem.
   b. History of being abused and no parenting role models.
   c. Coping problems with daily activities.
   d. Unrealistic expectations and attitudes toward the child.
   e. No friends or distrust of others.
   f. Weak coping skills when faced with a crisis.
   g. Personal needs are lacking, such as food, housing, and employment.
   h. Significant illness or the birth or presence of a child with special needs.
   i. Little or no support from spouse.
   j. Inadequate financial resources.

WEB SITES

Child Trauma Academy
  http://www.childtrauma.org
Prevent Child Abuse America
  http://www.preventchildabuse.org
Child Welfare League of America
  http://www.cwla.org
Child Welfare Information Gateway
  http://www.childwelfare.gov

VIOLENCE IN THE SCHOOLS

PEER HARASSMENT AND BULLYING

I. Definition

A. Peer harassment and bullying are repeated hurtful actions directed at one person or group by another person or group. It is repeated oppression of a weaker or less stable individual or group that affects the physical, emotional, or psychological well-being of its victims. Bullying may run the gamut from casual teasing, name calling, and exclusion to threatening physical safety.

II. Etiology

A. Peer competition, aggression, and conflict commonly are expressed in the form of teasing, taunting, name calling, rumor mongering, scapegoating, threats, intimidation, hitting, stealing of items, and minor nonverbal actions, such as scowls, negative finger movements, and social ostracism or physical isolation.

B. Victims of peer harassment and bullying (PH&B) are often those students who are small of stature, overweight, passive and quiet, socially isolated or nonconformist, new or transient, ethnic or racially diverse, or disabled. Victims are often physically weaker than their peers, insecure, and unlikely to defend themselves. Their parents are usually overprotective. Peer pressure precludes reporting of incidences to adults and teachers, and parents are perceived as ineffective.

C. Studies have indicated that students at low risk include those who are popular, from intact families, high achieving, academically or athletically proficient, and those recognized, rewarded, and liked by school staff.

D. Bullies have higher rates of tobacco and alcohol use, and bullying is an early sign of future antisocial behavior. Bullies may come from homes where corporal punishment is used; parents or guardian may not show empathy or may lack warmth. Bullies may appear to have a strong self-esteem but are defiant toward authority, and they like the feeling of power. Research concludes that boys are more likely to bully or be bullied. Although physical aggression is more prevalent among boys, incidence is rapidly increasing among girls. Generally, however, boys use physical aggression and girls use psychological combat, such as ridicule, social isolation, or malicious gossip.

III. Characteristics

A. Increased absenteeism by student victim and internalizing disorders, such as acute anxiety (fears, phobias, and panic attacks), depression, and psychosomatic illness (headaches, stomachaches, and muscle ailments). A nationwide study reports that bullying behavior in American schools affects 1 in every 3 children (Nansel et al, 2001). Bullying is reported at 26% of primary schools, 43% of middle schools, and 25% of secondary schools (DeVoe et al, 2005).

IV. Health Concerns and Emergencies

A. Treat injuries, both physical and emotional.

B. Follow emergency care and school procedures in cases of violent aggression with use of firearms.

V. Effects on Individual

A. Victim.
1. Feigns illness to avoid school. May have recurring unexplained physical symptoms while at school.
2. May cry, display sadness or fright, or become depressed.
3. May experience enuresis.
4. Shows signs of low self-esteem or may exhibit behavioral changes, such as going from passive and withdrawn to aggressive.

5. Exhibits signs of injury.
6. Avoids particular people, situations, or places and displays signs of fear when questioned about circumstances.
7. Frequently missing money or personal possessions.
8. Experiences decrease in academic performance.
9. Suffers from social isolation and insomnia; may become suicidal.
   B. Bullies.
   1. Want attention.
   2. Often do not assume responsibility for their actions.
   3. Have a need to win.
   4. Observe their victim and choose a person they can intimidate or tyrannize.
   5. Have low self-esteem; at risk for depression or suicide.
   6. Sixty percent of childhood male bullies have an arrest record by the time the reach their twenties (Fox et al, 2003).

VI. Management/Treatment

NOTE: Be aware of individual state laws for prevention and reporting.

Because bullying has been common in public and private schools for generations, school staff have not given the necessary attention to prevention, intervention, and postvention. The recent alarming research has been a wake-up call for educators, counselors, and nurses to design and manage a positive, proactive, school-wide culture of cooperation and care for all students. As the health care member of the school staff, the nurse can collaborate with staff to initiate the following practices:

   A. Take health histories to target PH&B.
   B. Solicit relevant information regarding PH&B when providing health care. Ask where it happens, when, what happens, and who is there.
   C. Assist student to increase self-esteem and confidence—encourage them to stand up straight, walk with confidence, maintain eye contact, develop skills for making and keeping new friends, and assign a student peer model.
   D. Provide timely and appropriate intervention when cruelty or discrimination is observed.
   E. Refer to counselor, social worker, principal, and parents. Discuss peer counseling and conflict resolution if not already used in the school.
   F. Prepare and distribute critical incident report to parents and staff.
   G. Educate staff regarding awareness of bullying. Discuss monitoring lunchroom, locker areas, and hallways; teach positive social skills; establish and post clear antibullying rules.
   H. Assist in follow-up counseling, discipline, and sanctions for the bully. A program called *Olweus Bullying Prevention Program* has had international success. Other programs can be found through Web sites on bullying in schools and through the Office of Community-Oriented Policing Services (COPS).

VII. Additional Information

   A. Cyberbullying is a new phenomenon that can include defamatory emails, text messaging, and postings in a chat room or on personal Web sites. These messages are often chronic and can be very hurtful. Bullying is done anonymously; there is no one to monitor the messages sent on computers or cell phones; and victims cannot escape the bullying, because it is omnipresent in their high-tech world, and these activities are usually undertaken apart from adult supervision. The victim is often afraid to report cyberbullying to parents for fear of losing access to the technology (e.g., cell phones, Internet). There are now ways to combat cyberbullying.

1. Saved messages can be used as evidence by police, your telephone company, or your Internet service provider (ISP). Save as much information as you can by copying the email with full header and forwarding it to your ISP. This information allows tracking of the perpetrator.
2. For chat room bullying, save the date, time, name, and web address of the chat room. Save the nickname and email address of the bully and a screen shot of the chat.
3. Do not erase or delete text messaging or reply to the cyberbully; the messages can be used as evidence. Similar words may be used that can be recognized as someone you know. Encourage students to tell an adult and get help.

WEB SITES

Bully Police USA
    http://www.bullypolice.org
Net Family News
    http://www.netfamilynews.org
Office of Community Oriented Policing Services (COPS)
    http://www.cops.usdoj.gov
Olweus Bullying Prevention Program
    http://www.clemson.edu/olweus
Stop Bullying Now: U.S. Health Resources and Services Administration (HRSA)
    http://www.stopbullyingnow.hrsa.gov
Wired Kids
    http://www.wiredkids.org

PHYSICAL AGGRESSION AND ASSAULT

Another category of school violence is the occurrence of hurt or harm from one student to another by pushing, shoving, hitting, kicking, biting, and pinching that leads to bodily injury and personal humiliation. Peer verbal abuse is a frequent antecedent to physical harm and assault. Physical assaults with weapons such as sticks, furniture, eating utensils, knives, and guns result in abrasions, lacerations, contusions, concussions, fractures, severe bleeding wounds, loss of consciousness, and death; so some of these injuries are beyond nursing care. This level of school violence leads to administrative action, school security intervention, primary health care provider services, emergency medicine, paramedic treatment, or emergency room care.

Recent statistics indicate a decrease in school violence. The rate of violent crime decreased in schools, from 48 per thousand in 1992 to 28 per thousand in 2003. However, violence is still widespread. In 2003 there were 740,000 violent acts committed against students ages 12 to 18 (DeVoe et al, 2005).

Students who are victims or witnesses of violent behaviors develop specific emotional and psychosocial distress symptoms, including pervasive fear, feelings of vulnerability, traumatic memories, and sleep disorders. Exposure to violence also has been associated with truancy, school avoidance, phobias, hypervigilance, inability to concentrate or learn, and school dropout. Frequent or severe student violence creates an atmosphere of insecurity and mistrust that lowers student body morale and motivation for academic achievement (Warner and Weist, 1996). Posttraumatic reactions are common for student victims, and some may experience PTSD.

School nurse interventions for physical aggression and assaults are the same as those listed for PH&B. Other effective violence-prevention practices and policies adopted countrywide for school sites include the following:

1. Vigilant adult supervision of the student body throughout the school day, especially in high-risk areas (e.g., restrooms, playgrounds, stairways), before and after school, and during transitions.
2. Staff development and training in critical incident management and crisis intervention.
3. Classroom training in anger management and conflict resolution.
4. Increased use of peer mediation, peer counselors, and helpers.
5. Additional uniformed security guards and supervisory staff on playgrounds and after school hours.
6. Hallway and classroom camera surveillance, better lighting, more open spaces.
7. Intensive mental health services for perpetrators and victims.
8. Zero tolerance for student violence; consequences may include suspensions, mandated counseling services, expulsion, and referral to educational and psychosocial treatment services.

WEB SITES

National Center for Juvenile Justice
    http://ncjj.servehttp.com/NCJJWebsite/main.htm
Office of Juvenile Justice and Delinquency Prevention Statistical Briefing Book
    http://www.ojjdp.ncjrs.org/ojstatbb/index.html

LIFE THREATS AND HOMICIDES

The most serious student violence consists of threats to human life and limb and actual incidences of homicides. Overall, homicide is the fourth leading cause of death for children ages 1 to 11, and it is the third leading cause of death for juveniles aged 12 to 17 (Snyder and Sickmund, 2005). Rates of violent crime have decreased substantially from 1992 to 2001, both in and away from school (DeVoe et al ,2006).

High-profile school shootings throughout the country have resulted in the identification of those at high risk for perpetrating violence. They have the following factors in common:

1. Boys and older students.
2. Victims of physical abuse, sexual abuse, or both.
3. A background of neglect.
4. Antisocial or delinquent histories.
5. Unpopular students and victims of bullying.
6. History of poor school relationships and academic failure.

7. History of substance abuse and access to firearms.
8. Depression and/or personality disorders (e.g., antisocial personality).
9. Those who threaten or resort to intimidation for control or power.
10. Heavy exposure to violence in the media.
11. Member of a hate group or cult.

Additional violence prevention and intervention practices and policies for homicides include the following:

1. Quick prosecution and sentencing for juvenile perpetrators of violence and crime.
2. Early detection and treatment for high-risk students.
3. Threat-appraisal teams and intervention services.
4. Available crisis intervention teams and posttraumatic support services.
5. Gun control enforcement and limited access to weapons.
6. Timely school cancellations in response to threats and campus-wide lockdown during violent episodes.

In developing effective and cost-efficient intervention strategies, no easy answers or certain solutions exist to prevent violence in the schools (Lamberg, 1998). Research concludes that positive policies and practices are more effective than punitive ones (Dusenbury et al, 1997); however, children and youths are still safer at school than in their homes or communities (DeVoe et al, 2005). School nurses should be careful not to generalize from past dramatic and sensational school violence episodes with catastrophic predictions and an ominous perspective. Nurses should join with other responsible school adults, concerned parents, and prosocial students to provide a protective shield and a caring ethos in the school setting.

GANGS

I. Definition

    A. A group of individuals, usually peers, that are bound together by camaraderie, loyalty, a common sense of purpose, and common clothing or colors. Gangs are cliques and groups with social and antisocial objectives. Studies estimate about 840,500 U.S. youths are in gangs (Youth Violence, Report of the Surgeon General, 1999).

II. Etiology

    A. Multiple long-term factors are involved, which can include poor parenting; lack of parental involvement, supervision, and support; low self-esteem and confidence; antisocial or aggressive behaviors with rejection by peers; poor school achievement; and increased truancy. Alcohol consumption, drug abuse, gambling, or combinations of these factors are common among gang members. Gangs are more common in urban schools (DeVoe et al, 2005).

III. Characteristics

    A. Informal social groups with unusual names.
    B. Signing, display of gestures.
    C. Representation by clothing, mannerisms, display of actions on one side of body (e.g., bandanna on one arm, cut across one eyebrow).
    D. Wearing colors that display gang allegiance.
    E. Possessing unexplained cash or goods.
    F. Breaks curfews, rules, and laws.

    G. Sacrifices morals and feelings for those of the gang.

    H. Developmental needs and goals are no different than those of youths who are not gang members.

    I. Gang is structured, secure, and protective.

    J. Most members drop out of gangs by age 20.

    K. Antisocial outcome factors associated with gang activity include drug availability in or near school; graffiti or tagging, which marks particular gang territory as a warning; presence of weapons; drive-by shootings; daytime burglaries; and an increased number of racially motivated incidences.

IV. Health Concerns/Emergencies

    A. Homicide.

    B. Bodily injury from violence, including rape.

    C. Disfigurement and risk of infection and disease (e.g., hepatitis B from tattoos and piercings).

    D. Incarcerations.

    E. Drug and alcohol use.

    F. Sexual activity.

V. Effects on Individual

    A. Lack of personal or academic success, school failure.

    B. Sense of belonging and purpose, although not socially acceptable.

    C. Negative peer pressure related to association with gangs or unpopular reference groups.

    D. Radical peer orientation contrary to parental bonding and family association.

    E. Change in personality and preference for nickname or street name.

    F. Outcomes can include violence recidivism, criminality, incarceration, and premature death.

    G. Effects extend to the community and society in general (e.g., increased financial liability, impact on criminal justice system, decreased individual safety and freedom, loss of life and productivity).

VI. Management/Treatment

    A. Start intervention early in life. Early prevention and intervention techniques include support techniques for good parenting skills, appropriate social and emotional support; referrals to centers for child care and management of behavioral, aggressive, and violence problems.

    B. Provide school-age support: school staff can be more tolerant of students who have different personal styles, ethnic backgrounds, and behaviors. All children need to be needed; tasks can be assigned in the school setting—nurse's assistant or runner for secretary—to increase self-esteem and provide sense of accomplishment, acceptance, and feelings of belonging.

    C. School security may profile known gang members and provide additional monitoring of these students.

VII. Additional Information

    A. Incarcerated youths have higher incidences of physical abuse, learning disabilities, psychiatric illness, lead toxicity, and early sexual activity.

    B. Much attention has been directed to school violence, including the use of guns and weapons by students on school sites across the country.

News stories are dramatic and shocking, but national incidences should not lead the school nurse to postulate that schools are unsafe places for students.

WEB SITES

Gang Resistance Education and Training (GREAT)
http://www.great-online.org
National Criminal Justice Reference Service
http://www.ncjrs.gov
Institute for Intergovernmental Research: National Youth Gang Center
http://www.iir.com/nygc
Youth Crime Watch of America
http:///www.ycwa.org

BIBLIOGRAPHY

American Psychiatric Association: *Diagnostic and statistical manual of mental disorders,* ed 4, text revision, Washington, DC, 2000, American Psychiatric Association.

Behrman R, Larner M, Stevenson C: Protecting children from abuse and neglect analysis and recommendations, *The Future of Children* 8(1), 1998, Packard Foundation.

Belsey B: *Cyberbullying: an emerging threat to the "always on" generation* (available online): www.cyberbullying.ca. Accessed June 2006.

Carpenito, L: *Nursing diagnosis: application to clinical practice,* Philadelphia, 2000, Lippincott Williams & Wilkins.

Centers for Disease Control and Prevention, National Center for Injury Prevention and Control: Sexual violence prevention (available online): www.cdc.gov/ncipc/factsheets/svfacts.htm. Accessed June 2006.

Child Welfare Information Gateway: *Long-term consequences of child abuse and neglect* (available online): www.childwelfare.gov/pubs/factsheets/long_term_consequences.cfm. Accessed June 2006.

Davidson R, Putnam K, Larson C: Dysfunction in the neural circuitry of emotion regulation: a possible prelude to violence, *Science* 289:591-594, 2006.

DeVoe JF, Peter K, Noonan M, et al: *Indicators of school crime and safety* (NCES 2006-001/NCJ 210697), US Dept of Education and Justice, Washington, DC, 2005, US Govt Printing Office.

Dusenbury L, Falco M, Lake A: Nine critical elements of promising violence prevention programs, *J Sch Health* 67(10):409-414, 1997.

Enserink M: Searching for the mark of Cain, *Science* 289:575-579, 2000.

Farrington DP, Loeber R: Epidemiology of juvenile violence. In Lewis DO, Yeager CA, eds: *Child and adolescent psychiatric clinic,* Philadelphia, 2000, WB Saunders.

Favazza A: The coming of age of self-mutilation, *J Nerv Ment Dis* 186(5):259-268, 1998.

Finberg L: *Saunders manual of pediatric practice,* Philadelphia, 2002, WB Saunders.

Fox JA, Elliott DS, Kerlikowske RG et al: *Bullying prevention is crime prevention,* Washington, DC, 2003, Fight Crime: Invest in Kids.

Giardino AP, Datner EM, Asher JB: *Sexual assault: victimization across the life span, a clinical guide,* St Louis, 2003, GW Medical.

Girardin BW, Faugno DK, Seneski PC et al, editors: *Color atlas of sexual assault,* ed 1, St Louis, 1997, Mosby.

Glaser D: Child abuse and neglect and the brain: a review, *J Child Psychol Psychiatry* 41(1):97-116, 2000.

Grunbaum J, Kann L, Kinchen S: Youth Risk Behavior Surveillance, United States, 2003. In *Surveillance summaries* (MMWR No SS-2), Atlanta, 2004, Centers for Disease Control and Prevention.

Violence

CHAPTER 7

Heim C, Newport DJ, Heit S: Pituitary-adrenal and autonomic responses to stress in women after sexual and physical abuse in childhood, JAMA 284(5): 592-597, 2000.

Hockenberry MJ, Wilson D, Winkelstein, ML, Kline, NE: *Wong's nursing care of infants and children,* St Louis, 2003, Mosby.

Kress V: Self-injurious behaviors: assessment and diagnosis, *J Counseling Dev* 81(4): 490-496, 2003.

Muelhlenkamp J, Gutierrez P: An investigation of differences between self-injurious behavior and suicide attempts in a sample of adolescents, *Suicide and Life-Threatening Behavior* 34(1):12-22, 2004.

Nansel TR, Overpeck M, Pilla RS: Bullying behaviors among U.S. youth: prevalence and association with psychosocial adjustment, *JAMA* 285(16):2131-2132, 2001.

Niehoff, D: *The biology of violence: how understanding the brain, behavior, and environment can break the vicious circle of aggression,* New York, 2002, Free Press.

Olweus D, Limber S, Mihalic S: Bullying prevention program. In Elliott DS, ed: *Blueprints for violence prevention: book nine,* Boulder, Colo, 1999, Center for the Study and Prevention of Violence.

Perry, BD: Childhood experience and the expression of genetic potential: what childhood neglect tells us about nature and nurture, *Brain Mind* 3:79-100, 2002.

Perry BD, Marcellus JE: *The impact of abuse and neglect on the developing brain,* Colleagues for Children 7:1-4, 1997. Missouri Chapter of the National Committee to Prevent Child Abuse.

Pollak SD, Cicchetti D, Hornung K: Recognizing emotion in faces: developmental effects of child abuse and neglect, *Dev Psychol* 35(5):679-688, 2000.

Post R, Weiss S: Emergent properties of neural systems: how focal molecular neurobiological alterations can affect behavior, *Dev Psychopathol* 9:907-929, 1997.

Rogeness G, McClure E: Development and neurotransmitter–environmental interactions, *Dev Psychopathol* 8:183-199, 1996.

Ross S, Heath N: Two models of adolescent self-mutilation, *Suicide Life Threat Behav* 33 (3):277-287, 2003.

Snyder HN, Sickmund M: *Juvenile offenders and victims: 2006 national report,* Washington, DC, 2006, US Dept of Justice, Office of Justice Programs, Office of Juvenile Justice and Delinquency Prevention.

Suyemoto K, Kountz X: Self-mutilation, *Prevention Researcher* 6(94):1-11, 2000.

Sylwester R: The neurobiology of self-esteem and aggression, *Educational Leadership* Feb:75-79, 1997.

Teicher MD: Wounds that time won't heal: the neurobiology of child abuse. *Cerebrum: the Dana forum on brain science* 2(4):50-67, 2000.

US Department of Health and Human Services, Administration for Children and Families: *Child maltreatment 2004,* Washington, DC, 2006, Government Printing Office (available online): www.acf.hhs.gov/programs/cb/pubs/cm04/index.htm.

US Department of Health and Human Services: *National strategy for suicide prevention goals and objectives for action: summary,* Washington, DC, 2001 (available online): www.mentalhealth.samhsa.gov/suicideprevention/strategy.asp.

US Department of Health and Human Services: *Youth violence: a report of the surgeon general,* Washington, DC, 1999: www.surgeongeneral.gov/library/youthviolence.

US Public Health Service: *The surgeon general's call to action to prevent suicide. 2006.* Available online: http://www.mentalhealth.org/suicideprevention/calltoaction.asp.

Warner BS, Weist MD: Urban youth as witnesses to violence: beginning assessments and treatment efforts, *J Youth Adolesc* 25:361-377, 1996.

Wolak J, Mitchell K, Finkelhor D: *Online victimization of youth: five years later,* 2006, National Center for Missing & Exploited Children (available online): www.missingkids.com/en_US/publications/NC167.pdf#search%22online%20victimization%20of%20youth%22.

CHAPTER 8

Adolescent and Gender-Specific Issues

*P*roviding comprehensive care to adolescents with an emphasis on preventive and proactive health care services is a strategic and challenging role for school nurses. Adolescents are an at-risk population for accidents, illness, and inconsistent health care, and they have a challenging lifestyle, often with inadequate nutrition, sleep deprivation, and poor physical fitness habits. Because they live for the moment, adolescents take their health for granted, unaware of the long-term implications of poor health habits. Subject to peer pressure that promotes experimentation with technology, toxic substances, and sexuality, they often become victims of accidents, illness, and addictions. Brain research adds a new reference to understanding adolescent behavior (see Chapter 1, Growth and Development Characteristics).

Nurses who work with middle school and high school students need resources to consistently and creatively provide health information. Health screening, diagnosis, management, and treatment of diseases should be accessible to adolescents, and the confidentiality provided by state laws should be respected. Nurses should involve families when possible.

Adolescents are peer oriented, and interventions centralized among teens as helpers and trainers result in optimal outcomes for adolescent compliance. The nurse should support and oversee programs such as peer tutoring, counseling, and safe-sex education, antidrug dramas and plays, and Students Against Destructive Decisions (SADD).

School health clinics on high school campuses throughout the United States have provided health education services since the late 1980s. These clinics often are staffed by school nurses, school nurse practitioners, or nurse practitioners with a specialty in adolescent medicine. Other health care staff may include adolescent primary care physicians, mental health practitioners, and other public health providers.

Every nurse requires up-to-date, reliable reference guides and manuals to access best practices for adolescent health care. This chapter addresses general health issues, gender-specific issues, sexually transmitted infections (STIs), and breast and testicular self-examinations. Some controversial and basic adolescent concerns are presented; these include tattooing, body piercing, steroid use, cosmetic-related skin care concerns, and oral health care. Other adolescent health issues are covered elsewhere in the manual; these include eating disorders, obesity, depression, rape, herpes I and herpes II infections, and suicide. The bibliography at the end of this chapter lists useful resources.

General guidelines and frames of reference for nurses serving adolescent students in middle schools and high schools include the following:

- Adolescence is a time of change, experimentation, and risk taking.
- Adolescents should be encouraged to pursue a positive, proactive lifestyle based on healthy choices regarding self-care and personal health.
- School nurses should affirm the decision-making and problem-solving capacities of the adolescent for self-determination in the context of confidential delivery of service.
- Adolescents have a great capacity for individual responsibility and can be supported and strengthened by personal grievance and treatment contracts with school nurses, teachers, and parents.
- Health care providers (HCPs) should assess risk factors to maximize the resiliency of the vulnerable adolescent.
- Given the effect of peer orientation on the adolescent, preventive health care efforts should promote a positive peer culture, whereby teenagers assume responsibility for the well-being of one another.
- Every effort should be made to strengthen the adolescent's resources within the family and the support they receive from parents or parent surrogates, such as foster parents and group home staff.
- The stage of adolescence is fundamental to the formation of attitudes and personal habits regarding health that have long-range effects on quality of life and the onset of diseases and disabilities.

The nurse should:
- Be skilled at using health history and high-risk inventories.
- Provide anticipatory guidance in social, sexual, peer pressure, nutrition, exercise, substance abuse, and risk-taking behavioral issues.
- Be aware of important mental health issues.
- Be able to say "I don't know, but I can find out and get back to you."

GENERAL CONDITIONS

ACNE VULGARIS

I. Definition
A. Chronic skin condition of the pilosebaceous units, well-developed sebaceous glands with miniature hairs, usually located on the face, neck, upper chest, shoulders, and upper back. Acne is the result of an interaction between keratin, sebum, and sometimes bacteria. When the opening of the follicle is tight, it appears to be white and is referred to as a *whitehead* (closed comedo); when the pore is open to the air, it appears black and is referred to as a *blackhead* (open comedo). The black color probably is due to the melanin pigment in the skin and does not represent dirt.

II. Etiology
A. The causes of acne include a strong genetic predisposition; increased secretion of hormones, specifically androgens, which trigger production of oil (sebum) on the skin; and plugged oil ducts that allow bacteria on the skin to multiply and produce redness and swelling. The exact mechanisms of acne are unknown.
B. Many adolescents (80%) develop some degree of acne (Darmstadt and Sidbury, 2004). No scientific link has been identified between diet and acne, but some individuals have acne breakouts after eating certain foods.

III. Characteristics
A. Usually observed between the ages of 12 and 17, but it can begin as early as age 8 and can last for 10 to 15 years.
B. Boys have more severe acne that lasts a shorter time, and girls have milder acne that lasts a longer time.
C. Whiteheads may resolve spontaneously or rupture, resulting in an inflamed pustule, or pimple.
D. Inflammation, redness, and swelling can occur and may result in pustules, papules, nodules, and cysts, some of which may cause scars.
E. Inflammation, slow healing, and possible scar formation may occur as a result of trauma (e.g., picking, wearing athletic gear).
F. Hormonal triggers, such as premenstrual flares, occur in about 25% to 50% of females with acne (Darmstadt and Sidbury, 2004).
G. Acne is aggravated and intensified by emotional stress or nervous tension.
H. Oil-based cosmetics may increase the likelihood of comedones; adolescents should avoid occlusive products, such as cocoa butter and vitamin E oil.

I. Acne is exacerbated by certain medications, such as androgenic oral contraceptives (e.g., Lo-Ovral, Nordette), barbiturates, hydantoin (Dilantin), corticotropin (Acthar), and oral and topical steroids.

J. Acne can be exacerbated by environmental factors where adolescents work (e.g., exposure to cooking oils in fast-food facilities, grease in auto repair shops).

IV. Health Concerns/Emergencies

A. *Excoriée des filles,* or *picker's acne,* is a superficial type of acne caused by compulsive picking of trivial facial lesions, which causes secondary damage and often leads to scarring. Picking is also seen in teens who abuse methamphetamines.

B. *Acne fulminans* is rare but occurs in adolescent boys and manifests with inflammatory nodules and plaques, which lead to severe pustules that leave large ulcerations. Onset is abrupt with fever, weight loss, anemia, and polyarthritis.

C. Differential diagnosis.

    1. Flat warts: skin-colored papules that spread with trauma.

    2. Rosacea, milia, folliculitis, and cosmetic, environmental, mechanical, or drug-induced acne. Acne clears with removal of causative factors.

V. Management/Treatment

A. Preventive health education or sex education and family education classes.

B. Student education should include the following recommendations:

    1. Wash face with a mild soap, such as Neutrogena; harsh and frequent scrubbing may irritate the skin.

    2. Do not pick, scrub, or squeeze acne

    3. Identify aggravating agents, such as oil-based cosmetics, face creams, hairspray, or mousse.

    4. Discuss psychosocial concerns.

    5. Encourage compliance with treatment regimen, because it takes months to clear acne; some teenagers believe particular foods are related to a flare-up, so recommend avoidance of those foods.

    6. Discuss lack of documentation that cola, chocolate, nuts, or french fries cause acne, but emphasize the importance of a well-balanced diet for healthy skin.

    7. Avoid sun when using tretinoin (Retin-A) or antibiotics (e.g., tetracycline [Achromycin], minocycline [Dynacin, Minocin]).

    8. If acne does not resolve, referral to a dermatologist for prescription medication is indicated.

C. Monitor side effects of medications.

D. Medications include topical agents (e.g., tretinoin, adapalene, acetylinic retinoid, benzoyl peroxide); systemic therapy to clear eruptions and prevent recurrence (e.g., tetracycline, clindamycin, minocycline, doxycycline, erythromycin); acne surgery, extraction of comedones, or incision and drainage; and peeling treatments, or cryotherapy with liquid nitrogen to remove superficial skin. Usually 6 to 8 weeks are required before significant improvement is noted with antibiotic treatment.

E. Isotretinoin (Accutane) is an important prescription antiacne treatment for severe nodulocystic acne that does not respond to antibiotic therapy. It is a major teratogenic drug and must not be taken during pregnancy or lactation. A pregnancy test must be performed before use, and parents of minors must sign a patient consent form regarding birth defects and Accutane. Girls who cannot take Accutane may be given a trial of hormonal therapy, which may include oral contraceptives.

F. Warnings for adolescents taking prescribed medications include the following:
1. When systemic antibiotics are prescribed, girls taking oral contraceptives should use a back up method of contraception for the first 2 weeks.
2. Effective contraception must be used 1 month before, during, and 1 month after therapy with isotretinoin for sexually active adolescents.
3. Sun exposure should be avoided, particularly with certain medications (e.g., tetracycline, tretinoin, isotretinoin).

WEB SITES

American Academy of Dermatology
   http://www.aad.org
MedlinePlus: Acne
   http://www.nlm.nih.gov/medlineplus/acne.html

COSMETIC-RELATED SKIN CARE CONCERNS

I. Definition
A. The regular use of products—specifically by teenage girls—to cleanse, enhance, beautify, or alter appearance may contribute to irritation, infection, and physical health problems.

II. Etiology
A. Cosmetic-related skin care concerns may be associated with the integrity of the skin or nails, predisposition, or family genetics. The type of product, amount used, frequency, and lack of adherence to recommended use also may contribute to skin care concerns. Product ingredients, such as fragrances and preservatives, may cause contact dermatitis and allergic reactions. Using outdated cosmetics or the sharing of products may cause adverse reactions. Table 8-1 lists potential risks of cosmetic products.

III. Characteristics
A. Health concerns usually develop within the first few applications of a cosmetic or skin care product but may develop after continual use.
B. Reaction to products depends on the skin condition and the immune system.
C. Open skin lesions may be irritated, or an allergic reaction to the product may occur.
D. Overly dry, sensitive, or oily skin may lead to obstructed pores.
E. Burning, itching, stinging, and redness are indicators of irritation.
F. Sunlight may potentiate the allergen or irritant in the product.

Adolescent and Gender-Specific Issues

CHAPTER 8

Table 8-1	*Potential Risks of Cosmetic Products*	
Products	**Risks**	**Comments**
Artificial nails	Fungal infection may lead to permanent nail loss. Nail may peel and crack with methacrylate-free glue. Methacrylate is an allergen.	May be avoided when complete seal is made between natural and artificial nail. Avoid methacrylate-free glue.
Nail polish	May cause rash on other parts of body that have been exposed before drying (face, eyelids, neck, fingers).	Avoid touching body, or try hypoallergenic polish.
Hair dye	Semipermanent and permanent dyes may cause contact dermatitis or immediate reactions that include hives and wheezing.	Be aware of personal allergens and avoid those ingredients. Temporary dyes usually are nonallergenic.
Hair shampoo	May irritate and dry skin or scalp.	Change product brand.
Hair permanents	Can damage hair and cause brittle, dry hair and scalp irritation.	Do not use more frequently than every 3 months; do not use on damaged or dyed hair without corrective products. Always follow instructions.
Aerosol sprays	Risk of fire. Contamination of food may occur. Inhalation may cause lung damage.	Avoid use while smoking or when near heat or fire. Keep away from foods. Avoid inhaling product.
Powders	Inhalation may cause lung damage.	Avoid when possible or apply gently to decrease airborne inhalation.

IV. Health Concerns/Emergencies

A. *Irritant contact dermatitis* may be caused by many products, including antiperspirants, soaps, detergents, cosmetics, moisturizers, shampoos, and permanent wave solutions.

B. *Allergic contact dermatitis* may be caused by cosmetic ingredients, such as fragrances and preservatives.

1. More than 5000 known additive fragrances are used in skin care products; hypoallergenic fragrances are available. By law, hypoallergenic products must be labeled, so users should check the label for indications that a product is fragrance-free. *Unscented* does not mean fragrance-free, because an additive may be used to disguise the chemical odor. Users must also check labels of products advertising natural ingredients to avoid plant or animal allergens.

2. Preservatives added to skin products are the second most common cause of contact dermatitis. These agents are added to preserve the

products from light and oxygen damage and to prevent bacterial and fungal growth that causes skin reactions. Preservatives must be added if a cosmetic contains water. Not all students will react to every preservative, and a reaction to one preservative does not imply that a reaction will occur to all preservatives.
   a. Preservatives include dimethylol dimethyl (DMDM) hydantoin, formaldehyde, imidazolidinyl urea, methylchloroisothiazolinone, phenoxyethanol, and quaternium-15.
 C. *Acne cosmetica* may be caused by the use of heavy, oil-based products. Check the product label for the term *noncomedogenic* or *nonacnegenic*; this means the product will not clog pores or cause acne.

V. Management/Treatment
 A. Discuss possible causes and available solutions with the student.
 B. Washing hands before applying cosmetics or performing skin care decreases contamination of skin and products. Bacteria in the products can contribute to skin irritation and decrease the effectiveness of the product.
 C. Use of products developed to maintain healthy skin—such as astringents, moisturizers, and sunscreens—may minimize potential concerns but also poses risks:
   1. Astringents may cause drying, itching, or burning of skin.
   2. Users may be allergic to some ingredients in moisturizers and sunscreens.
 D. Discuss proper use of cosmetics and skin care products:
   1. Makeup should be discarded if color or odor changes.
   2. Liquid should never be added unless indicated in the instructions.
   3. Containers should be stored away from sunlight and tightly closed to maintain active preservatives.
   4. Eye makeup should never be used if wearer has an active eye infection, such as conjunctivitis.
   5. Contaminated products should be discarded.
   6. Cosmetics should not be shared.
   7. Check expiration date on products, especially eye products.

WEB SITES

American Academy of Dermatology
   http://www.aad.org
Environmental Working Group
   http://www.cosmeticsdatabase.com

HOMOSEXUALITY
I. Definition
 A. Homosexuality is the persistent attraction to a member of the same sex. Same-sex attractions may have their onset in late elementary and early adolescence and may involve some homosexual experimentation.
II. Etiology
 A. The etiology of homosexuality is unknown. Several theories are associated with the cause of homosexuality: *genetic* (gene and twin

studies), *hormonal* (prenatal effects of sex hormones on the brain), *psychosocial circumstances* (learned behavior, lack of heterosexual exposure), *neurological* (prenatal development of brain structures and genitalia), and *combinations* (complex interplay of many theories).

III. Characteristics

A. Sexual identity is formed gradually over time and becomes more dominant in late adolescence and young adulthood.

B. Feeling of being different.

C. Acknowledgment of same-sex attraction.

D. Guilt and embarrassment regarding feelings.

E. Strives to change feelings by adapting behaviors and thoughts.

F. Unable to alter sexual preference.

G. Exploration of homosexual lifestyle.

H. May experiment with both sexes until preference or orientation is established.

I. Commitment to a lifestyle and pursuit of a positive image.

IV. Health Concerns/Emergencies

A. At risk for sexually transmitted infections (STIs); traumatic injuries related to intercourse should be assessed based on sexual behavior, not sexual orientation.

B. At risk for hepatitis A, B, and C and human immunodeficiency virus (HIV).

C. May have psychosocial problems adjusting to identity.

D. Increased risk for depression, substance abuse, and suicide.

E. Health care may not be adequate; some health care professionals lack understanding of special health issues and concerns involved with same-sex attraction and fear of HIV.

F. Documentation could jeopardize confidentiality and compromise a student's ability to obtain insurance or certain types of employment.

G. Concern for physical danger due to homophobia.

V. Management/Treatment

A. Listen to adolescents and encourage them to articulate concerns and fears about sexual orientation.

B. Screen and immunize for hepatitis A and B.

C. Recommend yearly testing for gonorrhea, syphilis, and chlamydia; encourage periodic HIV testing for students who are sexually active or substance abusers; discuss safe-sex practices.

D. Listen to and support parents; provide contact for support groups, such as the local chapter of Parents, Family, and Friends of Lesbians and Gays (PFLAG).

VI. Additional Information

A. Some heterosexual teens will engage in homosexual activity in certain environments (e.g., incarceration facilities, summer camps, military or boarding schools) but revert to heterosexual activities when environment changes. These experiences may lead to confusion and panic, especially when the teenager enjoys the activity.

B. Decisions made for a child with ambiguous genitalia may have been incorrect. Genitalia, genes, internal gender structures, and feelings may not match sexual assignment, causing inner confusion, guilt, and discontent (see Ambiguous Genitalia in Chapter 4).

C. Bisexual students are attracted to both sexes and engage in both heterosexual and homosexual behaviors. These sexual behaviors place them at increased risk for STIs and HIV.

WEB SITES

Sex, etc.: A Web Site by Teens for Teens
 http://www.sexetc.org
KidsHealth
 http://www.kidshealth.org/teen

DENTAL CARIES
I. Definition
A. Dental caries is the term used for progressive loss of tooth mineral caused by a bacterial infection, particularly *Streptococcus mutans*. It is the most common health problem for the school-age child.
II. Etiology
A. Formation of dental caries depends on dietary sucrose or fermentable carbohydrates that are broken down into sugar in the mouth. Bacteria in plaque feed on the sugar-producing organic acids, which demineralize the tooth.
III. Characteristics
A. Caries may begin in toddlers with bedtime bottle use and frequent intake of sugary drinks and foods.
B. Cavity-causing bacteria, *Streptococcus mutans,* may be spread from person to person (e.g., a mother or father with cavities may pass the bacteria to the baby through kissing).
C. Children's early cavities begin as white spots on the four upper front teeth, which is an indicator of demineralization.
D. Left untreated, cavities progress and cause pain, infection, and tooth loss.
IV. Health Concerns/Emergencies
A. Large holes in teeth, pain, inflammation with or without fistulas, or draining abscesses on gums in root area of teeth.
B. Premature loss of primary teeth can affect nutrition, speech, self-esteem, resulting in crowding of permanent teeth.
V. Management/Treatment
A. Refer for dental checkups beginning at age 1.
B. Biannual dental examinations.
C. Provide fluoride supplements in areas with nonfluoridated water supply up to age 18.
D. Brush twice a day and floss between teeth daily.
E. Limit intake of sweet, sticky foods and drinks, especially at snack time; provide fruits and vegetables.
F. Use a pea-sized amount of fluoride toothpaste daily as early as age 1 and a larger amount for adolescents.
G. Apply sealants on permanent molars when they erupt, around 6 years for first molars and 12 years for second molars (see Appendix D, Dental Development).

Adolescent and Gender-Specific Issues

CHAPTER 8

WEB SITE

American Dental Association
   http://www.ada.org

MALOCCLUSION, ORTHODONTIA, AND BRACES

I. Definition
  A. Orthodontics concern the diagnosis, prevention, and correction of malocclusion and irregularities of the teeth. Most orthodontic appliances exert continuous pressure to modify teeth positions and move or keep teeth aligned for an extended period of time. A variety of appliances are used, including fixed, removable, intraoral, and extraoral devices.

II. Etiology
  A. A common cause of malocclusion is genetics, but thumb sucking, tongue thrusting, trauma, dental disease, or early loss of primary or permanent teeth may be contributory factors.

III. Characteristics
  A. Malocclusion.
    1. Includes overbite, underbite, crossbite, rotated or twisted teeth, or an overcrowded mouth.
    2. May cause self-consciousness or embarrassment because of appearance of teeth.
    3. Chewing may be painful and ineffective.
    4. May interfere with speech.
    5. Could contribute to dental disease.
  B. Orthodontic appliances.
    1. May be uncomfortable, especially after initial placement and adjustments.
    2. Braces may be metal, attached with adhesives; clear and attached to outside surfaces; ceramic, appearing like natural teeth; minibraces; or invisible, which are fixed to the inside of the teeth.
    3. Head or neck gear is ordered when extra tension outside the mouth is needed; worn during the day, at night, or evening.
    4. Appliances may be needed from 6 months to 2 years or longer.

IV. Health Concerns/Emergencies
  A. Inability to brush teeth well may cause dental disease.
  B. Orthodontic wires may come loose and harm oral tissue.

V. Management/Treatment
  A. Assessment of pain for medication or referral to orthodontist.
  B. Analgesics: ibuprofen (Motrin) or acetaminophen (Tylenol) may be needed to relieve discomfort and pain. Never place medication directly on gums.
  C. Encourage wearing of orthodontic devices during lengthy treatment regimen and after treatment, if retainer devices are prescribed.
  D. First aid for broken braces and wires.
    1. If the damaged appliance can be removed, take it out.
    2. If unable to remove the appliance, cover sharp or protruding points with cotton balls, gauze, wax, or chewing gum.

3. If wire is stuck in the gums, cheek, or tongue, do not remove it; immediately refer student to a dentist or orthodontist.
4. Broken or loose appliance: usually does not need immediate attention unless it is bothersome.

VI. Additional Information
A. After appliances are removed, the teeth are cleaned thoroughly, and more x-ray films and impressions of the teeth may be taken. Monitor growth of wisdom teeth for possible extraction. Retention treatment may be needed to maintain teeth position and prevent shifting and moving of teeth until gums, bones, and muscles adapt to the change. Retainers may be ordered to be worn on a daily basis for a few months to several years. Retainers prevent shifting of teeth back to their prior position.

WEB SITE

American Dental Association
   http://www.ada.org

PERIODONTAL DISEASE
I. Definition
A. Periodontal disease, often called *gum disease,* refers to a pathological condition of the tissues surrounding and supporting the teeth.
II. Etiology
A. Periodontal disease usually is caused by plaque, a sticky film of bacteria that continuously forms on teeth. When the plaque is not removed, gums become irritated, inflamed, and begin detaching from teeth to form pockets, where bacteria can be harbored. When untreated, this process can destroy bone and other important tooth-supportive tissues, eventually leading to tooth loss.
III. Characteristics
A. Early stage.
   1. Called gingivitis.
   2. Gums are red, swollen, and bleed easily.
   3. Normally reversible through better brushing, flossing, and routine professional cleanings.
B. Late stage.
   1. Called periodontitis.
   2. Gums and bone that are supportive structures of the teeth are seriously damaged; pockets form, and gums recede or pull away from teeth.
   3. Teeth become loose and fall out or must be extracted.
C. Warning signs.
   1. Bleeding of gums while brushing.
   2. Tender, red, or swollen gums.
   3. Pulling away of gums from teeth.
   4. Separating or loose teeth.
   5. Pus between gums and teeth.
   6. Changes in the way teeth fit together when biting.

Adolescent and Gender-Specific Issues

CHAPTER 8

7. Pain usually is not present.
8. Persistent bad breath.

IV. Health Concerns/Emergencies

A. Inflammatory process can destroy bone and healthy tissue in and around the teeth.
B. Plaque or bacteria create toxins that can damage gums.
C. Bacteria or inflammatory response from gum disease may be associated with systemic problems, such as bacterial pneumonia, cardiovascular disease, or stroke.
D. Loss of teeth.

V. Management/Treatment

A. Brushing and flossing twice a day and use of proximal brush between teeth daily.
B. Routine dental assessments.
C. Avoidance of tobacco.
D. Eating a balanced diet.

VI. Additional Information

A. When plaque hardens, it becomes a porous, rough deposit called *tartar* or *calculus*. When hardened, plaque can be removed only by a dentist or dental hygienist. An instrument called a *periodontal probe* is used to measure the gingival sulcus depth around each tooth, and the space between the gums and teeth, to determine whether pockets are present. The normal depth between healthy gums and teeth is 3 mm or less.

WEB SITE

American Dental Association
   http://www.ada.org

TATTOOING AND BODY PIERCING

I. Definition

A. *Tattoos* are permanent body designs made by inserting a needle containing pigment into the dermal layer of the skin; this includes permanent facial makeup, such as eyebrow and lid-lining, and lip augmentation.
B. *Body piercing* is a creation of a hole anywhere in the body for placement of adornments. Areas commonly pierced include ears, eyebrows, nose, lip, tongue, breasts, navel, and genitalia on both males and females. Both tattoos and body piercing are considered body art.

II. Etiology

A. Tattoos and body piercing may express commitment to a significant other, or they may be an expression of individuality or beauty enhancement. They also may be symbols of loyalty to a particular group, such as gangs, motorcyclists, or military affiliations.

III. Characteristics

A. May be observed on various body areas.
B. Both procedures present a risk for infection. Box 8-1 and Box 8-2 describe care for new tattoos and body piercings to prevent infection.

Box 8-1 *New Tattoo*

- Leave dressing on for 2 to 12 hours or overnight; remove by gently soaking or showering.
- Clean with antibacterial or mild soap and pat dry.
- Do not use alcohol (drying) or hydrogen peroxide (cytotoxic) for cleaning.
- Do not use petroleum jelly; may cause heavy scabbing and will dull the tattoo.
- Apply antibiotic (Bacitracin) ointment for around 5 days, unless allergic reaction occurs.

- Do not disturb scab when applying antibiotic ointment.
- Application of cream or ointment can promote the healing process and help preserve color.
- Avoid sun exposure for approximately 4 weeks.
- Do not use tanning bed during healing.
- Avoid soaking in a hot tub, swimming, or taking hot baths for about 1 week, or until peeling has stopped.

Box 8-2 *New Body Piercing*

- Requires routine wound care.
- Wash at least twice daily with antibacterial soap and water; some oozing and edema are anticipated; if scabbing occurs, remove with a wet swab.
- Do not use alcohol (drying) or hydrogen peroxide (cytotoxic) for cleaning.
- *Navel piercing*: To minimize irritation, do not wear tight clothing over area. Navel piercings heal the slowest.
- *Tongue piercing*: After all meals and snacks, rinse with antibacterial mouthwash that

does not contain alcohol. If bad breath occurs or tongue color changes, the natural mouth bacteria may have been destroyed; change to salt water rinses. Ice reduces swelling; once healed, avoid smoking and use dental dams for dental work. Jewelry should be left in place until healing is complete, even if signs of infection occur, because removing jewelry may result in an abscess. Jewelry may need to be removed if an allergic reaction occurs.

C. Signs of infection include pain, redness, swelling or edema, and purulent discharge.

D. Signs of allergic reaction include swelling and itching. Box 8-3 lists the potential risks of piercing and tattooing.

E. Piercing is less permanent than tattooing.

F. Average age of first tattoo is 14 years; for first body piercing, average age is 15 years, but it does occur at younger ages.

G. Teenagers may like the shock value of tattooing or piercing in unusual places.

H. Table 8-2 lists the healing times for body piercings in various areas of the body.

IV. Health Concerns/Emergencies

A. Improper follow-up care by students.

B. Infections and hygienic concerns.

C. Swelling, inflammation, crusting, or scabs at tattoo or piercing site can occur.

D. Allergic reaction to tattoo dye.

| **Box 8-3** | *Potential Risks of Piercing and Tattooing* |

General
Bloodborne pathogen transmission
Risk of tetanus
Severe inflammation and swelling

Piercing
Allergic reaction to jewelry
Nerve or soft tissue damage; keloids
Dental fracture; speech impediments
Swelling of tongue and airway occlusion

Pain or impaired healing when jewelry is
  improperly sized
Aspiration of jewelry (oral piercings)
Prolonged bleeding (tongue piercings)
Easily infected (navel or oral piercing)

Tattooing
Severe allergic reaction to dyes
Sarcoidlike granuloma
Magnetic resonance imaging (MRI) com-
  plications; rare with short-term effects

| **Table 8-2** | *Healing Times for Body Piercing* |

Site and Tissue	Healing Time
Ear cartilage	4-12 mo
Earlobe	6-8 wk
Eyebrow	6-8 wk
Nostril	1-4 mo
Nasal septum	6-8 mo
Lip	2-3 mo
Tongue	4-8 wk
Nipple	2-6 mo
Navel	4-12 mo
Female genitalia	3-10 wk
Male genitalia	1-6 mo

    E. Should not donate blood for a year after receiving a tattoo or piercing.
    F. Possibility of serious infection from nonsterile needles and piercing equipment. Infections may include tetanus, hepatitis, and HIV infection.
    G. Potential complications can occur with piercing, including excessive bleeding, development of keloids, nerve and soft tissue damage, or speech impediment.
    H. Tattooing is typically done by unlicensed personnel. Permanent facial makeup usually is done by licensed personnel.

V. Management/Treatment
    A. Discuss with adolescents the possible health risks and stigma attached to piercings and tattooing particular body parts, and the fact that adolescents are doing these procedures.
    B. Suggest to adolescents that they:
        1. Talk with peers who have tattoos or piercings.
        2. Discuss expense, healing time, pain, and complications.
        3. Consider individuality and independent decision making.
        4. Suggest that they delay or change their decision.

C. If a decision to proceed is made, follow up with how to select a professional tattoo artist or piercer. Suggest they:
1. Use recommendations from peers or family.
2. Visit shops to observe room lighting, cleanliness, techniques for sterilization of equipment, and to talk with the piercer or tattooist.
3. Observe for hand washing, use of gloves, use of unopened ink containers and sterile, packaged equipment.
4. Use stainless steel, niobium, titanium, or 14K gold jewelry immediately after piercing.
5. When a piercing gun is used, be aware of potential tissue damage and lack of adequate sterilization that could lead to infection.
D. Treatment of infection includes the use of dicloxacillin (Diclox) or cephalexin (Keflex).
E. Check date of last tetanus injection.
VI. **Additional Information**
A. Many notable historical figures and celebrities who serve as role models for teenagers have tattoos and piercings. Body embellishment has been a tradition in many cultures. Late-nineteenth-century Victorian royalty preferred nipple and genital piercing, and Lady Randolph Churchill had a snake tattooed around her wrist. Most types of body adornment sought by adolescents have been done in earlier periods of history.
B. Adolescents may use *fake body jewelry* on the eyebrow, nose, tongue, eyelid, and other areas. This practice allows for the appearance of piercing with the advantage of easy removal in social situations not accepting of this practice.
C. *Tattoo removal* usually is possible but can be very expensive and is done over a long period. A laser is used, which may cause permanent discoloration in some cases.
D. During MRI scanning, tattoos and permanent makeup may cause burning or swelling in the affected area that may distort the clarity of the image (Mayo Clinic, 2006).

WEB SITES

American Dental Association: Oral Piercing
    http://www.ada.org
Mayo Clinic
    http://www.mayoclinic.com
KidsHealth
    http://www.kidshealth.org

GENDER-SPECIFIC CONDITIONS

NOTE: Teach students correct anatomy and physiology; many have no idea how the reproductive system works.

AMENORRHEA

I. **Definition**
A. *Primary amenorrhea* is failure to start menstruation by age 17; a medical examination is recommended if no secondary characteristics develop

by age 15, or if menarche does not occur within 2 years of development of secondary sexual characteristics. *Secondary amenorrhea* is the absence of menses for 6 months or 3 cycles after menarche has been established when pregnancy has been ruled out.

II. Etiology

A. The cause of primary amenorrhea may be genetic (e.g., Turner syndrome, structural abnormal X), or it may be caused by dysfunction of the hypothalamus, pituitary gland, ovary, uterus, or the congenital absence, malformation, or surgical removal of the uterus or both ovaries. May also be caused by medication.

B. Use of drugs such as marijuana, cocaine, heroin, tricyclic antidepressants, metoclopramide, cimetidine, and some contraceptive methods.

C. *Secondary amenorrhea* is the cessation of an established menstrual cycle caused by extreme weight loss or gain, systemic illness, extreme physical activity, or increased stress.

III. Characteristics

A. Primary amenorrhea.

   1. Absence of menses by age 17, absence of breast bud development by age 13, absence of menses more than 4 years after breast bud development, height and weight below 3% for age, cyclic lower abdominal pain without menses.

B. Secondary amenorrhea.

   1. Abrupt cessation of menstrual cycles, oligomenorrhea (scant, infrequent periods), or pregnancy symptoms.

IV. Management/Treatment

A. Complete reproductive history, including the following:

   1. Age of menarche, frequency and length of periods, amount of flow, presence of cramps, use of tampons or pads, last menstrual period (LMP).

   2. Family history of dysmenorrhea and gynecological problems.

   3. Past medical history, including hospitalizations or surgery, chronic illnesses, bleeding disorders.

   4. Medications, contraceptives, substance abuse.

   5. Related health issues, such as weight changes, nutrition, exercise, sports, emotional symptoms, and eating disorders.

B. Counsel student regarding extreme exercise and diet as appropriate. Supplementation, such as with calcium and protein, may be considered.

C. Referral for endocrine evaluation, which may include bone age, determination of follicle-stimulating hormone (FSH), luteinizing hormone (LH) levels, and karyotyping.

D. Oral contraceptives may be used to treat secondary amenorrhea and establish normal ovulatory cycles.

WEB SITES

Children's Hospital Boston, Center for Young Women's Health,
Sports and Menstrual Periods: The Female Athlete Triad
    http://www.youngwomenshealth.org/triad.html
TeensHealth: Coping with Common Period Problems
    http://www.kidshealth.org/teen/sexual_health/girls/menstrual_problems.html

DYSMENORRHEA

I. Definition

A. Dysmenorrhea is cramping and lower abdominal pain during menses. *Primary dysmenorrhea* incapacitates girls for 1 to 3 days, whereas *secondary dysmenorrhea* varies depending on the etiology. This is the most common cause of short-term school absenteeism for girls. The prevalence of dysmenorrhea is 38% at age 12 and 66% to 77% at age 17 (Slap, 2003).

II. Etiology

A. *Primary dysmenorrhea* occurs when no evidence of a pelvic pathological condition exists; however, a familial factor is associated. *Secondary dysmenorrhea* is caused by an underlying pathological condition, such as pelvic inflammatory disease (PID), endometriosis, uterine fibroids, polyps, or anatomical abnormalities. A higher level of prostaglandin release leads to strong uterine contractions and results in pain; this occurs in both primary and secondary dysmenorrhea.

B. For both types of dysmenorrhea, a cultural or family behavioral component influences the nature and extent of the adolescent response to menstrual discomfort.

III. Characteristics

A. Primary dysmenorrhea.
   1. Pain is crampy or spasmodic, bilateral, symmetrical, and may be referred to the lower back or anterior thighs. Pain may be accompanied by nausea, vomiting, and diarrhea.
   2. Obesity, longer menstrual periods, and use of intrauterine devices (copper) may contribute to increased dysmenorrhea.
   3. Pain lasts from a few hours to 3 days before and during start of menses.

B. Secondary dysmenorrhea.
   1. Pain may be dull and constant, accompanied by nausea, vomiting, and diarrhea.
   2. Dyspareunia.
   3. Pain may occur at menarche, or onset may be 3 or more years later.
   4. History of abnormal discharge, infection, intermenstrual bleeding, or menorrhagia.

IV. Management/Treatment

A. Complete reproductive history, including the following:
   1. Age of menarche, frequency and length of periods, amount of flow, presence of cramps, use of tampons or pads, and last menstrual period (LMP).
   2. Family history of dysmenorrhea and gynecological problems.
   3. Past medical history: hospitalizations or surgery, chronic illnesses, bleeding disorders.
   4. Medications, contraceptives, illicit drug use.
   5. Related health issues: weight changes, poor nutrition, excessive exercise, eating disorders, and school absenteeism.
   6. Sexual history: sexual activity, method of contraception, STDs, number of sexual partners, age of first coitus, types of sexual contact, sexual abuse.

Adolescent and Gender-Specific Issues

CHAPTER 8

B. Primary dysmenorrhea.
   1. Assure adolescent that pain is a normal occurrence with primary dysmenorrhea.
   2. Primary palliative treatment: use of pads instead of tampons, application of mild heat to abdomen, warm herbal teas, avoidance of salt, and increased exercise to increase endorphins.
   3. Muscle relaxation may be enhanced with use of supplements such as magnesium and calcium.
   4. Fluid retention may be reduced by vitamin B6.
   5. Mild pain may be treated with nonsteroidal antiinflammatory drugs (NSAIDs) such as ibuprofen (Motrin), naproxen (Naprosyn), or ketoprofen (Orudis). NSAIDs inhibit prostaglandin and provide relief for some women, if NSAIDs are started 1 to 3 days before menstruation and continued through the first few days of menses.
   6. More severe pain may be treated with oral contraceptives, which are 90% effective in controlling pain.
   7. Complementary treatments include use of transcutaneous electrical nerve stimulation (TENS), a battery-powered device that reduces pain by transmitting an electrical impulse to underlying nerves.
   8. Primary dysmenorrhea generally decreases with age and after childbirth.
C. Secondary dysmenorrhea.
   1. Symptomatic treatment is the same as for primary dysmenorrhea.
   2. Refer for evaluation and treatment of underlying cause.

V. Additional Information
A. General health may have an effect on dysmenorrhea. Encourage exercise, proper nutrition, not smoking, and weight loss if indicated.

WEB SITES

KidsHealth
   http://www.kidshealth.org
Mayo Clinic
   http://www.mayoclinic.com/health/menstrual-cramps/DS00506

ENDOMETRIOSIS

I. Definition
A. *Endometriosis* is the implantation and growth of endometrial tissue on pelvic and abdominal organs, such as the uterus, bladder, ovaries, fallopian tubes, and ligaments that support the uterus, the lining of the pelvic cavity, and the internal area between the vagina and rectum.

II. Etiology
A. Endometriosis is rare but occurs in one half of adolescents with refractory dysmenorrhea or chronic pelvic pain. The condition is believed to be familial.
B. Endometriosis affects about 5 million women, preadolescents, and adolescents in the United States. Often it is misdiagnosed in the teenage years.

III. Characteristics

A. Complicated by increased prostaglandin release by the endometrium and endometrial implants, resulting in severe dysmenorrhea.

B. Ectopic implants become larger with each cycle, and pain increases over time.

C. Severe pelvic pain in the lower abdominal area.

D. Pain may be occasional, constant, or associated with menses.

E. Student often misses school, social, or sports activities because of pain.

F. Pain may increase during exercise or during sexual activity.

G. Heavy menstrual flow, constipation, or diarrhea.

IV. Management/Treatment

A. Refer student to HCP.

B. Complete reproductive history, including the following:

 1. Age of menarche, frequency and length of periods, amount of flow, presence of cramps, use of tampons or pads, LMP.

 2. Family history of dysmenorrhea and gynecological problems.

 3. Past medical history, including hospitalizations or surgery, chronic illnesses, bleeding disorders.

 4. Medications, contraceptives, substance abuse, and the misuse of prescription medication.

 5. Related health issues: weight changes, nutrition, exercise, sports, emotional symptoms, and eating disorders.

C. Discuss the type of pain experienced—location, duration, intensity—and whether anything is used to treat pain.

D. Suggest keeping a diary of symptoms.

E. Avoidance of sugar, wheat, dairy products, and caffeine may reduce discomfort.

F. Use of over-the-counter (OTC) pain relievers may be helpful.

G. Oral contraceptives may be prescribed; these are known to reduce painful menstrual periods.

V. Additional Information

A. A confirming diagnosis is made by laparoscopy. Endometriosis can cause infertility and chronic pelvic pain. Medical and surgical options are available, but recurrence is common and may occur from 6 months to years later.

WEB SITES

U.S. Department of Health and Human Services,
National Women's Health Information Center
 http://www.womenshealth.gov
Healthfinder
 http://healthfinder.gov

DYSFUNCTIONAL UTERINE BLEEDING

I. Definition

A. *Dysfunctional uterine bleeding (DUB)* is described as abnormal uterine bleeding that occurs in the absence of a pathological condition or disease. DUB is a diagnosis of exclusion and should be considered only after other causes have been ruled out.

Adolescent and Gender-Specific Issues

CHAPTER 8

II. Etiology

A. DUB usually occurs at the beginning and end of a woman's reproductive years. The most severe DUB occurs shortly after the onset of menstruation. Adolescents with sustained anovulation—competitive athletes and those who are pregnant or have eating disorders, chronic illness, or endocrine disorders—have a higher incidence of DUB. Anovulatory DUB is caused by an imbalance in hormones. Approximately 95% of DUB in adolescents is caused by anovulation, but anovulation does not always lead to DUB (Bravender and Emans, 1999).

B. When a woman does not ovulate, the ovaries do not receive the signal to produce progesterone. Without progesterone, the endometrium continues to grow until it breaks down and is rejected in a very heavy period. Irregular or prolonged bleeding occurs when the endometrium is shed irregularly and incompletely.

III. Characteristics

A. DUB may be mild, moderate, or severe and usually is painless.

B. DUB can result in a variety of menstrual patterns, including the following:
   1. Hypermenorrhea: exceptionally heavy bleeding during a normal-length period; synonymous with menorrhagia.
   2. Metrorrhagia: periods that occur at irregular intervals, or frequent bleeding of varying amounts that is not heavy.
   3. Menometrorrhagia: frequent, excessive, and prolonged bleeding that occurs during menses and at irregular intervals.
   4. Oligomenorrhea: menstrual intervals of more than 5 weeks for longer than 6 months.
   5. Polymenorrhea: frequent, regular periods that occur more often than every 21 days.

C. DUB is common in overweight girls who have increased endogenous estrogen from both peripheral conversion of androgens to estrogens and fat storage.

IV. Management/Treatment

A. Treatment depends on the underlying mechanism.

B. Initially, concern is for the amount of blood loss and symptoms; observe student and reassure her.

C. Obtain a complete reproductive history (see Amenorrhea).

D. Assess orthostatic blood pressure, pulse changes, height and weight changes, hirsutism, and thyroid enlargement or nodules.

E. Assess number of pads or tampons saturated in a 24-hour period, which may or may not be typical, and history of previous three menstrual cycles.

F. Refer to parent for HCP assessment.

G. Treatment consists of bleeding control, prevention of endometrial hyperplasia and recurrence, and prevention and treatment of anemia.

H. Treatment is based on the intensity and timing of bleeding.

I. Hormonal regulation is the most effective treatment for those with anovulatory bleeding.

V. Additional Information

A. Most unusually heavy uterine bleeding has no underlying anatomical cause and is considered DUB. However, many possible underlying problems could cause the same symptoms. Diagnosis of DUB usually involves elimination of more serious causes.

WEB SITE

MedlinePlus: Dysfunctional Uterine Bleeding
http://www.nlm.nih.gov/medlineplus/ency/article/000903.htm

PREMENSTRUAL SYNDROME

I. Definition

A. Premenstrual syndrome (PMS) is a pattern of physical and emotional symptoms that occur in the second half of the menstrual cycle, usually appearing after ovulation (day 14) and resolving with the onset of menses. Symptoms disrupt daily living and must be present for at least two to three cycles to establish diagnosis.

II. Etiology

A. The cause of PMS is unknown, but research links the symptoms to an unusual response to normal hormonal changes. Research also has demonstrated a connection between PMS and low levels of serotonin (Stenchever et al, 2001). Approximately 40% of women who menstruate have some symptoms of PMS, but only 2% to 10% have symptoms severe enough to interfere with school, work, and social life (Freeman et al, 2000).

III. Characteristics

A. Symptoms are cyclical, appearing and resolving about the same time every month.

B. Discomfort starts about the middle of the cycle and intensifies in the last days before menses.

C. Rapid relief occurs with start of menses.

D. Days 4 through 12 of the cycle are symptom-free.

E. More than 150 physical and emotional symptoms are linked to PMS; they may be mild, moderate, or severe (Stenchever et al, 2001).

F. Physical symptoms:
   1. Abdominal bloating and swollen breasts, hands, and feet.
   2. Backache, lower abdominal pain, headache.
   3. Joint or muscle pain.
   4. Exhaustion.
   5. Upset stomach or constipation followed by diarrhea.
   6. Increased appetite or anorexia.
   7. Acne.

G. Emotional/behavioral symptoms:
   1. Mood swings, anxiety, depression, and irritability.
   2. Tearfulness, withdrawal from usual activities.
   3. Changes in sexual desire.
   4. Difficulty in concentrating and handling stress.
   5. Feelings of being out of control.

IV. Management/Treatment

A. Complete reproductive history, including the following:
   1. Age of menarche, frequency and length of periods, amount of flow, presence of cramps, use of tampons or pads, LMP.
   2. Family history of dysmenorrhea and gynecological problems.
   3. Past medical history, including hospitalizations or surgery, chronic illnesses, bleeding disorders.
   4. Medications, contraceptives, substance abuse.
   5. Related health issues: weight changes, nutrition, exercise, sports, emotional symptoms, and eating disorders.
B. Establish pattern by keeping a diary or calendar of symptoms.
C. Eliminate common offending foods and substances.
   1. Sugars: fructose, sucrose, syrups, and honey.
   2. Artificial sweeteners.
   3. Caffeine (chocolate, coffee, and colas).
   4. Cigarettes and alcohol.
D. Avoid foods that may exaggerate symptoms.
   1. Salty or smoked foods.
   2. Dairy products.
E. Increase intake of foods that will diminish symptoms of PMS.
   1. Whole grains (bread, pasta, brown rice).
   2. Dried beans and nuts.
   3. Fresh fruits and vegetables, especially spinach.
F. Establish rigorous exercise routine; aerobic exercise is especially helpful.
G. Practice stress reduction through deep breathing, meditation, naps, walking, hot baths, or massage.
H. Consider using supplements, but discuss with HCP.
   1. Multivitamin containing vitamins B6 and E, calcium, and magnesium.
   2. Evening primrose oil (available in health food stores).
   3. l-tryptophan, an amino acid.

V. Additional Information

A. Treatment is symptomatic; antidepressants, such as selective serotonin reuptake inhibitors (SSRIs) and tricyclics, have been helpful in relieving emotional symptoms. Other pharmacological treatments include diuretics, oral contraceptives, progesterone, thyroid hormone, and prostaglandin inhibitors.

WEB SITES

Mayo Clinic
   http://www.mayoclinic.com
U.S. Health and Human Services
   http://www.womenshealth.gov

VAGINITIS, VULVITIS, AND VULVOVAGINITIS

I. Definition

A. *Vaginitis* refers to a discharge with irritation and pruritus of the vagina. *Vulvitis* refers to erythema and pruritus of the vulva. *Vulvovaginitis* refs to inflammation, generally with a discharge, from infection or irritating substances that involve the vulva and vagina.

II. Etiology

A. An infection in the vagina caused by an overcolonization of bacteria normally found in the vaginal flora or by the introduction of pathological organisms. A small amount of vaginal mucus, which is usually clear, is normal; mucus production in adolescent girls generally increases during ovulation and before the onset of menses. This normally does not cause discomfort.

III. Additional Information

A. This is an opportunity to teach girls about personal hygiene: correct toileting habits (i e , wiping from front to back), changing underclothes daily, and washing hands frequently. Protective measures include avoiding bubble baths, perfumed powder, lotions or soap, shampoo in bath water, and residual bleach and fabric softener in clothes. Use mild soaps, such as Neutrogena, Dove, or Basis, and double rinse clothes during laundering. Human development and sexuality, including the importance of an evaluation when unusual vaginal discharge occurs, is also a part of health education. History of sexual activity is part of the health teaching on an individual level (see Table 8-3 for more information on the different types of vaginitis and vulvitis).

WEB SITES

MedlinePlus: Vaginal Discharge
    http://www.nlm.nih.gov/medlineplus/ency/article/003158.htm
MedlinePlus: Vulvitis
    http://www.nlm.nih.gov/medlineplus/ency/article/001445.htm

CERVICAL CANCER

I. Definition

A. Cancer of the uterine cervix is a neoplasm that can be detected in the early developmental stages. The Papanicolaou (Pap) smear is a diagnostic test to detect and diagnose early stage cancers of the cervix and other organ tissues. It usually is performed at an annual, routine pelvic examination, beginning at 18 years of age or younger if sexually active.

II. Etiology

A. Risk factors for cancer of the cervix include young age at first coitus, multiple sex partners, partners who have had sex with someone who has had cervical cancer, human papillomavirus (HPV) infection, exposure to diethylstilbestrol (DES), and smoking and oral contraceptive use. Current data are unclear regarding how these risk factors may lead to cancer. Some research suggests that sexually transmitted viruses cause cervical cells to begin developmental changes that can result in cancer.

III. Characteristics

A. Cervical cancer usually is asymptomatic and develops slowly.
B. Vaginal bleeding.
C. Abnormal-appearing cervix.

Table 8-3   Vaginitis and Vulvitis: Types and Clinical Information

Type	Etiology	Characteristics	Discharge	Treatment and Care
Bacterial	*Streptococcus, Escherichia coli, Shigella, Staphylococcus,* or other bacteria; usually sexually transmitted	Often asymptomatic	Green, malodorous; bleeding may occur	Penicillin, erythromycin, broad-spectrum antibiotic
Candidiasis	Diabetes, pregnancy, recent antibiotic, contraceptive, systemic corticosteroid use, or depressed immunity	Abrupt onset Severe itching, erythema, edema, dysuria, dyspareunia	Thick, white, cottage cheeselike, except in pregnancy; odorless	Miconazole (Monistat) or clotrimazole (Gyne-Lotrimin) cream nightly for 1 week; ketoconazole (Nizoral) orally or single-dose fluconazole (Diflucan); oil-based preparations may weaken condoms or diaphragms
Chemical irritant	Bubble bath, lotion, perfumed soap, tampons, deodorant pads, sand or dirt, tight-fitting clothing	Erythema, itching, vulvar inflammation, dysuria	White to yellow, small amount	Topical steroids, removal of irritant
Gardnerella	Gram-negative bacteria *G. vaginalis;* nonspecific; sexually transmitted; among mostcommon contagious bacterial STIs	No itching or mucosal irritation; no symptoms	Thin, gray, fishy smelling discharge	Metronidazole (Flagyl), clindamycin (Cleocin HCl) may be taken orally or applied as topical cream; concurrent treatment of sexual partner
Nonspecific	Poor hygiene, irritating substances	Itching and burning, dysuria; varied vulvitis	Foul smell, scant to copious, mucoid, brown to green in color	Topical antibiotics or estrogen, removal of irritating substances
Trichomonas	*Trichomonas vaginalis,* a parasitic protozoan; usually sexually transmitted	Often asymptomatic, self-limiting in males; vulvo-vaginal soreness, dysuria	Vaginal discharge	Metronidazole for 7 days, or as a single dose (is best for adolescents); concurrent treatment of sexual partner

IV. Management/Treatment
A. Complete reproductive history, including the following:
1. Age of menarche, frequency and length of periods, amount of flow, presence of cramps, use of tampons or pads, LMP.
2. Family history of dysmenorrhea and gynecological problems.
3. Past medical history, hospitalizations or surgery, chronic illnesses, bleeding disorders.
4. Medications, contraceptives, and misuse of prescribed medications.
5. Related health issues: weight changes, nutrition, exercise, sports, emotional symptoms, eating disorders, and substance abuse.
6. Sexual history: sexual activity, method of contraception, STIs, number of sexual partners, last sexual contact, types of sexual contact, sexual abuse.
B. Two types of Human Papillomavirus (HPV) cause 70% of cervical cancers. They can be prevented with the HPV vaccine (CDC, 2006).
C. Discuss the need for a yearly Pap smear if the adolescent is or has ever been sexually active.
D. Yearly chlamydia and gonorrhea testing, if adolescent is sexually active.
E. Treatment options are individualized and based on the adolescent's history and likelihood of continuous follow-up.
F. Pap smear findings are grouped descriptively into classes:
1. Class I: only normal cells seen.
2. Class II: atypical cells consistent with inflammation.
3. Class III: mild dysplasia.
4. Class IV: severe dysplasia, suspicious cells.
5. Class V: carcinoma cells seen.

WEB SITES

MedlinePlus: Pap Smear
http://www.nlm.nih.gov/medlineplus/ency/article/003911.htm
Women's Health Queensland, Student Fact Sheet: Cervical Cancer
http://www.womhealth.org.au/studentfactsheets/cervicalcancer.htm

UNDESCENDED TESTIS (CRYPTORCHIDISM)
I. Definition
A. *Cryptorchidism* is an undescended testis that does not enter the scrotum and cannot be manipulated into it; may be unilateral or bilateral.
II. Etiology
A. The testes usually descend into the scrotum by the eighth month of fetal life; less than 1% have not descended by the ninth month. Undescended testes also can be a result of retractile testes or anorchia, the absence of testes. Anorchia is categorized according to location: *abdominal, canalicular,* or *ectopic.*
III. Characteristics
A. Fertility is severely affected if cryptorchidism is bilateral and is not corrected by age 6.

B. A small percentage of testicular cancers occur in men with a history of undescended testes. Cancer is more common with an intraabdominal testis.

C. Testes undescended into scrotum.

D. Rarely causes discomfort.

E. All or one side of scrotum appears smaller than normal with incomplete development.

F. Undescended testis usually is softer and smaller than descended one.

G. Retractile testes can be manipulated back into the scrotum; usually bilateral.

H. Distinction between a lymph node and an undescended testis is made by its elastic nature. A testis can be manipulated down into the scrotum but will spring back into the inguinal canal.

I. No evidence exists that testes will descend with puberty, unless they are retractile and not truly undescended.

IV. Management/Treatment

A. Refer to parent for HCP assessment.

B. Hormone therapy trial may be initiated.

C. Corrective surgery between 1 and 2 years of age.

D. Teach testicular self-examination to adolescent students.

WEB SITE

MedlinePlus: Undescended Testicle
   http://www.nlm.nih.gov/medlineplus/ency/article/000973.htm

TESTICULAR CANCER

I. Definition

A. Development of a malignant neoplasm in the testicle. Testicular cancer occurs most frequently in the 15- to 34-year-old age group. It can occur anytime after age 14.

II. Etiology

A. The cause of testicular cancer is unknown, but a tenfold to fortyfold greater risk exists with a history of ectopic or undescended testes, even if the testes have been descended surgically. Most solid tumors in males younger than age 30 are testicular tumors and may be benign or malignant, but most testicular masses in adolescents are malignant. Testicular cancer is the cause of one in seven deaths among late adolescent and young adult males. It is approximately five times more common in white American men than in African-American men, and white men have twice the risk of Asian-American men (National Cancer Institute, 2005).

III. Characteristics

A. Risk factors include the following:

1. Late descended testes or undescended testes, even if they were corrected surgically.

2. Family history of testicular cancer.

3. Abnormal testicular development.

4. Inguinal hernia.

5. Klinefelter syndrome.

B. Usually asymptomatic, although localized pain or a dull ache may be present in the back or lower abdomen, or a sudden collection of fluid may occur in the scrotum.

C. Detected as a heavy, hard, unilateral lump, usually about the size of a pea but may be as large as an egg. Palpable on the anterior or lateral part of the testis (see Testicular Self-Examination).

D. May be found after an injury, but injury is not believed to be a causative factor. Pain and tenderness may be due to hemorrhage into the tumor.

E. Develops more commonly in the right testicle. Involved testis often hangs lower.

F. Mass does not transilluminate unless associated with a hydrocele, which is present in 10% of malignancies.

G. May metastasize to lymph nodes, liver, or lungs before detection.

H. Later stages include pulmonary symptoms, ureter obstruction, gynecomastia (enlarged breasts), or an abdominal mass.

I. Early discovery and treatment leads to a 95% survival rate. Approximately 70% of men with advanced testicular cancer can be cured (National Cancer Institute, 2005).

IV. Management/Treatment

A. Depends on type of tumor and the stage. Three stages of testicular cancer exist:
   1. Stage 1: Malignancy is confined to the testicle.
   2. Stage 2: Disease has spread to retroperitoneal lymph nodes.
   3. Stage 3: Cancer has spread to remote sites in the body, such as the lungs and liver.

B. First line of treatment is orchiectomy of the affected testicle.

C. Radiation, chemotherapy, and bone marrow transplantation are other treatments.

D. Sexual function and fertility usually are unaffected, since the remaining testicle can produce sperm. More extensive surgery may cause infertility but does not affect ability to have erections or orgasms. A prosthesis can be inserted to provide a normal appearance.

E. Teach anatomy and physiology prior to teaching testicular self-examination to adolescents.

WEB SITES

National Cancer Institute: Testicular Cancer
   http://www.cancer.gov/cancer_information/cancer_type/testicular
MedlinePlus: Testicular Cancer
   http://www.nlm.nih.gov/medlineplus/ency/article/001288.htm

---

SEXUALLY TRANSMITTED INFECTIONS

NOTE: Sexually transmitted infection (STI) has a broader meaning than sexually transmitted disease (STD). A person can be infected and infect others but not have signs or symptoms of disease.

Adolescent and Gender-Specific Issues

CHAPTER 8

The role of the school nurse in meeting with students with suspected or confirmed STIs involves the following:
1. Discuss safe-sex practices, including abstinence, condoms, spermicidal barriers, and the risks associated with multiple partners. Table 8-4 provides more information on the various types of contraceptives.
2. Complete reproductive history assessment for girls:
   - Age of menarche, frequency and length of periods, amount of flow, presence of cramps, use of tampons or pads, LMP.
   - Family history of dysmenorrhea and gynecological problems.
   - Past medical history, including hospitalizations or surgery, chronic illnesses, bleeding disorders.
   - Medications, contraceptives, substance abuse.
   - Related health issues: weight changes, nutrition, exercise, sports, emotional symptoms, and eating disorders.
3. Sexual history (boys and girls):
   - Sexual activity, method of contraception, STIs, number of sexual partners, last sexual contact, types of sexual contact, sexual abuse.
   - Collect data regarding physical health and social, emotional, and sexual developmental history; include Tanner stages of development (see Growth and Development, Chapter 1).
4. Maintain student confidentiality and awareness of state laws. The American Academy of Pediatrics (AAP) has a policy statement on confidentiality and adolescent health care.

CHLAMYDIA

I. Definition
A. Chlamydia is the most common bacterial STI and the fastest spreading STI in the United States.

II. Etiology
A. *Chlamydia trachomatis* is a gram-negative bacterium contracted through vaginal sex, oral–genital contact, and perinatally. *C. trachomatis* infection may occur in the eye with exposure to contaminated body fluid.

III. Characteristics
A. The *incubation period* is poorly defined but probably is 7 to 14 days or longer.
B. Chlamydia often is asymptomatic, thus making it difficult to diagnosis.
C. Symptoms:
   1. A white or yellowish vaginal discharge, dysuria, burning or itching in the vagina, dyspareunia, and pelvic or abdominal pain.
   2. Discharge from penis, urethral pain, dysuria, swollen testicles; may be able to express discharge from the urethral meatus; rectal infections usually are asymptomatic.
D. Reiter syndrome (conjunctivitis, disseminated arthritis, and dermatitis).
E. Untreated chlamydia can cause infection of the urethra, inflammation of the cervix, or dysfunctional uterine bleeding and pelvic inflammatory disease (PID), which can lead to infertility.

Table 8-4   Contraceptives

Method	Efficacy of Actual Use (%)	Benefits	Disadvantages
Natural Methods			
Abstinence	100	Prevents pregnancy and STIs	High motivation by both partners required, peer pressure involved
Rhythm method Avoidance of intercourse during time of ovulation (fertile period)	Rate similar to barrier methods	No prescription needed, no side effects from medication	No protection from STIs, requires a predictable menstrual cycle
Withdrawal Withdrawal prior to ejaculation	High failure rate	No prescription needed, no medication side effects	No STI protection, ejaculation prior or during withdrawal may result in seminal fluid entering vagina
Hormonal Methods			
Oral contraceptives Estrogen/progesterone preparation inhibits ovulation	95% to 99% When used correctly	Nothing required before sex, simple method, decreased dysmenorrhea and acne	Requires prescription, expensive, requires consistent use, no STI protection, some weight gain, regulates menstrual cycle
Transdermal patch Hormonal patch to deliver norelgestromin and ethinyl estradiol suppresses ovulation	88% when used appropriately	Visible reminder of contraceptive device, applied once a week, three times a month; regulates menses	May cause breast tenderness, nausea, headaches, and weight gain; risk of blood clots in legs and lungs
Vaginal ring NuvaRing delivers estrogen and progestin to inhibit ovulation	99% if used correctly	Predictable and lighter menses, inserted once a month for three weeks, less premenstrual discomfort, no weight gain	No STI prevention; tender breasts; mood alterations; ring may be felt by individual or partner; device can fall out; headaches, nausea, vaginitis, and break-through bleeding

Continued

Table 8-4 *Contraceptives—cont'd*

Method	Efficacy of Actual Use (%)	Benefits	Disadvantages
Barrier Methods			
Condom *Male:* Traps sperm in penile covering *Female:* Single use, inserted into vagina, fits against cervix	86%	No prescription needed, easy methods, inexpensive, accessible, decreases STI risk, no side effects	Must apply correctly, must use consistently; motivation by both partners required, may interfere with sexual pleasure; use polyurethane condom if allergic to latex
Diaphragm Cervical covering to prevent sperm from entering, use with spermicidal jelly, three types: *flat, arching spring, and coiled wire*	80%	Decreases PID, bacterial, and viral infection but not HIV and herpes virus; can reuse; usually not felt by either partner	Can increase UTIs, must be prescribed and fitted by HCP, must be used correctly; messy; can be placed in vagina up to 1 hr before and stay in place 6 to 8 hr after; can be left in up to 24 hr, requires cleaning, do not use if allergic to latex or spermicide
Cervical caps and cervical shield A soft cap with a firm ring that fits over the cervix, the shield has an air valve to provide a snug fit and a loop to aid in removal, spermicide recommended for both	80%	Usually not felt by partner, immediately effective, does not interfere with natural hormones, no latex allergy concerns with cervical shield made from silicone, make sure products are latex free for those with latex sensitivity	May be difficult to insert, must see clinician for fitting and directions for use

Intrauterine devices (IUDs) T-shaped intrauterine devices are inserted into the uterus to prevent the sperm from fertilizing the egg. Mirena releases progestin, which inhibits the sperm's ability to fertilize the egg, and ParaGard slowly releases copper, which in turn inactivates the sperm.	99%	The devices once in place stay there, Mirena lasts for 5 years, ParaGard lasts for 10 years	Increases risk for PID and sterility, both must be fitted and inserted by an HCP, menstrual cramps may increase, periods may be heavier and longer, no protection against STIs, not recommended for teens
Emergency contraception Oral contraceptive given within 72 hr of unprotected sex and again 12 hr later	75%	Useful for method failure or unplanned sexual intercourse	Nausea, vomiting; must take within 72 hr; not for continual use; no STI protection

IV. Additional Information

A. Newborns can be infected in the birth canal, so ophthalmic prophy-laxis is used after birth.

WEB SITES

MedlinePlus: Chlamydia
    http://www.nlm.nih.gov/medlineplus/ency/article/001345.htm
TeensHealth: Chlamydia
    http://www.kidshealth.org/teen/sexual_health/stds/std_chlamydia.html

GONORRHEA

I. Definition

A. *Neisseria gonorrhoeae,* or gonorrhea (GC), is a bacterial infection of the urethra and genital tract. It is the most frequently reported com-municable disease in the United States.

II. Etiology

A. *N. gonorrhoeae* is a gram-negative coccus that is contracted perina-tally and through oral, vaginal, or anal sexual contact.

III. Characteristics

A. The *incubation period* varies between men and women; infection usually occurs in 2 to 14 days.

B. GC may be asymptomatic in women but is often symptomatic in men.

C. Symptoms:
   1. A yellowish-green vaginal discharge and pelvic pain; other symp-toms include burning or itching around the vagina, odor from the vagina, dysfunctional uterine bleeding, menstrual irregularities, or dysuria. Women often exhibit no symptoms but learn about the presence of STI from their partner.
   2. Men have urethral pain, burning, dysuria, and a thick, greenish, purulent discharge from the penis.
   3. Occasionally pharyngitis and conjunctivitis occur.

D. Untreated infection increases risk for damaged heart valves, chronic infection of the genital tract, disseminated arthritis-dermatitis syn-drome (fever, chills, arthritis, skin lesions), meningitis, and peritonitis.

E. GC can cause pelvic inflammatory disease.

IV. Additional Information

A. Guidelines from the Centers for Disease Control and Prevention (CDC) recommend treatment with a single dose of a 400 mg tablet or a suspension of cefixime (Suprax) or a single dose injection of 125 mg ceftriaxone (Rocephin). The treatment of choice used to be penicillin, but many strains of GC have become resistant. Some an-tibiotics are available in one-dose preparations. Concurrent treat-ment for chlamydia is recommended with doxycycline, unless chla-mydia infection has been ruled out.

B. Newborns can be infected in the birth canal, so ophthalmic prophy-laxis is used after birth.

WEB SITES

eMedicine.com: Gonorrhea
    http://www.emedicine.com/ped/topic886.htm
TeensHealth: Gonorrhea
    http://www.kidshealth.org/teen

HUMAN PAPILLOMAVIRUS

I. Definition

A. Human papillomavirus (HPV) causes a variety of skin and mucosal lesions, including distinct-appearing warts; genital–anal tract lesions can be benign or malignant. The National Cancer Institute (2006) states HPVs are a major cause of cervical cancer.

II. Etiology

A. HPV infection is spread by sexual activity. The warts are found on any part of the female and male genitalia and occur as single or multiple soft, generally painless growths. To date, 100 different genotypes have been identified, and more than 30 types are sexually transmitted (CDC, 2004). HPV types 6 and 11 are associated with 90% of visible genital warts (Jenson and Baltimore, 2006; National Cancer Institute, 2006). HPV 16 and 18 are responsible for about 70% of all cervical cancers; types 31, 33, 35, and possibly others, are associated with cervical neoplasia (Jenson and Baltimore, 2006).

III. Characteristics

A. Most types of HPV infection are asymptomatic.

B. In women warty lesions are commonly found on the vulva, cervix, vagina, or rectum.

C. In men, the lesions usually occur on the shaft of the penis but also appear on the meatus, scrotum, rectum, or anus.

D. Condom use can decrease transmission.

E. *Condyloma acuminata* warts are described as cauliflower-like in appearance.

F. Untreated lesions grow larger and multiply; when condyloma affects the cervix, it can lead to cervical cancer.

G. Smoking can increase the risk of cervical cancer.

H. Large warts can obstruct the birth canal.

I. Newborns can develop warts on the larynx from exposure in the birth canal.

IV. Additional Information

A. The treatment goal is to decrease transmission to partners and alleviate symptoms; no cure exists. Treatment includes laser therapy, cryotherapy (liquid nitrogen), catheterization, and surgical excision. Chemical agents (topical ointments) are used to treat low-level lesions of the cervix; these agents should not be applied to healthy tissue.

B. To eliminate cancer, sexually active females should have annual pelvic examinations and Pap smears when atypical warts are observed.

C. Gardasil was approved by the FDA in 2006 as a vaccine to prevent cervical cancer and venereal warts caused by HPV. It is effective against HPV subtypes 6, 11, 16, and 18. It is licensed for girls and women 9 through 26 years of age and is a series of three vaccines given over a 6-month period. Research is being conducted to investigate the effectiveness in older women and in men.

WEB SITES

MedlinePlus: Genital Warts
> http://www.nlm.nih.gov/medlineplus/ency/article/000886.htm

Planned Parenthood: HPV and Genital Warts
> http://www.plannedparenthood.org/health-topics/stds-hiv-safer-sex/hpv.htm

PELVIC INFLAMMATORY DISEASE

I. Definition

A. Pelvic inflammatory disease (PID) is an acute, progressive infection of the upper genital tract—uterus, fallopian tubes, or surrounding structures—that usually is caused by ascending microorganisms from the vagina or endocervix.

II. Etiology

A. PID usually is a result of polymicrobial infections, mainly gonorrhea and chlamydia. It is more common in women under age 25.

III. Characteristics

A. Asymptomatic if associated with chlamydia.

B. Lower abdominal tenderness, pain, or dysfunctional uterine bleeding (DUB).

C. Fever, chills, gastrointestinal (GI) symptoms (e.g., nausea, vomiting, anorexia).

D. Lower-quadrant pain that worsens with movement or sexual intercourse.

E. Foul-smelling vaginal discharge.

F. Malaise, weakness, and dizziness.

G. Recurring PID is associated with infertility, ectopic pregnancy, or chronic pelvic pain.

IV. Additional Information

A. Treatment includes a course of antibiotics. It is important to be diagnosed and treated early to prevent damage to the reproductive organs.

B. Hospitalization may be recommended if an infected woman is pregnant or does not respond to oral medication, if severe illness results, or if an abscess in the fallopian tube or ovary occurs.

C. Women can take precautions against PID; these include abstinence, early treatment for STIs, and use of condoms. CDC recommends yearly testing for all sexually active females age 25 and younger.

WEB SITES

MedlinePlus: Pelvic Inflammatory Disease
> http://www.nlm.nih.gov/medlineplus/ency/article/000888.htm

TeensHealth: Pelvic Inflammatory Disease
> http://www.kidshealth.org/teen/sexual_health/stds/std_pid.html

Centers for Disease Control
   http://www.cdc.gov/std/PID/STDFact-PID.htm

SYPHILIS

I. Definition
   A. Syphilis is a bacterial STI; when untreated, it progresses through four clinical stages: *primary, secondary, latent,* and *tertiary.*

II. Etiology
   A. Syphilis is caused by the *Treponema pallidum* spirochete and is contracted through oral, vaginal, or anal sexual activity; transplacentally or perinatally; and by contact with open infected lesions, body fluids, and secretions of infected individuals. It is more prevalent in women than men. The *T. pallidum* spirochete can survive almost anywhere in the body.

III. Characteristics
   A. *Incubation period* is approximately 3 weeks with a range of 10 to 90 days.
   B. The majority of cases are asymptomatic.
   C. Symptoms:
      1. Primary stage. Syphilis begins with a painless sore (chancre) at the site of infection, on the sex organs, or in the mouth. It may be accompanied by swollen glands in that region. The sore appears as a flat ulcer with rolled, raised edges. The sore often is believed to be a cold sore, so treatment is not sought. Untreated chancres can last 3 to 6 weeks and then disappear. Without treatment, the disease will progress to the secondary stage.
      2. Secondary stage: A rash (papular, macular, or annular) may appear anywhere on the body, including the palms of the hands, the soles of the feet, or on mucous tissue. Generalized adenopathy and viruslike symptoms occur. These symptoms can clear spontaneously with or without treatment. Without treatment the STI can progress to the latent stage.
      3. Latent stage: If untreated, no symptoms of the disease may exist, but test results will be positive, indicating that the spirochetes are still active in the body.
      4. Tertiary stage: Onset is usually 5 to 20 years after the primary stage. This stage is rarely seen in adolescents. The spirochetes spread all over the body and affect the skin, subcutaneous tissue, bone, heart, brain, and other vital organs.

IV. Additional Information
   A. Treatment is a one-time injection of benzathine penicillin (Bicillin) for the primary, secondary, and early latent syphilis stage. For tertiary syphilis or latent syphilis of unknown duration, treatment is three injections at 1-week intervals (Jenson and Baltimore, 2006). Penicillin has remained effective because T. pallidum bacteria have not developed resistance. Assessment of the effectiveness of treatment requires blood testing at 3, 6, and 12 months, followed by additional therapy if indicated.
   B. During pregnancy, transmission to the fetus approaches 100%. Fetal and perinatal death occur in 40% of cases (Azimi, 2004). Early prenatal

screening is mandated in all states, and some states require screening at delivery.

WEB SITES

MedlinePlus: Syphilis
>http://www.nlm.nih.gov/medlineplus/ency/article/001327.htm

TeensHealth: Syphilis
>http://www.kidshealth.org/teen/sexual_health/stds/std_syphilis.html

BREAST AND TESTICULAR SELF-EXAMINATIONS

BREAST SELF-EXAMINATION

Monthly breast self-examination (BSE) and palpation of breasts should be done, preferably 7 to 10 days after the beginning of the menstrual cycle. If cycles are irregular, the BSE should be performed on the same day each month and at the same time of day. If any abnormalities are noticed, adolescents should report them to a parent, HCP, or both.

 I. Self-Inspection
   A. Stand or sit in front of a mirror with arms relaxed at sides.
   B. Note size, color, shape, and direction of breasts and nipples; one breast may be slightly larger than the other; this is normal.
   C. Examine breasts for dimples or discoloration in the skin, nipple changes, or discharge.
   D. Raise arms overhead and examine breasts while turning slowly from side to side.
   E. Place hands on hips and, pressing firmly, move shoulders forward; look at each breast separately.

 II. Palpation, or Examination by Feeling
   A. In front of mirror, apply firm pressure with the pads of three middle fingertips just below the collarbone; make small circles over the breast area in a pattern to cover all of the breast; palpation should be circular, up and down, or in spokes.
   B. Extend the examination to the underarm area.
   C. Change hands and complete the BSE on the opposite breast.

 III. Additional Information
   A. Breast cancer is extremely rare in adolescents, but BSE helps them become comfortable and familiar with their breasts and establishes a pattern of preventive care.

WEB SITES

National Women's Health Information Center: Breast Self-Exam
>http://www.4woman.gov/faq/bsefaq.htm

Teens Health
>http://www.kidshealth.org/teen/sexual_health/girls/bse.html

TESTICULAR SELF-EXAMINATION

Testicular self-examination (TSE) is a monthly inspection and palpation of the testes for detection of testicular cancer. TSE should be performed after a warm bath or shower, because heat relaxes the scrotum and increases the chance of spotting an abnormality. If any abnormalities are noticed, the adolescent should report them to a parent, HCP, or both.

I. Self-Inspection

A. Stand in front of a mirror and look for any swelling on the skin of the scrotum or any discoloration or changes in the testicle.

B. One testicle may be *slightly* larger than the other, but a significant difference in size should be checked.

C. Look at the entire penis and note bumps or blisters, open sores, warts, or drainage that may be signs of an STI.

II. Palpation

A. Stand with the right leg elevated on the toilet or a stool.

B. Support the testicle in the left hand and feel it with the right hand.

C. Gently roll the testicle between the thumb and the fingers.

D. Separate the epididymis—the soft, tubular structure covering the back and bottom of the testicle—from the testicle to palpate the testicle itself.

E. The testicle should be firm and smooth but not hard; no lumps or bumps should be present.

F. No pain should exist.

G. Repeat for the left testicle, elevating the left leg instead.

III. Additional Information

A. Testicular cancer is one of the most common tumors in boys and men younger than age 40. It usually develops between ages 15 and 44.

WEB SITES

MedlinePlus: Testicular Self-Exam
   http://www.nlm.nih.gov/medlineplus/ency/article/003909.htm
Teens Health: Testicular-Self Examination
   http://www.kidshealth.org/teen

BIBLIOGRAPHY

American Dental Association, Division of Communications: Oral piercing and health, *J Am Dent Assoc* 132:127, 2001.

Armstrong ML, Ekmark E, Brooks B: Body piercing: promoting informed decision making, *J School Nurs* 11(2):20-25, 1995.

Azimi P: Syphilis. In Behrman RE, Kliegman RM, Jenson HB, editors: *Nelson textbook of pediatrics*, Philadelphia, 2004, Saunders.

Bravender T, Emans SJ: Adolescent gynecology, part 1, common disorders, *Pediatr Clin North Am* 46(3):543-553, 1999.

Centers for Disease Control and Prevention: *HPV vaccine questions and answers*, Available at: http://www.cdc.gov/std/hpv/STDFact-HPV-vaccine.htm#hpvvac7. Accessed July 13, 2007.

Centers for Disease Control and Prevention: *Genital HPV infections*, CDC fact sheet (available online): www.cdc.gov/std/HPV/STDFact-HPV.htm. Accessed July 13, 2007.

Darmstadt GL, Sidbury R: The skin. In: Behrman RE, Kliegman RM, Jenson HB, editors: *Nelson textbook of pediatrics*, Philadelphia, 2004, Saunders.

Ehrman W, Matson SC: Adolescents and sexually transmitted diseases. In Osborn LM, DeWitt TG, First LR, Zenel JA, editors: *Pediatrics*, Philadelphia, 2005, Mosby.

Freeman EW, Sondheimer SJ, Polansky M: Predictors of response to sertraline treatment of severe premenstrual symptoms, *J Clin Pschiatry* 61(8):579-574, 2000.

Herron M, Vanderhooft SL: Acne. In Osborn LM, DeWitt TG, First LR, Zenel JA, editors: *Pediatrics,* Philadelphia, 2005, Mosby.

Howard PJ: *The owner's manual for the brain: everyday application from mind-brain research,* Austin, Tex, 2006, Bard Press.

Jenson HB, Baltimore RS: Infectious diseases. In Kliegman RM, Marcdante KJ, Jenson HB, Behrman RE, editors: *Nelson essentials of pediatrics,* Philadelphia, 2006, Saunders.

Kollar LM: Physical health problems of adolescence. In Hockenberry MJ, Wilson D, editors: *Wong's nursing care of infants and children,* Philadelphia, 2007, Mosby.

Lembo R: Dermatology. In Kliegman RM, Marcdante KJ, Jenson HB, Behrman RE, editors: *Nelson essentials of pediatrics,* Philadelphia, 2006, Saunders.

Mayo Clinic: *Tattoos and body piercing: what to know beforehand* (available online): www.mayoclinic.com/health/tattoos-and-piercings/MC00020. Accessed July 12, 2007.

Mosby's dictionary of medicine, nursing, and health, St. Louis, 2006, Mosby.

National Cancer Institute: *Human papillomaviruses and cancer: questions and answers* (available online): www.cancer.gov/cancertopics/factsheet/Risk/HPV. Accessed July 14, 2007.

National Cancer Institute: *Testicular cancer: questions and answers* (available online): www.cancer.gov/cancertopics/factsheet/sites-types/testicular. Accessed July 13, 2007.

Schwab N, Gelfman M: *Legal issues in school health services: a resource for school administrators, school attorneys, school nurses,* Lincoln, Neb, 2005, Authors' Choice Press.

Slap GS: Menstrual disorders in adolescence, *Best Pract Res Clin Obstet Gynecol* 17(1):75-92, 2003.

Stenchever MA, Droegemueller W, Herbst AL et al: *Comprehensive gynecology,* St Louis, 2001, Mosby.

U.S. Department of Health and Human Services: *Healthy people 2010, vol I,* Washington, DC, USDHHS (available online): www.health.gov/healthypeople. Accessed July 17, 2007.

U.S. Department of Health and Human Services: Sexually transmitted diseases treatment guidelines, *Morb Mortal Wkly Rep (MMWR 55, RR11)* August 4, 2006:1-94, Centers for Disease Control (available online): www.cdc.gov/mmwr/preview/mmwrhtml/rr5511a1.htm. Accessed July 17, 2007.

U.S. Preventive Service Task Force: *Screening for chlamydial infection* (available online): www.ahrq.gov/clinic/uspstf/uspschlm.htm. Accessed July 17, 2007.

CHAPTER 9

Special Education

Chapter Outline

School nurses, teachers, psychologists, and professional educators face the growing challenge and responsibility of providing exceptional children and young adults with an appropriate education. Individuals with disabilities attend public schools whenever possible. Support services are available that enhance the chances for students with disabilities to reach their maximum potential. Special education is now a large and integral part of the U.S. educational system as it identifies and attempts to meet each student's unique needs.

The primary reason that more than 6.6 million students ages 3 to 21 years are receiving special education is passage of Public Law (PL) 94-142, Section 504, the more current PL 108-446 (2004), and the revised Individuals with Disabilities Education Improvement Act (IDEA or IDEIA). These laws detail educational rights of the disabled and provide funding to help states cover the costs of providing for these rights (National Center for Education Statistics, 2005). This chapter discusses the changes and main components of this legislation and cites the 13 handicapping conditions. Table 9-1 summarizes some of the significant changes to IDEA.

As more children and young adults with disabilities are integrated into community life, important implications affect nursing in all fields. An awareness of the effect of the disability on the child, family, and siblings enables

Table 9-1	*Significant Issues Addressed by IDEA 2004*
Significant Issues	**Changes and Additions**
Alignment with No Child Left Behind (NCLB)	• Ensures equity, accountability, and excellence • Applies NCLB *highly qualified* requirement to special education teachers
Provide earlier identification and eligibility	• Removes requirement that student must exhibit severe discrepancy between IQ and achievement for eligibility in learning disability category • Parent can initiate request for initial evaluation
Early Intervening Services (EIS) K-12	• Services for students not identified for special education, but who need academic or behavioral support to succeed in general education • Reduces need to determine student has a disability before providing support • Emphasis for services is on K-3
Private schools (Parent-placed child with disability)	• Must provide Child Find activities and fund proportionate amount for special education services as in public schools
School nurse services	• Expanded and renamed *school health services* and *school nurse services* • *School nurse services* are provided by a qualified school nurse • *School health services* may be provided by a qualified school nurse or other qualified person
Medication	• Prohibits schools from requiring medication (covered by the Controlled Substance Act) for attendance, evaluation, or for services in schools
Adaptive devices	• Must ensure that hearing aids are working properly • Must ensure that external components of surgically implanted medical devices (e.g. cochlear implants) are functioning adequately • Not responsible for postsurgical maintenance, programming, or replacement of the medical device
Individualized education program (IEP) More relevant to student progress Reduces paperwork	• Removes requirement of objectives • Must contain annual goals and description of how progress will be measured and reported • Team members may be excused if area is not being modified; parents and school agree in writing; written information is shared before the IEP meeting • May use alternative methods for IEP meeting, such as conference call or video conference • Minor changes can be made by conference call or letter, without meeting, if all parties agree

Table 9-1	Significant Issues Addressed by IDEA 2004—cont'd
Significant Issues	Changes and Additions
Time limits	• 60-day time line for initial evaluation starts when consent form for evaluation is signed or per state guidelines
Part C: Birth to age 3 services	• Must be based on scientifically based research • Recognizes significant brain development in first 3 years of life • Recommends training of personnel in emotional and social development of young children • States may opt to offer extension of Part C services to kindergarten age • Promotes collaboration among Early Head Start, early education, child care programs, and Part C services
New Child Find referral sources	• Expands program for referral sources to include homeless family shelters, clinics, and child welfare system • Children involved in substantiated child abuse and neglect or prenatal drug exposure (PDE) must be screened to determine need for referral to early intervention
Discipline for students with disability	• Serious bodily injury added to drugs and weapons as reason for 45-day removal from school

the nurse not only to develop a special personal understanding but facilitates the acceptance of the individual into community and school settings.

The chapter concludes with specialized health care procedures. Many students, either in regular classrooms or special classes, require specialized procedures. The techniques used in a school setting frequently differ from those used in a hospital. The school nurse now may need to delegate certain health care procedures to licensed and unlicensed personnel and must provide teaching and monitoring for effective management. The nurse retains the responsibility for the delegated procedures. The needs of exceptional children are complex and require multiple treatment modalities and assistance in some form throughout their academic lives.

THE LAW

The right to a free and appropriate public education (FAPE) for children with disabilities from 5 to 21 years of age was established in 1975 with the enactment of PL 94-142, the Education for All Handicapped Children Act (EHA). This law addresses identification, evaluation, placement, and education of children with disabilities. In 1986, PL 99-457 amended EHA and provided a phase-in mandate for states to provide special education services to children ages 3 to 5 years. EHA provided grants for states to establish programs for children with developmental delays from birth to age 3.

The title of EHA was changed to the Individuals with Disabilities Education Act (IDEA) in 1990, and special education services for 3- to 5-year-olds were mandated in all states. In 1993, Part C of IDEA offered every state the opportunity to apply for federal funding for the implementation of a statewide, comprehensive, coordinated, multidisciplinary, interagency system of early intervention services for infants and toddlers with developmental delay and their families. These early intervention services for children from birth through 2 years of age are provided through various public agencies (e.g., Department of Health, Department of Education), private agencies, or any combination of public and private sources, depending on state laws and the state's lead agency. The individualized educational program (IEP), birth to 3, is written as the individualized family service plan (IFSP). The bulk of this chapter applies to Part B, ages 3 through 21.

The first major revision of PL 94-142 occurred in 1997 with passage of PL 105-17, referred to as *IDEA '97*. The 1997 amendments provided a new emphasis on improving educational results for children with disabilities by ensuring they have meaningful access to the general curriculum through improvements in the IEP. A full educational opportunity goal was established to include students with disabilities in the general education reform efforts related to accountability and improvement of teaching and learning.

Major issues addressed by IDEA '97 include the following:

1. Focusing on the IEP as the primary tool for enhancing the child's involvement and progress in the general curriculum. The IEP goals must relate more clearly to the general curriculum that children receive in regular classrooms.
2. Provision of regular progress reports to parents as often as reports are provided for other children.
3. Inclusion of students in state and district assessments, with accommodations and appropriate modifications if necessary, and establishment of alternate assessments as needed.
4. Inclusion of at least one regular education teacher on the IEP team. Decisions regarding participation by regular education teachers are made on a case-by-case basis.

These changes in IDEA establish high expectations for children with disabilities, and they exceed merely providing access to an education—they promote an optimal education. Parental involvement at all levels is encouraged, and full inclusion is emphasized.

I. Thirteen Disabling Conditions Defined in IDEA

   A. *Autism* is a developmental disability that significantly affects verbal and nonverbal communication and social interaction, generally evident before age 3, which adversely affects a child's educational performance.

   1. The term does not apply if a child's educational performance is adversely affected primarily because the child has an emotional disturbance (see paragraph D of this section).
   2. A diagnosis of autism can be made in a child who manifests the characteristics of autism after age 3, if the criteria above are satisfied.

B. *Deaf-blindness* indicates concomitant hearing and visual impairments, the combination of which causes such severe communication and other developmental and educational needs to the extent that affected children cannot be accommodated in special education programs established solely for children with deafness or children with blindness.

C. *Deafness* is a hearing impairment so severe that the child is impaired in processing linguistic information through hearing, with or without amplification, and such impairment adversely affects educational performance.

D. *Emotional disturbance** means a condition exhibiting one or more of the following characteristics over a prolonged period, and to a marked degree, that adversely affects a child's educational performance.

    1. Inability to learn that cannot be explained by intellectual, sensory, or health factors.

    2. Inability to build or maintain satisfactory interpersonal relationships with peers and teachers.

    3. General pervasive mood of unhappiness or depression.

    4. Tendency to develop physical symptoms or fears associated with personal or school problems.

    5. Inappropriate behaviors or feelings under normal circumstances.

E. *Hearing impairment* means impairment in hearing, whether permanent or fluctuating, that adversely affects a child's educational performance but that is not included under the definition of deafness in this section.

F. *Mentally retarded* indicates significantly subaverage general intellectual functioning concurrent with deficits in adaptive behavior manifested during the developmental period that adversely affects a child's educational performance.

G. *Multiple disabilities* means concomitant impairments (e.g., mental retardation and blindness, mental retardation and orthopedic impairment), the combination of which causes such severe educational problems that the child cannot be accommodated in special education programs set up solely for one of the impairments. The term does not include deaf-blindness.

H. *Orthopedic impairment* means a severe orthopedic impairment that adversely affects a child's educational performance. The term includes impairments caused by congenital anomaly (e.g., club foot, absence of limb), impairments caused by disease (e.g., poliomyelitis, bone tuberculosis), and impairments from other causes (e.g., cerebral palsy, amputations, and fractures or burns that cause contractures).

I. *Other health impairment* means limited strength, vitality, or alertness—including a heightened alertness to environmental stimuli—that results in limited alertness with respect to the educational environment. Must meet both of the following conditions:

    1. Is related to chronic or acute health problems, such as asthma, attention-deficit disorder or attention-deficit/hyperactivity disorder,

Special Education

CHAPTER 9

---

*The term includes schizophrenia. The term does not apply to children who are socially maladjusted unless they have an emotional disturbance.

diabetes, epilepsy, heart condition, hemophilia, lead poisoning, leukemia, nephritis, rheumatic fever, sickle cell anemia, and Tourette's syndrome.
2. Adversely affects a child's educational performance.
J. *Specific learning disability* is defined as follows:
   1. A disorder in one or more of the basic psychological processes involved in understanding or using language, spoken or written, that may manifest as an imperfect ability to listen, think, speak, read, spell, or do mathematical calculations. This includes conditions such as perceptual disabilities, brain injury, minimal brain dysfunction, dyslexia, and developmental aphasia.
   2. The term does not include learning problems that primarily result from visual, hearing, or motor disabilities; mental retardation; emotional disturbance; or environmental, cultural, or economic disadvantage.
K. *Speech or language impairment* indicates a communication disorder—such as stuttering, impaired articulation, language impairment, or a voice impairment—that adversely affects a child's educational performance.
L. *Traumatic brain injury* means an acquired injury to the brain caused by an external physical force—resulting in total or partial functional disability, psychosocial impairment, or both—that adversely affects a child's educational performance. The term applies to open or closed head injuries that result in impairments in one or more areas, such as cognition; language; memory; attention; reasoning; abstract thinking; judgment; problem solving; sensory, perceptual, and motor abilities; psychosocial behavior; physical functioning; information processing; and speech. The term does not apply to brain injuries that are congenital, degenerative, or caused by birth trauma.
M. *Visual impairment including blindness* refers to a visual impairment that, even with correction, adversely affects a child's educational performance. The term includes both partial sight and blindness.

II. Components of IDEA
A. *Those served* are from birth through 21 years of age.
B. An effort must be made to *screen and identify all children* who are in need of special education and related services.
C. The *environment* must be the *least restrictive*. That is, children with disabilities are to be educated with children who are not disabled. Special education classes, separate schooling, or other arrangements that remove children with disabilities from regular education occur only when the disability is so severe that the student cannot be included in regular education, when provided with supplementary aids and services. In Part C, for children from birth to age 3, if children cannot be served in their natural environment, justification for a restricted placement must be stated on the IFSP. The *natural environment* is defined as anyplace a typical child of this age may be found (e.g., home, day care, Early Head Start, play group).

D. The *program options* within the special education system include the following:
1. Regular class with supplementary aids and services.
2. Related services.
3. Resource specialists.
4. Special day classes.
5. Special schools.
6. Nonpublic schools.
7. Residential facilities, hospitals, home.
E. *Classroom placement* is decided on an individual basis. Certain mandated attendees for the initial placement meeting include the following:
1. One member of the evaluation team.
2. A representative of the public agency.
3. The teacher.
4. A person knowledgeable about evaluation procedures and results.
5. One or both parents or a representative.
6. Other people as appropriate.
F. The *Individualized Education Program (IEP)* is a written plan for each student that guarantees appropriate services. Every special education student must have an IEP at least once a year. The IEP is developed by a team that comprises the following:
1. Parents of the child.
2. Not less than one regular education teacher if the child is, or may be, participating in a regular education environment.
3. Special education teachers or special education providers.
4. A public agency representative who has certain specific knowledge and qualifications.
5. An individual who can interpret instructional implications of evaluation results; may also be one of the other listed members.
6. Other individuals with knowledge or expertise regarding the child, chosen at the parents' or educational agency staff's discretion.
7. The child, when appropriate.
G. The IEP includes statements of the following:
1. Present levels of educational performance and how the individual's disability affects progress in the general curriculum.
2. Measurable annual goals for meeting the student's needs to enable the student to be involved and progress in the general curriculum.
3. Specific special education services, related services, and supplementary aids to be provided for the student; program modifications or supports to school personnel, so the student can participate in regular educational programs and activities as much as possible.
4. An explanation of the extent, if any, to which the child will not participate with nondisabled children in regular education.
5. Modifications needed to participate in state and district assessments; if not participating in a particular state or district assessment, a statement of why that assessment is not appropriate for the child, and how the child will be assessed, must be provided.

Special Education

CHAPTER 9

6. Statement of anticipated frequency, location, and duration of services and modifications.
7. Beginning at age 16, a statement of transition service needs a plan that promotes movement from school to postschool activities.
8. Statement of how the student's progress will be measured and how parents will be regularly informed (e.g., report card).

H. *Student and parent rights* are defined.
1. Parents must receive detailed, written notice in their language whenever the school plans to change, or refuses to change, the identification, assessment, or educational placement of their child.
2. Parents have a right to one independent educational assessment at public expense each time the parent disagrees with an assessment conducted by the public agency. Parents have a right to review and inspect all educational records, give written consent to the assessment plan, give written consent before the child is placed, and refuse to consent to an assessment.
3. Evaluation and tests must be conducted in the student's own language or mode of communication; a variety of achievement tests and teacher recommendations, as well as assessments of physical condition and social or cultural background, are used for placement procedures; regulations prohibit more than one reevaluation in a single year, unless both school district and parents agree; triennial evaluation may be waived when parents and public agency agree the reevaluation is unnecessary.

I. Regarding *confidentiality,* results of assessment data and placement must be kept confidential, and parents or guardians must have access to inspect and obtain copies of information regarding their child. An educational agency receiving federal monies must allow parents to inspect, challenge, and correct their child's records. Students 18 years and older also have the same rights regarding their records. Parents are to be notified when unneeded records are to be destroyed.

J. *Related services* as required to help the child with a disability benefit fully from special education. Services are not limited to the following list, and other services may be included, provided they help the child benefit from special education. Exception: services that apply to children with surgically implanted devices, including cochlear implants (e.g. optimization of the device [mapping] or replacement of the device). Routine checking of external parts of such devices is required. Such children are eligible for all other individual-related services. Public agencies are responsible for monitoring and maintaining medical devices that are needed for the health and safety of the child; these include devices for breathing, nutrition, or operation of other bodily functions, and this responsibility applies when the child is transported to and from school or is at school. Individual-related services:
1. Audiology.
2. Counseling services.
3. Early identification and assessment of disabilities in children.
4. Interpreting services.
5. Medical services (diagnostic and evaluation services only).

6. Occupational therapy.
7. Orientation and mobility services.
8. Parent counseling and training.
9. Physical therapy.
10. Psychological services.
11. Recreation, including therapeutic recreation.
12. Rehabilitation counseling.
13. School health services and school nurse services.
14. Social work services.
15. Speech and language pathology services.
16. Transportation.

K. *Discipline and safety.*
1. IDEA clarifies how school disciplinary rules apply to children in special education. IDEA specifically states that children who need special education must receive instruction and services to help them follow the rules and behave in school. The law recognizes that if students with disabilities bring illegal drugs or weapons to school, or if students cause serious bodily injury, schools have the right to remove the children to an alternative educational setting for up to 45 days. The law also acknowledges the right of schools to report crimes to law enforcement or judicial authorities. While under suspension or expulsion, the student should still receive special education services in an appropriate setting.

SECTION 504 OF THE REHABILITATION ACT OF 1973

This legislation defines disability more broadly than IDEA, which is limited to 13 categories of eligibility. Children with mental or physical disabilities that affect their ability to care for themselves, perform activities of daily living, or participate in educational activities may not be excluded from general school programs or denied special services because they do not have one of the eligible disabilities. Section 504 does not require a student to be enrolled in special education to receive related services. Accommodations and services must be provided to support the maximum educational opportunities possible (e.g., modifications in student assignments, physical adaptations of the school building, peer assistance).

Students are deemed eligible for services through an individualized evaluation by a multidisciplinary team. Students do not need an examination by a physician to qualify for Section 504, unless it is required by school administration. Under Section 504, a *handicapped person* means an individual with a mental or physical impairment that substantially limits one or more major life activities (e.g., breathing, self-care, walking, seeing, hearing, speaking, performing manual tasks, learning). Examples of students who may be eligible for Section 504 include those with attention-deficit disorder (ADD), diabetes, alcohol and drug addiction, asthma, obesity, and acquired immunodeficiency syndrome (AIDS).

Section 504 is a civil rights statute that prohibits discrimination on the basis of disability. States must comply with the regulations of Section 504 if they are to continue to receive federal financial assistance, but they do not receive federal funds for services provided under Section 504. The Office of Civil Rights (OCR) is responsible for monitoring compliance with Section 504 regulations.

Special Education

CHAPTER 9

WEB SITES

Building the Legacy: IDEA 2004
    http://idea.ed.gov/
National Information Center for Children and Youth with Disabilities, State Resource Sheets
    http://www.nichcy.org/states.htm
Office for Civil Rights
    http://www.ed.gov/about/offices/list/ocr/index.html
Offices of Special Education and Rehabilitation Services
    http://www.ed.gov/about/offices/list/osers/index.html

SPECIALIZED HEALTH CARE PROCEDURES AND RELATED ADAPTATIONS

State, county, and district guidelines, procedures, and policies for administering specialized health care procedures (SHCPs) may vary but should include the following components:

1. HCP's authorization for procedure.
2. Parents' written request for the procedure.
3. Waiver signed by parent if procedure is to be performed by nondistrict personnel.
4. Universal precautions.

The main purpose of providing SHCPs in the school is to maintain the student in the school environment. Whether the SHCPs are performed in the student's classroom or another location, one objective is to minimize disruption in educational programming. Other objectives are to address the privacy issues and health needs of the student and their classmates, to address the social and emotional effects surrounding exposure to procedures executed in the classroom, and to address the distraction from classroom work for all students.

When possible the nurse should:

1. Discuss with parents the possibility of doing the procedure before or after school.
2. Provide the procedure at the least disruptive time, if flexible schedule allowed.
3. Minimize the student's time out of the classroom.
4. Have necessary equipment ready and medication available.
5. Use the procedure as an opportunity to teach health and secondary prevention.

The SHCP should be included in the student's IFSP, IEP, IHCP, or Section 504 plan. The plan should reflect information in the SHCP, such as health treatment necessary during school, frequency, personnel involved, and the educational plan for school participation and optimal health. Include goals and objectives as appropriate.

ALLERGIES
Latex Allergies

Allergic reactions and sensitivity to latex proteins have risen dramatically during the past 15 years. The term *latex* is used here to describe products made from *natural rubber latex,* not *synthetic latex* (e.g., latex paint). Children who undergo frequent surgeries or bladder catheterization and individuals who regularly wear latex gloves are at the greatest risk for developing latex allergies. People with allergic rhinitis or other allergies also have a higher risk. Up to 68% of children with spina bifida and 8% to 17% of health care personnel have latex sensitivity, but the figure is less than 1% for the general population (American Latex Allergy Association, 2007).

The extensive use of latex gloves to prevent the spread of human immunodeficiency virus (HIV) and hepatitis B virus is believed to have contributed to the increase and awareness of latex sensitivity. This awareness has led to the education of health care providers regarding the potential health hazards and the necessity to minimize latex exposure.

Symptoms of latex allergy include flushing of the skin or an itchy skin rash, edema, watery or itchy eyes, hives, and wheezing. Anaphylactic shock can also occur. A more severe reaction is likely when latex contacts moist skin, mucous membranes, the airway, or bloodstream.

Cross-reactivity may occur in individuals with latex sensitivity, because they may react to certain foods with a similar protein (see Box 9-1). This cross-reactivity occurs when the immune system mistakes a similar protein or chemical composition for an allergen. Not all foods containing latexlike proteins affect everyone with latex allergies. An allergist can help identify foods and items that will cause an allergic reaction. Most common manifestations of latex-food syndrome are hives, facial edema, rhinitis, and conjunctivitis. Box 9-2 lists items that may contain latex.

Prevention is the best treatment; people who have latex allergy, or who are at high risk, should avoid latex products and foods with latexlike proteins. Those with an allergic reaction to the foods listed in Box 9-1 should discuss a possible latex allergy with their HCP.

I. Procedure
   A. Develop an individualized emergency care plan (IECP) in consultation with the student's parents and HCP.
   B. Educate school staff regarding IECP, and have a plan readily available.
   C. Indicate latex allergy alert on school records.
   D. Use latex-free products when providing nursing care.
   E. Educate staff and student regarding identification of latex products and allergic reaction.
   F. Promote use of personal medical identification (MedicAlert) bracelet.
   G. Discuss availability of injectable epinephrine in all settings (e.g., home, school, car, sports events, day care).

Box 9-1	*Foods with Latexlike Proteins*

• Avocados*	• Mangos	• Peanuts
• Bananas*	• Melons	• Pineapples
• Celery	• Nectarines	• Plums
• Chestnuts*	• Papaya	• Shellfish
• Figs	• Passion fruit	• Strawberries
• Kiwifruit*	• Peaches	• Tomatoes

*Most common allergies.

Special Education

CHAPTER 9

Box 9-2	*Items That May Contain Latex*

- Adhesive tape
- Ambu bags
- Art supplies (markers, glue, paint)
- Baby bottle nipples
- Balloons
- Balls, rubber mats, racquet handles
- Adhesive bandages (Band-Aids) or similar products
- Beach toys
- Blood pressure cuffs (bladder and tubing)
- Bulb syringes
- Chewing gum
- Colostomy pouch
- Condoms and condom urinary collection devices
- Diaphragm
- Elastic bandages

- Eye shields/patches
- Foam rubber padding on wheelchairs, lining on splints and braces
- Gloves—examination and sterile
- Pacifier
- Racquet handles
- Raincoats/gear
- Rubber bands
- Shower cap/swimming cap
- Stethoscope tubing
- Stomach and gastrointestinal tubes
- Swimming fins
- Tennis/squash shoes
- Tourniquets
- Urinary catheters
- Underwear
- Wheelchair tires

WEB SITE

American Latex Allergy Association
  http://www.latexallergyresources.org

ELIMINATION
Urinary Self-Catheterization (Clean, Intermittent)

I. Definition

   A. Self-catheterization is the introduction of a catheter through the urethra into the bladder. It is performed using a clean technique by students with a neurogenic bladder resulting from spinal cord dysfunction or neuromuscular disease. Self-catheterization is important, because it promotes independence.

II. Purpose

   A. The purpose of self-catheterization is to allow an individual who has no bladder control, or the student using a bladder-training program, to empty the bladder at appropriate intervals. It relieves bladder distention that can lead to discomfort, overflow, and dribbling. It also control odors, prevents skin breakdown, and decreases susceptibility to urinary tract and bladder infections by reducing residual urine.

III. Equipment

   A. Catheter, as prescribed by HCP.
   B. Mirror for initial female instruction.
   C. Water-soluble lubricant, if ordered.
   D. Cleansing agent and 4-inch gauze squares or cotton balls.
   E. Clean, disposable, nonlatex gloves, when student does not perform the procedure.

    F. Container for urine, if individual is unable to use the toilet or for measurement of urine.

    G. Storage container for catheter (jar, plastic bags, make-up bag).

NOTE: Facilities often are not available for adequate cleansing of the catheter, in which case the individual may carry extra catheters and two containers: one marked "dirty" and one marked "clean."

    H. Storage container for all of the equipment, labeled with the student's name.

IV. Instructions

    A. Before urinary catheterization:

      1. Wash hands thoroughly.

      2. Clean table surface or place clean protective paper on the table.

      3. Place catheter and a small amount of lubricant on a paper towel on a clean surface.

      4. Position of student varies according to gender and disability.

      5. Use gloves when nurse or designated individual performs procedure.

    B. Female student:

      1. The student should lie down or be in a sitting position; catheterization may be easier if the student sits facing backward on the toilet or stands with one foot on the toilet edge.

      2. Expose and cleanse urethral area, wiping from front to back; use a cotton ball for each stroke.

      3. Identify location of urethral meatus by beginning at clitoris and applying pressure with finger until urethral indentation is felt.

      4. Holding the catheter 3 inches (7.5 cm) from the tip, lubricate the tip and insert it through the meatus 1 to 2 inches, downward and back, until urine appears; rotate gently if resistance is felt; the other end of the catheter should be placed in a collection container or in the toilet.

      5. When the urine flow stops, advance the catheter slightly. If no more urine passes, withdraw the catheter slightly, and rotate to ensure drainage of all areas of the bladder.

      6. When the bladder is empty, pinch the catheter and withdraw it slowly.

    C. Male student:

      1. Individual should sit on the toilet or in a chair until the technique has been learned.

      2. Hold penis up at 45 to 90 degree angle. If not circumcised, retract foreskin, and wash glans with soapy cotton balls or with student-specific supplies; begin at urethral opening and proceed in a circular manner, washing away from the meatus.

      3. Gently insert the catheter until urine returns; place the other end of the catheter in a collection container or toilet. If resistance is felt at the external sphincter of the bladder, have student breathe deeply or slightly increase the traction on the penis and apply gentle, steady pressure on the catheter. When urine has been obtained, insert the catheter about an inch farther, and rotate it so that the catheter openings have reached all areas of the bladder.

Special Education

CHAPTER 9

    4. Slowly remove the catheter when urine ceases to flow. When the bladder is emptied, pinch the catheter and withdraw it.

D. After urinary catheterization:
1. Nurse: remove gloves, wash hands, and don clean gloves.
2. Wash, rinse, dry, and store catheter.
3. Rinse and dry urine receptacle, if appropriate.
4. Remove gloves and wash hands.
5. Document time, approximate amount of urine, and any signs of infection such as an off color, odor, or change in appearance of urine.
6. Help student with any difficult clothing items and transfers if needed.
7. Encourage student to assume responsibility for procedure as appropriate.

Other Elimination Adaptations

I. Urinary Diversions

A. Urinary diversion procedures, continent and incontinent, may be used for a neurogenic bladder, urinary strictures, birth defects, damage resulting from trauma, or chronic infections that have led to ureteral and renal damage. These procedures are used to divert urine from the bladder to another location, most commonly an opening on the skin.

B. *Vesicostomy* is a relatively uncomplicated procedure whereby the bladder is sutured to the abdominal wall; an opening is made through the abdominal wall into the bladder wall, creating a stoma on the skin surface for urinary drainage. Diapers are worn high, or absorbent pads are used to cover the stoma; these must be changed frequently to avoid skin irritation from the continuous urinary drainage. A vesicostomy usually is a temporary solution, usually performed on children under age 5, but it may be used in older children also.

C. One of the most common procedures for continent urinary reconstruction is the *appendicovesicostomy.* This involves using the appendix to join the bladder to the wall of the abdomen. The appendix provides a conduit for catheterization, and a one-way valve is created to prevent urinary leakage. The location of this opening on the abdomen is convenient for catheterization, especially self-catheterization, at routine intervals to maintain continence. In some situations, the bladder is augmented with bowel or stomach tissue to increase bladder size and reduce spasticity. Appendicovesicostomy is also called the Mitrofanoff catheterizable channel.

D. Another urinary diversion is a *Kock pouch,* in which an artificial bladder is created surgically from a section of the small intestines, or an *Indiana pouch,* using the large intestine. The stoma is located on the skin, which allows for periodic catheterization. This pouch is an adaptation of the one used for bowel incontinence.

E. Other urinary diversions involve use of a collection bag or pouch. *Urostomy* is the general term used for the surgical technique to divert urine from the bladder. One of the oldest procedures is the *ileal conduit (loop),* which is made by implanting a ureter into a 12 cm loop of ileum or sigmoid colon that is brought out to the abdominal wall for urinary drainage. Urine is collected in an ileostomy bag or pouch. A variety of appliances are available, and most last 3 to 7 days before leaking develops.

II. Bowel Diversions

A. *Colostomy* is the surgical procedure to make an opening from the large intestine to the abdomen with a stoma on the skin. The stoma should be shiny and pink to bright red. The colostomy may be temporary or permanent and also is differentiated by the part of the colon brought to the surface of the abdomen. The *sigmoid or descending colostomy* is the most common type, and the stoma is on the lower left side of the abdomen. A *transverse colostomy* results in one or two stomas in the upper, middle, or right side of the abdomen. A *loop colostomy* has two stomas and usually is found in the transverse colon; one stoma is for stool, and the other is for mucus. A loop colostomy usually is a temporary procedure. Colostomies may be irrigated to establish a regular evacuation pattern.

B. An *ileostomy* involves bringing the small intestine to the abdomen and creating a stoma that may be temporary or permanent. Contents of the ileum are semiliquid fecal material that seeps continuously, so routine bowel habits are impossible. Skin care is especially important. Other surgical procedures are used to develop internal pouches that can be drained by a tube or catheter, such as the *ileoanal pouch*. See Box 9-3 for more information on urinary and stool collection systems care.

C. *Appendicostomy,* also known as the Malone Antegrade Continent Enema (MACE), is a procedure allowing bowel control through the use of a daily enema in a stoma created on the abdomen that connects to the proximal colon. These are often confused with a urinary stoma, because they are similar in appearance and location. The student sits on the toilet while the stoma is irrigated with normal saline, a procedure generally done once a day.

III. Stoma Complications

A. *Infection* of stoma site can occur due to bacteria or fungus on the skin or cross-contamination. Symptoms include redness around the site, pain, loss of appetite, nausea, vomiting, and fever. Mild infections can be treated with topical ointment, but more serious infections require oral antibiotics.

B. *Stomal stenosis* may be caused by infection, hypergranulation of the stoma, or by scarring. Dilatation of the stoma may be urgently needed; if untreated, stenosis may lead to surgical revision.

C. *Bladder perforation* may result from forceful or traumatizing catheterization. Symptoms include suprapubic or abdominal pain, a vague illness with nausea, vomiting, and abdominal distention.

D. *Hypergranulation* occurs when there is growth of tissue beyond the level of the stoma that may bleed easily and ooze fluid; the surrounding skin appears red. Hypergranulation may be caused by friction or excess moisture. Treatment is usually cauterization with silver nitrate or surgical intervention.

Box 9-3   *Urinary and Stool Collection Systems Care*

- Pouching systems attach to the abdomen with an adhesive back and use a bag, which fits over the stoma to collect the diverted output, either urine or stool. The backing may be one piece (face-plate) or two pieces (flange).
- The bag may be open-ended for required drainage; a closing device such as a clamp, clip, or wire closure is used.
- The sealed type bag is used most commonly for individuals who are undergoing irrigation for control or have a regular elimination pattern.
- Meticulous skin care is needed to prevent peristomal skin breakdown and maintain a good seal.
- Ivory soap removes oils from the skin so that the pouch will adhere better.
- Use of a skin barrier (e.g., tincture of benzoin, Stomahesive, or Stomaguard) helps protect the skin and aids in adhesion. The barrier may be in liquid form or barrier wipes. Some pouches have a built-in skin barrier.
- Skin barrier paste can be used to fill crevices or folds in the skin, thus creating a better seal.
- Special tapes are available to help support the adhesive backing and for waterproofing.

- Ostomy belts that circle the abdomen and attach to the pouch may be used for support or as an alternative to adhesives.
- The bag should be emptied when about one-third full to prevent the weight from pulling it off the skin.
- Most systems will last 3 to 7 days without leaking.
- Colostomy bags usually are changed every 2 to 4 days.
- Adhesive remover is useful for removing residue when the system is changed.
- Reusable appliances should be rinsed in warm water and soaked in a 3:1 solution of water and white vinegar, or a commercial cleaner, for 30 minutes.
- Rinse the appliance with tepid water and dry away from direct sunlight to avoid drying out the material, which may lead to cracking.
- Certain foods (e.g., eggs, cheese, asparagus) give a strong odor to urine.
- Specific foods—such as cabbage, onions, and fish—increase stool odors. Some foods, such as spinach and parsley, help fight odors.
- Some systems have an odor barrier; a liquid deodorizer or a few drops of diluted vinegar may be added to the bag to help fight odors.

WEB SITE

United Ostomy Associations of America
http://www.uoaa.org

FEEDING

Gastrostomy and Jejunostomy Feedings

I. Definition

A. A gastrostomy is an artificial opening through the abdominal wall with a tube extended directly into the stomach; with a jejunostomy, the tube extends directly into the jejunum (i.e., the small intestine between the duodenum and the ileum).

B. Feeding by a *gastrostomy* or *jejunostomy* is performed by passing a nutrient solution, medication, or both through a tube inserted directly into a skin-level device or attached to an external tube at the abdominal site or stoma. Several types of skin-level (button) devices are available.

C. Feeding by a gastrostomy, or G tube, may be by bolus (about 15 to 20 minutes), by gravity, or by slow drip through a pump. The jejunostomy feeding is best tolerated as a continuous slow drip.

D. The jejunostomy, or J tube, may be in a separate stoma. If a student has *both* a J tube and a G tube, both tubes may be in the same stoma; or one tube (gastrojejunal) with several ports may be used (J port, G port, medication port, or balloon inflation limb). The combination tubes are used for students who require gastric decompression during the J feeding because of an obstruction in the gastric outlet.

II. **Purpose**

A. Gastrostomy and jejunostomy feedings provide total or supplemental nutritional support, hydration, and administration of medication when the oral route is not feasible or adequate.

III. **Equipment**

A. Catheter-tipped syringe, 60 ml for irrigation and feeding by gravity or bolus.

B. Feeding bag or bottle for slow drip-feeding.

C. Prescribed formula, medication, or both at room temperature; check expiration date. Opened formula usually is good for 24 hours when refrigerated and 4 hours when not.

D. Water for flushing and hydration, as prescribed.

E. Catheter plug, clamp, or rubber band.

F. Gauze pads (2 or 3 inch squares) and scissors.

G. Nonlatex, disposable gloves.

H. Extension tube or adapter if skin-level device is being used.

I. Decompression tube may be needed for some skin-level devices with an antireflux valve or two-way valve to vent when abdominal distention occurs. The decompression tube should be in place no longer than 5 to 10 minutes; frequent prolonged use may prematurely weaken the valve.

J. Hook on the wall or a stand to suspend the formula for feeding.

K. Feeding pump, if prescribed.

L. Pacifier for a baby during feeding.

IV. **Instructions**

A. Refer to HCP's prescription for specific recommendations or adaptations to the following procedure. Students with a feeding tube need written permission from their HCP to be given any oral foods. The order should include the texture and amount of oral foods tolerated. Box 9-4 describes some problems with enteral feedings.

1. The student should be in high Fowler's position if possible; the back should be well supported. Some students may tolerate feeding while semireclined or lying down; lying on the right side is optimal.

2. Wash hands and don gloves.

3. With G tube: assess bowel sounds, check for abdominal distention, and check for residual prior to feeding (gastrostomy feedings only). Follow HCP's orders for instructions.

4. When tube placement is confirmed, connect the syringe to the external tube or extension tube for skin-level device. Fill extension tube with formula before connecting it to the button.

Box 9-4   *Problems Associated With Enteral Feedings*

Follow specific instructions found in HCP orders, IHCP, and state, county, or district policies and procedures.

If tube is forcefully pulled out:

1. If bleeding occurs, press on the site with clean gauze pads until bleeding stops.
2. Maintain ostomy by inserting catheter 2 to 3 in and secure with tape; if Foley catheter is used, inflate balloon and pull Foley catheter back to ensure balloon is inflated adequately. Follow HCP's instruction for reinsertion if skin-level device is dislodged. Do not attempt replacement unless tube is well established.
3. New gastrostomy tubes (<3 weeks) should be replaced within 3 hours to prevent closure of stoma. Established tubes will remain patent for a longer period and are easier to replace.
4. Jejunostomy tubes must be replaced within 3 to 4 hours; longer delays may result in tract closure.

If vomiting or diarrhea occur:

1. For formula intolerance, try another formula.
2. Try formulas with texture, which may help alleviate diarrhea.
3. Dry heaves may also occur.
4. Could be caused by gastrointestinal virus.

If excessive leakage occurs around stoma:

1. Occurs when the tube pulls away from the interior abdominal wall.
2. Occurs when stoma is enlarged so that the button or tube does not fit properly; may need larger button or tube; changes in student's weight (gain or loss) may necessitate adjustment of tube length and space between balloon and fixation device to maintain appropriate tension.
3. Occurs when balloon is not sufficiently inflated to maintain appropriate tension on stoma to prevent leakage (too loose); but may cause necrosis if too tight; tension is appropriate when tube

is flush with the abdomen and the tube fixation device can be easily rotated. Skin-level feeding device should be one-eighth inch above the skin.

4. Is treated with stoma adhesive powder or skin barrier (DuoDerm) cut and placed around stoma.

If peristomal area redness with increased tenderness, swelling, and purulent drainage occur:

1. May result from excessive leakage of caustic gastric juices from stoma.
2. Is cleaned with soap and water and dried thoroughly, check temperature, and notify parent.
3. May have prescribed daily application of antibiotic ointment and placement of gauze dressing around the stoma.
4. May be prevented by keeping peristomal skin dry and rotating button during stoma care to prevent skin breakdown.

If hypergranulation tissue is present:

1. May increase with leakage, although granulation (proud flesh) occurs normally during the healing process of the stoma.
2. May be cauterized with silver nitrate.
3. May decrease in amount or skin may heal with application of moisture barrier (Calmoseptine), sucralfate powder, or foam dressing (Hydrasorb).

If tube/button is occluded:

1. May occur after feeding or administration of medication if irrigation is insufficient.
2. May be prevented by cleaning inside of feeding button with moist, cotton-tipped applicator to help maintain patency.
3. May be irrigated with 2 to 3 ml of water in a 10 ml syringe while gently trying to dislodge plug. *Do not force.* Notify parent, HCP, or both.

If tube or button must be replaced frequently:

1. May need larger tube or button.

5. With MIC-KEY, line up black lines of the skin-level button and extension tubing, lock into place by turning extension tubing a quarter-turn clockwise. Do not turn past the stop point, because this will break the lock.
6. Pour feeding into tilted syringe, unclamp the filled tubing, and let fluid flow into the stomach; tilting of syringe lets air bubbles escape and not enter the stomach.
7. Regulate the flow rate by raising or lowering the syringe and tubing.
8. Decompression may be needed before, during, or after feeding to relieve excessive gas.
9. Continuous decompression is provided by using a Y tube (opened) while feeding.
10. For gravity or slow-drip feeding, place the bag on a hook at the height needed to achieve ordered flow, pour in formula, and allow tubing to fill before attachment to the feeding button. The flow may be 2 to 3 ml/min.
11. After each feeding, flush the tube with 10 to 30 ml of water, unless a larger amount is prescribed; clamp or insert plastic stopper before water drains from the tubing.
    a. Water will keep the tube clean and prevent clogging.
    b. Air will not enter the stomach with next feeding.
    c. If a clamp is used, a small gauze dressing can be placed over the tube opening to keep it clean.
12. Tubing should be secure; an abdominal binder or netting can be used.
13. Wash feeding equipment and store in a clean area. Equipment can be placed in a zippered plastic bag and refrigerated to inhibit bacterial growth.
14. Remove gloves and wash hands.
15. Feed with other students whenever feasible; use of a pacifier with infants may provide oral stimulation, improve oral function, and facilitate absorption of nutrients.
16. Refer to general orders for activity level after feeding.
17. Document date and time of procedure, amount and type of formula and irrigant, and tolerance level of procedure.

V. **Complications and Treatment for Gastroesophageal Reflux Disease**

A. *Gastroesophageal reflux disease (GERD)* occurs when the lower esophageal sphincter is weak or relaxes inappropriately, allowing reflux of gastric contents into the esophagus. The exact cause is unknown, but GERD may occur with prematurity, bronchopulmonary dysplasia, neurological disorders, asthma, cerebral palsy, and tube feedings. Reflux may lead to esophagitis, recurrent respiratory infections, aspiration pneumonia, or reflux-associated apnea and bradycardia.

B. *Symptoms of GERD* include restlessness, irritability, spitting up, frequent respiratory tract infections, vomiting, and weight loss.

C. Treatment includes frequent, smaller feedings of thickened liquids or formula. Reflux may be reduced by feeding the student in a semi-Fowler's position, avoiding slumping, and remaining in semireclining position for 30 minutes after eating. Medications to improve gastric motility (e.g., metoclopramide [Reglan]) or neutralize gastric acid (e.g., ranitidine hydrochloride [Zantac]) and proton-pump inhibitors (e.g., omeprazole [Prilosec]) may be prescribed.

VI. Surgical Options for Gastroesophageal Reflux Disease

A. If reflux persists, *fundoplication* surgery is considered. In this procedure, the upper portion of the stomach (fundus) is wrapped around the lower part of the esophagus to prevent reflux; it may involve a partial wrap to a full 360-degree wrap. A tight wrap prohibits vomiting, and the child may gag or develop respiratory distress when overfed or when intestinal flu is present. With a gastrostomy, a decompression tube can be used to release gas or stomach contents, thus relieving pressure on the diaphragm and lungs. If fundoplication is performed without a gastrostomy, pressure is relieved by insertion of a nasogastric tube. Over time, the fundoplication may loosen, and vomiting will again be possible.

B. Newer, less invasive alternatives than fundoplication are available. The Stretta device is inserted by endoscopy. The device coagulates the tissue in the gastroesophageal junction, making it resistant to reflux. Several treatments are required for this procedure. The EndoCinch is a tool inserted by endoscopy wherein stitches create a pleat in the sphincter at the gastroesophageal junction, which reduces the backflow of acid from the stomach into the esophagus. The Plicator procedure utilizes a tool that grasps, folds, wraps, and fixates tissue at the junction between the esophagus and the stomach to minimize reflux.

WEB SITES

International Foundation for Functional Gastrointestinal Disorders, About Kids' and Teens' GI Health
> http://www.aboutkidsgi.org

Gastrostomy Information and Support Society (GISS)
> http://www.scopcvic.org.au/therapy_advisory_giss.html

United Ostomy Associations of America
> http://www.uoaa.org

ORTHOPEDIC
Crutches

I. Definition

A. Crutches are devices used as temporary or permanent aids for walking, when an injury or disability is too severe for a cane but not severe enough for a wheelchair. A *crutch gait* is achieved by alternately bearing weight on one or both legs using the crutches. The condition, functional level, and physical abilities of the student determine the gait selected to teach. *Crutch gaits* include two-point, three-point, four-point, swing-through, and swing-to gaits. The term *point* refers to the number of points in contact with the floor during ambulation.

II. Purpose
A. Crutches are used by students to prevent weight bearing on the affected limb, to move gait control to the arms and hands, or to support and balance while walking with braces. Crutches free the student from dependence on others as much as possible.

III. Equipment
A. A variety of crutch types exist, and the student's specific condition and physical ability determine their use.
   1. *Axillary crutches* are the most common for short-term assistance.
   2. *Forearm crutches* generally are used when permanent assistance is anticipated. The *Lofstrand crutch* has a cuff that fits around the forearm supporting the weight on a handbar, thus allowing the student to release the hand and grasp objects or a handrail without dropping the crutch.
   3. *Trough crutches* allow body weight to be assumed by the elbow.

IV. Instructions
A. Crutches or any assistive devices used by children (e.g., cane, walker) must be fitted properly to prevent crutch pressure on the axilla, develop a stable and normal gait, maintain safety, and ensure good posture during ambulation. This fitting is commonly done by a physical therapist, whereas the nurse manages the procedure at school, and often in the home.
   1. When using axillary crutches, the student's weight is on the hands with crutches pressed against side of the chest wall.
   2. Crutches should not be pressed into the axilla, because pressure can damage the brachial plexus nerves.
   3. For a gross check of measurement, have the student stand in good balance with crutches and assess the following points:
      a. Standing base is with crutch tips about 4 to 8 inches in front of and 4 inches to sides of the student; taller individuals need a wider base.
      b. Bend in elbows is between 20 and 30 degrees.
      c. Crutch pads are 1½ inches below axilla.
   4. Observe for difficulty in grasping horizontal handpiece.
   5. For security, crutch tips should be wide and provide good suction.
   6. Check tips and replace worn tips promptly to prevent slipping.
   7. Take extra precautions in rainy weather to avoid slipping.
   8. Screws and nuts often become loose on mechanical aids; properly maintained equipment increases student's safety.
   9. Designate a place in the classroom for crutches to be kept when not in use, because they can be a safety hazard to other students; often the custodian is willing to install a hook or other form of crutch holder in a convenient spot.
   10. A backpack is useful for students who use crutches or other assistive devices, because it allows the student to maintain maximum independence; discuss with student and caregiver the proper packing and distribution of weight and total weight for backpack. See Chapter 10 for Backpack Complications.

11. Student should wear appropriate nonskid shoes.
12. Consult physical therapist or occupational therapist as needed.

Orthoses

A variety of orthoses are available and may be used to prevent deformity, control alignment, increase efficiency of gait, or stabilize weakened or paralyzed extremities.

Orthoses *must* be well fitted and maintained to promote ambulation; if not, they can disturb balance, create a safety hazard, produce muscle stress, and cause tissue breakdown. See Box 9-5 for precautionary considerations for skin and orthoses. If long-term use is necessary, ongoing adjustment and replacement by an orthotist is required.

Four common types of lower-limb orthoses are used. They are characterized by the joints controlled by the specific device. An *ankle–foot orthosis (AFO)* is used to support the ankle and foot in an appropriate position for standing and walking; prevent foot-drop caused by trauma, paralysis of flexor muscles, or bed rest; or prevent heel-cord tightening after heel-cord-lengthening surgery. AFO devices promote optimal motion and are designed to maintain a rigid ankle, but they may allow for some flexibility. They are made in distinct lengths for specific ankle and foot conditions, and they can be ordered in a variety of colors and patterns.

Box 9-5 | *Precautionary Considerations for Skin and Orthoses*

Skin

1. Skin requires meticulous care.
2. Check skin every 4 hours, if decreased sensation in limb occurs or orthosis is new, check more frequently.
3. When placing orthoses, check skin for redness and make sure area is clean and dry; greaseless lotions can be used, preferably not before placement of device.
4. Check to ensure orthoses are on correct limbs with proper heel positioning, back and down.
5. Stockinette or sock worn under device is recommended, which allows for skin protection; should be clean, dry, and without wrinkles to prevent skin breakdown.
6. With any redness lasting more than 20 minutes, or if raw or sore spots are present, report to parent and HCP or orthotist.
7. If child complains of burning sensation, check skin; if complaint continues, contact parent and HCP or orthotist.

8. With blister or open skin, cover area with sterile dressing; avoid orthoses until healed.
9. When prolonged healing time occurs, contact parent and HCP or orthotist.

Orthoses

1. Clean plastic area with damp cloth, no soap, and dry thoroughly.
2. Oil joints of device periodically with three-in-one oil or WD-40, and check screws for tightness.
3. Clean once a month or more: unscrew joints, clean, oil, and reassemble; apply saddle soap to leather.
4. Clean thoracolumbosacral orthosis (TLSO) once a week with soap and water and rinse; must dry completely.
5. Keep away from heat or flame (e.g., hot surfaces, direct sunlight, warm radiator), because device is usually made of temperature-sensitive material that may melt or lose shape.
6. Misaligned or nonfunctioning brace should be reported immediately to parent and HCP or orthotist.

The *knee–ankle–foot orthosis (KAFO)* is used to redistribute weight, control motion at the knees, control functional gait, and improve general safety during ambulation. It is used in the event of paralysis or weakness of the quadriceps muscle, knee extension, or to limit weight bearing. The KAFO supports the knee, ankle, and foot and may have locked or unlocked knee joints.

The *hip–knee–ankle–foot orthosis (HKAFO)* is used to provide control of all joints from the hip down. The hip and knee design may be unlocked, allowing both sitting and standing, or it may allow for standing only.

The *reciprocal gait orthosis (RGO)* is similar to the HKAFO but allows paraplegic children to walk in a reciprocal fashion. RGOs are useful for children with spina bifida, sacral agenesis, or spinal cord injury.

The *thoracolumbosacral orthosis (TLSO)* is used to prevent the continuation of spinal curvature caused by scoliosis. The device is molded individually to fit snugly around the trunk or body, thus placing pressure on the ribs and back to support the spine in a straight position. The *Boston brace* is the commonly used brace for scoliosis and is made of polypropylene. It provides the necessary torso support for a paraplegic child, presents fewer difficulties with dressing, and is more comfortable than the leather-and-metal bracing. The *Jewett Hyperextension brace* may be used to provide support to the spine and trunk during ambulation to prevent compression for individuals who have had a spinal column fracture.

RESPIRATORY
Postural Drainage and Percussion
  I. **Definition**
   A. *Postural drainage* is positioning of a student to enhance gravity drainage of secretions from specific segments of the bronchi and major lung segments into the trachea. Coughing generally removes secretions from the trachea. Different positions are required to accomplish complete segmental drainage. The number of positions placed during each session is individualized and depends on the student's age and tolerance level.
   B. *Percussion* is placing the hand in a stiffened, cupped position and striking the student's chest in a rhythmic motion by flexing the wrist. The air pocket enclosed in the cupped hand strikes the chest; a clopping, not a slapping, sound should be heard. Percussion is performed over the rib cage and should be painless.
   C. Newer modes of providing chest percussion therapy (CPT) are available and are effective in clearing mucus. The Vest airway clearance system is an inflatable vest with hoses connected to a high-frequency pulse generator. As the air circulates, the vest causes vibrations that loosen secretions. The Flutter mucus clearance mechanism and the positive expiratory pressure (PEP) mask are other methods that allow independent chest percussion therapy, but they are more difficult to perform and require more discipline.
  II. **Purpose**
   A. Maintains maximum lung capacity by facilitating drainage and expectoration of secretions. Percussion is used in chronic pulmonary conditions that produce thick mucous secretions, such as cystic fibrosis, and

paralytic conditions, such as cerebral palsy and muscular dystrophy. It is most effective after other respiratory therapy (e.g., nebulization, bronchodilator therapy) and usually is administered three to four times a day before mealtimes.

III. Equipment
    A. Pillows.
    B. Tissues.
    C. Percussion cup, if used.
    D. Suction machine and necessary materials, if ordered.
    E. Wastebasket with plastic liner.

IV. Instructions
    A. Refer to HCP prescription for specific recommendations or adaptations.
       1. Have all necessary materials available before starting.
       2. Be alert to the need for suctioning if mucous plug or thick secretions are produced and occlude the airway.
       3. If percussion is to be used, percuss 1 to 5 minutes over appropriate lobe; time varies according to student and specific recommendations.
       4. Follow HCP prescription or use instructions for drainage and percussion of an infant or young child (Figure 9-1).
       5. Use the positions shown in Figure 9-2 for drainage and percussion of students who weigh more than 40 lb; a darkened area in the figure indicates percussion areas.
    B. Figure 9-1 and Figure 9-2 are anatomical, not functional, drawings. These positions promote drainage of secretions in the necessary pulmonary areas.
    C. Physician recommendations should be followed and usually are based on radiographic studies. Length of percussion time generally is 5 minutes for each position, but it may vary.
    D. The illustrations show approximate percussion points and body positions chosen to cover specific lobes of the lungs while minimizing fatigue or irritability in the infant or young child and diminishing disruptions in the educational programming for older children. Parents and caregivers are more inclined to do postural drainage on a consistent basis when fewer positions are taught, and these will provide the necessary action.

Tracheostomy Care

I. Definition
    A. A tracheostomy is a surgical method of providing an artificial airway through an opening into the trachea. The opening is made between the second and fourth tracheal rings. The inner cannula of the tracheostomy and stoma must be cleaned periodically to maintain a patent airway. The inner cannula is removed and cleaned, and the outer cannula remains in place.
    B. Plastic inner cannulas are cleaned every 8 hours or as needed. Metal inner cannulas are cleaned every 4 hours or as needed. Many plastic or silicone elastic (silastic) tracheostomy tubes do not have inner cannulas, because such tubes resist crusting and do not require daily cleaning.

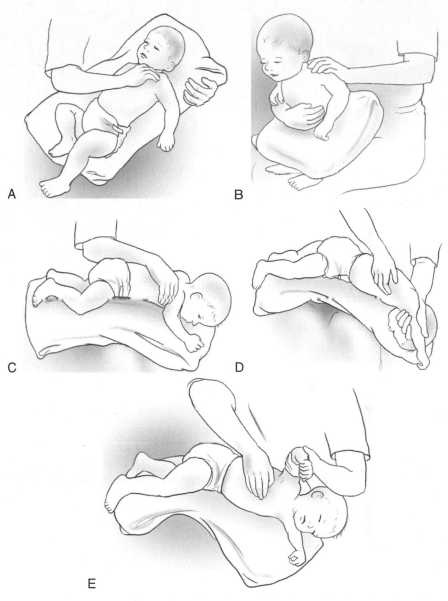

FIGURE 9-1 Postural drainage and percussion positions for infants and young children. **A,** Left upper lobe, apical and anterior segments. Same position, hand moves to right side to percuss right upper lobe, apical and anterior segments. **B,** Left upper lobe, posterior segment. Same position, hand moves to right side to percuss right upper lobe, posterior segment. **C,** Right lower lobe, superior segment and posterior basal segment. Same position, hand moves to left side to percuss left lower lobe, superior segment, and posterior basal segment. **D,** Right lower lobe, lateral basal segment. Reverse position and percuss on left for left lower lobe, lateral basal segment. **E,** Right lower lobe, anterior basal segment, and right middle lobe. Reverse position and percuss on the left side for left lower lobe, anterior basal and lingular segments.

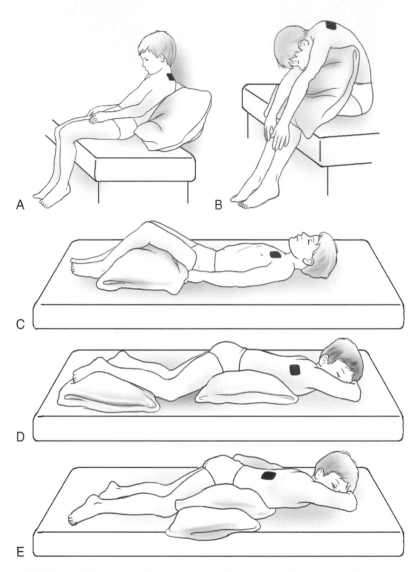

FIGURE 9-2 Postural drainage and percussion positions for students who weigh more than 40 pounds. **A,** Left and right upper lobes, anterior apical segments. Percuss at shoulders with fingers extending over collarbone in front. Percuss right side and left side**. B,** Right and left upper lobes, posterior apical segments. Percuss with hands on shoulders and fingers extending slightly over the shoulder. Percuss right side and left side. **C,** Right and left upper lobes, anterior segment. Percuss between clavicle and nipple. Percuss right side and left side. **D,** Right and left lower lobes, superior segments. Percuss at lower scapula. Percuss right side and left side. Have student lie flat with single pillow under stomach and lower legs. **E,** Left and right lower lobes, posterior basal segments. Percuss over lower ribs, avoid kidney area. Percuss right side and left side. Elevate hips 12 to 16 in.

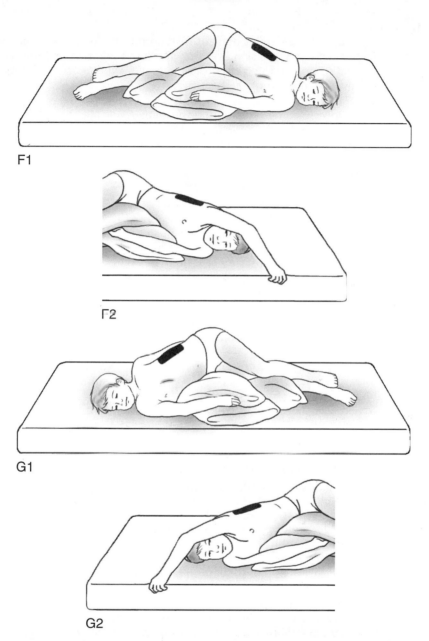

F1

F2

G1

G2

FIGURE 9-2, cont'd **F1,** Right middle lobe and lower lobe, anterior basal segment. Elevate hips 12 to 16 in. With student lying on left side, rotate one quarter turn backward. Percuss over ribs on right side of chest beneath armpit to end of rib cage. **F2,** Right lateral basal lobe. Rotate one quarter turn forward and percuss over ribs beneath armpit to end of rib cage. **G1,** Left lower lobe and lingular segment. Elevate hips 12 to 16 in. With student lying on left side, rotate one quarter turn backward. Percuss over ribs on left side of chest beneath armpit to end of rib cage. **G2,** Left lateral basal lobe. Rotate one quarter turn forward and percuss over left lower ribs beneath armpit to end of rib cage to drain.

II. Purpose
A. Tracheostomy care helps prevent irritation of the tissue surrounding the tube and prevents skin breakdown around the tracheostomy site to avoid secondary infections, and it removes exudate and secretions to prevent occlusion of the lumen.

III. Equipment
A. The following materials should be available:
1. Four nonwaxed paper cups.
2. Suction equipment and sterile or clean catheter.
3. Oxygen equipment if needed.
4. Half-inch twill tape or hook-and-loop (Velcro) ties.
5. Six to eight cotton-tipped applicators.
6. Pipe cleaners, doubled for cleaning.
7. Sterile saline solution, water, or both.
8. Hydrogen peroxide (H_2O_2); do not use with sterling silver tracheostomy tubes, because it may pit the surface.
9. Scissors, if tracheostomy ties are to be changed.
10. Clean, disposable, nonlatex gloves.
11. Plastic bag for waste.
12. Paper towels.
13. Replacement tracheostomy tube, one size smaller than the one in place if needed for reintubation.

IV. Instructions
A. Refer to HCP's prescription for specific recommendations or adaptations to the following procedure. Do not leave student unattended during procedure.
1. Explain procedure to student and allow participation as appropriate.
2. Wash hands.
3. Position student.
   a. Infant: place small towel roll under shoulders, since neck is short; this will provide optimal access to trachea. Elbow restraints may be necessary to keep child from reaching for the tube; or wrap the child in a towel or sheet.
   b. Older child: position with tracheostomy area exposed; if possible, place in Fowler's position to prevent any solution from seeping into stoma.
4. Place cotton applicators and pipe cleaners on paper towel.
5. Put four paper cups on the paper towel, labeled and filled with the following solutions:
   a. Hydrogen peroxide to cover inner cannula.
   b. Sterile saline solution to soak one half of cotton applicators.
   c. Sterile saline solution to soak inner cannula.
   d. Sterile saline solution to rinse inner cannula.
6. Wash hands and don gloves.
7. Perform tracheostomy suctioning as needed (see Tracheostomy Suctioning in the next section).
8. Turn latch that holds inner cannula in place, and slowly remove inner cannula with outward and downward semicircular movement of wrist.

9. If student is receiving mechanical ventilation, use one of the following methods:
   a. Plug tracheostomy opening and encourage student to ventilate by glossopharyngeal breathing.
   b. Attach ambulatory manual breathing unit (ambu bag) to outer cannula, and have another person assist by compressing bag.
10. Place inner cannula in cup with hydrogen peroxide and soak 1 to 5 minutes.
11. Roll soaked cotton applicators over skin surrounding stoma:
    a. Use circular motion, cleaning next to stoma first, then work outward to at least 1 inch (2.54 cm) beyond outer cannula.
    b. Clean each area of skin only once with each applicator; discard each soiled applicator into waste bag.

NOTE: Normal secretions are clear and white with no odor; odor and green or yellow drainage may indicate infection.

12. Dry skin with dry applicators.
13. Remove inner cannula from hydrogen peroxide and remove secretions with pipe cleaners
14. Place cannula in cup with saline solution to soak.
15. Remove cannula and pour clean saline solution over and through cannula to rinse thoroughly.
16. Shake excess water from cannula; cannula may be dried with clean gauze.
17. Replace inner cannula and secure lock.
18. Pour out solutions and discard cups, pipe cleaners, and so forth.
19. If suction of outer cannula is necessary, complete before replacing inner cannula.
20. Remove gloves and wash hands.
21. Change tape as necessary, using twill or Velcro tapes.
    a. Have another person help keep child still or wrap infant "mummy style."
    b. Keep old ties secured and push to top of holes on tracheostomy flange.
    c. Tie new tapes.
    d. Secure with knot at side of neck; rotate knot occasionally to prevent redness or breakdown of skin.
    e. Tie snugly while neck is flexed; ensure that tie is loose enough to allow one or two fingers underneath.
    f. Remove old tapes after new tapes are in place.
    g. Wash hands.
22. Offer student water for hydration.
23. Document procedure, including amount of secretions, color, odor, any complications, and student's tolerance of procedure.
24. Research demonstrates that hydrogen peroxide is cytotoxic, so it is not recommended as an antiseptic on human tissue (Jacobson, 2004).

Special Education

CHAPTER 9

Tracheostomy Suctioning (Sterile Technique)

I. Definition

A. Tracheostomy suctioning is the aspiration of excessive secretions from the trachea by insertion of a catheter into the tracheostomy opening.

II. Purpose

A. Suctioning maintains an open airway and adequate ventilation when the student is unable to cough and clear the airway.

III. Equipment

A. The following materials should be available for suctioning:
   1. Suction machine.
   2. Sterile suction catheter, no more than half the internal diameter of the tracheostomy tube.
   3. Sterile gloves.
   4. Sterile, normal saline solution.
   5. Sterile water.
   6. Sterile syringes.
   7. Clean paper cup (nonwaxed).
   8. Tissues.
   9. Plastic bag for contaminated tissues and materials used in suctioning.
   10. Replacement tracheostomy tube, one size smaller than tracheostomy tube currently in place.

IV. Instructions

A. Refer to HCP's prescription for specific recommendations or adaptations to the following procedure:
   1. Wash hands.
   2. On clean paper towel, place paper cup filled with sterile water, sterile syringe filled with sterile saline solution, sterile gloves, and sterile catheter suctioning packages that have been opened carefully so as not to contaminate the contents.
   3. Position student.
      a. Position depends on student's condition.
      b. HCP may give specific orders.
      c. *Infants and young children:* place small towel roll under shoulders, because neck is short, and this will provide optimal access to trachea.
      d. *Older child:* position with tracheostomy area exposed; if possible, place in Fowler's position to prevent any solution from seeping into stoma.
   4. Wash hands and don sterile gloves. The dominant hand remains sterile, whereas the other hand becomes nonsterile.
   5. Remove catheter from opened package with sterile gloved hand, taking precautions to avoid contamination.
   6. Hold suction connection tubing in nonsterile hand and connect catheter suction tubing with sterile hand.
   7. Turn on suction machine with nonsterile hand.
   8. Dip catheter end into cup of sterile water, and draw water through briefly.
   9. Proceed with suctioning.

a. Leaving vent of catheter open, gently insert the catheter into the tracheostomy tube just beyond the end of the premeasured tracheostomy tube (usually 4 to 5 in), then withdraw catheter slightly. Use a calibrated catheter or measure against extra tracheostomy tube; mark with thumb and insert until thumb reaches stoma.

    (1) Depth of suctioning may be specified by physician.

    (2) Tissue damage may occur with suctioning beyond tip of tracheostomy tube.

    (3) Never force catheter.

b. Place thumb of nonsterile hand over vent of catheter intermittently; and with sterile hand, gently rotate catheter between thumb and forefinger while slowly withdrawing catheter from trachea.

c. If student begins to cough, withdraw catheter.

d. Suction intermittently, but do not suction longer than 5 to 10 seconds at a time; allow 30 seconds to 1 minute between periods of suctioning.

    (1) If catheter is not withdrawn intermittently, hypoxia can occur from occlusion of airway.

    (2) Prolonged suctioning can precipitate vagal stimulation with cardiac arrest.

10. If secretions are thick, irrigation with sterile saline solution may be prescribed. This practice is controversial, because it may cause lower airway infections by washing organisms from the tracheostomy tube into the lower airway.

11. Suction water through the catheter between suctionings and when finished to clear.

12. Discard catheter, cup, syringe, and gloves; wash hands.

13. Document procedure, including amount of secretions, color, odor, and any change in secretions. Note tolerance of procedure and complications.

GLOSSARY OF SPECIAL EDUCATION TERMS

Adapted physical education A program of specially designed activities, games, sports, rhythms, and dance for students who demonstrate a developmental delay in motor skills. May be conducted in a special education class or regular classroom.

Affect Outward manifestation of an individual's emotional tone or feeling in presentation of self.

Agnosia Inability to process information through any of several major sensory systems: auditory, visual, olfactory, gustatory, or tactile. May result from organic brain damage and may be partial or complete.

Agraphia Inability to express thoughts in writing.

Anomia Inability to name objects or recognize names; creates a significant reading and writing problem; a form of aphasia caused by a lesion in the temporal lobe of the brain.

Apgar score Objective way to assess and describe the extrauterine adaptation by rating five areas—appearance (color), pulse, grimace (response to stimulation), activity (muscle tone), and respiratory effort. Rating is done at 1 and 5 minutes after birth, sometimes at 10 minutes, assigning scores from 0 to 2 in each area. Named for Virginia Apgar, anesthesiologist. The Apgar score assesses the need for immediate intervention but is a poor predictor of later developmental outcomes.

Aphasia Disturbance or loss of ability to understand or communicate in spoken or written language or by gesturing. May be complete or partial and most commonly is a mixture of incomplete receptive and expressive aphasia. May be transient or permanent.

Apraxia Inability to plan and carry out a particular act. Apraxia of speech is caused by brain damage and results in the inability to move speech muscles necessary to produce understandable speech.

Assessment Multifaceted systematic process of looking at an individual's behaviors and achievements. In the nursing process, assessment includes systematically collecting data on an individual's health status, analyzing the information collected, and determining the information's implications for nursing actions and student learning.

Associated movements (overflow) Extra motor activity that accompanies a certain motor performance; involuntary movements occurring in one area of the body when a voluntary movement occurs in another part of the body.

Ataxia Impairment in ability to coordinate voluntary muscular movement. May manifest as a staggering gait or postural imbalance caused by a lesion in the spinal cord or cerebellum.

Auditory association Ability to draw relationships from what one hears and then respond orally in an appropriate manner.

Auditory closure Ability to make a word or sound into a whole when parts of the word or sound have been omitted.

Auditory discrimination Ability to distinguish differences in sounds.

Auditory figure ground Ability to select relevant sound stimuli from a background of environmental stimuli.

Auditory learner Individual who acquires knowledge and skills primarily by listening.

Auditory memory Ability to remember auditory information presented verbally as sounds or in the form of sound symbols.

Auditory reception Admission of information by auditory avenues; however, this does not necessarily mean that comprehension has been achieved.

Auditory sequential memory Ability to retain in the correct order a sequence of information presented verbally.

Behavior modification Method using behavior concepts and laws to produce a positive change in behavior.

Bruxism Unconscious, compulsive grinding or clenching of teeth; bruxism primarily occurs during sleep but also may occur in waking hours, reflecting extreme stress or release of tension. May cause headache, muscle spasms, chronic pain in face and jaw, and damage to teeth.

Choreiform Involuntary, irregular, purposeless movements.

Cognitive style Mode by which the student appears to learn the best; the mode may be visual, auditory, or kinesthetic. See *learning styles*.

Cortical thumb Fisting with thumb flexed inside the clenched palm. May indicate hypertonicity; neurologically normal up to age 3 months.

Decoding   Process whereby the brain changes symbols into sounds. Examples of such processes are reading, the interpretation of the spoken word, facial expressions, and social cues.

Diadochokinesis/diadochokinetic rate   Ability in speech to produce a rapid rate of repetitive oral movements; the rapid production of sounds using different parts of the mouth. Used to assess dyspraxia or dysarthria by noting how quickly the child is able to produce sounds using different parts of the mouth.

Diagnostic tests   Tests that provide a finer analysis than a screening device so that strengths and weaknesses in skill development can be identified more specifically.

Dominance   Tendency to prefer using one side or part of the body over the other.

Dysarthria   Difficulty in articulating words because of impairment in the control of articulation muscles, usually caused by central or peripheral motor system damage; aphasias result from cortical damage.

Dyscalculia   Inability to perform mathematical functions.

Dysgraphia   Inability to produce the motor movements necessary for handwriting; may be part of a language disorder caused by an impairment of the motor system or the parietal lobe.

Dyslexia   An inability to read, spell, or write; can see and identify letters, but may reverse letters and have a poor sense of left and right; possible genetic association.

Dyspraxia   Partial loss or failure to develop ability to perform skilled, coordinated movements; not explained by any motor or sensory dysfunction or mental retardation.

Echolalia   Meaningless repetition of what is heard, both words and phrases. Occurs normally in early language development; seen in Tourette syndrome, catatonic schizophrenia, and neurological disorders such as transcortical aphasia.

Encoding   Process whereby ideas are changed into symbols for the specific purpose of communication. Such processes include body gestures, sign language, and spoken or written words.

Familial   Occurrence in members of the same family more than what might be anticipated by chance.

Figure ground disturbance   The inability to distinguish the figure from the background.

Fine motor function   Ability to use small muscle groups efficiently, smoothly, and quickly; usually parallels gross motor development.

Form constancy   Ability to perceive words or objects as basically the same; unaware of the differences in their presentation or occurrence.

Glossopharyngeal breathing   Method of forcing air into lungs with the pharynx and tongue. May be used by individuals dependent on mechanical ventilation to maintain adequate oxygenation during suctioning.

Graphesthesia   Ability to discriminate shapes, symbols, words, numbers, or letters drawn on the skin, particularly the palm of the hand, when the eyes are closed. Believed to have a relationship with intersensory integration.

Gross motor function   Ability to move large muscles in a coordinated and efficient manner.

Special Education

CHAPTER 9

Gustatory   Pertaining to sense of taste.

Hyperactivity   Excessive activity or restless motor movement, impulsivity, or both. It is an atypical behavior beyond the ability of the student to regulate well.

Impulsivity   Tendency to act without considering the consequences.

Intonation   Rise and fall in the pitch of the voice during speech.

Kinesthetic   Sense by which the individual is aware of the position, weight, and movement of various body parts in space.

Language   Communication of ideas through symbols that are used according to grammatical and semantic rules.

Laterality   The superior development of one side of the brain or body; use of one hand in preference over the other. Often referred to as preferential use; dominance or mixed preference, such as left-eyed, right-handed, right-legged.

Lateralization   The ability of one section of the brain to take the lead in organizing and processing a certain behavior or mental process; functional specialization of the brain occurring mainly in the right hemisphere, such as in the perception of spatial and visual relationships.

Learning disability   A disorder manifest by significant difficulties in learning, speaking, reasoning, reading, writing, or doing mathematical calculations. Often occurs in an individual with normal or above-average intelligence. May result from psychological or organic causes. Specific testing is used to identify.

Learning styles/intelligence factor   Eight intelligence/learning styles have been theorized, including visuospatial, verbal/linguistic, logical/mathematical, bodily/kinesthetic, musical/rhythmic, interpersonal, intrapersonal, and naturalistic (Gardner, 1998). Emotional intelligence is another theoretical concept.

Manifestation determination   If a student with a disability is removed from school for misbehavior for more than a total of 10 days in one school year, the school must hold a *manifestation* meeting to determine the cause. This means a team must determine whether the student's behavior is a result of the disability, failure to implement the IEP, or is inappropriate behavior.

Mirror movements   Phenomenon in which associated movements occur on the opposite side.

Neurodevelopmental examination   Assessment of the student's nervous system maturation level and developmental status in a variety of areas, including fine and gross motor function, visual perceptual function, and auditory language ability.

Nonacademic services   Extracurricular services for students with disabilities (e.g., clubs, athletics, recreational activities, transportation).

Obturator   A device used to guide a tracheostomy tube or gastrostomy button into position without causing trauma to tissue. The obturator is removed once the tracheostomy tube or gastrostomy button is in place.

Occupational therapist   Registered professional who evaluates and treats those who have difficulty with activities of daily living, play, fine motor skills, oral motor function, and other activities. Services include design and fabrication of adaptive equipment, assessment and treatment of sensory integration problems, adaptation of physical environment for the disabled, consultation with classroom teacher or staff, and prevocational evaluation. Licensed in some states.

Orthosis   A special brace or device to correct, control, or compensate for muscle or bone deformities.

Orthotics   The design and manufacture of external devices used to promote a specific motion, correct a deformity, or support a paralyzed limb.

Parent   Biological, adoptive, or foster parent; guardian or person legally responsible for a child.

Perception   Recognition and appropriate interpretation of stimuli received in the brain.

Percutaneous endoscopic gastrostomy (PEG)   Placement of a gastrostomy tube into the stomach from the abdomen with the guidance of an endoscope. A small incision is made, usually with the patient under light sedation or local anesthetic. Generally heals quickly.

Peristomal   Area of skin around a stoma.

Perseveration   Continuation of an activity, response, or reply after the causative stimuli has ceased. A student may continue with one activity long after a new task is offered.

Phonation   Controlling the breath flow to produce the sounds of speech.

Phoneme   Smallest sound unit in a language, which vary from language to language. The English language ranges from 40 or more different phonemes.

Phonetics   Study of speech sounds.

Physical therapist   Licensed professional who evaluates, plans, and implements a therapy program that promotes self-sufficiency. Assesses abilities in gross motor skills, motor planning, balance and equilibrium, postural tone, gait, and kinesthesia. Designs and develops adaptive equipment and provides assistance and information on the use of mechanical aids (e.g., wheelchairs and braces).

Praxis   The ability of the brain to process, organize, and perform unfamiliar actions. Children who have difficulty planning and carrying out motor activities are said to be *apraxic* or *dyspraxic*.

Projective test   Standardized assessment performed to elicit information concerning an individual's personality, subconscious feelings, and sources of conflicts; testing protocols may include the Thematic Apperception Test (TAT) or Rorschach or inkblot test.

School psychologist   Licensed professional who uses the science of psychometrics to evaluate a student's need for special services and assess the student's educational progress. A school psychologist interprets interpersonal behavior, assists students in coping with their environments, and helps teachers and staff in behavior management techniques.

School social worker   Licensed professional who is a member of the multidisciplinary team providing counseling to students and consultation to teachers; a liaison to the families of students in the educational setting, they network with community agencies and social support systems that can advance students' educational achievement and psychosocial functioning.

Screening   Identifying potential deviance (e.g., vision and hearing screenings). When indicated, assessment, diagnosis, and then treatment follow screening.

Self-esteem   The personal estimation or evaluation that the student has about himself or herself; includes emotional and value-based assessments.

Special Education

CHAPTER 9

Self-esteem has variations and is on a continuum of strong or weak, low or high, and worthy or unworthy.

Semantics   Study of language that deals with the meanings of words or symbols and rules for use.

Soft neurological signs   Slight or mild neurological abnormalities that are difficult to detect or interpret; may indicate immature or ineffective function of the central nervous system.

Sound blending   Ability to combine separate parts of a word and produce the complete word.

Spatial relationships   Ability to determine size, right and left, distance, and how one object is related to another.

Speech and language pathologist/speech therapist   Licensed professional who screens, evaluates, diagnoses, and treats those with communication disorders.

Stimulus   Anything that incites the individual to function, become active, or respond; stimuli may be physical, chemical, biological, or social.

Stoma   A surgically created opening of an internal organ on the surface of the body, (e.g., ileostomy, colostomy, gastrostomy, vesicostomy, tracheostomy).

Supplementary aids and services   As defined in IDEA, includes instructional assistants, services, and other supports that are provided in regular education classes or other education-related settings to enable children with disabilities to be educated with nondisabled children to the maximum extent appropriate.

Syntax/grammar   How words are put together in sentences according to established rules.

Tactile   Pertaining to sense of touch.

Testing   Presentation of a collection of predetermined tasks or questions to which predetermined responses exist.

Travel training   As defined in IDEA, providing instruction to children with significant cognitive or other disabilities to enable them to develop an awareness of the environment in which they live; teaching the skills necessary to move effectively and safely within that environment (e.g., in school, at home, in the community).

Visual aphasia   Inability to comprehend the meaning of written or printed words and sentences, usually caused by brain lesions. Also called *text blindness* or *word blindness*.

Visual association   Ability to see the relationship between various visual symbols.

Visual closure   Recognition of shapes, objects, or words when the visual presentation is incomplete.

Visual discrimination   Detection of differences in letters, forms, objects, or words.

Visual figure ground   Ability to separate a figure or object from its background.

Visual learner   Individual who acquires knowledge and skills primarily through vision.

Visual reception   Ability to look at symbols—words, letters, and so forth—and interpret their meaning.

Visual sequential memory   Ability to store, retrieve, and reproduce visual information from memory.

Visuomotor function   Ability to coordinate vision with movements of the body or body parts.

Visuoperceptual disability   Difficulty in organizing and interpreting visual sensory stimuli.

ACRONYMS USED IN SPECIAL EDUCATION

ADD Attention deficit disorder
ADHD Attention deficit-hyperactivity disorder
APE Adapted physical education
AT Assistive technology
CEC Council for Exceptional Children
CH Communicatively handicapped
CLD Council for Learning Disabilities
CSPD Comprehensive System of Personnel Development
DB Deaf-blind
DHH Deaf and hard of hearing
EHA Education of the Handicapped Act
EIS Early intervention services (K-12)
EPSDT Early periodic screening, diagnosis, and treatment
ESA Educational Service Agency
ESEA Elementary and Secondary Education Act of 1965
ESL English as a second language
FAPE Free and appropriate public education
FBA Functional behavioral assessment
FERPA Family Educational Rights and Privacy Act
HCP Health care provider
HI Hearing impaired
HIPAA Health Insurance Portability and Accountability Act
IAES Interim alternative educational setting
ICC Interagency Coordinating Council
IDEA Individuals with Disabilities Education Act
IEE Independent educational evaluation
IEP Individualized education program
IFSP Individualized family service plan
ILS Integrated life skills
LD Learning disability
LEA Local Education Agency
LEP Limited English proficiency
LRE Least restrictive environment
MFE Multifaceted evaluation
MIC-KEY Skin-level gastrostomy button that turns and locks into place
MR Mentally retarded
NICHCY The National Dissemination Center for Children with Disabilities; previously known as the National Information Center for Handicapped Children and Youth.
NPRM Notice of proposed rulemaking
O&M Orientation and mobility
OH Orthopedically handicapped
OHI Other health impaired
OMB Office of Management and Budget
OSEP Office of Special Education Programs
OSERS Office of Special Education and Rehabilitative Services
OT Occupational therapy
PE Physical education

CHAPTER 9   Special Education

PH Physically handicapped
PT Physical therapy
RSP Resource specialist program
R-T-I Response to intervention
SEA State educational agency
SH Severely handicapped
TDD Telecommunications device for the deaf
TPA Total parenteral alimentation
TPN Total parenteral nutrition
VH Visually handicapped
VI Visually impaired

GENERAL WEB SITES

Council of Educators for Students with Disabilities (CESD)
    http://www.504idea.org
Council for Exceptional Children (CEC)
    http://www.cec.sped.org
Education Resources Information Center (ERIC)
    http://www.eric.ed.gov
Exceptional Parent Resource Guide
    http://www.eparent.com
National Dissemination Center for Children with Disabilities (NICHCY)
    http://www.nichcy.org
SCOPE Disability Means Possibility
    http://www.scopevic.org.au

BIBLIOGRAPHY

American Latex Allergy Association: *Latex allergy statistics* (available online): www.latexallergyresources.org/topics/LatexAllergyStatistics. Accessed Jan 2007.

Council of Educators for Students with Disabilities (CESD): *Special education laws* (available online): www.504idea.org. Accessed Jan 2007.

Gardner H: A multiplicity of intelligences, *Sci Am* 9 (4):18-23, 1998.

Gardner H: *Frames of mind: the theory of multiple intelligences,* New York, 1983, Basic Books.

Gray EH, Blackington J, White GM: Stoma care in schools, *J Sch Nurs* 22(2):74-80, 2006.

Jacobson S: Errors in emergency practice: the wrong solution, *Emerg Med* 36 (8):13, 2003 (available online): www.emedmag.com/html/pre/err/0804.asp. Accessed Jan 2007.

Kliegman RM, Marcdante KJ, Jenson HB, Behrman RE: *Nelson essentials of pediatrics,* Philadelphia, 2006, WB Saunders.

Leier JL, Cureton VY, Canham DL: Special day class teachers' perception of the role of the school nurse, *J Sch Nurs* 19(5):294-300, 2003.

Mosby's Dictionary of Medicine, Nursing, and Health, St Louis, 2006, Elsevier Mosby.

Moses M, Gilchrest C, Schwab NC: Section 504 of the Rehabilitation Act: determining eligibility and implications for school districts, *J Sch Nurs* 21(1):48-59, 2005.

National Center for Education Statistics (NCES): *Digest of Education Statistics: 2005* (available online): http://nces.ed.gov/programs/digest/d05/tables/dt05_052.asp. Accessed Nov 2006.

Osborn LM, DeWitt TG, First LR, Zenel JA: *Pediatrics,* Philadelphia, 2005, Elsevier Mosby.

Schwab N, Gelfman M: *Legal issues in school health services: a resource for school administrators, school attorneys, school nurses,* Lincoln, Neb, 2005, Authors Choice Press.

Silkworth CK, Arnold MJ, Harrigan JF, Zaiger DS: *Individualized healthcare plans for the school nurse: concepts, issues and applications for school nursing practice,* North Branch, Minn, 2005, Sunrise River Press.

CHAPTER 10

Twenty-first Century Health Challenges

*E*merging incidences and prevalence of certain developmental variations and behavioral disorders are becoming more common in the school setting. This chapter includes frequently discussed and documented occurrences by school nurses and other staff on elementary and secondary school campuses. These issues affect the health and learning ability of students at all ages.

The conditions in this chapter are presented in two different formats. Backpack Complications and Computer Ergonomics are presented in the manual's traditional outline format. The other health-related issues are in paragraph format with the nursing management processes listed for quick access. These issues, some of which are new, are current health challenges for the nurse in the school setting and include school start time and adolescents, computer-related exploitation, commercialism of public schools, media and health, schools as community health centers, home schooling and alternative education, youth gambling, and precocious puberty.

BACKPACK COMPLICATIONS

I. Definition

A. Backpacks are used by the school-age student to carry schoolbooks and supplies, other articles, and equipment. Students often carry between 10 and 40 lb, sometimes more, on their backs to and from school and between classes. Backpacks should not weigh more than 15% of a student's body weight. Table 10-1 provides backpack weight limits, and Figure 10-1 demonstrates correct and incorrect ways to wear a backpack.

Table 10-1	*Backpack Weight Limits*
Student's Weight (lb.)	**Backpack Maximum Weight (lb.)**
60	5
70	10
100	15
125	18
150	20
200 or more	25*

*25 pounds is the maximum suggested safe limit.
Adapted from American Chiropractic Association (ACA) and American Physical Therapy Association (APTA).

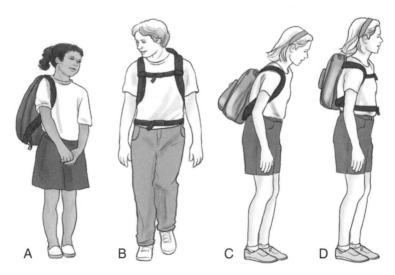

FIGURE 10-1 Appropriate and inappropriate backpack positioning. **A,** Incorrect. Wearing the backpack over one shoulder tends to make one side of the body bear all the weight. This can cause an asymmetry of the spine and potential back pain, shoulder and/or neck strain, and loss of balance. **B,** Appropriate. Both shoulders bear the weight of the backpack load. Reduces symptoms of a heavy, unbalanced pack. **C,** Incorrect. Leaning forward with shoulders bending inward is observed when the pack is too low on the back and the load is not distributed evenly, producing bad posture, improper spine alignment, causing fatigue and/or back and neck strain. **D,** Appropriate. The backpack should rest evenly in the middle of the curve of the back. Wear chest straps and waist belt for appropriate weight distribution, stabilization, and reduction of potential pain or injury. See Box 10-1 for further information on backpack safety.

II. Etiology

    A. Human beings have used their backs for centuries to carry heavy loads, and mothers often carry infants and babies on their backs. Now, backpacks can be a threat to the health of students when the load is too heavy and when these loads are packed, lifted, or worn improperly, or if these factors are combined. Students carry their backpacks in a variety of positions that can adversely affect the spinal column and other bone structures that are not fully developed (APTA, 2006). Studies on children discuss the use of backpacks and their relationship to back or shoulder pain (Siambanes et al, 2004).

B. Wearing backpacks alters the mobility of the spine, leading to passive movement—involuntary movement from an outside force—which is a risk factor for back pain (AOTA, 2006; Vacheron et al, 1999). Low back pain during the adolescent years can result in low back pain in adulthood (Salminen et al, 1999). Adjusting to a heavy load leads to incorrect postures that include bending forward, leaning to one side, or arching the back; all of these can lead to improper spinal alignment. This misuse may impede functioning of the discs that provide shock absorption to the system (APTA, 2006). Long-term incorrect, heavy, and chronic backpack use may trigger back pain in students that may continue into adulthood,even more so in individuals with a genetic predisposition or an existing disease process.

III. Characteristics
A. Poor posture.
B. Tingling or numbness in arms.
C. Headache, fatigue, or both.
D. Low back pain that may become chronic.
E. Discomfort, pain, or both in the neck and shoulders.
F. Muscle spasms of the neck and shoulders.
G. Redness, pressure sores, or blisters on the back or shoulders from strap wear resulting from heavy or inappropriately packed loads.

IV. Health Concerns/Emergencies
A. Heavy backpacks.
  1. May cause chronic health issues resulting from soreness, fatigue, and neck, shoulder, and back pain.
  2. Improper positioning and weight of backpack may cause muscles and soft tissue to work harder, leading to back strain.
  3. Headaches, red marks, neck and low back pain, numbness, and tingling in the upper arm area.
  4. Heavy backpacks interfere with balance and may cause falling.

V. Effects on Individual
A. Poor posture and pain resulting from leaning forward with neck thrust forward.
B. Shoulder and arm strain from dragging a backpack.
C. Strain and stress on one side of the body caused by using only one shoulder strap.
D. Fatigue.
E. Prepubescent girls appear to be most vulnerable to postural imbalance, specifically the forward head position, when a backpack weighs over 15% of body weight (APTA, 2006).

VI. Management/Treatment
A. Teach the proper techniques for packing, lifting, and carrying backpacks; warn of health concerns resulting from improper use. Determine maximum backpack load.
B. Warn against using a backpack as a weapon; encourage storage of backpack in a safe area to prevent injuries from tripping.
C. Teach back-strengthening exercises.

Twenty-first Century Health Challenges

CHAPTER 10

D. Always choose a lightweight backpack; look for one with padding in the back and multiple compartments to facilitate distribution of weight and for organization. Consider reflective strips or lights to increase visibility at night. Backpacks are now available with an inflatable air chamber to reduce pressure on the back and protect it.

E. Briefcases and backpacks on wheels for heavy loads are helpful but may be difficult to use in schools with multiple floors.

F. Use care when moving about in tight spaces, such as on a school bus, to avoid hitting others with the backpack.

G. Discuss safety hazards and placement of backpacks during evacuation of school buildings with administration and staff. See Box 10-1 for further information on backpack safety.

VII. Additional Information

A. Several conditions have arisen from backpack use that may cause complications:

1. Students are multitasking from early morning until late evening, causing them to carry not only their classroom needs, but also items ranging from food to sports equipment to computers.

2. The short time intervals between classes do not permit students to go to their lockers.

3. Some schools have eliminated lockers because of security, safety, or budget constraints.

B. Occasionally, students may need special accommodations or assistance carrying supplies. They may need to leave class early to go to their lockers, or they may require a second set of books to meet their individualized needs. Some schools require that backpacks be made of see-through vinyl or mesh to discourage the transport of weapons, alcohol, or drugs. This demand seems to forgo the adolescent's need for privacy but focuses on safety.

Box 10-1   *EUPAC: Encourage Use of Proper Packing and Caution*

1. Encourage weighing the pack and contents, limiting weight to no more than 15% of body weight to prevent neck and back strain.

2. Use wide and padded shoulder straps to avoid shoulder pressure and possible nerve damage.

3. Avoid slinging pack over one shoulder, which can cause loss of balance, muscle spasms, and low back pain.

4. A waist belt and chest straps provide good support and help with weight distribution and stabilization: fasten them. Adjust straps to allow arms to move freely.

5. Pack should not be longer than the distance between the shoulders and hips and not wider than the rib cage. It should rest in the curvature of the back.

6. Proper packing puts heaviest items close to the body and lighter items farther away or in small sections to distribute weight evenly, ease carrying, and prevent injury and strain.

7. Keep pack high up on the back. Do not wear low near the hips, because this shifts posture forward, producing back and neck strain.

8. Use caution when lifting a backpack. If the pack is very heavy, it should be placed on a desk or table before pulling it onto the back. Only pack what is needed for the day.

C. New technology may eliminate the need to carry heavy books between classes and to and from home. Small technological devices (e.g., USB flash drives, CDs) are available to store and transfer data to a home computer. Computerized textbooks are available for use on a lightweight device similar to a laptop computer, allowing students to highlight and take notes as they would with a textbook.

WEB SITES

American Occupational Therapy Association (Consumer tip sheets)
    http://www.aota.org
Backpack Safety America
    http://www.backpacksafe.com
International Chiropractic Pediatric Association, Research Foundation
    http://www.icpa4kids.org/index.htm
American Physical Therapy Association
    http://www.apta.org

COMPUTER ERGONOMICS

I. Definition
   A. Ergonomics is the science that uses current knowledge of human abilities and limitations to design or organize systems, products, machines, or tools for efficient, comfortable, and safe use by human beings.
   B. The computer monitor and workstation are used for academic learning, communication, and entertainment. Computers include both desktop and laptop styles. The physical arrangements (i.e., ergonomics) in the computer environment can have a negative impact on visual health and body mechanics.

II. Etiology
   A. Using a computer workstation poses a threat to the individual's health because of stress and fatigue from inappropriate body positioning, work environment, and repetitive activity. Health hazards from inappropriate or cumulative use of computers include carpal tunnel syndrome, back and neck pain, and computer vision syndrome (CVS).
      1. CVS symptoms occur as a result of a variety of factors: glare or reflections, failure to blink frequently enough to maintain moisture on the surface of the eyes, increased tear evaporation, corrective lenses that are inappropriate for the individual's distance and position from the screen, minor visual defects that manifest after intense computer use, and poor body positioning in relationship to the monitor or workstation.
      2. See Box 10-2 for tips on how to avoid eyestrain and body fatigue.

III. Characteristics
   A. Visual symptoms:
      1. Temporary myopia.
      2. Eye fatigue and strain.
      3. Blurry vision at near and far distances.
      4. Dry, watery, or irritated eyes (itching, burning).
      5. Sensitivity to light.

Twenty-first Century Health Challenges

CHAPTER 10

Box 10-2	*Tips to Avoid Eyestrain and Body Fatigue*

1. Blink frequently to moisten eyes.
2. Wear computer glasses, as needed.
3. Focus on distant objects periodically.
4. Use relaxation and stretching exercises.

5. Move away from the computer occasionally.
6. Follow 20/20/20 rule: Every 20 minutes, take 20 seconds and look 20 feet.
7. BBB Rule: Blink, breathe, and break.

20/20/20/ Rule and BBB Rule: From Dr. Jeff Anshel, personal conversation, Jan 25, 2007.

    6. Trouble refocusing from screen to paper or book work.

    7. Double vision.

  B. Physical symptoms:

    1. Neckaches, backaches, muscle spasms.

    2. Headaches.

    3. Carpal tunnel syndrome with chronic use; development of this type of injury may take 5 to 10 years to manifest.

  C. Referral:

    1. If any of these symptoms persist, refer to parent, HCP, eye specialist, or physical therapist.

IV. Health Concerns/Emergencies

  A. Delayed socialization skills can result from computer use that begins at too early an age. Supervision by an adult is especially critical for children younger than age 7 to establish appropriate and healthy ergonomics. Software is now available for infants.

  B. Temporary damage to vision or upper body muscles, nerves, or tendons.

  C. No *current* data suggest permanent visual damage.

  D. No *current* evidence exists that indicates computer displays emit hazardous radiation (ultraviolet or ionizing radiation), nor do data suggest a health risk from exposure to electromagnetic fields associated with monitor use (Occupational Safety and Health Administration [OSHA], 2005).

V. Effects on Individual

  A. Complaints of aching or pain, tenderness, swelling, cracking, numbness or tingling, loss of strength, decreased coordination in the injured area, or loss of joint movement of the fingers, shoulders, back, or neck; strain is most commonly seen in the hand, wrist, or arm. These complaints usually are called *repetitive strain injuries (RSIs*; see Additional Information).

  B. In young children, excessive computer use may impede the development of critical skills, such as creativity, imagination, and attention span; a decrease in pretending skills, motivation, and desire to persevere may also be evident. Select high-quality developmental software versus rote learning or drill-and-practice software.

  C. Weight gain can be an issue at all ages. Excessive time at the computer without set limits or exercise breaks can be a contributing factor to becoming overweight. Software programs and other tools are available to assist parents in limiting electronic media time and providing exercise breaks (e.g., Stretch Break for Kids, http://www.paratec.com/sbform/kidsform.htm).

VI. Management/Treatment

A. For home or school:

1. Students should wear prescribed eyeglasses. Computer glasses may be ideal when computer use lasts several hours per day.

2. Determine and record extent of computer use during vision screening.

3. Check display screen position for viewing without neck tilted either backward or forward. If screen position is too high, the individual will tip the neck backward; if the screen is too low, the individual will bend forward for easier viewing (see Figure 10-2 for suggested computer workstation positioning).

4. Maintain glare-free screen and reposition computer screen as appropriate for each child. Screen should be at a right angle to windows, and awning or blinds can be used to decrease glare. Check for glare by turning the screen off and observing any reflection of lights or lightly colored objects on the screen. Adjust the brightness of room lighting or use an antiglare filter approved by the American Optometric Association (AOA) or a three-sided computer hood. Clean the screen often with antistatic cloth.

5. Use a document holder. Place the text document or book in the holder and move it as close to the screen as possible. Maintain sufficient light on any paper documents by using a freestanding, adjustable-brightness task light. The light should not be exposed directly to the eyes. Light in the work area within 25 degrees of the screen should be approximately the same as the background illumination of the screen.

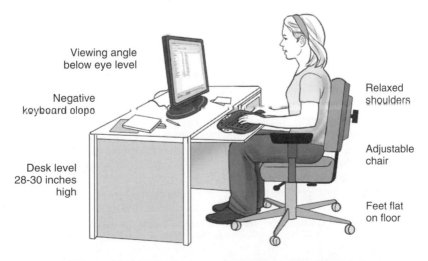

Viewing angle below eye level

Negative keyboard slope

Desk level 28-30 inches high

Relaxed shoulders

Adjustable chair

Feet flat on floor

FIGURE 10-2 Suggested computer workstation positioning.

CHAPTER 1)   Twenty-first Century Health Challenges

6. Ensure that appropriate workstation equipment and furniture are used. Use a height-adjustable chair with good back support. The work surface should be stable. Use a negative-slope or tilt-down keyboard system or a height-adjustable mouse or keyboard platform. The keyboard and mouse should be appropriate for the child's or adult's hand size; smaller hands need a smaller keyboard (e.g., LittleFingers keyboard).

7. Schedule timely work breaks, because postural problems associated with computer use depend on the length of continual use time. Breaks every 20 to 30 minutes are ideal for younger students. Software can be programmed to remind the user to take a break by providing on-screen alerts (see Web Sites); many provide guidance on simple exercises. Adolescents can focus on a distant object for about 2 minutes. Frequent blinking of the eyes also is necessary. Computer users should stretch frequently (e.g., make a fist and spread fingers wide apart for 10 seconds; tilt head to shoulder, side to side; turn head to each shoulder and hold for 10 seconds; lean over and put hands on the floor while seated; clasp hands together overhead and move arms side to side).

8. Apply ergonomic guidelines for computer use (see Web Sites). The neutral work posture applies to children, adolescents, and adults. It ensures comfortable and ergonomically correct computer use. Applying principles of ergonomics (i.e., fitting the workspace to the individual's body) can alleviate many of the health risks associated with computer use.

B. Problem postures and keyboard positions:
1. An upward-sloping keyboard increases muscle loads in upper arms, shoulders, and neck. Positioning the keyboard on the desk makes maintenance of neutral position difficult, because the forearms tire and sag. This puts the wrists into greater extension. The elbows, usually flexed, compress the median and ulnar nerves at the elbow, thus restricting blood flow to the hands.

C. Laptop computer use:
1. Keyboard and screen cannot be adjusted, making decisions about head and neck posture and hand and wrist position difficult, because one or the other will be compromised using a laptop.
2. Use a wireless or detachable keyboard to allow for proper positioning of keyboard and screen.
3. Tip screen back 100 to 110 degrees; a desktop screen is typically at 90 degrees; print will become more crisp.
4. When transporting a laptop, be aware of other items placed in bag and the overall weight. Carry only computer items needed.

VII. Additional Information
A. The effects of computer use on infants and young children are unknown, and research in this area is limited.
B. RSIs involve muscles, tendons, and nerves that are overused or misused. The damage is caused by repetitive tasks, forceful movements, awkward or fixed postures, or insufficient relaxation time between activities. RSIs may include carpal tunnel syndrome, ganglionic cysts, tendonitis, tenosynovitis and epicondylitis (tennis elbow),

trigger finger, thoracic outlet syndrome, De Quervain's disease (a painful condition affecting the tendons at the base of the thumb), and computer vision syndrome.

WEB SITES

Computer Ergonomics for Elementary School
    http://www.orosha.org/cergos/index.html
Cornell University Ergonomics Web
    http://ergo.human.cornell.edu
Corporate Vision Consulting
    http://www.cvconsulting.com
Stretch Break for Kids (Computer Ergonomics Exercises)
    http://www.paratec.com/sbform/kidsform.htm

SCHOOL TRENDS AND PHENOMENA

SCHOOL START TIME AND ADOLESCENTS

Adolescents experience a shift in circadian rhythms, the natural cycle of sleep–wake patterns, which causes a change in the secretion of the hormone melatonin. This change causes the adolescent to stay awake later at night and sleep later in the morning (National Sleep Foundation, 2006). Early school start times reduce the amount of sleep for most adolescents, and this lack of sleep impairs their cognitive and motor functioning, eye–hand coordination, accuracy, concentration, and short-term memory; it also shortens attention span and lengthens reaction time. Sleep deprivation affects specific areas of the brain and impacts how people learn. The brain needs more sleep than any other part of the body; during sleep, information received during the day is sorted out and consolidated (Peigneux et al, 2004; Spencer, Sunm, and Ivry, 2006). Lessons taught and learned at school—that is, new neuronal connections—are strengthened during sleep.

An adolescent requires 8.5 to 9.25 hours of sleep each night to function adequately (National Sleep Foundation, 2006). The most recent National Sleep Foundation Study reports that only 20% of adolescents get 9 hours of sleep, and almost 50% state that they get less than 8 hours, making them sleep deprived. Twelfth graders report that they get only 6.9 hours of sleep a night, making the senior year a particularly difficult time for adequate rest and sleep. Students find various coping mechanisms for sleep deprivation: 38% of high school students report taking at least two naps per week, they sleep later on weekends, and they frequently consume caffeine to stay awake—31% drank two or more caffeine drinks per day. Another sad consequence is that many give up exercising; they report being too sleepy or tired to do it. More than half (51%) of students who drive have driven while drowsy (National Sleep Foundation Study, 2006).

Sleep deprivation causes a negative mood: behavior and attitude of students lacking sleep show signs of anxiety, depression, hopelessness, and acting-out behaviors. They also have decreased focus, attention, and concentration in the classroom; 28% of students fall asleep during class at least once a week; 14% arrive late for morning class, skip that class, or miss school altogether. Most schools start between 7 A.M. and 8 A.M., so the average adolescent's day starts between 6 A.M. and 7 A.M. (National Sleep Foundation Study,

Twenty-first Century Health Challenges

CHAPTER 10

2006). More than half of all high school students (55%) go to bed after 11 P.M. on school nights, robbing them of many needed hours of sleep. Those with optimal sleep (20%) receive more A and B grades (34%), and those with less sleep generally achieve lower grades (National Sleep Foundation Study, 2006).

Over 80 school districts throughout the United States (e.g., Minnesota, Massachusetts, Rhode Island, Iowa) have a delayed start-time in high school. They found attendance improved, daytime alertness increased, and tardiness decreased. Students also reported less depression, fewer trips to the school nurse's office, more frequent breakfasts, and the ability to complete more of their homework during school hours (Wahlstrom, 2002). Sleep is one factor among many that affects learning.

If advocating for later school start times, it is imperative that the school nurse:

1. Be aware of the research and current data in support of a later-start school day.
2. Gather data regarding school start times, sports, extracurricular activities, and transportation schedules.
3. Look at attendance rates, tardiness, and rates of skipping first classes as a rationale for change.
4. Recognize sleep-deprived adolescents and know symptoms exhibited (e.g., depression, mood changes, anxiety, frequent visits to nurse's office). If sleep deprivation is suspected, take a sleep history, or ask the student to record sleep history in a log.
5. Educate parents and adolescents on changing sleep patterns related to learning.
6. Educate teachers and staff regarding sleep deprivation in adolescents.

WEB SITES

National Sleep Foundation, Sleep for All Ages
    http://www.sleepfoundation.org

COMPUTER-RELATED CHILD EXPLOITATION

Computers are a common, almost mandated, educational modality in all schools throughout the country. Students in early elementary grades are trained to use the Internet, e-mail, and chat rooms for educational and entertainment pursuits. Preschool programs even have cyberspace access for the youngest of children, and software is produced for infants as young as 9 months. Internet connectivity makes every American youth a world citizen and world traveler to all the commercial, educational, and entertainment sites available to adults throughout the world.

Like other technology developed in the twentieth century—such as the telephone, television, cellular phones, video games, and handheld devices—the computer is a wonderful and novel communication tool for children. As with all technology, cyberspace has a downside: an antisocial, destructive potential in its application. Conscientious parents, health providers, and political leaders increasingly are sounding the alarm about exploitation of children by pornographers, predators, and peddlers who place them at risk for abuse, disease, and disorders that can end tragically, even in death. An increasing proportion of unwanted solicitations are from persons known to the youth: 3% in 2000 and 14% in 2005 (Wolak, Mitchell, and Finkelhor, 2006). In 2005 the Youth Internet Safety Survey II (YISS II), sponsored by the National Center for Missing and Exploited Children, documented that 14% of teens had face-to-face meetings with individuals they met on the Internet. Most online solicitation (79%) occurs on home computers. The survey results show that when parents and guardians talk with their teens about Internet safety, the teen's exposure to potential threats and harm declines, and they make safer decisions about activity online. *Parents do make a difference.*

Internet exploitation of children and youth is becoming a national public health problem. Examples include the solicitation of expensive products for sale, display of soft- and hard-core pornography, invitation to associate with sexual predators and criminals, and access to antisocial peer group norms by way of chat rooms. E-mail provides unlimited and diverse communication with people whose belief systems and values may conflict with those of family, character-building organizations, and religious affiliations.

Continued, excessive, and even compulsive use of the Internet by children has been documented by clinicians and educators to have a deleterious effect on personality development and mastery of age-appropriate social skills. These effects can lead to symptoms of depression, fear, strong anxiety reactions, traumatic memories, and schizoid behavior. Some clinical studies have documented sexual addictions resulting from habitual use of pornographic Web sites, especially in older adolescents.

Recommendations for nurses and other educational leaders for safe, secure, and healthy Internet use by children and youths include the following:

1. Parents need to teach their young children discriminatory and critical thinking skills, so the child can make responsible decisions on their own.
2. Promote closer adult monitoring and supervision of Internet use in the home. Encourage computer placement in living areas shared by the entire family.
3. Support closer adult monitoring and supervision of Internet use in school and in all community access areas (i.e., libraries).
4. Endorse safety through commercial software that restricts violence, pornography, nudity, and other sexually explicit images.
5. Promote use of video games depicting common approaches to child abduction with parents and teachers supervising for student safety.
6. Use of home page with links only to child-friendly Web pages.
7. Train children and youth about safe communication that includes not providing personal identification information, not sending photographs, and not agreeing to meet people on the Internet without parental consent.
8. Warn youths that taking sexually explicit photos of anyone under 18 years of age is a federal crime under child pornography laws.
9. Address adolescent needs for companionship, love, and romance that may make them vulnerable to online solicitations masked as supportive overtures.
10. Support membership in national cyberspace protective organizations for youths.

Twenty-first Century Health Challenges

CHAPTER 10

11.   Encourage and support parents and students to report any Internet exploitation incidents to law enforcement immediately through http://www.CyberTipline.com or their toll free number, 800-843-5678.

WEB SITES

iSAFE: The Leader in Internet Safety Education
    http://www.isafe.org
National Center for Missing and Exploited Children
    http://www.missingkids.com
NetSmartz Workshop
    http://www.netsmartz.org
Web Wise Kids
    http://www.wiredwithwisdom.org

COMMERCIALISM OF PUBLIC SCHOOLS

Over the last two decades, corporate businesses have contracted with local school boards or school educational groups to provide services and products for the benefit of the students. In exchange for promoting services and products, schools receive monetary contributions toward operating budgets, equipment, and supplies. The most recent marketing strategy is for companies to provide over 50% of the cost of a new school or building contingent upon having naming rights to that school.

The most documented and widespread agreements are with Channel One (Primedia), which offers a daily, in-school news and advertising program to 7 million students—about 30% of America's middle and high school students (Primedia, 2006). Students are obligated to watch television every day, and in exchange, Channel One provides the school with electronic and digital equipment. The daily television viewing includes 10 minutes of fast-paced, flashy infotainment and 2 minutes of advertisements (Austin et al, 2006). Advertisers pay Channel One for the opportunity to market to this captive audience. One study found that most students believe the commercials were approved by the administrative staff, and 25% believe teachers approved the commercials (Austin et al, 2006). Channel One promotes their program as enhancing the student's curriculum; unfortunately, the primary reason for the school administration to use Channel One is for the equipment (Austin et al, 2006). Consequently, low-income schools are a target for commercialism of products and services that do not promote responsible student health or good education.

Opposition by parents and educators to the commercialization of schools by Channel One is growing and has resulted in a decrease of students involved, from 40% in 2002 to 30% in 2007 (Primedia, 2006). A study by the American Academy of Pediatrics (AAP) found that students tended to remember the commercials more than the educational content, and their purchases were influenced by the ads (Austin et al, 2006). The AAP study found that there were some positive effects of the programming that were enhanced when students were provided media literacy training (critical thinking) and discussed the programming with teachers and parents. Generally, commercialism in schools promotes materialism, a sense of entitlement, dissatisfaction, and an attitude that it is not who you are but what you have that matters. The notion of promoting commercialism and advertising in schools has been found to be not in the best interest of the health or education of students (Molnar, 2006).

The biggest corporate commercial contracts with schools across the country are with the three largest soft-drink beverage companies: Coca-Cola, Pepsi, and Cadbury Schweppes (makers of Dr. Pepper and Snapple), which together control 90% of school sales. The growing concern about increasing obesity has resulted in changes in products made available in school vending machines. Under pressure of lawsuits and state legislation, beverage companies agreed to voluntarily replace sodas with diet sodas, low-caloric juice drinks, and sports drinks, a practice that started in the fall of 2006. Some states and cities have even more restrictive regulations that allow only water, low-fat milk, and 100% fruit juice. This is a voluntary agreement, and the onus is on the school administration to initiate the change.

Other commercial and advertising enterprises related to public schools include *Appropriation of Space,* such as school bus advertisements and book covers showing ads for name-brand products; *Sponsorship of Programs and Activities*, such as high school assemblies sponsored by drug companies on National Depression Screening Day; *Incentive Programs* that use brand-name products, such as pizza, to reward student reading programs; *Sponsored Educational Materials* that utilize curricula or lesson plans with commercial interests included; *Fund Raising* that requires students to sell name-brand products; and *Electronic Marketing*, which occurs through the use of a particular brand of computers (Molnar, 2006; Center for Commercial-Free Public Education, 2000). BusRadio is another recent strategy, in which radios on buses provide music, programming, and advertising from the sponsor (BusRadio, 2007).

As an advocate for wellness, it is imperative for the school nurse to:
1. Be aware of the ages and stages when students are most impressionable; middle and high school students may be less vulnerable than students under age 8, who have little, if any, critical thinking skills (American Pyschological Association Task Force, 2004).
2. Teach students to be media literate, that is, increase critical thinking and skepticism regarding advertising.
3. Take the lead in educating school administrators regarding unhealthy lifestyles that may result from the promotion of certain products.
4. Encourage a commercial-free environment in the classroom and at school.
5. Promote and support legislation for responsible consumerism at school sites by contacting legislators, local newspapers, and trade journals as appropriate.
6. Make educational literature available to students, their families, and faculty.
7. Be proactive in seeking information on how to curtail or limit commercialism in the school environment, or at least make it more beneficial and profitable for the student and school versus the commercial entity. The Web sites for the Center for Commercial-Free Public Education and the Council for Corporate and School Partnerships offer more information.

WEB SITES

Arizona State University Commercialism in Education Research Unit (CERU)
    http://epsl.asu.edu/ceru
The Center for Commercial-Free Public Education
    http://www.ibiblio.org/commercialfree
Center for Media Literacy
    http://www.medialit.org
The Council for Corporate and School Partnerships
    http://www.corpschoolpartners.org

MEDIA AND HEALTH

Media includes television, radio, computers, Internet, handheld devices, movies, videos, video games, CDs, newspapers, books, magazines, and any organized method that affects the vast majority of the public. It provides fact, opinion, bias, and entertainment. Mass media messages influence attitudes, values, behaviors, and knowledge on a daily or even hourly basis. Adolescents believe that media affects everyone but themselves; this is called the "third person effect" (Buckingham, 2000). Consequently, when teaching or discussing the impact of media information, it may need to be related not to the adolescent but to members of the teen's family, younger siblings, or friends. This approach may prevent a defensive reaction from the teen.

Children ages 8 to 18 spend an average of 44.5 hours a week, or 6.5 hours a day, in front of a computer, TV, or game screen; this is more time than they spend engaged in any other activity except for sleeping (Rydeout, Roberts, and Foehr, 2005). This decreases physical activity, independent thinking, and often reduces family and peer face-to-face relationships. This technology is socializing the child and adolescent. The use of computers, TV, and other media should be made a family time by keeping these items in the family living area to encourage family sharing and interaction and to learn appropriate media-viewing skills.

Media has become a leader in *sex education* for children and youths; it is being used as a source of information for birth control and broader sexually explicit information when kids are reluctant to talk with their parents or other adults (Strasburger, 2005). Such information can be found 24/7 on the Internet, in chat rooms, on bulletin boards, electronic mailing lists, and Web pages. Sexual images are all pervasive in the media, which provides an environment that can influence sexual attitudes, moral values, and sexual activity—and it may contribute to sexual violence. Sex in the media is often depersonalized by portraying it as only an activity; rarely are the consequences of sex shown. Only 14% of shows with sexual content talk about any of the responsibilities or risks associated with sex (Strasburger, 2005).

Students may be intentionally or inadvertently exposed to pornography that may adversely affect older adolescents and boys, especially those already at risk for aggressive behaviors. A Kaiser Family Foundation Study (2001) found that 70% of 15- to 17-year-olds have inadvertently visited a pornography site. Having a warm, open parent-child relationship is one of the best ways parents can deal with the challenges of living in a sexualized culture.

Excessive television viewing in childhood and adolescence negatively impacts academic achievement and may have long-lasting adverse effects on socioeconomic status (Hancox, Milne, and Poulton, 2005). Viewing TV and movies and playing video games during the week has a more detrimental affect on school performance than time spent on these activities on weekends. This supports the displacement theory that media can replace time needed for school assignments due the next day (Sharif and Sargent, 2006). Sharif and Sargent also found that exposure to adult content had the greatest and most consistent adverse effect on school performance.

Children view more that 40,000 television ads in a year. Studies have shown that children under the age of 8 lack the critical skills to question the accuracy of the messages, and often young children believe such ads are truthful and unbiased (American Psychological Association Task Force, 2004). Advertisement of items such as beer, alcohol, and tobacco are generally promoted in a positive light. Advertisements influence kids by using models who are cool, sexy, and doing something smart and fun, intentionally leaving out the detrimental effects of these products. Ads make an impact: for instance, the top three cigarette brands advertised are the three most popular with teens (American Academy of Pediatrics, 2006).

Girls and boys of all ages worry about their weight and dieting. This worry often starts at a young age, and yet there is an epidemic of obesity among children and adolescents. The media contributes to obesity by promoting unhealthy foods that contain large amounts of fat and sugar. Conversely, many ads depict young, thin, girls and women and buff young men, making one believe it is easy to be thin and have a beautiful body. In reality, the pictures and photos are usually airbrushed or enhanced with computer graphics. Media further contributes to obesity, because watching TV and playing video games lowers children's metabolic rate (Klesges, Shelton, and Klesges, 1993). Children exercise less, snack frequently while using media devices, and eat less healthy meals while watching TV; all of these factors result in poor nutrition and increased weight (see Chapter 4, Chronic Conditions, Obesity).

Over a thousand studies, and another 2500 reviews, demonstrate that media violence has a significant impact on children and youth (Wartella, Olivarez, and Jennings, 1998). Children are affected by violence at any age, but younger children are the most vulnerable; and their attitudes about violence, once established, are difficult to change. They become desensitized to violence and become aggressive, tending to solve conflicts by physical means, rather than using self-control. Media is not the only contributor to violent behavior; other factors include poverty, abuse, racism, and personality traits. However, approximately 10% to 30% of violence in society can be attributed to the influence of media violence (Comstock and Strasburger, 1993; Strasburger and Wilson, 2002). Violent video games can teach aggressive behaviors and decrease caring or helping attitudes toward peers. Some have said that "first person" shooter games are "murder simulators"; the player is the aggressor, who is rewarded for successful violent behaviors. Repeated exposure to media violence is associated with physical and mental health problems that include anxiety, depression, sleep disturbances, and post-traumatic stress disorder (AAP, 2001). As they play the games, young people cannot tell the difference between virtual reality and real life; they cannot tell the fake from the real.

Interpersonal violence, whether as perpetrator or victim, is a greater health risk factor for children, adolescents, and young adults than is cancer, infectious disease, or congenital disorders (Strasburger and Wilson, 2002). Firearms are the second-leading cause of death, after motor vehicle accidents, for young people 19 years and younger in the United States (CDC, 2005).

Despite all of the negative influences, there are positive aspects of media. Media can instruct, encourage, and even inspire students when used with positive intention and discrimination. Educational and informational (E/I) programs such as Sesame Street, Between the Lions, and Mr. Roger's Neighborhood promote school readiness and success. The Children's Television Act requires broadcasters to provide at least three hours of E/I programming per week per channel and recently (2005) it was mandated that the E/I logo remain on the screen throughout the program. The Internet allows instant access to unlimited resources for educational purposes, and computer software expands creative skills. Media can promote prosocial behaviors (e.g. altruism, empathy, cooperation, and friendship) in programs and in advertising. Entertainment provides health information through the integration of health conditions and diseases into soap operas, sitcoms, Public Service Announcements (PSAs), and entire channels dedicated to health issues.

School nursing practice has expanded and become more active in the media health of children. Thus, the school nurse must:

1. Become familiar with research on the effects of media on young people; acknowledge positive as well as negative influences.
2. Assume a strategic role in promoting the teaching of media literacy (critical thinking and viewing).
3. Take a media history as an avenue to discuss media with parents and students.
4. Expand their job description to include classroom teaching regarding controversial and sensitive issues.
5. Present greater visibility in the school and community in a healthy approach to the current media crisis with students.
6. Have materials readily available that define the health risks of particular products, such as tobacco and alcohol.
7. Refer students to school social worker, psychologist, and mental health professional if needed.
8. Serve on school district policy development committees to address and promote health issues related to media exposure.

WEB SITES

Children Now
> http://www.childrennow.org

The Henry J. Kaiser Family Foundation
> http://kff.org

American Academy of Pediatrics,
Media Matters: A National Media Education Campaign
> http://www.aap.org/advocacy/mmcamp.htm

SCHOOLS AS COMMUNITY HEALTH CENTERS

Although public schools are not designed primarily to provide health services, for many years the movement to identify the school as a health center has been advocated by parent organizations, educators, health and mental health associations, and political parties. Recently the Department of Health and Human Services (DHHS), the National Association of School Nurses (NASN), the National Association of Pediatric Nurse Practioners (NAPNAP), and other prominent health care organizations have issued position statements promoting the expansion of school-based and school-linked health centers into community-based health care systems.

The National Assembly on School-Based Health Care found that there are 1700 school-based health centers, serving almost 2 million students in 44 states (NASBHC, 2007). Centers provide a wide range of services that include health education (e.g., nutrition and exercise), diagnosis and treatment of acute and chronic illness, and mental health services (e.g., grief therapy, suicide prevention, coping tools for peer pressure and bullying).

In January 2001, the American Academy of Pediatrics (AAP) issued the School Health Centers and Other Integrated Health Services policy statement. The objectives of the AAP are to enhance accessibility, provide quality health care, link children to a medical home, be financially sustainable, and address both long- and short-term wellness needs of children and adolescents. In other words, the school reform movement in the area of health and human services would provide a seamless web of services from the school to the home for all children and their families.

The school as a community health care facility has been a longstanding operational reality throughout the country, but no uniform model of the ideal health service system exists in any local school district. Many school districts do not offer conventional health services, such as school nursing, immunization clinics, or preventive screening programs. More innovative and progressive school districts offer greater comprehensive services, such as school-based clinics and mental health services, home health education, and collaboration with hospitals and community clinics.

School nursing practice will expand and become more challenging in the twenty-first century, given the community collaboration and centralization of health care services at the school site and purposed legislation and foundation contributions. Thus school nurses:

1. Must assume a strategic role in influencing and shaping the medical ecology of school staff, students, and families
2. Need to expand their job description to include increased case management, networking, monitoring, evaluation, and research to keep pace with the partnership of community health care providers (HCPs) and health care systems.
3. Must present greater visibility, because they are required to be in the community and away from the school campus as representatives of the educational sector of services.
4. Be innovative and progressive in determining the "right size" of comprehensive services, such as school-based clinics, home health education, and collaboration with hospitals and community clinics. A "one size fits all" approach to a school health care delivery system is not possible.

CHAPTER 10   Twenty-first Century Health Challenges

5. Increase proficiency in information and communication technology (e.g., computer, Internet, e-mail).
6. Ensure provision of adequate funding for these services.

WEB SITES

The Center for Health and Health Care in Schools
   http://www.healthinschools.org
National Assembly on School-Based Health Care
   http://www.nasbhc.org

HOME SCHOOLING AND ALTERNATIVE EDUCATION

The societal phenomenon of educating children at home with the parents as the primary, if not exclusive, educators is a cherished tradition in the United States. In the 1980s and 1990s, the home was promoted and advocated as an alternative to both public and parochial schools. As of 1993, home schooling was made legal in all 50 states, and reports indicate the number of students in home schooling has almost tripled since then. Various state and national surveys estimate that 1.7 to 2.1 million children in 2003, in grades equivalent to Kindergarten through twelfth grade, were being taught by their parents (National Home Education Research Institute, 2006); this number represents a small percentage of the country's 50 million students. However, the numbers are increasing, from 1.7% in 1999 to 2.2% in 2003 (National Center For Education Statistics [NCES], 2006).

Public policy debate among educators and politicians is ongoing regarding the benefits and detriments of this societal trend. However, parents of all socioeconomic and ethnic groups continue to assert their prerogative and exercise more control over their children's education and socialization. Home schooling is popular with and provided more often by white, middle-class, and traditional two-parent families.

The reported reasons for the tremendous growth of home schooling in the past and its continuing increase in all socioeconomic and ethnic groups are varied:

1. School environment, including the concerns about bullying, aggression, substance abuse, negative peer pressure, and sexual harassment or assault (31%).
2. Provision of religious or moral instruction (30%).
3. Dissatisfaction with academic instruction in public education (16%).
4. Other reasons, including transmission of a distinct belief system and values to children; stronger filial bonds for nurturing and socialization; controlled and positive peer interactions; personal instruction and quality learning of academics; education of gifted children and those with special needs, and protection from antisocial influences (NCES, 2006).

With recent research documenting higher academic achievement and strong prosocial character development of children who are home schooled, parents have an added motivation to keep their children at home despite the personal sacrifices and financial limitations associated with home schooling (Home School Legal Defense Association, 2004).

No epidemiological studies have implicated the home school movement in inadequate medical care or at-risk health status of the children. Home-schooled children receive home health care and community services from public health agencies, clinics, and hospitals funded by private and public insurance.

Recommendations for nurses include the following:
1. Identify students receiving home schooling.
2. Assume a strategic role in providing required health screening to home-schooled students of all ages.
3. Be innovative and collaborative in determining approaches to the provision of health-related education and collaboration with the student, parents, or both (e.g., on school site, by e-mail, one-on-one meetings, home visits).
4. Data gathering for research is necessary and valuable for this population of students.

WEB SITES

National Association of Catholic Homes and Educators
  http://www.nache.org
National Home Education Research Institute
  http://www.nheri.org
National Home Education Network
  httpi//www.nhcn.org

SCHOOL SOCIAL ISSUES

YOUTH GAMBLING

The generation born in the 1990s is the first in modern American history to grow up with gambling considered legal and culturally acceptable. With gambling more widespread throughout the United States in state lotteries, at casinos, and on the Internet, more adults are gambling than ever before. This increase has been accompanied by an increased prevalence of problem gambling and pathological gambling among the adult population. Youth practices follow those of the adult population in social behavior such as smoking, alcohol use, drug abuse, and games of chance.

Gambling is putting something of value, such as money, at risk in anticipation of getting something of more value. Youth in America have traditionally engaged in social and informal gambling, such as sports betting, lottery tickets, and bingo. Recently, young people have increased gambling through unlawful access to casinos and the Internet. Most illegal gambling for American youth occurs through the Internet, done anonymously or deceptively, by posing as adults (Wilber and Potenza, 2006).

Only in the last 10 years have systematic and reliable studies on youth gambling been conducted. According to researchers at the Harvard Medical School in Children's Hospital Boston, between 60% to 90% of youth engage in gambling (Shaffer and Hall, 2001). The earlier a person starts gambling, the more likely they are to develop a serious problem. The average for beginning gambling is 12 years of age, which is a younger age than the first use of alcohol, tobacco, or other drugs (Jacobs, 2004). Research shows that rates of pathological gambling for adolescents is two to four times that of adults: 4% to 8% of high school students are pathological gamblers, and an additional 10% to 14% are at risk for problematic gambling (Griffiths, 2003; Hardoon, Derevenisky, and Gupta, 2003).

Twenty-first Century Health Challenges

CHAPTER 10

The National Gambling Impact Study Commission issued a summary of several studies that revealed adolescent pathological gambling to be associated with low grades, truancy, alcohol and drug abuse, problematic parent gamblers, and involvement in unlawful activities to finance their gambling (NGISC, 1999). Studies cite the reasons for *problematic gambling* as enjoyment, excitement, and a motivation to win money. *Pathological gamblers* cite enjoyment and excitement but also want to escape, relieve depression, and cope with loneliness; winning money is not the key motivator (Bergevin et al, 2006). These two terms are often used interchangeably. Among young gamblers, boys gamble three to four times more than girls (Wilber and Potenza, 2006). High school students gamble more than junior high school students, and male high school students prefer sports gambling, whereas female high school students prefer gambling with lottery tickets and bingo.

Educational and school health implications vary. Young people with problematic gambling issues are often involved in illegal and unlawful behavior, and they bring such activity to the school site. This practice contributes to an antisocial culture and an environment that requires more adult supervision, school security surveillance, and administrative discipline. Gambling youths tend to lose interest in academic and regular study to achieve passing grades. The lure of quick and easy money is a disincentive for youth to invest in educational approaches to later vocational and career opportunities as an adult. Truancy and school dropout are more likely with gambling youth in pursuit of more pleasurable activity. Often the associated personality and behavior disorders are untreated and therefore create complicated health and mental health problems (e.g., depression, conduct disorders, obsessive–compulsive disorders).

Action plans for the school nurse and other staff include the following:
1. Awareness of risk factors for problem gambling that include parents with gambling problems, earlier age of first gambling, and greater impulsivity.
2. Work together to develop a uniform and integrated gambling-prevention strategy that includes teaching more effective coping strategies in place of gambling.
3. Develop a positive discipline code and an array of corrective and remedial services that can be implemented throughout the school district.
4. Recommend detection of high-risk youths.
5. High-risk youths should be given more targeted services for recovery and resiliency.
6. Serve as advocate for more community, statewide, and national remedies to prevent access to adult gambling sources.

PRECOCIOUS PUBERTY

Precocious puberty is the development of secondary sexual characteristics before age 9 in boys and before age 8 in Caucasian girls, earlier in Hispanic girls, and as early as age 6 in black girls. This atypical variation has been reported in girls as young as 3 years. Development of breasts and growth of axillary and pubic hair in 5- to 8-year-old children are not isolated phenomena or statistical outliers but actual concerns of parents, nurses, HCPs, and other school professionals. Other characteristics include accelerated development of external genitalia and changes in behavior. Girls experience increased moodiness and irritability, whereas boys may develop a sex drive and become more aggressive and hyperactive than their peers. Boys develop more body mass, body hair, and have deeper voices.

Precocious puberty may occur as a result of an underlying condition, such as a hypothalamic tumor or disorder of the adrenal glands; but the cause generally is unknown. The recent increase in idiopathic precocious puberty causes alarming concern for physical, psychological, and social effects in the child, because all developmental stages take an upward spiral from the norm. The increase is so new that etiological research lags, although several theories exist. These theories include improper nutrition; an association between weight gain and early development; the presence of hormones found in milk and meat; exposure to dichlorodiphenyldichloroethylene (DDE), a by-product of the chemical dichlorodiphenyltrichloroethane (DDT), banned in 1972; polychlorinated biphenyls (PCBs), which are chemicals used in electrical equipment as a flame retardant; or contact with phthalates and bisphenol A, chemicals found in certain plastics.

Regardless of the cause, evaluation of precocious puberty for possible treatment is necessary. When no underlying cause is found, assessment of bone age determines the need for treatment. Children with precocious puberty with advanced bone age experience early rapid growth that plateaus in adolescence. If untreated, males typically do not exceed 5 feet 2 inches as an adult, and females usually are only about 5 feet tall. Treatment consists of medication including gonadotropin-releasing hormone (GnRH agonists; brand name is Lupron or Synarel). Medication is by injection or a drug depot under the skin, which is replaced every three months. This treatment is extremely expensive, but early treatment will halt progression of puberty and optimize the child's adult height.

In middle elementary students, precocious puberty is an antecedent to a host of psychosocial and relational issues affecting age-appropriate self-care and mastery of social skills, moral conduct, and peer group acceptance. These issues have been documented in the health literature as it relates to females, including reference to negative body images; engaging in sexual activity and acting out behavior; negative mood and depression; and a greater risk for eating disorders. Precocious female development differs by racial group; white adolescents experience a greater decrease in self-worth than African-American females (Rosenthal, Lewis, and Biro, 2000).

Precocious puberty for both boys and girls increases their risk for early sexual activity, sexual harassment, transmission of sexually transmitted diseases, and childhood pregnancy. Marginal peer relationships and exposure to older adolescent and adult relationships also contribute to confusing sex, romance, intimacy, and love issues. Boys face issues of masculine identity, whereas both sexes face premature readiness for exclusive dating and committed relationships with the opposite sex and the prospect of assuming parenting obligations before attaining the necessary personal, educational, and economic resources.

School nurse practice focuses on supporting and providing health care and knowledge to students with advanced psychosexual development. Services provided to the students include the following:

1. Education about sexual hygiene and self-care according to students' developmental age, not grade level.
2. Monitoring of growth anthropometry.

3. Provision for safe-sex education for children if and when sexual experimentation and activity occur.
4. Sensitization of school staff to the implications and consequences of precocious puberty.
5. Prevention and intervention for sexual harassment within or outside of peer group, including verbal and socially discriminatory behaviors.
6. Provision of adult guidance regarding issues related to precocious puberty.
7. Referral of the student to social and family counseling and mental health services as needed.

WEB SITE

The Magic Foundation for Children's Growth
http://www.magicfoundation.org

BIBLIOGRAPHY

American Academy of Pediatrics: Policy statement: children, adolescents, and television, *Pediatrics* 107(2):423-426, 2001.

American Academy of Pediatrics: Understanding the impact of media on children and teens, *Children's Health Topics: Violence Prevention* (available online):www.aap.org/healthtopics/violprev.cfm. Accessed Feb 20, 2006.

American Chiropractic Association: *American Chiropractic Association offers backpack safety checklist* (available online): www.amerchiro.org/press_css.cfm?CID=1834. Accessed Aug 2006.

American Occupational Therapy Association: *Backpack strategies for parents and students:pack it light, wear it right* (available online): www.promoteot.org/AI_BackpackStrategies.html. Accessed Sept 23, 2006.

American Physical Therapy Association: *Is your child's backpack making the grade?* (available online):www.apta.org/AM/Template.cfm?Template=/CM/HTMLDisplay.cfm&ContentID=32647. Accessed Aug 24, 2006.

American Psychological Association Task Force: *Television advertising leads to unhealthy habits in children,* 2004 (available online): www.apa.org/releases/childrenads.html. Accessed April 14, 2008.

Anshel J: *Smart medicine for your eyes: a guide to natural, effective, and safe relief of common eye disorders,* New York, 2007, Square One.

Austin EW, Chen Y, Pinkleton BE et al: Benefits and costs of Channel One in a middle school setting and the role of media-literacy training, *Pediatrics* 117(3):e423-e433, 2006 (available online): http://pediatrics.aappublications.org/cgi/content/full/117/3/e423. Accessed April 14, 2008.

Bergevin T, Gupta R, Derevensky J et al: Adolescent gambling: understanding the role of stress and coping, *J Gambl Stud* 22:195-208, 2006.

Brindis CD, Klein J, Schlitt J et al: School-based health centers: accessibility and accountability, *J Adolesc Health 32* (6):Supplement 98-107, 2003.

Buckingham D: *After the death of childhood: growing up in the age of electronic media,* Cambridge, England, 2000, Polity Press.

BusRadio: *BusRadio program,* 2007 (available online): www.busradio.org. Accessed April 14, 2008.

Centers for Disease Control and Prevention: *Emergency preparedness and response,* 2001 (available online): www.bt.cdc.gov. Accessed April 14, 2008.

Cergo S: *Computer ergonomics for elementary school,* Department of Consumer and Business Services, Oregon, 2006, OSHA (available online): www.orosha.org/cergos. Accessed April 14, 2008.

Comstock GA, Strasburger, VC: Media violence, *Adolesc Med Clinc* 4:495-509, 1993.

CUErgo: *Workstation ergonomics guidelines for computer use by children,* Cornell University Ergonomics Web (available online): http://ergo.human.cornell.edu. Accessed April 14, 2008.

Griffiths M: Adolescent gambling. In Romer D, editor: *Reducing adolescent risk: toward an integrated approach,* Thousand Oaks, Calif, 2003, Sage.

Grimmer KA, Williams MT, Gill TK: The association between adolescent head-on-neck posture, backpack weight, and anthropometric features, *Spine* 24(21): 2262-2267, 1999.

Guilday P: School nursing practice today: implications for the future, *J School Nurs* 16(5):25-31, 2000.

Hancox RJ, Milne BJ, Poulton R: Association of television viewing during childhood with poor educational achievement, *Arch Pediatr Adolesc Med* 159(7):614-618, 2005.

Hardoon K, Derevensky J, Gupta R: Empirical vs. perceived measures of gambling severity: Why adolescents don't present themselves for treatment, *Addictive Behavior* 28:1-14, 2003.

Henderson DA, Inglesby TV, Bartlett JG et al: Smallpox as a biological weapon: medical and public health management, Working Group on Civilian Biodefense, *JAMA* 281:2127-2137, 1999.

Home School Legal Defense Association: Academic statistics on homeschooling, *Legal Research Supplement,* 2004 (available online): www.hslda.org/docs/nche/000010/200410250.asp. Accessed April 14, 2008.

Jacobs DF: Youth gambling in North America: long term trends and future prospects. In Derevensky JL, Gupta R, editors: *Gambling problems in youth: theoretical and applied perspectives,* New York, 2004, Klewer Academic/Plenum Publishers.

Kaiser Permanente Medical Group: *Anthrax update: revised October 31, 2001* (available online): www.kpcmi.org/guideline_anthrax_mas.pdf. Accessed April 14, 2008.

Klesges RC, Shelton ML, Klesges LM: Effects of television on metabolic rate: potential implications for childhood obesity, *Pediatrics* 91:281-286, 1993.

Meyers-Walls J: Terrorism and children, *Purdue Extension,* Sept 2001 (available online): www.ces.purdue.edu/terrorism/children/terrorism.html. Accessed April 14, 2008.

Molnar A: School commercialism and adolescent health, *Adolesc Med Clin* 16(2): 447-461, 2005.

National Assembly on School-Based Health Care: *Capitol hill briefing explains school-based health centers' role as first responders to students in crisis,* Jan 2007 (available online): www.nasbhc.org/Jan07/nationalrelease1%2025.pdf. Accessed Sept 20, 2006.

National Association of Pediatric Nurse Practitioners: *Position statement: school-based and school-linked centers,* June 2004 (available online): www.napnap.org/index.cfm?page=54&sec=74. Accessed April 14, 2008.

National Association of School Nurses: *Position statement: backpacks,* Revised 2006 (available online): www.nasn.org/Default.aspx?tabid=204. Accessed April 14, 2008.

National Association of School Nurses: *Position statement: the role of the school nurse in school-based health centers,* Revised 2001 (available online): www.nasn.org/Default.aspx?tabid=245. Accessed April 14, 2008.

National Center for Education Statistics: *Homeschooling in the United States: 2003,* Feb 2006 (available online): http://nces.ed.gov/pubs2006/homeschool/index.asp.

National Center for Missing and Exploited Children: *Internet-related child exploitation,* 2000 (available online): www.missingkids.com. Accessed April 14, 2008.

National Gambling Impact Study Commission: *Final report,* Aug 1999 (available online): http://govinfo.library.unt.edu/ngisc/. Accessed Feb 20, 2007.

National Sleep Foundation: *NSF 2006 Sleep in America poll* (available online): www.sleepfoundation.org/site/c.huIXKjM0IxF/b.2425081/k.63D9/Americas_Sleepy_Teens.htm. Accessed April 14, 2008.

Occupational Safety and Health Administration: *Computer workstations: hazards and solutions,* 2005 (available online): www.osha-slc.gov/SLTC/computerworkstation/solutions.html. Accessed Jan 14, 2007.

Twenty-first Century Health Challenges

CHAPTER 10

Peigneux P, Laureys S, Fuchs S: Are spatial memories strengthened in the human hippocampus during slow wave sleep? *Neuron* 44 (3): 535-545, 2004.

Primedia: *Channel one* (available online): www.primedia.com/divisions/channelone. Accessed Dec 12, 2006.

Rideout V, Roberts DF, Foehr UG: *Generation M: media in the lives of 8- to 18-year-olds,* A Kaiser Family Foundation Study, 2005 (available online): www.kff.org/entmedia/upload/Executive-Summary-Generation-M-Media-in-the-Lives-of-8-18-Year-olds.pdf. Accessed April 14, 2008.

Rosenthal S, Lewis L, Biro F: Psychosexual development. In Coupey SM, editor: *Primary care of adolescent girls,* Philadelphia, 2000, Hanley & Belfus.

Salminen J, Erkintalo MO, Pentti J et al: Recurrent low back pain and early disc degeneration in the young, *Spine* 24(13):1316-1321, 1999.

Saltzman, A: *Stretch break for kids: kids window version 6.0* (available online): www.paratec.com/sbform/kidsform.htm. Accessed Jan 23, 2007.

Shaffer HJ, Hall MN: Updating and refining prevalence estimated of disordered gambling behavior in the United States and Canada, *Can J Public Health* 92(3):168-172, 2001.

Sharif I, Sargent JD: Association between television, movie, and video game exposure and school performance, *Pediatrics* 118(4):e1061-e1070, 2006.

Siambanes D, Martinez JW, Butler EW et al: Influence of school backpacks on adolescent back pain, *J Pediatr Orthop* 24(2):211-217, 2004.

Spencer RM, Sunm M, Ivry RB: Sleep-dependent consolidation of contextual learning, *Curr Biol* 16(10):1001-1005, 2006.

Strasburger VC: Risky business: what primary practitioners need to know about the influence of the media on adolescents, *Primary Care: Clinics in Office Practice* 33(2):317-348, 2006.

Strasburger VC, Wilson BJ, Jordan A: *Children, adolescents, and the media,* Thousand Oaks, Calif, 2007, Sage.

Vacheron JJ, Poumarat G, Chandezon R et al: Changes of contour of the spine caused by load carrying, *Surg Radiol Anat* 21(2):109-113, 1999.

Wahlstrom K: Bridging the gap between research and practice: what will adolescents' sleep/wake patterns look like in the twenty-first century? In Carskadon MA, editor: *Adolescent sleep patterns: biological, social, and psychological influences,* Cambridge, United Kingdom, 2002, Cambridge University Press.

Wartella E, Olivarez A, Jennings N: Children and television violence in the United States. In: Carlsson U, von Feilitzen C, editors: *Children and media violence,* Goteborg, Sweden, 1998, UNESCO International Clearinghouse on Children and Violence on the Screen.

Wilber MK, Potenza MN: Adolescent gambling: Research and clinical implications, *Psychiatry* 3(10):40-48, 2006.

Wolak J, Mitchell K, Finkelhor D: *Online victimization of youth: five years later,* National Center for Missing & Exploited Children, 2006 (available online): www.missingkids.com/en_US/publications/NC167.pdf#search=%22online%20victimization%20of%20youth%22. Accessed April 14, 2008.

CHAPTER 11

Emergency and Disaster Preparedness

Chapter Outline

*A*lthough there have been historical sporadic events of terrorism and emergency situations in schools both within America and abroad, traditionally schools are thought of as a safe place to be. Given the increased threat of terrorism, natural disasters, and school violence, school administrators must create an emergency plan for a school crisis. All school staff must be aware of what to do during a potentially violent situation or disaster.

For the purpose of this chapter, emergency is defined as a threatening event that can be generally managed by local resources. This might include bomb threats, incidents with hazardous materials, gas leaks, student unrest, and intruder or hostage situations. A disaster is defined as an event that overwhelms local management capacity, causes considerable loss of human life and economic resources, and necessitates a request for state and national support (Doyle and Loyacono, 2007). Disasters can include earthquake, weather-related events, radiological and chemical exposures, and a pandemic. The National Association of School Nurses has published a resource, *Disaster Preparedness Guidelines for School Nurses* (Doyle and Loyacono, 2007), which is helpful in disaster planning.

Given the large population of students and the many hours spent in school, the potential physical and psychosocial fallout of an emergency or disaster must be addressed. By virtue of education and experience, the school nurse is a valuable resource for disaster prevention, response, and recovery.

Should a disastrous event occur, the physical safety, emotional well being, and moral integrity of the school population are at risk. As a member of the emergency preparedness team and crisis response team at the school, the school nurse is prepared to work collaboratively with community agencies. A central focus of this service includes crisis management for physical injuries and psychosocial trauma resulting from the critical incident. Every county and district school office has been called upon to organize system-wide responses to emergencies and disasters. The school nurse can be involved as a policy maker and health care practitioner in this organized endeavor. This chapter provides the school nurse with suggestions, guidelines, and resources to use.

PREPARATION FOR EMERGENCIES AND DISASTERS

EMERGENCY SAFETY AND SECURITY MEASURES

The School Emergency Planning Team has a number of areas to develop and include in the emergency preparedness plan. Box 11-1 provides suggestions of key points to address.

The school team should identify and define the following immediate response measures: *evacuation; duck, cover, and hold; hit the deck; shelter-in-place;* and *lockdown.*

Box 11-1   *Preparedness Plan For Schools*

- Identify and involve community stakeholders, including parents and community emergency responders.
- Review existing plan.
- Establish what crises the plan will cover by considering local hazards, such as earthquakes or tornadoes.
- Identify and define immediate response measures (e.g., evacuation, lockdown).
- Assign appropriate duties to personnel and assign backups.
- Train personnel for specific tasks, including triage, first aid, and search and rescue.
- Obtain adequate supplies and equipment and identify appropriate storage space.
- Make plans for students with physical, sensory, motor, developmental, or mental challenges; include provisions for those with limited English.

- Develop accountability and student release procedures and forms.
- Convey details of the plan with families, especially procedures for reuniting.
- Create a plan to overcome communication difficulties with staff, students, and families both during and after the incident.
- Conduct emergency drills and crisis exercises on a routine basis with students, staff, and emergency responders.
- Prepare the school to be used as an emergency shelter for others in the community.
- Address policies to deal with terror threats and hoaxes.
- Prepare for recovery issues related to ongoing physical and psychosocial well being of students, staff, and parents.

Modified from US Dept of Ed, Office of Safe and Drug-Free Schools: *Practical information on crisis planning: a guide for schools and communities,* Washington, DC, 2007 (available online): www.ed.gov/admins/lead/safety/emergencyplan/crisisplanning.pdf. Accessed April 20, 2008.

Evacuation

Evacuation is an emergency measure to protect building inhabitants from fire and injury resulting from structural damage and hazardous materials. Alternate evacuation routes need to be in place in the event that the normal route is not useable. In the case of intentional terrorism, when the same routes are used repeatedly, they may become a target for an attack. Make plans for a buddy system so that two classes evacuate together with one teacher in the lead and the other teacher trailing behind the students. The lead teacher can pass information about barriers or dangers down the line so that injuries can be prevented. If one teacher is injured, the other one can take over both classes. One may need to remain with injured students, while the other evacuates the rest of the students. A memorandum of understanding should be made with a nearby school or other suitable facility in the neighborhood for a safe evacuation site in case the campus is unsafe for students. This site also would become the pick-up location for parents. Arrangements for student transportation must be made for both the school site and the alternate location.

Duck, Cover, and Hold

Duck or drop down on the floor and take cover under desks or tables; hold on to the furniture, and be prepared to move with it. If no sturdy furniture is available, seek cover against an interior wall or in a corner of supporting walls. Avoid dangerous features inside a building, such as windows, hanging objects, tall furniture, or mirrors. Protect the head and neck by covering them with your arms. Stay in place until a teacher gives the all-clear signal. The first person to duck, cover, and hold must be the teacher, who must provide help for students after an earthquake or explosion. Be prepared for aftershocks, and plan where to take cover.

Special education students in wheelchairs need to stay in place, lock the chair, and hold on. Leaning forward to protect the head and neck is not always possible because the individual may not be able to bend down to the knees. The wheelchair back does not provide sufficient protection (Doyle and Loyacona, 2007). Students with impaired mobility who are not in a wheelchair also need guidelines. Children with special needs should have practice prior to the drill.

Hit the Deck

Hit the deck, and do not look up or move: play dead, and use shallow breathing. This technique is used during gunfire.

Shelter-in-Place

Shelter-in-place is an emergency measure to protect students from hazardous airborne chemicals and radiation release, when there is no time to evacuate the site safely. Direct students and staff to their classrooms or to the closest building. Seal windows and doors with plastic and duct tape, close down ventilation systems, lock exterior doors, and leave one door unlocked with signs posted to direct individuals arriving on campus. Shelter-in-place is a short-term measure, usually for minutes to hours, not for days. Public safety officials will determine when school is safe or if evacuation is needed, and they will evaluate the situation for cleanup.

Lockdown

During a lockdown, all students must be inside a building and sitting against an inside wall or flat on the floor. All doors are locked and windows are covered. Lockdown is used for an intruder or sniper. Remain until the all-clear signal is given. A code word or phrase should routinely be used with the all-clear signal indicating to all staff that the danger really is over (Arizona Department of Education, 2006). During a real event or drill, if the word or phrase is not used, it could indicate the all-clear signal is being given under duress (e.g., at gunpoint).

NOTE: Notification should be given to parents of all procedures regarding school preparedness. Communications to parents explaining the emergency and disaster preparations made at school, how parents are to be involved, and what they can provide will make the plan more efficient. Additional information may need to be provided to parents of special needs students.

EMERGENCY PLANNING

Preparedness plans for schools include five phases: *prevention, preparedness, response, recovery* and *mitigation.* Prevention strategies are used to avoid an incident, and preparedness activities reduce the secondary consequences of an incident. The outcome of the disaster directly reflects the comprehensiveness and execution of the plan (Doyle and Loyacono, 2007). *Frequent emergency drills and updates keep the plan current and workable.*

When selecting team members, consider their level of motivation, leadership qualities, ability to communicate, calm attitude, organization skills, and empathy. Strategic duties are varied and include administration, security, medical management, psychosocial counseling, and communication with a variety of people and agencies. Below is one example of assignment of tasks. Also included in this section are boxes and data listing forms, procedures, supplies, equipment, and other staff information.

NOTE: During emergency drills, check expiration dates of supplies.

ORGANIZATIONAL PERSONNEL

   I. Incident Commander (IC): Head Administrator on Site
      A. Evaluates incident and potential harm to life or property.
      B. Coordinates and manages all other teams in the event of an emergency.
      C. Controls internal and external communications.
      D. Accounts for the presence of all students and staff.
      E. Authorizes release of students to parents.
   II. Public Information Officer (PIO): Usually Assistant Principal or Administrator
      A. Collects all communication and reports to IC.
      B. Signs in media personnel and functions as school spokesperson.
      C. Responds to and corrects media misinformation immediately.
   III. Student Management Team: Usually Teachers
      A. Takes attendance and reports missing students on teacher report form to Incident Command Center.
      B. Supervises students until release to parents.

IV. **First-Aid and Health Team: School Nurse and Trained Staff Members**
   A. Under supervision of school nurse and team leaders, provides first aid according to triage procedures and manages acute and chronic health problems.
   B. Documents treatment and disposition of students and staff on nurse emergency forms.
V. **Security Team: Can Be Custodians**
   A. Secures and patrols all entrances to the site.
   B. Shuts off gas, water, and electricity.
   C. Prevents community members from entering site without permission.
   D. Directs emergency vehicles and parents to reunion gate.
VI. **Search and Rescue Teams: Can Be Teachers or as Assigned**
   A. Rescue the injured.
   B. Check for and control dangerous situations resulting from the disaster.
VII. **Reunion Team: Can Be Clerical Staff**
   A. Reunites students with parents and documents all releases.
NOTE: Prepare grab-and-go box that can easily be taken to incident command site. See Box 11-2 for contents.

FORMS AND PROCEDURES

I. **Emergency Health Cards for Students and Staff, Including Health Information and Contact Numbers**
II. **Documentation Forms**
   A. Teacher report forms.
   B. Nurse emergency forms.
   C. Release forms—to whom and where.
III. **School Site Map with Locations Marked as Listed Below**
   A. Incident Command Center.

Box 11-2   *Grab-and-Go Box*

Each school needs to prepare a box that can easily be taken to the incident command site during an emergency or crisis. The box contains equipment and critical student and school information; it should be lightweight and portable.

1. List of current students and staff
2. Photographs of students and staff (recent yearbook)
3. Bus lists
4. List of health problems (students and staff)
5. Student emergency cards
6. Medication lists (students and staff)
7. Critical medications (3-day supply)
8. First-aid flip chart
9. Local and district phone directories
10. Evacuation plans
11. Blueprint plans of school and yard areas
12. Flashlight with extra batteries
13. Walkie-talkie, megaphones, mobile phones
14. Whistle
15. Master keys for buildings
16. Pens, markers, legal paper pads, name tags

During emergency drills, check expiration dates of supplies.
Modified from Fitzpatrick B: Emergency management, crisis response, and the school nurse's role. In Selekman J, editor: *School nursing: a comprehensive text*, Philadelphia, 2006, FA Davis.

Emergency and Disaster Preparedness

CHAPTER 11

B. Emergency assembly areas (students).

C. First-aid area.

D. Reunion gate.

E. Morgue.

F. Location of emergency equipment and shut-off valves for gas, water, electricity.

STAFF RESPONSIBILITIES

I. Personal Preparation

A. Prior arrangements should be made for care of family members in case of emergency, because staff may need to remain on the school site for up to 72 hours. Staff should maintain personal supplies in a classroom or another designated area, such as in their vehicle (except medications). The following items should be available:

1. Change of clothing, sturdy shoes, and warm jacket.
2. Blanket.
3. Water and food supplies.
4. Heavy gloves.
5. Flashlight and batteries.
6. Eyeglasses and/or materials to care for contact lenses.
7. Medications for three days.

II. Student Comfort Packs

A. Request comfort pack from parents for each child at beginning of school year. Send home a gallon-zippered plastic bag with list of suggested items to include food options (high-protein foods, hard candies; avoid salty snacks), pictures of family members, a favorite book, a small package of facial tissue, and a short comfort note written by parent for elementary or younger students. Include note from parent indicating any allergies and regular medications taken at home. A 3-day supply of medications should include medication orders for a 24-hour period and parent permissions; these should be kept in the nurse's office. The comfort bag and medications should be returned home at the end of the school year. Comfort packs are kept in a classroom emergency supply container.

SUPPLIES FOR THE WHOLE SCHOOL

NOTE: The nurse plays an integral part in the preparation of all school emergency planning. Provision of disaster supplies should be coordinated between the nurse and school staff.

I. Water

A. Paper cups and a gallon of water per day per person should be provided (2 qt for drinking and 2 qt for food preparation). Fifty-gallon drums of water are available for purchase.

B. Water purification methods:

1. Empty bleach bottles—add water without rinsing; expires in 1 yr.
2. Water purification tablets—follow directions (available at sporting goods stores and drug stores).
3. Unscented bleach—add 16 drops per gal or 1 tsp per 5 gal of water.
4. Rolling boil for 10 minutes.

II. First-Aid Supplies*

A. 4 × 4-in compresses: 1000 per 500 people.
B. 8 × 10-in compresses: 150 per 500 people.
C. Kerlix bandaging: 12 per 500 people.
D. Elastic (Ace) wrap bandage: 2 in, 12 per campus; 4 in, 12 per campus.
E. Triangular bandage: 24 per campus.
F. Cardboard splints: 24 each—small, medium, large.
G. Cardiopulmonary resuscitation (CPR) pocket masks, deluxe.
H. Ice packs, instant.
I. Tapes: 1-in cloth, 50 rolls per campus; 2-in cloth, 24 per campus.
J. Water in small, sealed containers for wound irrigation.
K. Antibiotic ointment: 144 squeeze packs per campus.
L. Wound closure strips, Steri-Strips, or butterfly bandages: 50 per campus.
M. Antiseptic.
N. Towelettes.
O. Unscented bleach, 1 bottle.
P. Paramedic scissors (for cutting through heavy materials): 4 per campus.
Q. Tweezers: 3 assorted per campus.
R. Triage tags: 50 per 500 people.
S. Oval eye patch: 50 per campus.
T. Dust masks: 25 per 100 people.
U. First-aid books: 2 standard and 2 advanced per campus.
V. Vinyl gloves: 100 per 500 people.
W. Heavy duty rubber gloves, 4 pairs.
X. Plastic basket or wire basket stretchers or backboards: 1.5 per 100 people.

NOTE: To disinfect rubber gloves, use 1 part bleach per 10 parts water.

III. Classroom Supplies: Keep in Clean Trashcans with Lids or in Large Backpacks

A. Current list of classroom students.
B. Student accounting forms, blank.
C. Permanent marker, pen, and note pads.
D. Masking tape to put name on each student.
E. Packaged hard candy (1 to 2 lb).
F. Flashlight and batteries.
G. Leather gloves: 1 pair.
H. Vinyl gloves: 6 pair.
I. Safety goggles: 1 pair.
J. Crow bar.
K. Duct tape, 3 rolls (for sealing doors and windows).
L. Scissors.
M. Whistle.
N. Sunscreen SPF 15 or higher.
O. Supplies for maintenance of body heat for each person (thermal or aluminum blankets or large garbage bags to wrap up in).
P. Tarp or ground cover.

---

*First-aid supplies must follow the laws related to the delivery of nursing care in each state.

    Q. Small first aid kit.

    R. Diapers and special feeding supplies for very young or disabled students.

    S. Large card identifying teacher, grade, and room number for display to facilitate reunification.

    T. Activities to keep students occupied.

IV. Sanitation Supplies

    A. One toilet kit per 100 people; include 1 portable toilet, 20 rolls of toilet paper, 300 wet wipes, 300 plastic bags with ties, and 10 large plastic trash bags.

    B. Soap and water or waterless hand gel, in addition to wipes, are recommended.

    C. Feminine hygiene supplies.

V. Tools and Other Supplies

    A. See Box 11-3.

VI. Food

    A. Non-perishable foods that are easy to serve and require no cooking or refrigeration. Especially important for those with diabetes,

---

Box 11-3　*Emergency Equipment*

- Job description clipboards for teams
- Stretchers: 1 for every 150 people
- Two-way radios to search area
- System to mark areas that have been searched (e.g., red tape on doorknob)
- Tables and chairs for emergency operations center and reunification teams
- Marking pens, paper, pencils
- Shovel
- Broom
- Short-handled ax
- Short-handled sledgehammer
- Set of screwdrivers
- Pipe wrench, 14 in
- 12-hour snap light (friction)
- One 5.5 lb fire extinguisher
- Gray tape, duct tape, barrier tape (3 rolls)
- Whistle, megaphone
- Box of safety matches in waterproof container
- Small votive candles
- Multipurpose pocket knife (e.g., Swiss army knife)
- Pliers
- Hammer
- Can opener

- AM/FM portable radio and batteries
- 50 ft braided nylon cord
- Individual, handheld, personal warmth packets (e.g., HotHands, Heatmax,): shake to activate
- Ground cover or tarps

Protective Items for Rescue Team Members

- Hard hats
- Vests to identify teams
- Flashlight with batteries
- Leather gloves and vinyl gloves
- Dust masks
- Safety goggles
- Tote bag to carry supplies

Items for Rescue Team (one team per 1000 people)

- Master keys
- First-aid kit
- Pliers
- Crowbar
- Hacksaw, small and collapsible
- Bolt cutters
- Hammer

American Red Cross: *Recommended emergency supplies for schools, 2003* (available online): www.redcross.org/disaster/masters/supplies.html. Accessed July 1, 2007.

hypoglycemia, and other specific health conditions; otherwise, food is a low priority. A supply of granola bars, power bars, or energy bars is recommended.

SCHOOL NURSE'S ROLE IN CRISIS SITUATIONS

One of the primary roles of the school nurse in disaster is *triage,* the making of ethical decisions based on the greatest good for the greatest number of victims. It begins by sorting victims where they are by using color-coded tags to identify those who can be rescued (see Box 11-4). Following the first triage, the second step is a more comprehensive assessment, made to determine the individual needs of each victim. A layperson can be taught to do the first screening, but a nurse or trained first-aid provider needs to do the second assessment. Box 11-5 lists activities that the walking wounded can help with. The procedure for the initial triage includes the following:

- Survey the scene for safety: What caused the incident?
- Put on protective equipment if necessary (e.g., vinyl gloves, goggles, boots).
- Work with a team member.

Box 11-4	*Simple Triage and Rapid Treatment (START)* **Tag system for injured and triage conditions**

Tag guidelines: Can be seen from a distance and cannot be damaged by liquids

Red: Immediate care, for correctable but life-threatening injuries

Delayed capillary refill (greater than 2 sec)
Unable to follow simple commands
Respirations present only after opening an airway or respiration faster than 30 breaths/min
Major lacerations with extensive hemorrhage
Open fractures of major bones
Critical injuries to respiratory tract or central nervous system (CNS)
Severe burns
Ionizing radiation

Yellow: Delayed care, for serious but not immediately life–threatening injuries; requires care beyond basic first aid within 1 to 3 hours

Any living injured person not fitting into red or green categories

Fractures or minor burns
Major lacerations without extensive hemorrhage

Green: Walking wounded, minimal care

All injured persons not requiring hospital intervention

Black: Dead and mortally wounded*

Legally dead or with injuries incompatible with life
No respirations present even after attempting to reposition the airway
State law may require that a body not be removed, searched, or undressed until released by the coroner, unless it presents a hazard or hinders the care of others.

*Caution: Modifications of START are needed for children, because they are more likely to sustain respiratory failure prior to cardiac arrest; thus, absence of breathing after repositioning does not indicate a fatal condition, as it does in adults. For children who are not breathing, if pulse is present, give five rescue breaths. Team Life Support: www.jumpstarttriage.com

| **Box 11-5** | *Activities for Walking Wounded: Older Students or Adults* |

- Find first aid supplies.
- Help establish area for first aid.
- Help move victims within triage area.
- Help calm victims.
- Write down names of individuals.

Doyle J, Loyacono TR: *Disaster preparedness guidelines for school nurses,* Silver Spring, Md, National Association of School Nurses, 2007; Romig LE: *The jump START pediatric MCI triage tool and other pediatric disaster and emergency medicine resources,* Team Life Support, Inc, 2006 (available online): http://www.jumpstarttriage.com. Accessed April 24, 2008.

- Call out "If you can walk, come forward" or "Move to the wall," depending on the situation.
- Keep uninjured, older students and adults nearby to help control urgent problems, such as bleeding and airway management.
- Assign someone to remove hysterical people, and assign someone else to stay with them.
- Assign a gatekeeper.
- Maintain a calm, controlled demeanor; use positive communications and language.
- Continue systematic triage, working in an outward pattern.
- Assess respiration, perfusion (blood flow), and mental states.
- Spend less than a minute on each individual.

A disaster or traumatic event usually precipitates several predictable signs of stress in both adults and children. Signs and symptoms are expressed in different ways in different children and it varies according to their developmental age. If symptoms persist or become extreme, professional help should be secured.

A survey sponsored by the National Association of Pediatric Nurse Practitioners (NAPNAP [2001]) showed that parents and children worry about parent–child relationships, depression, anxiety, self-esteem, and coping with stress (Melnyk et al, 2001). We must pay attention to all students who have suffered a traumatic event or emergency in their lives to provide services both during and after the incident.

Knowing how children and adolescents react to stress is important in planning appropriate strategies to avoid long-term sequelae. Reactions to trauma are usually age-related and vary by individual temperament. The emotional reactions to the emergency or disaster often manifest in changes in behavior. Signs and symptom may appear immediately after the event or even many weeks later. If reactions last longer than expected, or if a condition worsens, a referral to a mental health professional may be needed (see Table 11-1). Box 11-6 lists typical reactions seen in children of all ages.

The parents are key in maintaining the optimal well being of their child. During a crisis, it is especially important for the school nurse to join with the family in assisting the child back to normal adaptation in the school setting. Furthermore, children usually mimic their parents' and older siblings' reactions to disaster. When parents cope well, their children generally cope well. When concerns are not brought forth and discussed openly, children may interpret this as a negative sign and may imagine the situation to be worse than it really is. Box 11-7 provides a list of helpful actions parents can take.

BIOTERRORISM AND PANDEMIC FLU

Given the threat of domestic terrorism in the United States, the school nurse is a resource for disaster prevention, preparedness, response, recovery, and mitigation for the entire school population, both students and staff. Should a man-made emergency or pandemic occur in the school, community, or even other regions of the country, the physical safety and emotional well being of the school population are at risk. As a member of the crisis response team at the school and in the community, the school nurse is prepared to work collaboratively with the public health department and local health care providers. A central focus of this service includes first aid and crisis management for the physical and psychosocial trauma that result from an act of terrorism or a pandemic.

The school nurse is a key person in early response to bioterrorism events or pandemic flu. The school nurse is involved with a large population of students and staff and may be the first to detect signs and symptoms indicative of a pandemic outbreak or a biological terrorist insult (For detailed data on biological agents, see Table 11-2 and Table 11-3 for detailed data on biological agents.) The school nurse often sees students and staff at the first sign of illness and prior to their seeking any other care. They are available to large numbers of people 6 to 10 hours a day, 5 days a week. Nurses are in a prime position to detect and assess risk and to make appropriate referrals, thus improving patient outcomes and curtailing the spread of disease. Due to the large number of children in a concentrated area, the school represents an important place of epidemic amplification. The National Association of School Nurses provides an informative position statement, "School Nurse Role in Bioterrorism Emergency Preparedness and Response, 2005."

PANDEMIC FLU

A *pandemic* is a global disease outbreak. A *flu pandemic* occurs when a new influenza virus emerges for which people have little or no immunity and for which there is no vaccine. There are three general conditions: 1) a new flu that is extremely pathogenic to humans; 2) a virus that is unique, in that people have no preexisting immunity; 3) a virus that transmits easily from human to human. The Avian (H5N1) virus meets the first two criteria but does not yet pass efficiently from person to person. Box 11-8 defines some flu terminology.

It is difficult to predict when the next influenza pandemic will occur or how severe it will be. When people have not been exposed to a new virus before, they have little or no immunity to it; therefore, serious illness and death are more likely to result than with a seasonal flu. The virus can sweep across the country and around the world in a very short time. Border closures and travel restrictions may delay arrival of the virus but cannot stop it. Depending on the category of the influenza, *social distancing* could be part of the implementation to minimize spread of the disease; schools may be closed, the work force could be staggered, and public gatherings could be limited.

Emergency and Disaster Preparedness

CHAPTER 11

Table 11-1   Students' Biological and Emotional Responses to Trauma and Interventions

Age	Physical	Behavioral and Emotional	Interventions
Preschool 3-5 years	Change in appetite Constipation Loss of bowel and bladder control Trembling Sleep disturbances	Strongly affected by parents' reactions Excessive clinging Whimpering Speech difficulties (stammering) Confusion Aimless motion Irritability Screaming Bed-wetting Night terrors Thumb sucking Fear of darkness, animals, strangers, being left alone, and abandonment Fear of being separated from parents	Utilize role playing, art, and play therapy to encourage expression of feelings Provide extra attention Give verbal reassurance and physical comfort Explain more carefully each transition and activity Discuss events at the appropriate developmental level
Elementary 5-12 years	Psychosomatic complaints: Headaches Abdominal pain Changes in appetite Sleep abnormalities	Increase in anger, fear, sadness, worries, and negative behaviors Irritability Clinginess Aggression Anxiety Emotionally labile Depression Withdrawal from friends and activities Perseveration of the event Decreased concentration and attention Changes in school performance Absenteeism Loss of control Angry outbursts	Listen to students Support expression of feelings Provide time for community grieving Provide for discussion and role playing with adults and peers Involve in peer support group Display patience and tolerance for mood swings Temporarily relax expectations Encourage activities to help students recover (e.g., memorial fund, planting trees) Rehearse prevention strategies for future disasters and emergencies

| Middle and High school 13-18 years | Tantrums
Increased sensitivity to sounds: loud noises, sirens, cars backfiring (depends on type of crisis)
Nightmares, night terrors, and fear of darkness
Psychosomatic complaints:
Vague aches and pains
Headaches
Stomachaches
Skin rashes and eruptions
Constipation
Diarrhea
Appetite and sleep disturbances
Amenorrhea or dysmenorrhea | Decreased attention or concentration, depression, anxiety
Academic performance changes
Hyperactivity
Agitation or reduced energy level
Withdrawal from or irritability with friends, family, teachers, events
Loss of interest in peer social activities
Irresponsible or delinquent behavior
Abrupt change in emancipation struggles over parental control
Anger, fear, sadness, worries, guilt
Fears of death and dying
Aware of and influenced by peer reactions | Allow time for grieving for both students and staff
Listen to students
Encourage discussion of disaster events with peers, family, and other adults
Reassure students that feelings will diminish over time and become easier to accept
Communicate with staff and parents about students' having extreme reactions and seek help
Give one-on-one-time when needed
Guide students into realistic understanding of event
Discuss safety and security and reinforce many times
Provide calming exercises such as deep breathing, quiet reflecting, art therapy
Consider facilitating a group art project
Remain aware of own emotions and reactions and seek help as needed
Keep students active by increasing physical education time and increasing time for group social activities
Relax expectations in class
Provide schoolwork requiring less concentration and limit new information
Encourage activities to help students recover (e.g., collecting money for families, designing cards) |

| **Box 11-6** | *Common Disaster Reactions of Children* |

- Fears of future disasters
- Loss of interest in school
- Regressive behavior

- Sleep disturbances and night terrors
- Fears of events associated with disaster

From Substance Abuse and Mental Health Services Administration, National Mental Health Information Center: *Reaction of children to a disaster,* 2003, (available online): http://mentalhealth.samhsa.gov/publications/allpubs/Ken01-0101/default.asp. Accessed April 24, 2008.

| **Box 11-7** | *Parent Hints for Helping Children Cope* |

- Offer physical comfort; hug and touch your child frequently.
- Be honest in discussing what has happened and what lies ahead.
- Share your feelings about the incident at the child's developmental level.
- Avoid frequent reexposure to the disaster via TV and newspapers.
- Encourage your child with the reassurance that you are safe and together.
- Allow children to grieve their loss of people, pets, or things.
- Reassure your child that their reactions are normal and will diminish over time.
- Help your child express their feelings through role playing, art, or play.

- Allow extra attention at bedtime.
- Promote physical activity.
- Communicate with your child's teacher or school nurse.
- Maintain family routines as much as possible.
- Prevent unnecessary separations from you and other significant caregivers.
- Increase your patience and tolerance for your child and yourself.
- Take good care of yourself; seek help if needed.
- Involve children in planning activities to help others in need.

In schools, having many children in a confined space contributes to the efficient transmission of disease. Young children are more susceptible to airborne viruses due to their rapid respiratory rate, smaller size, and less well-developed immune system. Schools can emphasize respiratory etiquette, provide tissues, teach thorough hand washing, and reinforce prevention strategies through student and staff education, posters, and reminders to families. School nurses must gain administrative support to enforce the health directive that sick children stay home.

Avian influenza is a flu virus that occurs naturally in birds; the birds usually do not get sick, but domesticated birds can become infected and frequently die. It is caused by one strain of avian virus, the H5N1 strain, and it is spread from bird to bird. Most human cases have resulted from direct contact with infected poultry or contaminated surfaces. The first human case was reported in 1997, and there are only 200 confirmed cases to date. To date, it has had a limited spread from person to person.

Table 11-2 *Characteristics of Anthrax*

Anthrax Type	Incubation Period	Transmission	Symptoms	Complications	Mortality Rate
Inhalational most severe form	2-7 days; may be up to 60 days	By inhalation of aerosolized or airborne spores Not known to be spread from person to person	Prodromal: brief, flulike respiratory symptoms, cough, fatigue, muscle aches (runny nose or discharge is rare), vomiting, possible chest pain, followed by development of dyspnea, low blood pressure, shock	Sepsis or meningitis	80% or higher Death can follow within 36 hr after occurrence of respiratory distress
Cutaneous	1-12 days	Through cut or opening in skin when in contact with infected animals or animal products Not known to be spread from person to person	Evolves from papule, to vesicle, to depressed eschar (black scab) Usually painless Other symptoms include fever, malaise, headache, and regional adenopathy Usually 3-7 days for eschar to develop	Can lead to sepsis, meningitis, thrombocytopenia, anemia, severe edema (head and neck), secondary bacterial infection, causing cellulitis and lymphadenitis	20% without treatment and less than 1% with antibiotic treatment

Continued

CHAPTER 11   Emergency and Disaster Preparedness

Table 11-2 *Characteristics of Anthrax—cont'd*

Anthrax Type	Incubation Period	Transmission	Symptoms	Complications	Mortality Rate
Gastrointestinal	1-7 days	Eating raw or under-cooked contaminated meat or drinking contaminated water Not known to be spread from person to person	Overall symptoms: severe abdominal pain, fever, signs of septicemia Oral pharyngeal forms: lesions at base of tongue, dysphagia, fever, regional lymph-adenopathy Abdominal form: nausea, loss of appetite, fever, abdominal pain, hematemesis, bloody diarrhea	Systemic toxicity, sepsis, shock, and meningitis	Estimated 25 to 75%

Note: Vaccine is available for military personnel, persons working in laboratories, or those working with potentially infected animal products.
Source: Centers for Disease Control and Prevention, 2005.

Table 11-3 *Other Biological Agents and Clinical Data*

Disease	Etiology and Incubation Period	Transmission	Symptoms and Complications	Treatment	Mortality Rate
Smallpox	Variola virus 7-17 days; virus is fragile and inactivated in 1-2 days Prior infection provides lifelong immunity	Infected saliva, from handling infected clothing or bedding; rarely airborne Most infectious 7-10 days after rash appears; risk of transmission lasts until all scabs are off	High fever, headache, body aches, malaise; flat lesions become pustules on face and/or torso; scabs develop and fall off in 3-4 weeks In early stages may be misdiagnosed as chickenpox Smallpox rash erupts quickly, beginning in mouth or throat and progressing downward; occurs on palms and soles of feet	Vaccination up to 4 days after exposure; no available pharmaceutical treatment New vaccine being developed	30%
Botulism	*Clostridium botulinum* bacillus Symptoms start 8-36 hrs after exposure, can be several days	Ingestion of improperly prepared or canned food Found in human feces; not spread person to person	Early signs are double or blurred vision, slurred speech, and muscle weakness; progressive limb paralysis	Antitoxins can stop progression Ventilator for respiratory failure	5-8%

Continued

Table 11-3 *Other Biological Agents and Clinical Data—cont'd*

Disease	Etiology and Incubation Period	Transmission	Symptoms and Complications	Treatment	Mortality Rate
Hemorrhagic fevers	Various viruses	Some spread by arthropods, others by infected humans or animals	Vary according to virus; fever, fatigue, muscle aches, loss of strength; can include coma, bleeding, and shock	No treatment for Ebola virus; antiviral ribavirin is often helpful with other viruses Ebola vaccine being researched	Varies
Pneumonic plague	*Yersinia pestis* bacillus Pulmonary exposure symptoms occur 1-3 days; flea-borne, 2-8 days	Spread by respiratory droplets person-to-person; known to be spread from infected rodents to humans by infected fleas	Headache, malaise, weakness, productive cough, chest pain, fever, chills, progressing to pneumonia in 2-4 days; septic shock, death. Early treatment is critical	Antibiotics Prophylactic antibiotics for 7 days to protect those exposed New vaccine is being developed	50-90% if untreated; 5% with diagnosis and treatment
Tularemia	*Francisella tularensis* bacillus One of the most infectious pathogenic bacteria Incubation 3-14 days	Bite of infective arthropod, handling infected animal tissues or fluids, direct contact with or ingestion of contaminated food, water, or soil; inhalation of infective aerosols Acquired through skin, mucous membranes, lungs, and gastrointestinal tract Not spread person to person	Fever, fatigue, chills, headache, sore throat, weakness, pharyngitis, bronchitis, and pneumonia	Antibiotics Vaccine is under review by FDA	5% for untreated inhalational; less than 1% when treated

Adapted from U.S. National Library of Medicine and National Institutes of Health, MedlinePlus, (available online): http://www.nlm.nih.gov/medlineplus. Accessed April 24, 2008.

Box 11-8	*Flu Terminology*

Seasonal flu is a respiratory illness that can be transmitted from person to person. Most people have some immunity, and a vaccine is available.

Avian or bird flu (AI) is caused by influenza viruses that occur naturally among wild birds. Low-pathogenic AI is common in birds and causes few problems. Highly pathogenic H5NI is deadly to domestic fowl, can be transmitted from birds to humans, and is deadly to humans. There is virtually no human immunity and human vaccine availability is very limited.

Pandemic flu is virulent human flu that causes a global outbreak, or pandemic, of serious illness. Because there is little natural immunity, the disease can spread easily from person to person. Currently, there is no pandemic flu.

From US Dept of Health and Human Services (available online): www.pandemicflu.gov. Accessed July 27, 2007.

Symptoms are flulike: fever, cough, sore throat, and muscle aches. Conjunctivitis, pneumonia, acute respiratory distress, and other severe and life-threatening complications have been reported. No vaccine is currently available. Two antiviral drugs, oseltamavir (Tamiflu) and zanamavir (Relenza), may be useful treatments for avian influenza.

WEB SITES

American Academy of Pediatrics: Children and Disasters
    http://www.aap.org/terrorism/index.html
American Psychological Association: Trauma
    http://www.apa.org/topics/topictrauma.html
American Red Cross
    http://www.redcross.org
Center for Effective Collaboration and Practice,
School Violence Prevention and Intervention
    http://cecp.air.org/school_violence.asp
Centers for Disease Control and Prevention,
Emergency Preparedness and Response
    http://www.bt.cdc.gov
Federal Emergency Management Agency (FEMA)
    http://www.fema.gov/index.shtm
Federal Emergency Management Agency (FEMA) for Kids
    http://www.fema.gov/kids
National Association of School Nurses
    http://www.nasn.org
National Association of School Psychologists
    http://www.nasponline.org
National Mental Health Information Center
    http://mentalhealth.samhsa.gov
National School Safety Center
    http://www.schoolsafety.us
National School Safety and Security Services
    http://www.schoolsecurity.org
Online Support for Bomb Threat Response Planning Tool
    http://www.threatplan.org

Emergency and Disaster Preparedness

CHAPTER 11

PandemicFlu.gov/AvianFlu.gov
    http://www.pandemicflu.gov
U.S. Department of Homeland Security,
Ready: Prepare. Plan. Stay Informed.
    http://www.ready.gov
U.S. Department of Education: Emergency Planning
    http://www.ed.gov/admins/lead/safety/emergencyplan/index.html
U.S. Environmental Protection Agency, Ground Water and Drinking Water,
Emergency Disinfection of Drinking Water
    http://www.epa.gov/safewater/faq/emerg.html

BIBLIOGRAPHY

Arizona Department of Education, Arizona Division of Emergency Management: *Arizona School Site Emergency Response Plan Template,* 2006 (available online): www.ade.az.gov/schooleffectiveness/health/schoolsafety/safetyplans/SitePlan.doc. Accessed July 20, 2007.

Bobo N, Hallenbeck P, Robinson J: Recommended minimal emergency equipment and resources for schools: national consensus group report, *J Sch Nurs* 19(3):150-56, 2003.

DeRanieri JT, Clements PT, Clark K et al: War, terrorism, and children, *J Sch Nurs* 20(2):69-75, 2004.

Doyle J, Loyacono TR: *Disaster preparedness guidelines for school nurses,* ed 2, Silver Spring, Md., National Association of School Nurses, 2007.

Ethier AM: Family-centered end-of-life care. In Hockenberry MJ, Wilson D, Editors: *Wong's nursing care of infants and children,* ed 8, St Louis, 2006, Elsevier Mosby.

Fein RA, Vossekuil B, Pollack WS et al: *Threat assessment in schools: a guide to managing threatening situations and to creating safe school climates,* Washington, DC, US Secret Service and US Dept of Ed, 2002 (available online): www.secretservice.gov/ntac/ssi_guide.pdf. Accessed July 2, 2007.

Fitzpatrick B: Emergency management, crisis response, and the school nurse's role. In Selekman J, Editor: *School nursing: a comprehensive text,* Philadelphia, 2006, FA Davis.

Johnson K: *Classroom crisis: the teacher's guide.* Alameda, Calif., 2004, Hunter House.

Melnyk BM: The KySS (keep your children and yourself safe and secure) campaign: A national effort to reduce psychosocial morbidities in children and adolescents, *J Pediatr Health Care* 15(2):31a-34a, 2001.

National Association of School Nurses: *Position statement: disaster preparedness—school nurse role,* 2006 (available online): www.nasn.org/positions/disasterpreparedness. htm. Accessed July 27, 2007.

National Association of School Nurses: *School nurse role in bioterrorism emergency preparedness and response,* 2005 (available online): www.nasn.org/positions/bioterrorism.htm. Accessed July 27, 2007.

Romig LE: *The jump START Pediatric MCI triage tool and other pediatric disaster and emergency medicine resources,* Team Life Support, Inc, 2006, (available online): http://www.jumpstarttriage.com. Accessed April 24, 2008.

Vossekuil B, Fein RA, Reddy M et al: *The final report and findings of the safe school initiative: implications for the prevention of school attacks in the United States.* Washington, DC, 2002, US Dept of Ed and US Secret Service, National Threat Assessment Center.

CHAPTER 12

First Aid

Chapter Outline

When student illness or injury occurs in the school setting, the school nurse is called on to provide leadership. The school nurse must be knowledgeable to provide the necessary care and to direct others in providing first aid daily and in emergency and disaster situations. A school emergency plan for all students and staff should be in place. Individualized health care plans (IHCP) and emergency care plans (ECP) should be available for all

First Aid

CHAPTER 12

medically involved students (e.g., diabetics, asthmatics). These plans allow the nurse to be free from all tasks except caring for the involved student, while others are helping with the necessary telephone calls and other duties. *Documentation* must follow all incidents regardless of severity. *Universal Precautions* must be followed when providing health and emergency care to students and staff.

This chapter provides information for basic first aid for numerous common emergency situations. Box 12-1 lists supplies that are useful for first-aid kits. When a nurse cannot be at the school site when an emergency arises, teachers or other school personnel must know how to handle such situations. The nurse can use this chapter as a teaching tool for training school staff, thereby ensuring provision of appropriate health care and sound advice. Nursing practices vary by state, county, and school district; so nurses must be aware of, and compliant with, individual school policies and procedures.

The following are used by school nurses under the direction of a health care provider (HCP) and with parents' signed consent:

1. Autoinjector pen with epinephrine (EpiPen, Twinject) and epinephrine solution and syringes.
2. Antihistamines such as diphenhydramine (Benadryl).
3. Acetaminophen.

Box 12-1   *Nurse's Health Office Supplies*

The Following Items Are Listed by A or B When Useful for the Following Kits:

    A *First-aid kit for classroom*
    B *First-aid kit for field trips*

First-aid manual for classroom or field trip (A, B)
Vinyl gloves (A, B)
Mild soap
Antiseptic solution
Sodium bicarbonate
Hypoallergenic adhesive tape, several sizes (B)
Elastic (Ace) wraps, 2- and 4-in (B)
Gauze rolls, stretch (B)
Gauze squares, different sizes
Triangular bandage
Adhesive bandages (Band-Aids), various sizes; Steri-Strips, butterfly bandages (A, B)
Cotton balls (A, B)
Cotton applicators
Tongue blades (A)
Combine dressings (ABD pads) for heavy bleeding (B)
Topical skin powders and adhesives for lacerations or wounds (B)

Splints: small, medium, and large
Tweezers
Cold packs, instant
Moistened towelettes
Antibacterial hand soap (B)
Sunscreen (B)
Eye cup
Eye pads
Bottle of eye irrigation solution
Contact lens case (B)
Paper cups
Red plastic bags
Small plastic bags, resealable plastic bag (A, B)
Scissors (A, B)
Thermometer
Matches
Penlight (B)
Blanket: lightweight and washable
Bleach
Sanitary napkins
Disposable protective gown or apron
Protective eyeglasses
Mouth-to-mouth resuscitator with one-way valve (A, B)

Some medications may be stored in a locked container in the classroom or carried on the student if requested and authorized by the parents. The nurse must check individual state, county, and school district policies regarding particular medications, storage methods, and disposal procedures.

ABDOMINAL PAIN

I. **Immediate First Aid**
   A. Have the student lie down; keep student warm and quiet.
   B. Obtain appropriate history regarding onset, circumstances, and duration of pain; note presence of fever, nausea, vomiting, guarding, abdominal rigidity, constipation, or diarrhea.
   C. Determine type of pain: dull, diffuse, sharp, localized, continuous, or intermittent.
   D. Do not give student anything to eat or drink.
   E. Notify parents and urge them to seek immediate medical care for their child if pain is severe, persistent, or if student health history indicates a pathological condition.

BEE, WASP, YELLOW JACKET, AND HORNET STINGS

Any stings by bees, wasps, yellow jackets, or hornets can present a life-threatening emergency; therefore, special precautions are necessary when administering first aid. If a child is known to be sensitive or allergic to bee stings, keep an emergency bee-sting kit at the school site, keep it available when students are outside, and take it on all field trips. Some students are allowed to keep an epinephrine injection, such as an Epipen or Twinject, with them. More than one individual, including the student, should be trained in the proper administration of the injection.

If a student is stung and has history of allergies or severe reaction, give injection and quickly activate EMS, especially if generalized or local symptoms continue after injection, such as throat and chest tightness, wheezing, swelling of the face, abdominal pain, or nausea and vomiting.

I. **Immediate First Aid**
   A. Remove stinger as soon as possible, keeping it intact by brushing it out as gently as possible with thumbnail, credit card, straight-edged object, or a piece of cardboard. Speed is essential. Do not delay removal, because it will prolong pain and venom will continue to enter the body.
   B. Pinching or using tweezers to remove a stinger may release more venom into the body.
   C. Wash with soap and water.

II. **Symptoms of Allergic Systemic Reaction: Mild Reaction**
   A. Flushed skin and itching.
   B. Stinging and swelling.
   C. Apply ice, ice water, cold washcloth, or paste of sodium bicarbonate (baking soda).
   D. Administer antihistamine, unless contraindicated on student health records; some states, school districts, or counties require a medical order that may be either generic or child-specific.
   E. Notify parents.

First Aid

CHAPTER 12

III. Symptoms of Systemic Allergic Reaction: Severe Reaction
A. Flushed skin, puffy face, mouth, or eyelids.
B. Hives or extensive skin rash.
C. Difficulty breathing or swallowing; hoarseness.
D. Sneezing, coughing, or asthmalike wheezing.
E. Gastrointestinal complaints.
F. Generalized swelling, dizziness, nausea, weakness, paleness, faintness, or confusion.
G. For severe reaction, call 911 and give epinephrine injection, unless contraindicated on student health records; some states, school districts, and counties require a medical order that may be either generic or child-specific.

IV. Prevention
A. If highly allergic to bees and insects, avoid wearing strong-smelling perfumes and carrying or standing near sweet drinks and foods that attract bees; trash containers on school playgrounds may attract bees. Allergic students should wear light-colored clothing.

WARM-BLOODED ANIMAL BITES

I. Immediate First Aid
A. Capture the animal, if this can be done safely; if not, have someone follow the animal so that authorities can capture it later. The animal must be kept under observation for 14 days to rule out rabies.
B. Wear gloves and use universal precautions. Rinse wound immediately under running water; scrub wound thoroughly with soap and water; repeat procedure three to four times. Cleaning the bite is important to wash the animal's saliva from the wound.
C. Notify parents; inform them of the importance of consulting their HCP.
D. Report the bite to a state or county health department and follow their instructions. The *incubation period* for rabies in humans is usually several weeks to months but it ranges from days to years (CDC, 2007).

HUMAN BITES

Wounds caused by human bites, especially if they are deep and penetrating, are extremely dangerous, because it exposes the person to bacteria and blood-borne pathogens.

I. Immediate First Aid
A. Wear gloves and use universal precautions.
B. If wound is bleeding freely, allow bleeding for 3 to 4 seconds, then irrigate the wound under running water.
C. Wash wound with water and soap, preferably antiseptic soap.
D. Let wound dry and apply sterile dressing.
E. Further treatment depends on hepatitis B immunization information for both individuals.
F. Human immunodeficiency virus (HIV) transfer is a threat; victim, perpetrator, or both may need testing, depending on county, district, or school policy or HCP's recommendation.

G. Notify parents and urge them to contact their physician; alert parents to signs of possible infection.

INSECT BITES

Bites from insects such as mosquitoes, fleas, and chiggers can cause swelling, irritation, and redness. Chiggers are tiny red mites that live in tall grass and weeds, and they are usually found on a person's legs and around the belt line; itching lasts 5 to 6 days but can persist for months. Impetigo can occur as a result of scratching the bites.

I. Immediate First Aid
  A. Wear gloves and use universal precautions.
  B. Wash with soap and water.
  C. If the bite is swollen or inflamed, cover it with an ice pack or cool compress.
  D. If no systemic allergic reaction occurs, follow procedures for bee and wasp stings.
  E. Notify parents.

TICK BITES

Ticks can transmit bacteria that cause several diseases, including Lyme disease, which has been diagnosed in almost every state (see Chapter 4, Chronic Disease). Another disease is Rocky Mountain spotted fever, which occurs in temperate zones: symptoms include headache, fever, and muscle pain followed by a skin rash.

Ticks are small, brown, blood-sucking mites (arachnids) that are found in shrubs, grasses, vines, brush and heavily wooded areas. They attach themselves to humans and animals and adhere tenaciously to the skin or scalp. All parts of the tick must be removed. If mouth fragments or proboscis are left in the skin, local symptoms will develop. Evidence suggests that the longer the infected tick remains attached, the greater the chance of disease transmission.

I. Immediate First Aid
  A. Carefully and quickly remove the tick with fine-tipped tweezers or gloved fingers in one motion; grasp close to the skin, and be certain to remove all parts of the insect. Save tick for identification if possible to identify the likelihood of serious disease transmission; place in a container of alcohol to kill and preserve the tick.
  B. Gently scrub the bite area with soap and warm water to remove any bacteria present on the skin.
  C. Do not apply heat (lighted match or cigarette) to the tick's body or cover it with any type of oil, alcohol, or other such liquids. These methods may leave tick parts in the wound, injure the victim's skin, or cause complications.
  D. If the student must stay in school, and the tick cannot be removed, cover it with a dressing. The tick should be removed as soon as possible, because the risk of infection increases between 24 to 72 hours after the tick attaches to the skin.
  E. Observe for rash, headache, fever, and difficulty walking.

First Aid

CHAPTER 12

F. Notify parents and educate them regarding disease transmission, signs of infection, and necessity of contacting HCP.

II. Prevention

    A. Wear hat, long sleeves, and pants; tuck pants into socks or boots and tuck shirt into pants.

    B. Use insect repellent; DEET, an active ingredient in many repellents, is safe and most effective repellent when instructions are followed (EPA, 2007).

    C. Examine for ticks after possible exposure, checking limbs, scalp, nape of neck, under arms, around waist, and on clothing.

    D. Wear white or light-colored clothing.

BLEEDING

I. Immediate First Aid

    A. Put on gloves and use universal precautions. If gloves are unavailable, use other protective material and wash hands thoroughly as soon as possible.

    B. Place thick, sterile gauze pad directly over wound; if sterile material is not available, use cleanest cloth or material.

    C. If bleeding is severe and continuous, apply pressure directly over the wound until bleeding stops; elevate wound above victim's heart level if possible.

    D. Do not remove impaled object.

    E. Never remove initial dressing; if additional dressings are needed, place them over the old dressing; continue direct hand pressure even more firmly if bleeding persists.

    F. Monitor for signs and symptoms of shock.

    G. Activate EMS for severe bleeding or bleeding that does not stop with first aid.

    H. Notify parents of injury; recommendations to parents depend on the extent of injury (e.g., immediate care for suturing or observation for infection).

BLISTERS

I. Immediate First Aid

    A. Put on gloves and use universal precautions.

    B. If blister has not ruptured, and surrounding area is clean, apply only gauze dressing; do not attempt to open blister.

    C. If area is dirty, clean blister and surrounding area with soap and water, rinse, and apply sterile dressing.

    D. If blister is open, clean surrounding area with soap and water, rinse, and cover with dressing.

    E. Notify parents; discuss with parents if area is red, swollen, or painful.

BRUISES

I. Immediate First Aid

    A. If skin is broken, wear gloves and use universal precautions.

B. Immediately apply cold compresses or ice pack to reduce swelling and relieve pain, but do not apply directly to skin. Elevate bruised area if possible.

C. Notify parents if swelling or severe pain persists, especially if no known reason can be found; recommend referral to HCP.

BURNS

First-degree burns are superficial and cause the skin to turn red (e.g., sunburn, scalding). Such burns may cause pain, mild swelling, and may blanch with pressure; they are not a major medical problem, because they heal rapidly and affect only the epidermis. Individuals with severe sunburn should receive medical care as soon as possible.

Second-degree burns are deeper than first-degree burns and are more painful, cause swelling, and split or blister the skin layers. The skin is red or mottled and blanches with pressure. The skin also may appear wet because of the loss of plasma through the damaged layers of skin. Second-degree burns affect the epidermis and dermis.

Third-degree burns destroy all layers of the skin and extend into deeper tissues. They are painless because nerve endings have been destroyed. These burns appear white and charred, swollen but dry, and do not blanch with pressure.

Put on gloves for any burn situation and follow universal precautions. Do not use ice on burns, because it can cause frostbite.

I. Immediate First Aid

A. First degree, superficial burn:
   1. Remove rings, bracelets, or any constricting jewelry before swelling occurs.
   2. Place burned area under cold running water, or put cold compresses on the area; cover compresses before placing them on injured skin.
   3. Repeat step 2 until pain stops.
   4. Cover burn with sterile gauze or clean dressing.
   5. Do not apply any ointments.
   6. Notify parents.

B. Second-degree, partial-thickness burn:
   1. Remove rings, bracelets, or any constricting jewelry before swelling occurs.
   2. Run cool water over burned area, or put cold compresses on the area until pain subsides.
   3. Cover with sterile gauze or clean dressing.
   4. If arms or legs are burned, elevate them above victim's heart level.
   5. Do not apply ointments or attempt to break blisters or remove tissue.
   6. Notify parents and recommend referral to HCP.

C. Third-degree, full-thickness burn:
   1. Activate EMS and notify parents.
   2. Remove rings, bracelets, or any constricting jewelry before swelling occurs.
   3. Do not attempt to remove garments that are clinging to the area; cut around them.
   4. Do not apply cold water, cold compresses, or ointments.

5. Cover area with sterile gauze or clean cloth.
6. If legs or arms are burned, elevate them above victim's heart level if possible.
7. Keep student warm, calm, and reassured.
8. If necessary, treat student for shock or administer CPR.
9. Check immunization records for current tetanus vaccine.

CHEMICAL BURNS

Chemical burns in schools can occur in chemistry, shop, photography, or automobile classes.

I. Immediate First Aid
A. Activate EMS if signs of shock are noted; if second degree burn has occurred; or if chemical is in eye, on hand, face, feet, groin, buttocks, or over a major joint. Notify parents.
B. Wear gloves and use universal precautions.
C. If chemical is a powderlike substance, brush off prior to flushing.
D. Run cool water over the area for at least 20 minutes.
E. If possible, immediately remove all contaminated clothing and jewelry.
F. Cover or wrap burn area with dry, sterile dressing or clean cloth.
G. If chemical container is available, follow instructions for first aid and send container with EMS.

CHEMICAL BURNS OF THE EYE

Alkaline burns to the eye can be caused by drain cleaner, laundry and dishwasher detergent, or chemistry lab chemicals; an eye may appear only slightly injured but later may become deeply inflamed and develop tissue damage with possible loss of sight.

I. Immediate First Aid
A. Flush eye with tap water for 15 minutes. While flushing the eye, activate EMS and notify parents.
B. If person is lying down, turn head to side and pour water into eye from inner corner of eye outward; hold eye open and do not wash chemical toward the other eye.
C. Immobilize the eye by covering it with dry dressing.
D. If possible, cover both eyes.

DISLODGED CONTACT LENS

I. Immediate First Aid
A. Gently push on eyelid to manipulate lens into proper position.
B. If necessary, use eye irrigation solution or sterile saline solution to facilitate free movement of the lens.

DIABETES MELLITUS

A child with diabetes may face two serious emergencies: *insulin reaction (hypoglycemia)* or *diabetic coma (hyperglycemia)*. Insulin reaction has a *rapid* onset, usually within minutes or a few hours; diabetic coma (acidosis) develops *gradually* over a few hours or days. Insulin reaction is the usual school emergency because of the sudden onset of symptoms. The two conditions must be distinguished, because two separate procedures should be followed (see Chapter 4, Diabetes).

Insulin reaction is caused by too much insulin, not eating enough food, an unusual amount of exercise, or a delayed meal. Diabetic coma is caused by too little insulin, failure to follow the proper diet, infection, fever, or emotional stress. Symptoms vary with individual students; often students are very familiar with their own symptoms.

I. **Signs of Insulin Reaction: Hypoglycemia, Rapid Onset**
   A. Excessive sweating, paleness, or faintness.
   B. Headache.
   C. Hunger.
   D. Increased heart rate, trembling, blurry vision.
   E. Irritability, personality change, confusion.
   F. Poor coordination, slurred speech.
   G. Seizures.
   H. Inability to waken.

II. **Immediate First Aid for Insulin Reaction**
   A. Give quick sugar source: any food containing sugar, such as juice, non-diet soda, candy, glucose tablets or gel, or tube frosting. Follow with protein and complex carbohydrate source, such as cheese and crackers.
   B. Do not give student insulin.
   C. Give glucagon if student loses consciousness or is having a seizure; place on side, and do not give foods or fluids by mouth. Glucagon is given per individual student's ECP, standing orders, Nurse Practice Act, state educational requirements.
   D. Activate EMS as needed and call parents.

III. **Signs of Diabetic Coma: Hyperglycemia, Slow Onset**
   A. Increased thirst and urination.
   B. Abdominal pains, centralized aches.
   C. Nausea, vomiting, blurred vision.
   D. Weakness, fatigue.
   E. Large amount of sugar and ketones in urine when urine is tested.
   F. Sweet-smelling breath.
   G. Labored breathing, confusion, extreme weakness, unconsciousness.

IV. **Immediate First Aid for Diabetic Coma**
   A. Activate EMS as needed and notify parents.

EYE INJURY

I. **Immediate First Aid**
   A. When an eye sustains a *severe blow or perforating wound*, do not attempt to open eye; put eye pad on affected eye and notify parents for immediate care.
   B. If student is cooperative, patch both eyes to restrict eye movement.
   C. Do not apply pressure.
   D. Treat bruises immediately with cold applications.
   E. If mild injury, assess for double or blurred vision, pain, or bleeding.
   F. If loss of vision, pain, or bleeding occur, call parents for immediate care.

First Aid

CHAPTER 12

FOREIGN BODY IN EYE

I. Immediate First Aid
A. Flush eye several times with saline solution or lukewarm water. Tilt head so that water runs from inner to outer aspect of eye.
B. If flushing does not remove the foreign body, close eye and apply eye pad; notify parents and advise immediate medical care.
C. If student will tolerate it, patch both eyes to control eye movement.
D. Encourage student to refrain from rubbing eyes.
E. If punctured or protruding object can be seen in the eye, do not attempt to remove it; do not attempt to rinse, but call parents and activate EMS.

FAINTING

Fainting is loss of consciousness lasting only a few moments. Fainting may occur from a sudden drop in blood pressure from prolonged standing, drug or alcohol use, blood loss, poisoning, severe allergies, heat exhaustion or heat stroke, fatigue, cardiac arrhythmias, or diabetic reaction. Symptoms include paleness, clammy skin, weakness, dizziness, lightheadedness, irregular pulse, or abdominal discomfort. Lightheadedness generally improves when lying down.

I. Immediate First Aid
A. Have student lie on back; if no injuries, slightly elevate legs and loosen any tight or constricting clothing.
B. Check for patent airway and observe for vomiting.
C. Check signs of circulation, breathing, heart rate, and pulse; if necessary initiate CPR and activate EMS.
D. Notify parents.

SEVERE FALL

I. Immediate First Aid
A. Keep student lying down, warm, and quiet.
B. Do not move student if any of the following signs are present:
   1. Severe headache.
   2. Inability to move extremities.
   3. Inability to perceive touch in any extremity.
   4. Severe neck or back pain.
   5. Altered mental status.
C. If any of these signs are present, activate EMS and notify parents.

FLESH WOUNDS/LACERATIONS

Flesh wounds may be minor, major, or puncture wounds. Minor flesh wounds include minor cuts, scratches, abrasions, and rug burns. Puncture wounds can be serious because of the danger of infection and tetanus. With any flesh wound, *put on gloves and use universal precautions.*

I. **Immediate First Aid**
A. Minor wounds:
 1. Gently cleanse wound with mild soap solution using applicator, cotton ball, or gauze.
 2. Rinse wound well, let dry, and then apply sterile gauze dressing.
B. Major wounds:
 1. Stop bleeding by applying direct pressure to the wound (see Bleeding section) and protect wound from further contamination.
 2. Notify parents and advise immediate care; sutures may be required.
 3. *Punctures:* Let wound bleed freely for several seconds to wash wound, then wash area around wound with mild soap solution and rinse well.
 4. Flush wound with running water, let the wound dry, and cover it with sterile dressing.
 5. Notify parents and remind them that tetanus booster or antitoxin may be needed; encourage parents to discuss this with their primary care provider.
 6. Check school immunization record for date of last tetanus immunization: it is effective for 10 years.
 7. If wound is deep or dirty, tetanus shot should be administered by HCP; if last injection was more than 5 years prior, a tetanus booster may be needed within 48 hours.

FRACTURES

Simple fractures (unopened wounds) are more common than *compound fractures* (open wounds); an x-ray is needed for accurate diagnosis. The following signs indicate a possible fracture:
 1. Edema, swelling, pain.
 2. Discoloration.
 3. Tenderness to the touch; crepitus tissue.
 4. Deformity or shortening of the limb.
 5. Inability to bear weight or inability to move. Even if doubt exists as to the presence of a fracture, provide first-aid measures for fracture to prevent aggravation of existing injuries.

I. **Immediate First Aid**
A. Keep student quiet and treat for shock if indicated (see Shock, page 523).
B. Notify parents and activate EMS if needed.
C. If paramedics or ambulance can arrive within short time, do not attempt to move victim unless in danger of fire, drowning, or other immediate harm. Do not attempt to set fracture or push back protruding bone.
D. If paramedic or ambulance service is not available, and student must be moved, apply splint and then elevate limb slightly. If student is unconscious, always lift and move as though neck and spine were injured.
 1. Make emergency splints from newspapers, rolled blankets, pillows, sticks, or boards. Splints should extend beyond the joint at either end of the suspected fracture.

First Aid

CHAPTER 12

    2. Another immobilization method involves tying or taping the injured leg to the uninjured leg or securing an injured arm to the chest or side. When possible, place padding between the affected limbs and the body and immobilize joints above and below the suspected fracture.

    3. Always check pulses distal to an injury before and after splinting.

    4. Loosen ties or tape if swelling, cyanosis, or numbness occurs, or if student complains of tingling sensation or is unable to move toes or fingers.

    5. If someone with a suspected neck or spinal injury must be moved, use three or four persons to lift the victim with all moving in unison and providing rigid support. Place the injured person on a firm and level surface (e.g., backboard or other similar surface). Do not use a blanket for lifting and carrying, because such support is not adequately firm.

E. If neck or spine injury is suspected, do not allow the head to move.

F. For *compound fracture* (open fracture), use the following measures:

    1. Call EMS and notify parents.

    2. Wear gloves and use universal precautions.

    3. Control hemorrhage by applying pressure with sterile or clean dressing over wound.

    4. Do not wash or probe wound.

    5. If bone is protruding, cover wound with sterile or clean bandage, compress, or pads.

    6. Do not attempt to replace bone fragments.

HEADACHE

A headache may represent the onset of illness, stress, vision concerns, reaction to medication, head injury, exposure to toxins, classroom avoidance, or it may be idiopathic. The nurse should determine the onset, location, type of pain (e.g., sharp, dull, pulsating), duration, frequency (continuous or intermittent), time of day, and associated symptoms or factors. If fever or other symptoms are identified, contact parents. If child is known for chronic visits with the same symptoms, further investigation is needed. If headache is described as the "worst pain ever," is accompanied by behavioral changes, altered mental status, or a combination of these symptoms, activate EMS.

HEAD INJURY

I. Symptoms of Possible Head Injury
A. Excessive drowsiness.

B. Nausea or persistent vomiting.

C. Unequal pupils.

D. Slurred speech or loss of speech.

E. Severe headache or dizziness.

F. Double vision.

G. Seizures.

H. Unsteady gait or lack of coordination of both arms and legs.

I. Paresthesia (numbness, tingling).

J. Behavioral changes with or without altered mental status.

K. Confusion or amnesia.

II. Immediate First Aid

A. Keep student quiet and lying down in a darkened room. Conduct initial assessment, and activate EMS and call parents if any of the above symptoms are present.

B. Maintain in cervical spine stabilization. Log roll if needed to prevent aspiration of vomit or saliva.

C. Never position student so that head is lower than the rest of the body.

D. Do not give fluids by mouth.

E. Do not attempt to clean scalp wound, because cleaning may cause more bleeding or cerebral infection if a fracture is present.

F. Control bleeding with sterile dressing or bandage.

EPISTAXIS (NOSEBLEED)

I. Immediate First Aid

A. Put on gloves and use universal precautions.

B. Have student sit with head erect, leaning slightly forward if possible to avoid drainage of blood into airway or esophagus.

C. Assess for trauma; if head injury, refer to Head Injury section.

D. Apply firm but gentle pressure over bleeding nostril for at least 10 minutes.

E. Apply cold compresses to bridge of nose and back of neck; do not apply ice directly to skin.

F. If bleeding does not stop within about 15 minutes, notify parents and urge immediate care; advise student to avoid blowing or picking nose for 1 to 2 hours to prevent dislodging clot.

FOREIGN BODY IN NOSE

I. Immediate First Aid

A. Do not attempt to remove object from nostril.

B. Try to keep student from sniffing; advise to breathe through mouth until object can be removed.

C. May instruct blowing of nose while holding uninvolved nostril to dislodge the object.

D. Notify parents and refer for care.

HEAT CRAMPS

Heat cramps are caused by sodium depletion after prolonged or excessive exercise during periods of high temperature and low humidity.

I. Symptoms of Heat Cramps

A. Profuse sweating.

B. Severe muscle cramps.

C. Blood pressure and pulse are usually normal.

D. Normal or slightly elevated temperature.

E. May be alert and oriented.

II. Immediate First Aid

A. Provide fluids (e.g., drinks with electrolytes, sports drinks, clear juice, or water).
B. Have student do gentle stretching and massage affected muscles.
C. Rest in a cool place.
D. If cramps are not gone in one hour, contact parents and urge further care.

HEAT EXHAUSTION

Heat exhaustion is caused by heat exposure and excessive sweating without necessary fluid replacement. The student may have water and/or salt depletion. First-aid measures are directed toward removal from heat source and replenishment of fluids.

I. Symptoms of Heat Exhaustion

A. Normal body temperature, rapid pulse.
B. Pale and clammy skin.
C. Profuse perspiration.
D. Anxiety, tiredness, and weakness.
E. Headache.
F. Cramps and muscle spasms.
G. Nausea, dizziness, and fainting.

II. Immediate First Aid

A. Take student to a cool, shaded, and well-ventilated area.
B. Remove or loosen clothing as much as possible, and have student lie down with feet elevated.
C. Apply cool, wet cloths or spray with water; fan student, or remove student to air-conditioned room.
D. If student is conscious, give sips of water with no ice or give sports drinks containing electrolytes.
E. If student is nauseated or vomits, do not give fluids; if no response to first-aid measures, activate EMS and notify parents.

HEATSTROKE/SUNSTROKE

Heatstroke or sunstroke occurs when body systems are overwhelmed by heat and are unable to compensate. Heatstroke or sunstroke can be immediate and life threatening. First aid is directed toward cooling the body quickly.

I. Symptoms of Heatstroke/Sunstroke

A. High body temperature (104 degrees F or higher).
B. Hot, red, and dry skin.
C. No sweating.
D. Rapid and strong pulse; fast or shallow breathing.
E. Anorexia, nausea, and vomiting.
F. Headache and fatigue.
G. Confusion and disorientation.
H. Can progress to coma and seizures.

II. Immediate First Aid

A. Activate EMS and notify parents.

   B. Take student into shade or cool room indoors; sponge with cool water or wrap in wet, cold sheets or use ice packs.

SHOCK

Determine the cause of symptoms, because shock can be secondary to a sudden illness or injury.

I. Symptoms of Shock
   A. Weakness, lethargy.
   B. Moist, clammy, pale skin.
   C. Rapid and weak pulse.
   D. Increased rate of breathing, which may be shallow, labored, irregular, or a combination of these.
   E. Possible anxiety and disorientation that later may progress to unresponsiveness and loss of consciousness.

II. Immediate First Aid
   A. Activate EMS and notify parents.
   B. Elevate legs 12 inches or more, unless injury contradicts such a position (e.g., head, neck, or chest injury); if elevation is contraindicated, keep student lying flat and quiet and loosen tight clothing.
   C. Assess and monitor respiratory and cardiac functioning; initiate CPR if necessary.
   D. Maintain warmth with blanket; keep victim warm but not hot.
   E. Give nothing by mouth.

SPLINTERS

I. Immediate First Aid
   A. Put on gloves and use universal precautions. If splinter is large and deeply embedded, leave it alone and notify parents.
   B. If splinter is near surface and protruding, gently remove splinter with tweezers, and cleanse area thoroughly with mild soap solution.
   C. Apply light, sterile dressing to keep area clean.
   D. Check for current tetanus immunization.

SPRAINS AND STRAINS

A *sprain* is an injury to the muscle and ligaments, tendons, or soft tissues around a joint. A *strain* is an injury caused by a muscle being overstretched. Differentiation of a sprain from a closed fracture usually is impossible without radiography; treat the injury as a possible fracture (see Fracture section).

A *stress fracture* is a small crack or weak spot in a bone due to repeated overuse. This can be observed during intensive training for school sports, such as running or basketball. There may be continuous foot pain and tenderness but no visible swelling.

I. Symptoms of Sprain or Fracture
   A. Swelling.
   B. Tenderness.
   C. Pain with motion.

First Aid

CHAPTER 12

D. Discoloration; black and blue.

E. Pain from use of the injured area, such as when walking.

II. Immediate First Aid

A. If possible, elevate injured part and apply cold compresses or ice pack.

B. Always place thin towel or cloth between skin and application of any cold treatment.

C. Immobilize injured area to prevent further injury. Tie injured part to a stiff object or secure it to another part of the body; tie loosely. Use elastic wrap, splint, or sling to immobilize.

D. Notify parents immediately and encourage them to seek further care.

TOOTH INJURIES

I. Immediate First Aid

A. Put on gloves and use universal precautions.

B. Notify parents and urge immediate dental care.

C. If permanent tooth has been avulsed as a result of trauma, it probably can be saved, if it is kept moist and promptly replaced.

    1. Gently wash dirt and debris from tooth; avoid touching or disturbing the root. Do not use running water because it may damage the root.

    2. If possible, place tooth into its socket if no risk to student, such as swallowing the tooth.

D. If replacement is impossible, place tooth in student's or parent's mouth next to cheek, or place in milk or normal saline solution. Do not use tap water.

E. If tooth is transported in saline solution or milk, it must be reimplanted within 1 hour; if left dry, tooth must be implanted within 30 minutes. Special containers are available to transport avulsed teeth.

F. If a baby tooth is avulsed, child should be seen by a dentist to determine if a spacer is needed.

G. If more severe facial or head injury has occured, activate EMS and send the tooth with the child.

WEB SITES

American Academy of Pediatrics: Safety and First Aid
    http://www.aap.org/healthtopics/safety.cfm
American Red Cross
    http://www.redcross.org
Mayo Clinic
    http://www.mayoclinic.com

BIBLIOGRAPHY

California Emergency Medical Services Authority: *Emergency first aid guidelines for California schools,* 2004, Sacramento, Calif.

Centers for Disease Control and Prevention, National Center for Infectious Diseases: *Rabies,* (available online); http://www.cdc.gov/ncidod/dvrd/rabies/natural_history/nathist.htm. Accessed April 17, 2008.

Environmental Protection Agency: *The insect repellent DEET,* Update March 2007, (available online): http://www.epa.gov/opp00001/factsheets/chemicals/deet.htm. Accessed April 17, 2008.

Kemper DW, Healthwise Staff, Kaiser Physicians and Staff: *Kaiser Permanente Healthwise handbook: a self-care guide for you and your family,* 2004, Boise, Id., Healthwise.

Krause-Parello CA: Tooth avulsion in the school setting, *J School Nurs* 21(5):279-282, 2005.

Mosby's Dictionary of Medicine, Nursing, and Health, St Louis, 2006, Elsevier Mosby.

Nemours Foundation: Kids health (available online): http://kidshealth.org/parent/ firstaid_safe. Accessed Jan 15, 2007.

Schwab N, Gelfman M: *Legal issues in school health services: a resource for school administrators, school attorneys, school nurses,* Lincoln, Neb., 2005, Authors' Choice Press.

Tarr J, Ford N, Henry J: *First aid guidelines for school emergencies,* Richmond, 1998, Virginia Department of Health (available online): www.vahealth.org/schoolhealth/ documents/appendixb.pdf. Accessed Jan 15, 2007.

APPENDIX CONTENTS

APPENDIX B: GROWTH MEASUREMENTS (ANTHROPOMETRY), 556

Body Mass Index, **556**
Growth Charts

APPENDIX C: IMMUNIZATIONS, 576

RESOURCES USED FOR APPENDIX

Behrman RE, Kliegman RM, Jenson HB: *Nelson Textbook of Pediatrics,* ed 17, 2004, WB Saunders.
Freedman DS, Dietz WH, Srinivasan SR, Berenson GS: The relation of overweight to cardiovascular risk factors among children and adolescents: the Bogalusa Heart Study. *Pediatrics* 103:1175-1182, 1999.
Siberry GK, Iannone R: *The Harriet Lane handbook,* ed 15, St Louis, 2000, Mosby.

APPENDIX A

Assessment Tools

As a member of the multidisciplinary team, having knowledge about assessment tools used in the evaluation of students aids the nurse in communicating with other professionals and with parents. Although the nurse may not always use many of these assessment tools, they may be helpful to gain understanding and communication skills. The assessment tools are used not only with special education students but also prior to qualifying for special education classes and for some observation methods.

ACHENBACH SYSTEM OF EMPIRICALLY BASED ASSESSMENT (ASEBA)

I. **Use**
   A. Assessment: behavior rating, early childhood.
II. **Ages**
   A. 1½ to 5 years.
III. **Purpose**
   A. Assesses adaptive and maladaptive behavior.
IV. **Areas Assessed**
   A. Two checklists are available to assess behavior problems: Child Behavior Checklists (CBCL) and Caregiver-Teacher Report Form (C-TRF).
   B. Emotional disturbance and psychopathology through assessment, reporting, and documentation.
   C. Six cross-informant syndromes determined using both checklists: emotionally reactive, anxious/depressed, somatic complaints, withdrawn, attention problems, and aggressive behavior.
   D. Sleep Problems syndrome derived from CBCL.
   E. Internalizing, externalizing, and total problems scales scored from both forms.

Box A-1 *Tester Qualification Rating Scale*

A: Completed at least one course in measurement, guidance, or related discipline or has equivalent supervised experience in testing and interpretation.
B: Completed graduate training in measurement, guidance, individual psychological assessment, or special training for specific test.
C: Completed recognized graduate training program in psychology and supervised practical experience.

Modified from *Standards for educational and psychological testing,* published by the American Educational Research Association (AERA), the American Psychological Association, and the National Council on Measurement in Education (NCME), 1999.

V. Additional Information

A. Administration time is about 10 to 15 minutes. Assessment is via teacher, parent, or report; direct or indirect observation. Can be scored electronically, software is on CD-ROM; available in Spanish.

B. CBCL includes Language Development Survey (LDS) for identifying language delays. DSM-orientated scales provided in addition to empirically based scales. Other scales are available for children 6 to 18 years.

VI. Tester Qualification: B

ADAPTIVE BEHAVIOR ASSESSMENT SYSTEM, SECOND EDITION (ABAS-II)

I. Use

A. Measurement of adaptive skills.

II. Ages

A. Birth to adult.

III. Purpose

A. Assesses independent behaviors that an individual actually can do. The adaptive skill measured is designed to correspond to the guidelines for evaluation of adaptive behavior according to the American Association on Mental Retardation (AAMR) and the Diagnostic and Statistical Manual of Mental Disorders, Fourth Edition (DSM-IV).

B. Helps determine treatment and training goals.

IV. Areas Assessed

A. Communication, community use, functional preacademics, home living, health and safety, leisure, self-care, self-direction, social skills, and motor skills.

V. Additional Information

A. The teacher and parent complete the forms. Teacher day care form is for ages 2 to 5; teacher form is for ages 5 to 21; parent form is for birth to 5 and from 5 to 21 years.

   1. Both English and Spanish protocols are available.

   2. Assesses individuals with autism, mental retardation, ADHD, learning difficulties, or other impairments.

VI. Tester Qualification: B

ASSESSMENT, EVALUATION, PROGRESS, AND SYSTEMS, SECOND EDITION (AEPS-II)

I. Use

A. Assessment.

II. Ages

A. Volume 1: Administration guidelines.

B. Volume 2: Assessment, birth to 3 years and 3 to 6 years.

C. Volume 3: Curriculum, birth to 3 years.

D. Volume 4: Curriculum, 3 to 6 years.

III. Purpose

A. Assesses and evaluates child's abilities in familiar environments (home, small group, or center-based program).

IV. Areas Assessed

A. Six developmental domains: fine motor, gross motor, adaptive, cognitive, social–communication, and social.

V. Additional Information
A. Generates a comprehensive profile of abilities. Can be used to develop goals, objectives, or both for IFSPs or IEPs; monitors progress.

VI. Tester Qualification: B

BATTELLE DEVELOPMENTAL INVENTORY, SECOND EDITION (BDI-2)

I. Use
A. Assessment.

II. Ages
B. Birth to 8 years.

III. Purpose
A. Screens, diagnoses, and evaluates early development; can be used for eligibility, reevaluation, and instructional planning.
B. Provides two types of tools: full assessment and screening.
C. Facilitates multidisciplinary work by team administration for a comprehensive picture of the child's skill level.

IV. Areas Assessed
A. Includes adaptive, personal–social, communication, motor, and cognitive domains.

V. Additional Information
A. Administration time for complete tool is 1 to 2 hours; screening test takes 10 to 30 minutes.
B. BDI-2 examiners can use any personal digital assistant (PDA) with 8 MB to collect data. A software program is available for PC or Mac, and scale is norm referenced.

VI. Tester Qualification: B

BAYLEY SCALES OF INFANT AND TODDLER DEVELOPMENT, THIRD EDITION (BAYLEY-III)

I. Use
A. Assessment.

II. Ages
A. From 1 to 42 months.

III. Purpose
A. Evaluates developmental function including auditory perception, behavior, motor, and social development.
B. Monitor progress, program evaluation, and intervention outcomes.

IV. Areas Assessed
A. Core battery of five scales. Cognitive, motor, and language scales are completed by interacting with the child; social–emotional and adaptive behavior scales are conducted with a parent questionnaire.

V. Additional Information
A. Administration time is 30 to 90 minutes, depending on age group. Scales are ideal for use by multidisciplinary teams and involve parents and caregivers in assessment and program planning. Data are provided for special needs students, are norm referenced, and software is available.
B. Bayley III Screening Test growth scores and growth charts are available.

VI. Tester Qualification: B

BECK DEPRESSION INVENTORY, SECOND EDITION (BDI-II)

I. **Use**
   A. Screening and diagnosis of depression.

II. **Ages**
   A. From 13 to 80 years.

III. **Purpose**
   A. Measures severity of depression and monitors therapeutic progress.

IV. **Areas Assessed**
   A. Twenty-one items that assess the severity of depression.

V. **Additional Information**
   A. Items conform to DSM-IV TR criteria and can be administered in 5 to 10 minutes.
   B. The BDI-Fast Screen uses seven self-report items that reflect cognitive and affective symptoms. It provides a quick assessment of depression in those with biological, medical, or substance abuse issues or a combination of these problems. Test is standardized.

VI. Tester Qualification: B

BEHAVIOR ASSESSMENT SYSTEM FOR CHILDREN, SECOND EDITION (BASC-2)

I. **Use**
   A. Evaluation.

II. **Ages**
   A. From 2½ to 19 years.

III. **Purpose**
   A. Measures behavioral and personality aspects including adaptive, problematic, and attention-deficit/hyperactivity disorder (ADHD).

IV. **Areas Assessed**
   A. Consists of five dimensions: teacher, parenting, and self-rating scales, student observation system, and structured developmental history. Areas rated include externalizing (aggression, hyperactivity, conduct problems), internalizing (anxiety, depression, somatization), school problems (attention, learning), and adaptive skills (adaptability, leadership, social, study).

V. **Additional Information**
   A. Administration time is 10 to 45 minutes, depending on the scale. English and Spanish are available, and audio is available in English for those who have difficulty reading.

VI. Tester Qualification: C

BENDER VISUAL–MOTOR GESTALT TEST, SECOND EDITION

I. **Use**
   A. Assessment (neuropsychology).

II. **Ages**
   A. Age 3 years and older.

III. **Purpose**
   A. Measures perceptual motor skills; assesses visual motor function and identifies developmental problems, regression, and organic brain defects.

IV. Areas Assessed

A. Perceptual maturation and neurological impairment: nine stimulus cards are shown; the student is asked to draw the figures, one at a time, on a blank sheet of paper; assesses concepts of form, shape, pattern, and orientation in space.

V. Additional Information

A. Untimed, about 10 minutes for an individual. Administration time for a group takes about 15 to 25 minutes. A nonthreatening test, it is often used as an introductory test in a larger battery of instruments.

VI. Tester Qualification: B

BOEHM TEST OF BASIC CONCEPTS: PRESCHOOL, THIRD EDITION

I. Use

A. Assessment.

II. Ages

A. From 3 to 5.11 years.

III. Purpose

A. Identifies children who lack understanding of relational concepts to provide early intervention for school success (oral language).

IV. Areas Assessed

A. Measures 30 basic concepts.

V. Additional Information

A. Administration time is 20 to 30 minutes. Includes an observation and intervention planning tool and modifying and adapting directions for testing children with varied abilities. Test is norm referenced and standardized on a representative sample. It is available in Spanish.

VI. Tester Qualification: B

BOEHM TEST OF BASIC CONCEPTS, THIRD EDITION (BOEHM-3)

I. Use

A. Assessment.

II. Ages

A. Kindergarten through second grade.

III. Purpose

A. Identifies students at risk for learning difficulty and determines need for further testing (oral language).

IV. Areas Assessed

A. Measures 50 key concepts occurring in kindergarten, first, and second grades that are necessary for achievement during the first years of school. It identifies concepts students know and those they need to know.

V. Additional Information

A. Administration time is 30 to 45 minutes for a classroom group. Results of pretest and posttest demonstrate progress as a result of intervention or teaching. A Spanish version is available.

VI. Tester Qualification: B

BRIGANCE INVENTORY OF EARLY DEVELOPMENT II

I. Use

A. Assessment.

II. Ages
   A. Birth to 7 years.
III. Purpose
   A. Assesses important skills, concepts, and behavior; identifies at-risk infants and preschoolers; provides information for planning purposes, a simple progress report, and an optional record monitors class progress.
IV. Areas Assessed
   A. Assesses 11 skill areas: motor, self-help, speech/language, social, emotional, reading, math, writing, general knowledge, comprehension, and readiness.
V. Additional Information
   A. Administration time is 10 to 15 minutes and is available for three age levels: pre-kindergarten, kindergarten, and grade 1. Easily administered by aides, volunteers, or tutors. These screening tools identify children who need immediate referral; evaluations are norm referenced and have scoring software.
VI. Tester Qualification: A

BRIGANCE COMPREHENSIVE INVENTORY OF BASIC SKILLS, REVISED (CIBS-R)
I. Use
   A. Assessment.
II. Ages
   A. Pre-kindergarten to grade 9.
III. Purpose
   A. Identifies specific areas of need that can be used for intervention, program planning, and IEP development.
IV. Areas Assessed
   A. Consists of 154 assessments of readiness, speech, listening, and research and study skills; assessments of spelling, writing, reading, and math can be chosen by the teacher according to student's individual needs.
V. Additional Information
   A. Can monitor progress of specific skills and has specific instructions to develop IEP goals and objectives. Options are included for group testing, and normed and standardized data are available.
VI. Tester Qualification: B

BRUININKS-OSERETSKY TEST OF MOTOR PROFICIENCY, SECOND EDITION (BOT-2)
I. Use
   A. Assessment.
II. Ages
   A. From 4 to 21 years.
III. Purpose
   A. Measures fine and gross motor skills.
IV. Areas Assessed
   A. Eight subtests include running speed and agility, balance, bilateral coordination, strength, upper limb coordination, fine motor precision, fine motor integration, and manual dexterity.

V. Additional Information

A. Administration time is 15 to 20 minutes for the short form and 45 to 60 minutes for the complete battery of tests. The test is used to develop and evaluate motor training programs.

VI. Tester Qualification: B

CAREY TEMPERAMENT SCALES

I. Use

A. Screening.

II. Ages

A. From 1 month to 12 years.

III. Purpose

A. Increases awareness of strengths and needs of a child; provides understanding of the child's behavioral style to clinicians and assesses the impact of the child's temperament on parents and caregivers.

IV. Areas Assessed

A. Addresses nine categories of behavior styles: activity level, rhythmicity, approach–withdrawal, adaptability, persistence–attention span, intensity of reaction, distractibility, threshold of responsiveness, and quality of mood.

V. Additional Information

A. Administration time is 20 minutes, scoring takes 15 minutes for hand scoring and 4 minutes for computer scoring. Forms are completed by a parent or caregiver that have a six-point rating scale to score questions regarding the infant or child's recent and current behavior.

VI. Tester Qualification: B

CHILDHOOD AUTISM RATING SCALE (CARS)

I. Use

A. Assessment.

II. Ages

A. From 2 years.

III. Purpose

A. Identifies and classifies children with autism.

IV. Areas Assessed

A. Fifteen items measure student's responses to various activities and situations in relation to people, imitation, emotional response, and body use.

V. Additional Information

A. Administration time is 5 to 10 minutes. A score is obtained using a seven-point scale to indicate the amount of variance from the norm on each item. The total score from all 15 items is computed and determines the presence and severity of autism.

VI. Tester Qualification: A

CHILDREN'S DEPRESSION INVENTORY (CDI)

I. Use

A. Assessment.

II. Ages

A. From 6 to 17 years.

III. Purpose
A. Provides self-reported key symptoms of depression, such as a child's feelings of worthlessness and loss of interest in activities; supports treatment planning and diagnosis.

IV. Areas Assessed
A. Assessment consists of seven scales and five-factor scores: negative mood, interpersonal difficulties, negative self-esteem, ineffectiveness, and anhedonia.
B. There are 27 items, each of which consists of three statements. The child is asked to select the statement for each item that best describes their feelings for the past two weeks. There is a total score and individual scale scores.

V. Additional Information
A. Administration time is 10 to 15 minutes, and the test takes about 10 minutes to score. There is a ten-item form that takes less time to administer; the reading level is first grade.
B. Test is norm referenced. The manual documents concurrent validity research, factor structure, test–retest, and internal consistency coefficients.

VI. Tester Qualification: B

CHILDREN'S MEMORY SCALE (CMS)

I. Use
A. Assessment.

II. Ages
A. From 5 to 16 years.

III. Purpose
A. Provides assessment of memory and learning as related directly to IQ.

IV. Areas Assessed
A. Six subtests include the following dimensions:
1. Verbal learning and memory.
2. Visual learning and memory.
3. Attention/concentration and working memory.
4. General or overall memory.
5. Immediate versus delayed memory.
6. Recall versus recognition.

V. Additional Information
A. Administration time for scoring is 20 minutes with a 30-minute delay, followed by 10 to 15 minutes for testing long-delayed memory. Memory and learning are compared with ability, achievement, and attention. Separate records are used for ages 5 to 8 and 9 to 16 years. The scale is standardized and normed on a U.S. representative sample.

VI. Tester Qualification: C

CLINICAL EVALUATION OF LANGUAGE FUNDAMENTALS: PRESCHOOL, SECOND EDITION (CELF PRESCHOOL-2)

I. Use
A. Assessment.

II. Ages
A. From 3 to 6 years.

III. Purpose
    A. Identify, diagnose, and follow-up on language deficits.
IV. Areas Assessed
    A. Language skills that include word meaning, word structure, sentence structure, expressive vocabulary, concepts, following directions, recall, basic concepts, word classes, and phonological awareness.
V. Additional Information
    A. Administration time is 15 to 20 minutes. This standardized test provides norm-referenced data, a four-level process model, and a scoring assistant is available.
VI. Tester Qualification: B

CLINICAL EVALUATION OF LANGUAGE FUNDAMENTALS, FOURTH EDITION (CELF-4)

I. Use
    A. Diagnostic and intervention planning.
II. Ages
    A. From 5 to 21 years.
III. Purpose
    A. Provides language age and percentiles for processing and production.
IV. Areas Assessed
    A. Level 1: Core Language score determines if a disorder exists and student qualifies for services.
    B. Level 2: Receptive and expressive language, language structure and content, working memory index scores, and direction.
    C. Level 3: Phonological awareness, rapid automatic naming, number repetition, familiar sequences, word associations, and working memory index.
    D. Level 4: Optional rating scale and pragmatics profile.
V. Additional Information
    A. Administration time is 30 to 60 minutes. The test is standardized and criterion referenced. It is sensitive to language difficulties of children with mental retardation or autism, and a Spanish version is available.
VI. Tester Qualification: B

COLUMBIA MENTAL MATURITY SCALE (CMMS)

I. Use
    A. Assessment.
II. Ages
    A. 3 years 6 months to 9 years 11 months.
III. Purpose
    A. Assesses general reasoning ability.
IV. Areas Assessed
    A. Assesses two categories: discrimination and classification.
V. Additional Information
    A. Administration time is 15 to 20 minutes; test is nonverbal and the student responds by pointing to figures on large cards. The test is useful for assessing students with severe developmental disabilities, particularly those with physical handicaps such as cerebral palsy.

VI. **Tester Qualification: C**

CONNER'S RATING SCALES, REVISED (CRS-R)

I. **Use**
   A. Assessment of ADHD.
II. **Ages**
   A. Parents and teachers of children and adolescents ages 3 to 17 and adolescent self-report for ages 12 to 17.
III. **Purpose**
   A. Helps assess ADHD and evaluates problem behavior in children and adolescents.
IV. **Areas Assessed**
   A. There are three versions: parent, teacher, and adolescent self-report. All have a short and long form.
   B. Scales include oppositional, cognitive problems/inattention, hyperactivity, anxious/shy, perfectionism, social problems, psychosomatic, Conner's global index, DSM-IV symptom subscales, and ADHD Index.
V. **Additional Information**
   A. Administration time for long version is 15 to 20 minutes; short version is 5 to 10 minutes. Reading level sixth to ninth grade and varies with each version. Standardized data are available.
VI. **Tester Qualification: B**

DENVER DEVELOPMENTAL SCREENING TOOL II (DDST-II)

I. **Use**
   A. Screening.
II. **Ages**
   A. Birth to 6 years.
III. **Purpose**
   A. Detects infants and children with social, motor, or language delays.
IV. **Areas Assessed**
   A. Assesses 125 items in the areas of personal–social, fine motor/adaptive, language, and gross motor development.
V. **Additional Information**
   A. Administration time is 15 to 20 minutes; test is nonverbal.
VI. **Tester Qualification: B**

DETROIT TESTS OF LEARNING APTITUDE, FOURTH EDITION (DTLA-4)

I. **Use**
   A. Assessment.
II. **Ages**
   A. From 6 to 17 years.
III. **Purpose**
   A. Isolates intraindividual strengths and weaknesses; identifies students with general deficiency or specific aptitude; measures intelligence and discrete ability areas.
IV. **Areas Assessed**
   A. Assesses linguistic, cognitive, attention, motor, and visual perception.

V. Additional Information

A. Administration time is 40 minutes to 2 hours and is useful for identifying learning disabilities and mental retardation. It produces a detailed profile of the student's abilities and deficiencies, and it is norm referenced. Cultural, gender, and racial bias have been minimized.

VI. Tester Qualification: B

DEVELOPMENTAL TEST OF VISUAL–MOTOR INTEGRATION, FIFTH EDITION (BEERY–BUKTENICA)

I. Use

A. Assessment.

II. Ages

A. Short form: 2 to 8 years; full form: 2 to 18 years.

III. Purpose

A. Assesses the integration of visual and motor skills and identifies problems that lead to future learning and behavior problems.

IV. Areas Assessed

A. Visual perception and motor coordination.

V. Additional Information

A. Administration time to individuals or a group is 10 to 15 minutes. Visual perception and motor coordination tests take 5 minutes each. The test is a developmental sequence of geometric forms that are copied with paper and pencil. It is norm referenced and standardized.

VI. Test Qualification: B

DRAW-A-PERSON TEST: SCREENING PROCEDURE FOR EMOTIONAL DISTURBANCE (DAP: SPED)

I. Use

A. Screening.

II. Ages

A. From 6 to 17 years.

III. Purpose

A. Assesses intellectual maturity and screens for emotional/behavioral disorders based on three drawings: a man, a woman, and the person taking the test.

IV. Areas Assessed

A. Fifty-five items are scored using 14 different criteria; areas are ability to perceive, abstract, and generalize.

V. Additional Information

A. Administration time is 15 to 20 minutes; test is standardized, provides an IQ score, and yields a standardized score; may be done individually or in groups.

B. DAP: Quantitative Scoring System (DAP: QSS) is a screening test measuring intellectual ability through figure drawing.

VI. Tester Qualification: B

GILLIAM ASPERGER'S DISORDER SCALE (GADS)

I. Use

A. Assessment.

II. Ages
A. From 3 to 22 years.

III. Purpose
A. Identifies children with Asperger's and distinguishes it from autism
B. Sets behavioral goals and documents behavioral progress.

IV. Areas Assessed
A. Assesses 32 items divided into four subscales that describe measurable behaviors.
B. Parents complete eight additional items related to first 3 years of life.

V. Additional Information
A. Administration time is 5 to10 minutes and must be completed by someone who knows the child well. A table is provided to help determine the likelihood of Asperger's disorder, and the assessment is norm referenced.

VI. Tester Qualification: B

GILLIAM AUTISM RATING SCALE, SECOND EDITION (GARS-2)

I. Use
A. Assessment.

II. Ages
A. From 3 to 22 years.

III. Purpose
A. Identifies individuals with autism and estimates the severity of the disorder.
B. Discriminates from other disorders, such as mental retardation and cognitive-delayed children.

IV. Areas Assessed
A. Three subscales include stereotyped behaviors, communication, and social interactions; there are 43 items divided into these subscales.

V. Additional Information
A. Administration time is 5 to 10 minutes and test is norm referenced. A separate booklet is available to develop goals and objectives.

VI. Tester Qualification: B

GRAY ORAL READING TEST, FOURTH EDITION (GORT-4)

I. Use
A. Assessment.

II. Ages
A. 6 through 18.11 years.

III. Purpose
A. Identifies oral reading proficiency, diagnoses specific reading strengths and weaknesses, and documents progress.

IV. Areas Assessed
A. Five scores are derived from assessment in three areas: reading rate, accuracy, and comprehension. The scores include reading rate, accuracy, fluency, comprehension, and overall reading ability.

V. Additional Information
A. Administration time is 20 to 30 minutes, and research is available.

VI. Tester Qualification: B

HAWAII EARLY LEARNING PROFILE (HELP)

I. Use
   A. Assessment and intervention.

II. Ages
   A. Birth to 3 years and 3 to 6 years.

III. Purpose
   A. Assesses, identifies areas of need, monitors progress, and provides sequential developmental activities.

IV. Areas Assessed
   A. Six areas are included: cognitive, language, gross and fine motor, social, and self-help.

V. Additional Information
   A. Administration time for initial assessment is 45 to 90 minutes but may be done in 15 to 20 minutes. Time to administer depends on the number of areas assessed and the age and behavior of the child.
   B. Best Beginnings: Helping Parents Make a Difference is a HELP assessment that provides anticipatory guidance for caregivers of children from birth to 3 years of age.

VI. Tester Qualification: B

HODSON ASSESSMENT OF PHONOLOGICAL PATTERNS, THIRD EDITION (HAPP-3)

I. Use
   A. Assessment.

II. Ages
   A. From 2 years and up.

III. Purpose
   A. Assesses children with unintelligible speech.

IV. Areas Assessed
   A. Speech sounds and phonological processes.

V. Additional Information
   A. Administration time is 15 to 20 minutes, and screening forms take about 5 minutes; test is norm and criterion referenced.

VI. Tester Qualification: B

HOME, EDUCATION, ACTIVITIES, DRUGS, SEX, SUICIDE (HEADSS FOR ADOLESCENTS)

I. Use
   A. Interview instrument.

II. Ages
   A. Adolescents at risk.

III. Purpose
   A. Provides information regarding adolescent psychosocial development; facilitates communication.

IV. Areas Assessed
   A. Seven areas assessed make the acronym: *h*ome, *e*ducation/vocation, *a*ctivities, *d*rugs, *s*exuality/identity, *s*uicide/depression.

V. Additional Information

A. Technique may take more than one meeting to complete, because it is a comprehensive interview format; open, accepting attitude is critical.

VI. Tester Qualification: B

HOME OBSERVATION FOR MEASUREMENT OF THE ENVIRONMENT (HOME)

I. Use

A. Assessment, parental guidance, and intervention.

II. Ages

A. From birth to 6 years.

III. Purpose

A. Samples the quantity and quality of certain social, emotional, and cognitive supports available to the child within the home; assesses person-to-person and person-to-object interactions that make up the infant or child's learning environment.

IV. Areas Assessed

A. Six subscales, birth to 3 years: parental responsiveness, acceptance of child, organization of environment, learning materials, parental involvement, and variety in experience.

B. Eight subscales, 3 to 6 years: learning materials, language stimulation, physical environment, parental responsiveness, learning stimulation, modeling of social maturity, variety in experience, and acceptance of child.

V. Additional Information

A. Administration time is 45 to 90 minutes. There are now scales for middle childhood (6 to 10 years) and early adolescence (10 to 15 years).

VI. Tester Qualification: B

HOUSE-TREE-PERSON (H-T-P) PROJECTIVE DRAWING TECHNIQUE

I. Use

A. Assessment, psychodiagnostic.

II. Ages

A. From 3 years and up.

III. Purpose

A. Assesses personality in individuals who are culturally different, educationally deprived, developmentally disabled, or non-English speaking.

IV. Areas Assessed

A. Three drawings are produced: a house, a tree, and a person. Individual is then asked to describe, define, and interpret these drawings.

B. This can be the first in a battery of psychodiagnostic tests.

V. Additional Information

A. Drawings can reduce tension in testing situation. The test is nonthreatening, fast, easy to use, and yields abundant information.

VI. Tester Qualification: B

KAUFMAN ASSESSMENT BATTERY FOR CHILDREN, SECOND EDITION (KABC-2)

I. Use

A. Assessment.

II. Ages

A. From 3 to 18 years.

III. Purpose

A. Establishes cognitive levels, an understanding of the individual's style of solving problems, and thought processes; measures intelligence separately from achievement.

IV. Areas Assessed

A. Twenty subtests are contained in five scales: sequential processing, simultaneous processing, planning, learning, and knowledge.

V. Additional Information

A. Administration time is 25 to 70 minutes, depending on tests used; test is standardized and designed with little cultural content, and one model excludes verbal ability.

VI. Tester Qualification: C

KAUFMAN BRIEF INTELLIGENCE TEST, SECOND EDITION (KBIT-2)

I. Use

A. Assessment.

II. Ages

A. From 4 years and up.

III. Purpose

A. Assesses both verbal and nonverbal intelligence.

IV. Areas Assessed

A. Verbal knowledge and riddles: both assess crystallized ability (knowledge of words and their meanings). Items cover both receptive and expressive vocabulary and do not require reading or spelling.

B. Nonverbal scale includes a matrix subtest that assesses fluid thinking and the ability to solve new problems by perceiving relationships and completing analogies. Items contain pictures and abstract designs rather than words.

V. Additional Information

A. Administration time is about 20 minutes, and test is easy to use.

B. Yields verbal and nonverbal scores and a composite IQ. Items are free of gender and cultural bias and are research based.

VI. Tester Qualification: B

KAUFMAN TEST OF EDUCATIONAL ACHIEVEMENT, SECOND EDITION (KTEA-II)

I. Use

A. Assessment.

II. Ages

A. Ages 4 through school age; comprehensive form or brief form.

III. Purpose

A. Assesses key academic skills in reading, math, written language, and oral language.

IV. Areas Assessed

A. Six subtests and composites: reading composite, reading-related subtests, math composite, written language composite, oral language composite, and comprehensive achievement composite.

V. Additional Information

A. Administration times:

1. Comprehensive form: Pre-K to K takes 30 minutes.
2. Grades 1 and 2 take 50 minutes.
3. Grades 3 and up take 80 minutes.

B. Provides a comprehensive achievement composite.

C. Grade-based standard scores (M=100, SD-15); age and grade equivalents, percentile ranks, and normal curve equivalents.

VI. Tester Qualification: B

KEYMATH R/NU—REVISED, NORMATIVE UPDATE

I. Use

A. Assessment.

II. Ages

A. Kindergarten through grade 12.

III. Purpose

A. Assesses mathematical skills.

IV. Areas Assessed

A. Thirteen subtests in three areas: basic concepts, operations, and applications.

V. Additional Information

A. Administration time is 35 to 50 minutes and does not require reading ability. The test can be used for program planning and evaluation, and software is available. Pretest and posttest forms are available, and test is norm referenced.

VI. Tester Qualification: B

LEITER INTERNATIONAL PERFORMANCE SCALE, REVISED (LEITER-R)

I. Use

A. Screening and assessment.

II. Ages

A. From 2 to 21 years.

III. Purpose

A. Test measures fluid intelligence (i.e., intelligence that is not significantly influenced by child's educational, social, and family experience) and provides composite IQ score and scores in each of the 20 subsets and numerous composites. It also measures visualization, reasoning, attention, and memory.

IV. Areas Assessed

A. Five subsets: IQ screening assessment, learning disability LD/ADHD screening assessment, gifted screening assessment, reasoning and visual battery, and memory and attention battery.

V. Additional Information

A. Administration time is 25 to 40 minutes. This nonverbal, standardized test is suitable for persons with speech, hearing, or motor impairments; those who are deaf or cognitively delayed; those with ADHD or autism; those who are disadvantaged, non–English-speaking, who use English as a second language, or who have sustained traumatic brain injury. The test can be used to determine whether low academic achievement is a result of low IQ or due to a specific neuropsychological cause, such as ADHD.

VI. Tester Qualification: B

McCARTHY SCALES OF CHILDREN'S ABILITIES (MSCA)

  I. Use
    A. Assessment.
  II. Ages
    A. 2.6 to 8.6 years.
  III. Purpose
    A. Evaluates general intelligence level and strengths and weaknesses in several ability areas.
  IV. Areas Assessed
    A. Eighteen separate tests and six scales are evaluated: verbal, perceptual performance, quantitative, memory, motor, and general cognitive.
  V. Additional Information
    A. Administration time is 45 minutes to test children younger than age 5 and 60 minutes with older children. May identify gifted children.
  VI. Tester Qualification: C

MODIFIED CHECKLIST FOR AUTISM IN TODDLERS (M-CHAT)

  I. Use
    A. Screening.
  II. Ages
    A. From 18 to 24 months.
  III. Purpose
    A. Early detection for autism.
  IV. Areas Assessed
    A. Contains 23 yes-or-no items with focus on communications and social relatedness.
  V. Additional Information
    A. Yes-and-no items list is completed by a parent or caregiver. Not all children who fail checklist meet the criteria for an autism spectrum disorder but should be further evaluated by a specialist.
  VI. Tester Qualification: A

MULLEN SCALES OF EARLY LEARNING

  I. Use
    A. Assessment.
  II. Ages
    A. Birth to 5.8 years.
  III. Purpose
    A. Assesses language, motor, and perceptual abilities and school readiness.
    B. Provides a baseline for a continuum of teaching methods and a foundation for interventions.
  IV. Areas Assessed
    A. Five scales: gross motor, visual reception, fine motor, expressive language, and receptive language.
  V. Additional Information
    A. Administration time is 15 to 60 minutes, depending on student's age. The test is standardized. Software is available for scoring and easy interpretation, and it includes developmental learning activities.

VI. Tester Qualification: B

NURSING CHILD ASSESSMENT SATELLITE TRAINING (NCAST)

I. Use
A. Assessment.

II. Ages
A. Feeding scale: birth to 1 year; teaching scale: birth to 3 years.

III. Purpose
A. Measures caregiver–child interaction during feeding and teaching situations; the scales are designed to assess problems in interaction and communication.

IV. Areas Assessed
A. Two scales: feeding and teaching, with six constructs:
  1. Four of the constructs—sensitivity to cues, response to distress, socioemotional growth fostering, and cognitive growth fostering—pertain to the caregiver.
  2. Two constructs—clarity of cues and responsiveness to the caregiver—pertain to the child.

V. Additional Information
A. Administration time depends on the age of the child and the instrument used. The tests can be administered together or separately.
B. Significant changes were made in 1994. Both scales have strong internal consistency and test–retest reliability for the caregiver and child total scores. The caregiver scores have predictive validity for later child cognitive scores; thus the tools can be used to promote early brain development. Positive quality interactions during early childhood promote development of intellectual and language capabilities and bonding with major caregivers.
C. The Nursing Child Assessment Sleep/Activity (NCASA) can be self-taught. This scale establishes methods to help caregivers record the activities of a child on a 24-hour/7-day form. The child's sleep pattern can then be evaluated. The Sleep Activity Manual explains interpretation of the record.

VI. Tester Qualification: B

PEABODY INDIVIDUAL ACHIEVEMENT TEST, REVISED/NORMATIVE UPDATE (PIAT-R/NU)

I. Use
A. Assessment and instructional planning.

II. Ages
A. From 5 to 22 years.

III. Purpose
A. Provides an overview of the student's individual scholastic achievement and identifies possible areas of weakness and learning disabilities.

IV. Areas Assessed
A. Six subtests include general information, reading recognition, reading comprehension, written expression, math, and spelling.

V. Additional Information
A. Administration time is 60 minutes. The revised version includes normative update. Software is available for scoring and comparison, and the test is norm referenced.

VI. **Tester Qualification: B**

PEABODY PICTURE VOCABULARY TEST, THIRD EDITION (PPVT-III)

I. **Use**
   A. Screening.

II. **Ages**
   A. 2.6 years and older.

III. **Purpose**
   A. Measures receptive vocabulary and screens verbal ability for standard American English.

IV. **Areas Assessed**
   A. Assesses auditory receptive language skills.

V. **Additional Information**
   A. Administration time is about 10 to 15 minutes. The test is useful as a pretest and posttest measurement for knowledge of simple words. Can be an initial screening device for bright, low-ability, and language-impaired students. Software is available, and test is norm referenced.

VI. **Tester Qualification: B**

PEDIATRIC SYMPTOM CHECKLIST (PSC)

I. **Use**
   A. Screening.

II. **Ages**
   A. From 4 to18 years.

III. **Purpose**
   A. Measures psychosocial dysfunction.

IV. **Areas Assessed**
   A. Three subscales: attention, internalizing, and externalizing.

V. **Additional Information**
   A. Two versions are available: Parent Completed Version for ages up to 11; Youth Self-Report for ages 11 and up.
   B. Attention subscale identifies ADHD; internalizing subscale screens for depression and anxiety; externalizing subscale screens for conduct disorder, oppositional disorder, rage disorder, and so on. It is a checklist that can be completed by parents, day care providers, or school staff. It is available in different languages.

VI. **Tester Qualification: A**

QUICK NEUROLOGICAL SCREENING TEST - II (QNST-II)

I. **Use**
   A. Screening.

II. **Ages**
   A. From 5 years through 18 years.

III. **Purpose**
   A. Assesses neurological integration as it relates to learning and identifies those with learning disabilities.

IV. **Areas Assessed**
   A. Motor development, skill in controlling large and small muscles, motor planning and sequencing, sense of rate and rhythm, spatial organization, visual perceptual skills, balance and cerebellovestibular functions, and attention disorders.

V. Additional Information
A. Administration and scoring take about 20 to 30 minutes. Does not label student as neurologically impaired; does not diagnose brain damage or dysfunction. Test includes latest research findings concerning the "soft" neurological signs associated with learning problems.

VI. Tester Qualification: B

RECEPTIVE–EXPRESSIVE EMERGENT LANGUAGE, THIRD EDITION (REEL-3)

I. Use
A. Assessment.

II. Ages
A. From birth through 3 years.

III. Purpose
A. Measures development in both receptive and expressive language.

IV. Areas Assessed
A. Two core subtests: expressive and receptive language.

V. Additional Information
A. Administration time is 20 minutes, and test provides information from child's caregiver. The manual offers interpretation information and reliability and validity data, and the test is norm referenced.

VI. Tester Qualification: B

SENSORY PROFILE

I. Use
A. Assessment.

II. Ages
A. From 3 to 10 years.

III. Purpose
A. Measures sensory processing abilities as they relate to functional performance.

IV. Areas Assessed
A. Long version comprises 125 items and short version comprises 38 items. Three areas are included: sensory process modulation, behavioral, and emotional responses. Nine factors are considered: sensory seeking, emotional reactivity, low endurance/tone, oral-sensory sensitivity, inattention/distractibility, poor registration, sensory sensitivity, sedentary, and fine motor perceptual skills.

V. Additional Information
A. Used in combination with other tests, because it is judgment based. Results can facilitate diagnosis and intervention planning. Sensory profile supplement is available to target effective intervention.

VI. Tester Qualification: A

STANFORD–BINET INTELLIGENCE SCALE, FIFTH EDITION (SB5)

I. Use
A. Assessment.

II. Ages
A. From 2 years to adult.

III. Purpose
  A. Assesses general mental ability, and the revised edition provides multiple IQ scores rather than a single IQ score.

IV. Areas Assessed
  A. Five factors of cognitive ability: fluid reasoning, knowledge, qualitative processing, visual–spatial processing, and working memory.

V. Additional Information
  A. Administration time is 5 minutes per subtest; there are 10 subtests. This is a highly standardized and reliable tool for measuring a child's intelligence. Scoring software is available.
  B. There is an Early Stanford-Binet, Fifth Edition (Early SB5) that is available for children to age 7.

VI. Tester Qualification: C

TEENSCREEN PROGRAM, COLUMBIA UNIVERSITY

I. Use
  A. Screening.

II. Ages
  A. From 11 through 18 years.

III. Purpose
  A. Identifies mental health issues and suicide risk.

IV. Areas Assessed
  A. Three screening instruments: Columbia Health Screen (CHS) for suicide risk; Diagnostic Predictive Scales (DPS) for anxiety, depression, and substance abuse; Columbia Depression Scale (CDS) for depression. When results are positive, an interview follows.

V. Additional Information
  A. Administration time for screening questionnaires is 10 minutes; interview is 20 to 30 minutes, and computers can be used to complete forms. Teachers and administrators cannot be involved with the program except for introduction and release from class for screening. The school nurse, psychologist, or counselor can be involved. Use is only by parent or caregiver permission.
  B. Training is offered free of charge through Columbia University; consultation, training, testing materials, and technical assistance are provided. Local school district must provide mental health professionals for interviews and follow-up. For information call 888-833-6727.
  C. Other screenings include Children's Depression Inventory (CDI) for ages 7 to 17; Suicidal Ideation Questionnaire, for grades 10 through 12. Assessment of Suicidal Risk in Children and Adolescents is a Web site that lists screening tools for suicidal risk and depression at http://www1.endingsuicide.com/TopicReq?id=1919.

VI. Tester Qualification: B

TEST OF ADOLESCENT AND ADULT LANGUAGE, THIRD EDITION (TOAL-3)

I. Use
  A. Evaluation.

II. Ages
  A. From 12 to 25 years.

III. Purpose
   A. Identifies students who may need intervention to improve language proficiency; determines language strengths and weaknesses; documents progress resulting from special intervention programs.
IV. Areas Assessed
   A. Ten subtests measure listening, speaking, reading, writing, spoken and written language, vocabulary, grammar, and receptive and expressive language skills.
V. Additional Information
   A. Administration time is about 40 to 60 minutes and may be administered individually or in groups. Internal consistency, test–retest, and reliability scores have been investigated.
VI. Tester Qualification: B

TEST OF EARLY READING ABILITY, THIRD EDITION (TERA-3)

I. Use
   A. Assessment.
II. Ages
   A. From 3 to 8 years.
III. Purpose
   A. Identifies children with reading problems and determines children's progress in learning to read.
IV. Areas Assessed
   A. Construction of meaning, knowledge about the alphabet, and conventions of written language.
V. Additional Information
   A. Administration time is 30 minutes. Standardized on a national level with norms available.
VI. Tester Qualification: B

TEST OF WRITTEN LANGUAGE, THIRD EDITION (TOWL-3)

I. Use
   A. Assessment.
II. Ages
   A. From 7½ to 18 years.
III. Purpose
   A. Identifies students who have difficulty in written expression and pinpoints specific areas of deficit.
IV. Areas Assessed
   A. Thematic, vocabulary, handwriting, spelling, word usage, and style.
V. Additional Information
   A. Administration time is 90 minutes Two equivalent forms are provided to administer the test individually or in small groups.
VI. Tester Qualification: B

THEMATIC APPERCEPTION TEST, CHILDREN AND ADULTS (TAT)

I. Use
   A. Assessment.
II. Ages
   A. Children and adults.

III. Purpose
A. Assesses presence of psychological needs by revealing emotions, sentiments, dominant drives, traits, and conflicts of a personality.

IV. Areas Assessed
A. Emotional and behavioral characteristics; a series of 31 pictures (with specific subtests recommended for male and female children and adults) is presented, and the student is asked to tell stories about the pictures.

V. Additional Information
A. Administration time can be as little as 15 minutes, depending on the version used. Nonstandardized and untimed but popular in school systems, because it provides quality information and is easy to administer as part of a battery of tests. Difficult for nonverbal students; not to be used alone for decision making. Results can be used for diagnosis, therapy, and research.

VI. Tester Qualification: C

VINELAND ADAPTIVE BEHAVIOR SCALE, SECOND EDITION (VABS-II)

I. Use
A. Assessment.

II. Ages
A. Interview: birth through 18 years 11 months and low-functioning adults.

B. Classroom: 3 years through 21 years 11 months.

III. Purpose
A. Assesses personal and social skills and responsibility for own needs.

IV. Areas Assessed
A. Four domains: communication (receptive, written, expressive), daily living skills (personal, domestic, community), socialization (interpersonal relationships, play and leisure time, coping skills), and motor skills (gross, fine). Maladaptive behavior index (internalizing, externalizing, and other) is optional.

V. Additional Information
A. Administration time is 20 to 60 minutes, depending on the form used.

B. Four forms provide flexibility. The Survey Interview Form is administered to caregivers and provides a general assessment of adaptive behavior; the Parent/Caregiver Rating Form is completed by parent or caregiver and covers the same content. The Expanded Interview Form provides a systematic basis for planning individual, educational, habilitative, or treatment programs. The Classroom Form teacher questionnaire assesses adaptive behavior in the classroom. Forms are available in Spanish, and software is available.

VI. Tester Qualification: C

VINELAND SOCIAL–EMOTIONAL EARLY CHILDHOOD SCALES (VINELAND SEEC)

I. Use
A. Assessment.

II. Ages
A. Birth to 5 years 11 months.
III. Purpose
A. Evaluates levels of social–emotional behavior for those with disabilities and how the disabilities affect their daily functioning; used to plan a program and monitor progress.
IV. Areas Assessed
A. Measures social–emotional adjustment with three scales: interpersonal relationships, play and leisure time, and coping skills.
V. Additional Information
A. Administration time is 15 to 25 minutes and is sometimes used in conjunction with the Mullen Scales. Software is available.
VI. Tester Qualification: C

WECHSLER INTELLIGENCE SCALE FOR CHILDREN, FOURTH EDITION (WISC-IV)
I. Use
A. Assessment.
II. Ages
A. From 6 to 7 years.
III. Purpose
A. Provides verbal, performance, and full-scale IQ scores.
IV. Areas Assessed
A. There are four index measurements: verbal comprehension, perceptual reasoning, working memory, and processing speed; there are 15 subtests.
V. Additional Information
A. Four scores are obtained, and a full-scale IQ is discerned from the total score. Core subtests take 65 to 80 minutes. Spanish version and software are available.
B. The two other standardized Wechsler intelligence measures are the Wechsler Adult Intelligence Scale, Third edition (WAIS-III), for children older than 16 years, and the Wechsler Preschool and Primary Scale of Intelligence, Third Edition (WPPSI-III), for children ages 2.6 through 7.3 years.
VI. Tester Qualification: C

WECHSLER PRESCHOOL AND PRIMARY SCALE OF INTELLIGENCE, REVISED (WPPSI-R)
I. Use
A. Assessment.
II. Ages
A. From 4 to 6½ years.
III. Purpose
A. Comprehensive measure of cognitive ability for preschoolers.
IV. Areas Assessed
A. Twelve subscales, six in the performance scale and six in the verbal scale. Five of the six subtests in each scale are designated as the standard subtests: object assembly, geometric design, block design, mazes, and picture completion are in the performance scale. Information,

comprehension, arithmetic, vocabulary, and similarities are in the verbal scale.

B. There are optional subtests in the performance scale and verbal scale.

V. Additional Information

A. Administration time is 50 to 75 minutes. Test provides verbal, performance, and full scale IQ and scaled scores for the subtests. A raw score on each subtest is converted to a scaled score within the child's own age group.

B. Test is norm referenced and research is available.

VI. Tester Qualification: B

WEISS COMPREHENSIVE ARTICULATION TEST (WCAT)

I. Use

A. Testing.

II. Ages

A. All ages.

III. Purpose

A. Provides diagnosis of articulation delays and disorders.

IV. Areas Assessed

A. Assesses articulation and misarticulation patterns.

V. Additional Information

A. Administration time is 20 minutes, and scoring time is 30 minutes. Scores obtained include articulation, age-equivalence, intelligibility, and stimulability. Test–retest reliability is available, and normative scores are based on test performance of 4000 children.

VI. Tester Qualification: A

WIDE RANGE ACHIEVEMENT TEST 4 (WRAT 4)

I. Use

A. Assessment.

II. Ages

A. From 5 years through adulthood.

III. Purpose

A. Identifies the need for basic academic skills.

IV. Areas Assessed

A. Areas assessed are spelling, reading, sentence comprehension, and math.

V. Additional Information

A. Administration time is 15 to 25 minutes for ages 5 to 7 and 35 to 40 minutes for ages 8 or older. Spelling and math tests may be administered to a group; reading and sentence comprehension tests are individually administered. Test is standardized.

VI. Tester Qualification: B

WIDE RANGE ASSESSMENT OF MEMORY AND LEARNING, SECOND EDITION (WRAML2)

I. Use

A. Assessment.

II. Ages

A. From 5 years through adulthood.

III. Purpose
A. Evaluates memory and learning.

IV. Areas Assessed
A. Six subtests, general memory index, plus three indexes with six subtests; verbal memory index (verbal learning, story memory); visual memory index (design memory, picture memory); and attention and concentration index (number/letter, finger/windows).

B. Three supplementary subtests and indexes are available for working memory and rapid memory decline.

V. Additional Information
A. Administration time is 60 minutes for the core battery; memory-screening form (four subtests) takes 10 to 15 minutes. Produces a general memory index plus three more specific index scores and six subtest scores.

B. Software is available.

VI. Tester Qualification: B

WOODCOCK–JOHNSON III TESTS OF ACHIEVEMENT (WJ III)

I. Use
A. Assessment.

II. Ages
A. From 2 years through adulthood.

III. Purpose
A. Measures intellectual abilities and academic achievement.

IV. Areas Assessed
A. Three oral tests, a diagnostic spelling test, and a measure of phonological awareness have been added to evaluate fluency in reading and math.

B. The WJ III battery and the WJ III Test of Cognitive Abilities (COG) are designed to measure general and specific cognitive functions. When administered together they demonstrate overachievement and underachievement and patterns of intraindividual discrepancies among cognitive or achievement areas. The batteries of WJ III COG and WJ III ACH are classified as standard.

V. Additional Information
A. Administration time is 60 to 70 minutes.

B. Test scores are helpful for determining the ability of nonnative speakers of English to function in informal and academic settings. Test can be used for educational, clinical, or research purposes; for diagnosis; educational programming; guidance; and program evaluation. Test has reliability and validity findings and is norm referenced.

VI. Tester Qualification: B

THE WORK SAMPLING SYSTEM

I. Use
A. Assessment.

II. Ages
A. Preschool to grade 6.

III. **Purpose**
   A. Documentation of student's skills, behavior, knowledge, academic achievement, and accomplishments across seven domains or curriculum areas on numerous occasions to enhance teaching and learning.
IV. **Areas Assessed**
   A. Personal and social development, language and literacy, mathematical thinking, scientific thinking, social studies, arts, physical development, and health.
V. **Additional Information**
   A. Provides an effective way to record student's progress to share with educators, families, and communities. Based on national and state standards. Research is available.
VI. **Tester Qualification: B**

WEB SITES

American Psychological Association (APA): Testing and Assessment
   http://www.apa.org/science/testing.html
Harcourt Assessments
   http://www.harcourtassessment.com
Pearson Assessments
   http://www.pearsonassessments.com
Western Psychological Services
   http://www.wpspublish.com

APPENDIX B

Growth Measurements (Anthropometry)

BODY MASS INDEX

Body mass index (BMI) is a convenient standard for estimating body fat. The World Health Organization (WHO) and the National Institutes of Health (NIH) have adopted standards for overweight and obese *adults* based on BMI standards. If BMI is more than 25, an individual is considered *overweight*. A BMI of 30 or more is considered *obese*. The U.S. Centers for Disease Control and Prevention (CDC) published revised growth charts for children in 2000 that include BMI charts. The CDC recommends that the BMI-for-age charts be used for all children 2 to 20 years of age in place of the weight-for-stature charts.

The International Task Force on Obesity has suggested new worldwide *pediatric standards* for overweight and obesity based on BMI. Data for the new study were collected globally using survey results from various locations, including the United States, Singapore, Brazil, Hong Kong, Great Britain, and the Netherlands, making the school nurse's weight monitoring of children from diverse cultures standardized.

Cardiovascular risk factors are associated with the BMI-for-age when they are at or above the 95th percentile. The Bogalusa Heart Study in 1999 found that approximately 60% of the 5 to 10 year olds with a BMI at or above the 95th percentile had at least one risk factor for cardiac disease, such as hypertension or elevated insulin level. Twenty percent of the children had two or more risk factors (Freedman et al, 1999).

BMI is a screening tool but is not diagnostic. A muscular athlete with a BMI over 95% does not necessarily reflect obesity. The student may have a high BMI because muscle weighs more than fat (CDC, 2007). Further assessment (e.g., skin fold measurements) may be needed to determine whether an individual has excess body fat.

BODY MASS INDEX FORMULAS

English Formula:
Weight in pounds ÷ Height in inches ÷ Height in inches × 703 = BMI
Metric Formula:
Weight in kilograms ÷ Height in meters ÷ Height in meters = BMI
For adults: BMI classification is read as calculated.
For children: BMI is calculated and plotted by age and sex. BMI changes substantially with age and differs among girls and boys. The BMIs by age for both normal weight and those with increased concern follow:

Underweight	BMI-for-age <5th percentile
Normal weight	BMI-for-age between 5th and 85th percentile
At risk of overweight	BMI-for-age ≥85th percentile
Overweight	BMI-for-age ≥95th percentile

Additional charts and a conversion calculator can be found at http://www.cdc.gov/nccdphp/dnpa/bmi/.

BOYS
Birth to 36 months
Weight-for-age percentiles

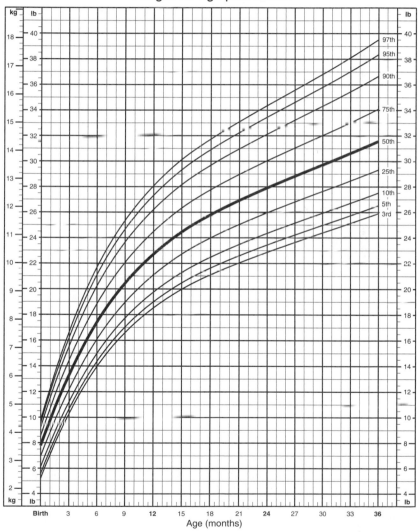

FIGURE B-1 From Centers for Disease Control and Prevention, National Center for Health Statistics. CDC growth charts: United States.

BOYS
Birth to 36 months
Length-for-age percentiles

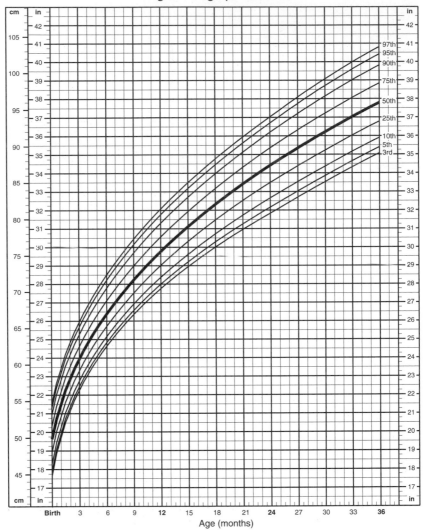

Figure B-2 From Centers for Disease Control and Prevention, National Center for Health Statistics. CDC growth charts: United States.

BOYS
Birth to 36 months
Weight-for-length percentiles

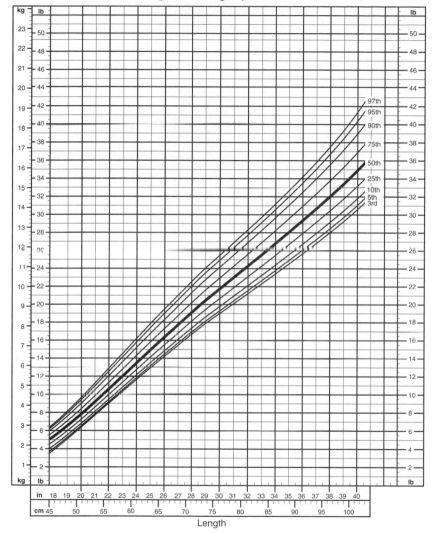

FIGURE B-3 From Centers for Disease Control and Prevention, National Center for Health Statistics. CDC growth charts: United States.

BOYS
Birth to 36 months
Head circumference-for-age percentiles

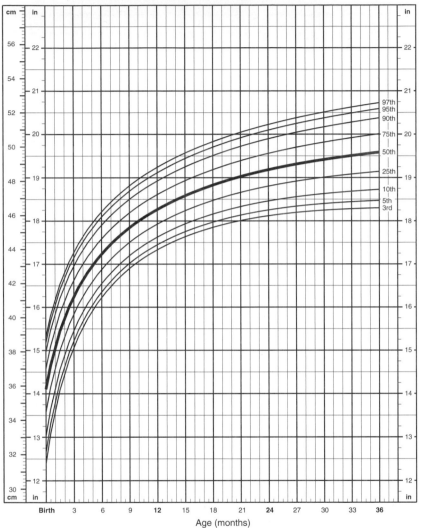

Figure B-4 From Centers for Disease Control and Prevention, National Center for Health Statistics. CDC growth charts: United States.

BOYS
2 to 20 years
Weight-for-age percentiles

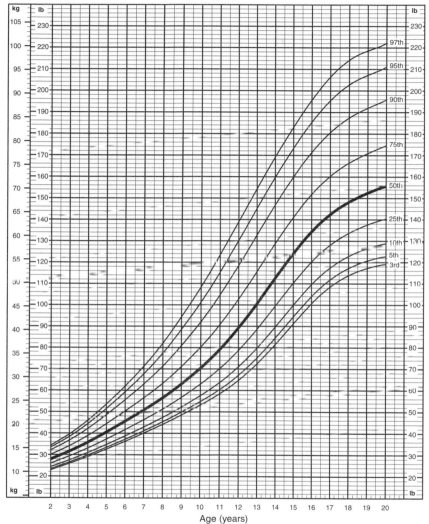

FIGURE B-5 From Centers for Disease Control and Prevention, National Center for Health Statistics. CDC growth charts: United States.

BOYS
2 to 20 years
Stature-for-age percentiles

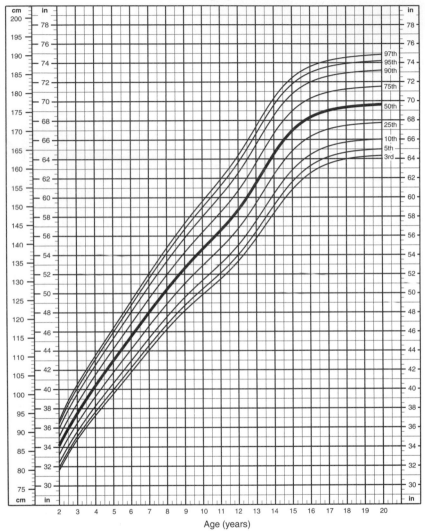

Figure B-6 From Centers for Disease Control and Prevention, National Center for Health Statistics. CDC growth charts: United States.

BOYS
2 to 20 years
Weight-for-stature percentiles

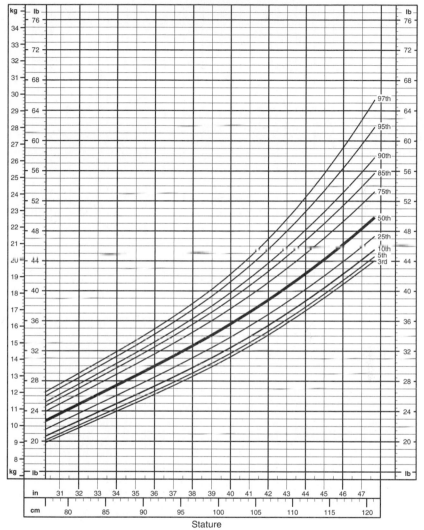

FIGURE B-7 From Centers for Disease Control and Prevention, National Center for Health Statistics. CDC growth charts: United States.

BOYS
2 to 20 years
Body mass index-for-age percentiles

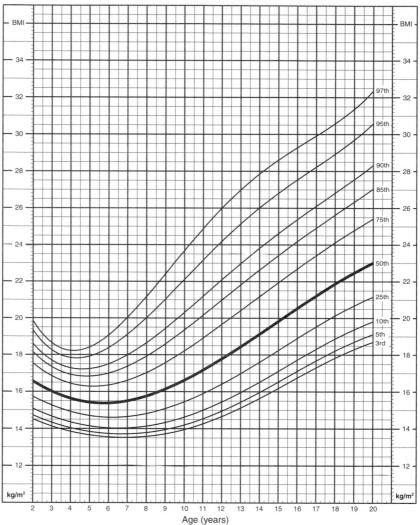

FIGURE B-8 From Centers for Disease Control and Prevention, National Center for Health Statistics. CDC growth charts: United States.

GIRLS
Birth to 36 months
Weight-for-age percentiles

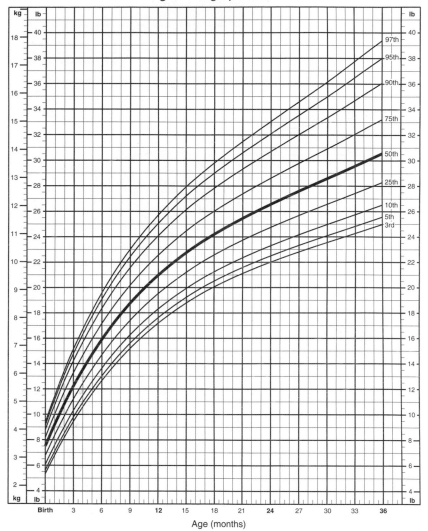

Age (months)

Figure B-9 From Centers for Disease Control and Prevention, National Center for Health Statistics. CDC growth charts: United States.

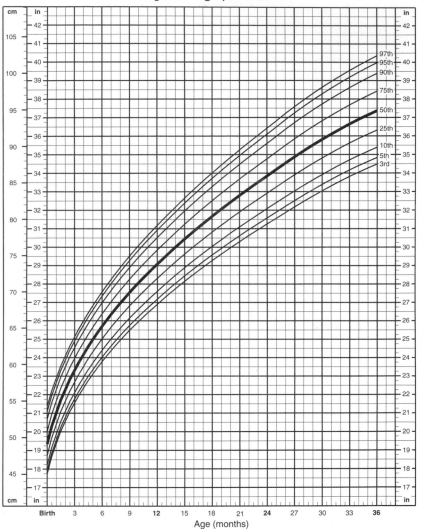

GIRLS
Birth to 36 months
Length-for-age percentiles

FIGURE B-10 From Centers for Disease Control and Prevention, National Center for Health Statistics. CDC growth charts: United States.

GIRLS
Birth to 36 months
Weight-for-length percentiles

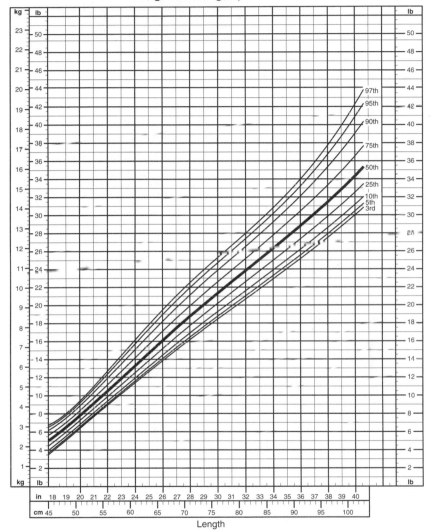

FIGURE B-11 From Centers for Disease Control and Prevention, National Center for Health Statistics. CDC growth charts: United States.

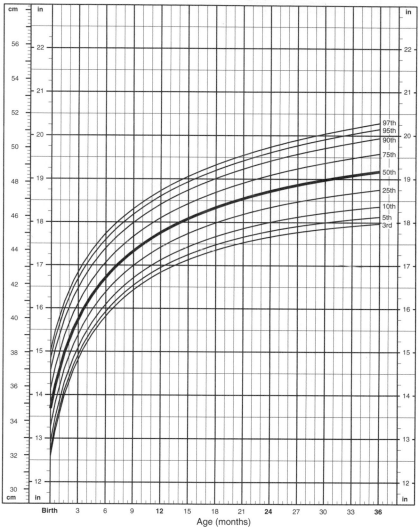

GIRLS
Birth to 36 months
Head circumference-for-age percentiles

FIGURE B-12 From Centers for Disease Control and Prevention, National Center for Health Statistics. CDC growth charts: United States.

GIRLS
2 to 20 years
Weight-for-age percentiles

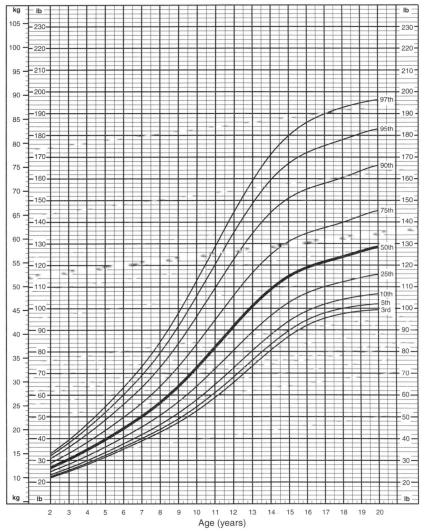

FIGURE B-13 From Centers for Disease Control and Prevention, National Center for Health Statistics. CDC growth charts: United States.

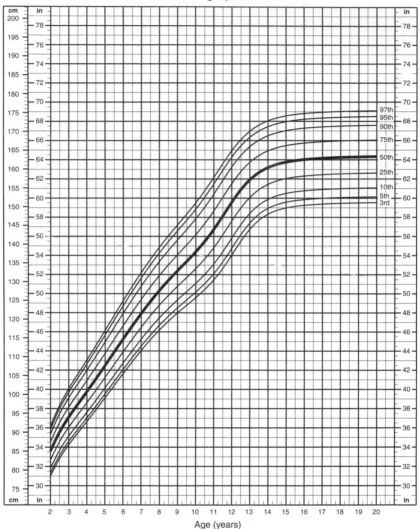

FIGURE B-14 From Centers for Disease Control and Prevention, National Center for Health Statistics. CDC growth charts: United States.

GIRLS
2 to 20 years
Weight-for-stature percentiles

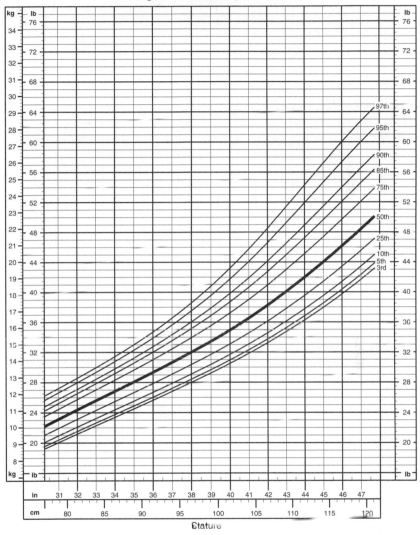

Figure B-15 From Centers for Disease Control and Prevention, National Center for Health Statistics. CDC growth charts: United States.

GIRLS
2 to 20 years
Body mass index-for-age percentiles

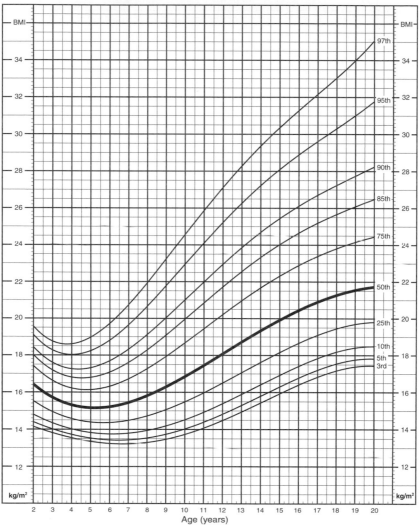

FIGURE B-16 From Centers for Disease Control and Prevention, National Center for Health Statistics. CDC growth charts: United States.

ACHONDROPLASIA
Height for boys with achondroplasia
from birth to 18 years

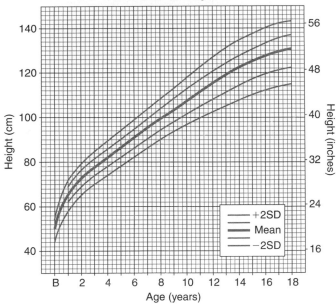

FIGURE B-17 From Horton WA, Rotter JI, Rimoin DL et al: Standard growth curves for achondroplasia, *J Pediatr* 93:435-438, 1978.

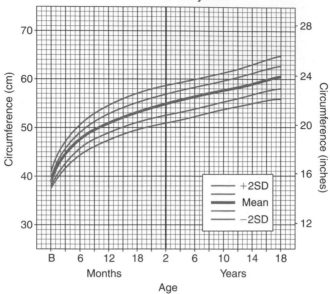

FIGURE B-18 From Horton WA, Rotter JI, Rimoin DL et al: Standard growth curves for achondroplasia, *J Pediatr* 93:435-438, 1978.

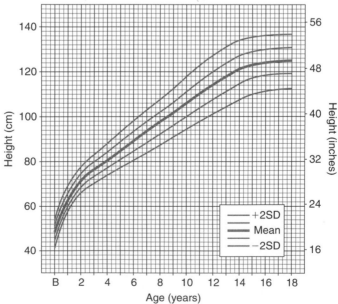

FIGURE B-19 From Horton WA, Rotter JI, Rimoin DL et al: Standard growth curves for achondroplasia, *J Pediatr* 93:435-438, 1978.

ACHONDROPLASIA
Head circumference for girls with achondroplasia from birth to 18 years

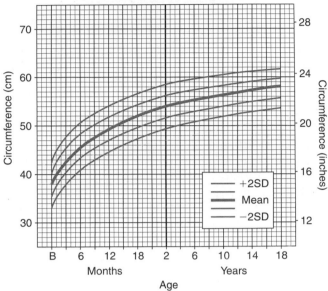

FIGURE B-20 From Horton WA, Rotter JI, Rimoin DL et al: Standard growth curves for achondroplasia, *J Pediatr* 93:435-438, 1978.

Immunizations

DEPARTMENT OF HEALTH AND HUMAN SERVICES • CENTERS FOR DISEASE CONTROL AND PREVENTION

Recommended Immunization Schedule for Persons Aged 0–6 Years—UNITED STATES • 2007

Vaccine ▼ / Age ▶	Birth	1 month	2 months	4 months	6 months	12 months	15 months	18 months	19–23 months	2–3 years	4–6 years
Hepatitis B[1]	HepB	HepB		see footnote 1	HepB				HepB Series		
Rotavirus[2]			Rota	Rota	Rota						
Diphtheria, Tetanus, Pertussis[3]			DTaP	DTaP	DTaP		DTaP				DTaP
Haemophilus influenzae type b[4]			Hib	Hib	Hib[4]	Hib					
Pneumococcal[5]			PCV	PCV	PCV	PCV				PCV	PPV
Inactivated Poliovirus			IPV	IPV		IPV					IPV
Influenza[6]						Influenza (Yearly)					
Measles, Mumps, Rubella[7]						MMR					MMR
Varicella[8]						Varicella					Varicella
Hepatitis A[9]						HepA (2 doses)				HepA Series	
Meningococcal[10]										MPSV4	

■ Range of recommended ages

■ Catch-up immunization

■ Certain high-risk groups

This schedule indicates the recommended ages for routine administration of currently licensed childhood vaccines, as of December 1, 2006, for children aged 0–6 years. Additional information is available at http://www.cdc.gov/nip/recs/child-schedule.htm. Any dose not administered at the recommended age should be administered at any subsequent visit, when indicated and feasible. Additional vaccines may be licensed and recommended during the year. Licensed combination vaccines may be used whenever any components of the combination are indicated and other components of the vaccine are not contraindicated and if approved by the Food and Drug Administration for that dose of the series. Providers should consult the respective Advisory Committee on Immunization Practices statement for detailed recommendations. Clinically significant adverse events that follow immunization should be reported to the Vaccine Adverse Event Reporting System (VAERS). Guidance about how to obtain and complete a VAERS form is available at **http://www.vaers. hhs.gov** or by telephone, **800-822-7967.**

FIGURE C-1 2007 Immunization Schedules. *(From Centers for Disease Control and Prevention, 2007. Available online at http://www.cdc.gov/vaccines/recs/schedules)*

1. Hepatitis B vaccine (HepB). *(Minimum age: birth)*

At birth:

- Administer monovalent HepB to all newborns before hospital discharge.
- If mother is hepatitis B surface antigen (HBsAg)-positive, administer HepB and 0.5 mL of hepatitis B immune globulin (HBIG) within 12 hours of birth.
- If mother's HBsAg status is unknown, administer HepB within 12 hours of birth. Determine the HBsAg status as soon as possible and if HBsAg-positive, administer HBIG (no later than age 1 week).
- If mother is HBsAg-negative, the birth dose can only be delayed with physician's order and mother's negative HBsAg laboratory report documented in the infant's medical record.

After the birth dose:

- The HepB series should be completed with either monovalent HepB or a combination vaccine containing HepB. The second dose should be administered at age 1–2 months. The final dose should be administered at age ≥24 weeks. Infants born to HBsAg-positive mothers should be tested for HBsAg and antibody to HBsAg after completion of ≥3 doses of a licensed HepB series, at age 9–18 months (generally at the next well-child visit).

4-month dose:

- It is permissible to administer 4 doses of HepB when combination vaccines are administered after the birth dose. If monovalent HepB is used for doses after the birth dose, a dose at age 4 months is not needed.

2. Rotavirus vaccine (Rota). *(Minimum age: 6 weeks)*

- Administer the first dose at age 6–12 weeks. Do not start the series later than age 12 weeks.
- Administer the final dose in the series by age 32 weeks. Do not administer a dose later than age 32 weeks.
- Data on safety and efficacy outside of these age ranges are insufficient.

3. Diphtheria and tetanus toxoids and acellular pertussis vaccine (DTaP). *(Minimum age: 6 weeks)*

- The fourth dose of DTaP may be administered as early as age 12 months, provided 6 months have elapsed since the third dose.
- Administer the final dose in the series at age 4–6 years.

4. *Haemophilus influenzae* type b conjugate vaccine (Hib). *(Minimum age: 6 weeks)*

- If PRP-OMP (PedvaxHIB® or ComVax® [Merck]) is administered at ages 2 and 4 months, a dose at age 6 months is not required.
- TriHiBit® (DTaP/Hib) combination products should not be used for primary immunization but can be used as boosters following any Hib vaccine in children aged ≥12 months.

5. Pneumococcal vaccine. *(Minimum age: 6 weeks for pneumococcal conjugate vaccine [PCV]; 2 years for pneumococcal polysaccharide vaccine [PPV])*

- Administer PCV at ages 24–59 months in certain high-risk groups. Administer PPV to children aged ≥2 years in certain high-risk groups. See *MMWR* 2000;49(No. RR-9):1–35.

6. Influenza vaccine. *(Minimum age: 6 months for trivalent inactivated influenza vaccine [TIV]; 5 years for live, attenuated influenza vaccine [LAIV])*

- All children aged 6–59 months and close contacts of all children aged 0–59 months are recommended to receive influenza vaccine.
- Influenza vaccine is recommended annually for children aged ≥59 months with certain risk factors, health-care workers, and other persons (including household members) in close contact with persons in groups at high risk. See *MMWR* 2006;55(No. RR-10):1–41.
- For healthy persons aged 5–49 years, LAIV may be used as an alternative to TIV.
- Children receiving TIV should receive 0.25 mL if aged 6–35 months or 0.5 mL if aged ≥3 years.
- Children aged <9 years who are receiving influenza vaccine for the first time should receive 2 doses (separated by ≥4 weeks for TIV and ≥6 weeks for LAIV).

7. Measles, mumps, and rubella vaccine (MMR). *(Minimum age: 12 months)*

- Administer the second dose of MMR at age 4–6 years. MMR may be administered before age 4–6 years, provided ≥4 weeks have elapsed since the first dose and both doses are administered at age ≥12 months.

8. Varicella vaccine. *(Minimum age: 12 months)*

- Administer the second dose of varicella vaccine at age 4–6 years. Varicella vaccine may be administered before age 4–6 years, provided that ≥3 months have elapsed since the first dose and both doses are administered at age ≥12 months. If second dose was administered ≥28 days following the first dose, the second dose does not need to be repeated.

9. Hepatitis A vaccine (HepA). *(Minimum age: 12 months)*

- HepA is recommended for all children aged 1 year (i.e., aged 12–23 months). The 2 doses in the series should be administered at least 6 months apart.
- Children not fully vaccinated by age 2 years can be vaccinated at subsequent visits.
- HepA is recommended for certain other groups of children, including in areas where vaccination programs target older children. See *MMWR* 2006;55(No. RR-7):1–23.

10. Meningococcal polysaccharide vaccine (MPSV4). *(Minimum age: 2 years)*

- Administer MPSV4 to children aged 2–10 years with terminal complement deficiencies or anatomic or functional asplenia and certain other high-risk groups. See *MMWR* 2005;54(No. RR-7):1–21.

Continued

DEPARTMENT OF HEALTH AND HUMAN SERVICES • CENTERS FOR DISEASE CONTROL AND PREVENTION

Recommended Immunization Schedule for Persons Aged 7–18 Years—UNITED STATES • 2007

Vaccine ▼ Age ▶	7–10 years	11–12 YEARS	13–14 years	15 years	16–18 years
Tetanus, Diphtheria, Pertussis[1]	see footnote 1	Tdap	Tdap		
Human Papillomavirus[2]	see footnote 2	HPV (3 doses)	HPV Series		
Meningococcal[3]	MPSV4	MCV4		MCV4[3] / MCV4	
Pneumococcal[4]		PPV			
Influenza[5]		Influenza (Yearly)			
Hepatitis A[6]		HepA Series			
Hepatitis B[7]		HepB Series			
Inactivated Poliovirus[8]		IPV Series			
Measles, Mumps, Rubella[9]		MMR Series			
Varicella[10]		Varicella Series			

Legend:
- Range of recommended ages
- Catch-up immunization
- Certain high-risk groups

This schedule indicates the recommended ages for routine administration of currently licensed childhood vaccines, as of December 1, 2006, for children aged 7–18 years. Additional information is available at **http://www.cdc.gov/nip/recs/child-schedule.htm.** Any dose not administered at the recommended age should be administered at any subsequent visit, when indicated and feasible. Additional vaccines may be licensed and recommended during the year. Licensed combination vaccines may be used whenever any components of the combination are indicated and other components of the vaccine are not contraindicated and if approved by the Food and Drug Administration for that dose of the series. Providers should consult the respective Advisory Committee on Immunization Practices statement for detailed recommendations. Clinically significant adverse events that follow immunization should be reported to the Vaccine Adverse Event Reporting System (VAERS). Guidance about how to obtain and complete a VAERS form is available at **http://www.vaers.hhs.gov** or by telephone, **800-822-7967.**

CS100131

1. Tetanus and diphtheria toxoids and acellular pertussis vaccine (Tdap).

(Minimum age: 10 years for BOOSTRIX® and 11 years for ADACEL™.)

- Administer at age 11–12 years for those who have completed the recommended childhood DTP/DTaP vaccination series and have not received a tetanus and diphtheria toxoids vaccine (Td) booster dose.
- Adolescents aged 13–18 years who missed the 11–12 year Td/Tdap booster dose should also receive a single dose of Tdap if they have completed the recommended childhood DTP/DTaP vaccination series.

2. Human papillomavirus vaccine (HPV). *(Minimum age: 9 years)*

- Administer the first dose of the HPV vaccine series to females at age 11–12 years.
- Administer the second dose 2 months after the first dose and the third dose 6 months after the first dose.
- Administer the HPV vaccine series to females at age 13–18 years if not previously vaccinated.

3. Meningococcal vaccine. *(Minimum age: 11 years for meningococcal conjugate vaccine [MCV4]; 2 years for meningococcal polysaccharide vaccine [MPSV4])*

- Administer MCV4 at age 11–12 years and to previously unvaccinated adolescents at high school entry (at approximately age 15 years).
- Administer MCV4 to previously unvaccinated college freshmen living in dormitories; MPSV4 is an acceptable alternative.
- Vaccination against invasive meningococcal disease is recommended for children and adolescents aged ≥2 years with terminal complement deficiencies or anatomic or functional asplenia and certain other high-risk groups. See *MMWR* 2005;54(No. RR-7):1–21. Use MPSV4 for children aged 2–10 years and MCV4 or MPSV4 for older children.

4. Pneumococcal polysaccharide vaccine (PPV). *(Minimum age: 2 years)*

- Administer for certain high-risk groups. See *MMWR* 1997;46(No. RR-8):1–24, and *MMWR* 2000;49(No. RR-9):1–35.

5. Influenza vaccine. *(Minimum age: 6 months for trivalent inactivated influenza vaccine [TIV]; 5 years for live, attenuated influenza vaccine [LAIV])*

- Influenza vaccine is recommended annually for persons with certain risk factors, health-care workers, and other persons (including household members) in close contact with persons in groups at high risk. See *MMWR* 2006;55 (No. RR-10):1–41.
- For healthy persons aged 5–49 years, LAIV may be used as an alternative to TIV. Children aged <9 years who are receiving influenza vaccine for the first time should receive 2 doses (separated by ≥4 weeks for TIV and ≥6 weeks for LAIV).

6. Hepatitis A vaccine (HepA). *(Minimum age: 12 months)*

- The 2 doses in the series should be administered at least 6 months apart.
- HepA is recommended for certain other groups of children, including in areas where vaccination programs target older children. See *MMWR* 2006;55 (No. RR-7):1–23.

7. Hepatitis B vaccine (HepB). *(Minimum age: birth)*

- Administer the 3-dose series to those who were not previously vaccinated.
- A 2-dose series of Recombivax HB® is licensed for children aged 11–15 years.

8. Inactivated poliovirus vaccine (IPV). *(Minimum age: 6 weeks)*

- For children who received an all-IPV or all-oral poliovirus (OPV) series, a fourth dose is not necessary if the third dose was administered at age ≥4 years.
- If both OPV and IPV were administered as part of a series, a total of 4 doses should be administered, regardless of the child's current age.

9. Measles, mumps, and rubella vaccine (MMR). *(Minimum age: 12 months)*

- If not previously vaccinated, administer 2 doses of MMR during any visit, with ≥4 weeks between the doses.

10. Varicella vaccine. *(Minimum age: 12 months)*

- Administer 2 doses of varicella vaccine to persons without evidence of immunity.
- Administer 2 doses of varicella vaccine to persons aged <13 years at least 3 months apart. Do not repeat the second dose, if administered ≥28 days after the first dose.
- Administer 2 doses of varicella vaccine to persons aged ≥13 years at least 4 weeks apart.

The Recommended Immunization Schedules for Persons Aged 0–18 Years are approved by the Advisory Committee on Immunization Practices (http://www.cdc.gov/nip/acip), the American Academy of Pediatrics (http://www.aap.org), and the American Academy of Family Physicians (http://www.aafp.org).

SAFER · HEALTHIER · PEOPLE™

Continued

Catch-up Immunization Schedule
for Persons Aged 4 Months–18 Years Who Start Late or Who Are More Than 1 Month Behind
UNITED STATES • 2007

The table below provides catch-up schedules and minimum intervals between doses for children whose vaccinations have been delayed. A vaccine series does not need to be restarted, regardless of the time that has elapsed between doses. Use the section appropriate for the child's age.

Vaccine	Minimum Age for Dose 1	Minimum Interval Between Doses			
		Dose 1 to Dose 2	Dose 2 to Dose 3	Dose 3 to Dose 4	Dose 4 to Dose 5
CATCH-UP SCHEDULE FOR PERSONS AGED 4 MONTHS–6 YEARS					
Hepatitis B[1]	Birth	4 weeks	**8 weeks** (and 16 weeks after first dose)		
Rotavirus[2]	6 wks	4 weeks	4 weeks		
Diphtheria, Tetanus, Pertussis[3]	6 wks	4 weeks	4 weeks	6 months	**6 months[3]**
Haemophilus influenzae type b[4]	6 wks	**4 weeks** if first dose administered at age <12 months **8 weeks (as final dose)** if first dose administered at age 12-14 months **No further doses needed** if first dose administered at age ≥15 months	**4 weeks[4]** if current age <12 months **8 weeks (as final dose)[4]** if current age ≥12 months and second dose administered at age <15 months **No further doses needed** if previous dose administered at age ≥15 months	**8 weeks (as final dose)[4]** This dose only necessary for children aged 12 months–5 years who received 3 doses before age 12 months	
Pneumococcal[5]	6 wks	**4 weeks** if first dose administered at age <12 months and current age <24 months **8 weeks (as final dose)** if first dose administered at age ≥12 months or current age 24–59 months **No further doses needed** for healthy children if first dose administered at age ≥24 months	**4 weeks** if current age <12 months **8 weeks (as final dose)** if current age ≥12 months **No further doses needed** for healthy children if previous dose administered at age ≥24 months	**8 weeks (as final dose)** This dose only necessary for children aged 12 months–5 years who received 3 doses before age 12 months	
Inactivated Poliovirus[6]	6 wks	4 weeks	4 weeks	**4 weeks[6]**	
Measles, Mumps, Rubella[7]	12 mos	4 weeks			
Varicella[8]	12 mos	3 months			
Hepatitis A[9]	12 mos	6 months			
CATCH-UP SCHEDULE FOR PERSONS AGED 7–18 YEARS					
Tetanus, Diphtheria/ Tetanus, Diphtheria, Pertussis[10]	7 yrs[10]	4 weeks	**8 weeks** if first dose administered at age <12 months **6 months** if first dose administered at age ≥12 months	**6 months** if first dose administered at age <12 months	
Human Papillomavirus[11]	9 yrs	4 weeks	12 weeks		
Hepatitis A[9]	12 mos	6 months			
Hepatitis B[1]	Birth	4 weeks	**8 weeks** (and 16 weeks after first dose)		
Inactivated Poliovirus[6]	6 wks	4 weeks	4 weeks	**4 weeks[6]**	
Measles, Mumps, Rubella[7]	12 mos	4 weeks			
Varicella[8]	12 mos	**4 weeks** if first dose administered at age ≥13 years **3 months** if first dose administered at age <13 years			

CS103164

1. **Hepatitis B vaccine (HepB).** *(Minimum age: birth)*
   - Administer the 3-dose series to those who were not previously vaccinated.
   - A 2-dose series of Recombivax HB® is licensed for children aged 11–15 years.

2. **Rotavirus vaccine (Rota).** *(Minimum age: 6 weeks)*
   - Do not start the series later than age 12 weeks.
   - Administer the final dose in the series by age 32 weeks. Do not administer a dose later than age 32 weeks.
   - Data on safety and efficacy outside of these age ranges are insufficient.

3. **Diphtheria and tetanus toxoids and acellular pertussis vaccine (DTaP).** *(Minimum age: 6 weeks)*
   - The fifth dose is not necessary if the fourth dose was administered at age ≥4 years.
   - DTaP is not indicated for persons aged ≥7 years.

4. **Haemophilus influenzae type b conjugate vaccine (Hib).** *(Minimum age: 6 weeks)*
   - Vaccine is not generally recommended for children aged ≥5 years.
   - If current age <12 months and the first 2 doses were PRP-OMP (PedvaxHIB® or ComVax® [Merck]), the third (and final) dose should be administered at age 12–15 months and at least 8 weeks after the second dose.
   - If first dose was administered at age 7–11 months, administer 2 doses separated by 4 weeks plus a booster at age 12–15 months.

5. **Pneumococcal conjugate vaccine (PCV).** *(Minimum age: 6 weeks)*
   - Vaccine is not generally recommended for children aged ≥5 years.

6. **Inactivated poliovirus vaccine (IPV).** *(Minimum age: 6 weeks)*
   - For children who received an all-IPV or all-oral poliovirus (OPV) series, a fourth dose is not necessary if third dose was administered at age ≥4 years.
   - If both OPV and IPV were administered as part of a series, a total of 4 doses should be administered, regardless of the child's current age.

7. **Measles, mumps, and rubella vaccine (MMR).** *(Minimum age: 12 months)*
   - The second dose of MMR is recommended routinely at age 4–6 years but may be administered earlier if desired.
   - If not previously vaccinated, administer 2 doses of MMR during any visit with ≥4 weeks between the doses.

8. **Varicella vaccine.** *(Minimum age: 12 months)*
   - The second dose of varicella vaccine is recommended routinely at age 4–6 years but may be administered earlier if desired.
   - Do not repeat the second dose in persons aged <13 years if administered ≥28 days after the first dose.

9. **Hepatitis A vaccine (HepA).** *(Minimum age: 12 months)*
   - HepA is recommended for certain groups of children, including in areas where vaccination programs target older children. See *MMWR* 2006;55(No. RR-7):1–23.

10. **Tetanus and diphtheria toxoids vaccine (Td) and tetanus and diphtheria toxoids and acellular pertussis vaccine (Tdap).** *(Minimum ages: 7 years for Td, 10 years for BOOSTRIX®, and 11 years for ADACEL™)*
    - Tdap should be substituted for a single dose of Td in the primary catch-up series or as a booster if age appropriate; use Td for other doses.
    - A 5-year interval from the last Td dose is encouraged when Tdap is used as a booster dose. A booster (fourth) dose is needed if any of the previous doses were administered at age <12 months. Refer to ACIP recommendations for further information. See *MMWR* 2006;55(No. RR-3).

11. **Human papillomavirus vaccine (HPV).** *(Minimum age: 9 years)*
    - Administer the HPV vaccine series to females at age 13–18 years if not previously vaccinated.

Information about reporting reactions after immunization is available online at **http://www.vaers.hhs.gov** or by telephone via the 24-hour national toll-free information line 800-822-7967. Suspected cases of vaccine-preventable diseases should be reported to the state or local health department. Additional information, including precautions and contraindications for immunization, is available from the National Center for Immunization and Respiratory Diseases at **http://www.cdc.gov/nip/default.htm** or telephone, **800-CDC-INFO (800-232-4636)**.

DEPARTMENT OF HEALTH AND HUMAN SERVICES • CENTERS FOR DISEASE CONTROL AND PREVENTION • SAFER • HEALTHIER • PEOPLE

APPENDIX D

Dental Development

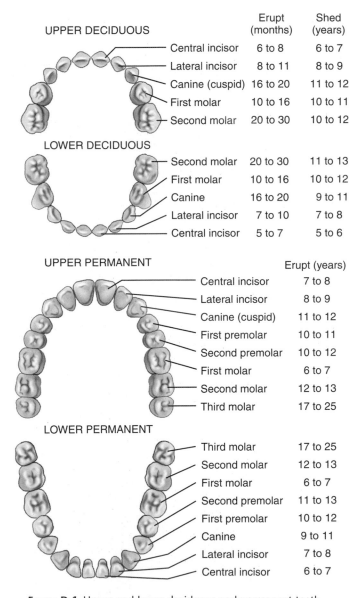

	Erupt (months)	Shed (years)
UPPER DECIDUOUS		
Central incisor	6 to 8	6 to 7
Lateral incisor	8 to 11	8 to 9
Canine (cuspid)	16 to 20	11 to 12
First molar	10 to 16	10 to 11
Second molar	20 to 30	10 to 12
LOWER DECIDUOUS		
Second molar	20 to 30	11 to 13
First molar	10 to 16	10 to 12
Canine	16 to 20	9 to 11
Lateral incisor	7 to 10	7 to 8
Central incisor	5 to 7	5 to 6

	Erupt (years)
UPPER PERMANENT	
Central incisor	7 to 8
Lateral incisor	8 to 9
Canine (cuspid)	11 to 12
First premolar	10 to 11
Second premolar	10 to 12
First molar	6 to 7
Second molar	12 to 13
Third molar	17 to 25
LOWER PERMANENT	
Third molar	17 to 25
Second molar	12 to 13
First molar	6 to 7
Second premolar	11 to 13
First premolar	10 to 12
Canine	9 to 11
Lateral incisor	7 to 8
Central incisor	6 to 7

FIGURE D-1 Upper and lower deciduous and permanent teeth.

APPENDIX E

Conversion Tables, Formulas, and Biostatistics

| Table E-1 | Weight Conversion Table |

Ounces	1 lb	2 lb	3 lb	4 lb	5 lb	6 lb	7 lb	8 lb
0	454 g	907	1361	1814	2268	2722	3175	3629
1	482	936	1389	1843	2296	2750	3204	3657
2	510	964	1418	1871	2325	2778	3232	3686
3	539	992	1446	1899	2353	2807	3260	3714
4	567	1021	1474	1928	2381	2835	3289	3742
5	595	1049	1503	1956	2410	2863	3317	3771
6	624	1077	1531	1985	2438	2892	3345	3799
7	652	1106	1559	2013	2466	2920	3374	3827
8	680	1134	1588	2041	2495	2948	3402	3856
9	709	1162	1616	2070	2523	2977	3430	3884
10	737	1191	1644	2098	2552	3005	3459	3912
11	765	1219	1673	2126	2580	3033	3487	3941
12	794	1247	1701	2155	2608	3062	3515	3969
13	822	1276	1729	2183	2637	3090	3544	3997
14	851	1304	1758	2211	2665	3119	3572	4026
15	879	1332	1786	2240	2693	3147	3600	4054

1 lb = 16 oz = 454 g; 1 kg = 2.2 lb. To convert pounds to grams, multiply by 454. To convert kilograms to pounds, multiply by 2.2.

Length and Weight Calculations

1. Length: To convert inches to centimeters, multiply by 2.54.
2. Weight (Table E-1): To convert pounds to kilograms, divide by 2.2.

Table E-2   Temperature Equivalents Table Celsius (Centigrade): Fahrenheit Scale

Celsius : Fahrenheit   °F = (°C × 9/5) + 32

°C	°F	°C	°F
− 50	− 58.0	49	120.2
− 40	− 40.0	50	122.0
− 35	− 31.0	51	123.8
− 30	− 22.0	52	125.6
− 25	− 13.0	53	127.4
− 20	− 4.0	54	129.2
− 15	+5.0	55	131.0
− 10	14.0	56	132.8
− 5	23.0	57	134.6
0	32.0	58	136.4
+1	33.8	59	138.2
2	35.6	60	140.0
3	37.4	61	141.8
4	39.2	62	143.6
5	41.0	63	145.4
6	42.8	64	147.2
7	44.6	65	149.0
8	46.4	66	150.8
9	48.2	67	152.6
10	50.0	68	154.4
11	51.8	69	156.2
12	53.6	70	158.0
13	55.4	71	159.8
14	57.2	72	161.6
15	59.0	73	163.4
16	60.8	74	165.2

Fahrenheit : Celsius   °C = (°F − 32) × 5/9

°F	°C	°F	°C	°F	°C
− 50	− 46.7	99	37.2	157	69.4
− 40	− 40.0	100	37.7	158	70.0
− 35	− 37.2	101	38.3	159	70.5
− 30	− 34.4	102	38.8	160	71.1
− 25	− 31.7	103	39.4	161	71.6
− 20	− 28.9	104	40.0	162	72.2
− 15	− 26.6	105	40.5	163	72.7
− 10	− 23.3	106	41.1	164	73.3
− 5	− 20.6	107	41.6	165	73.8
0	− 17.7	108	42.2	166	74.4
+1	− 17.2	109	42.7	167	75.0
5	− 15.0	110	43.3	168	75.5
10	− 12.2	111	43.8	169	76.1
15	− 9.4	112	44.4	170	76.6
20	− 6.6	113	45.0	171	77.2
25	− 3.8	114	45.5	172	77.7
30	− 1.1	115	46.1	173	78.3
31	− 0.5	116	46.6	174	78.8
32	0	117	47.2	175	79.4
33	+0.5	118	47.7	176	80.0
34	1.1	119	48.3	177	80.5
35	1.6	120	48.8	178	81.1
36	2.2	121	49.4	179	81.6
37	2.7	122	50.0	180	82.2
38	3.3	123	50.5	181	82.7
39	3.8	124	51.1	182	83.3

17	62.6	75	167.0	40	4.4

Table (pairs of index / value):

No.	Value
17	62.6
18	64.4
19	66.2
20	68.0
21	69.8
22	71.6
23	73.4
24	75.2
25	77.0
26	78.8
27	80.6
28	82.4
29	84.2
30	86.0
31	87.8
32	89.6
33	91.4
34	93.2
35	95.0
36	96.8
37	98.6
38	100.4
39	102.2
40	104.0
41	105.8
42	107.6
43	109.4
44	111.2
45	113.0
46	114.8
47	116.6
48	118.4

No.	Value
75	167.0
76	168.8
77	170.6
78	172.4
79	174.2
80	176.0
81	177.8
82	179.6
83	181.4
84	183.2
85	185.0
86	186.8
87	188.6
88	190.4
89	192.2
90	194.0
91	195.8
92	197.6
93	199.4
94	201.2
95	203.0
96	204.8
97	206.6
98	208.4
99	210.2
100	212.0
101	213.8
102	215.6
103	217.4
104	219.2
105	221.0
106	222.8

No.	Value
40	4.4
41	5.0
42	5.5
43	6.1
44	6.6
45	7.2
46	7.7
47	8.3
48	8.8
49	9.4
50	10.0
55	12.7
60	15.5
65	18.3
70	21.1
75	23.8
80	26.6
85	29.4
86	30.0
87	30.5
88	31.0
89	31.6
90	32.2
91	32.7
92	33.3
93	33.8
94	34.4
95	35.0
96	35.5
97	36.1
98	36.6
98.6	37.0

No.	Value
125	51.6
126	52.2
127	52.7
128	53.3
129	53.8
130	54.4
131	55.0
132	55.5
133	56.1
134	56.6
135	57.2
136	57.7
137	58.3
138	58.8
139	59.4
140	60.0
141	60.5
142	61.1
143	61.6
144	62.2
145	62.7
146	63.3
147	63.8
148	64.4
149	65.0
150	65.5
151	66.1
152	66.6
153	67.2
154	67.7
155	68.3
156	68.8

No.	Value
183	83.8
184	84.4
185	85.0
186	85.5
187	86.1
188	86.6
189	87.2
190	87.7
191	88.3
192	88.8
193	89.4
194	90.0
195	90.5
196	91.1
197	91.6
198	92.2
199	92.7
200	93.3
201	93.8
202	94.4
203	95.0
204	95.5
205	96.1
206	96.6
207	97.2
208	97.7
209	98.3
210	98.8
211	99.4
212	100.0
213	100.5
214	101.1

Table E-3 Conversion of Pounds and Ounces to Grams for Newborn Weights*

| | Ounces | | | | | | | | | | | | | | | |
Pounds	0	1	2	3	4	5	6	7	8	9	10	11	12	13	14	15
0	—	28	57	85	113	142	170	198	227	255	283	312	340	369	397	425
1	454	482	510	539	567	595	624	652	680	709	737	765	794	822	850	879
2	907	936	964	992	1021	1049	1077	1106	1134	1162	1191	1219	1247	1276	1304	1332
3	1361	1389	1417	1446	1474	1503	1531	1559	1588	1616	1644	1673	1701	1729	1758	1786
4	1814	1843	1871	1899	1928	1956	1984	2013	2041	2070	2093	2126	2155	2183	2211	2240
5	2268	2296	2325	2353	2381	2410	2438	2466	2495	2523	2551	2580	2608	2637	2665	2693
6	2722	2750	2778	2807	2835	2863	2892	2920	2948	2977	3005	3033	3062	3090	3118	3147
7	3175	3203	3232	3260	3289	3317	3345	3374	3402	3430	3459	3487	3515	3544	3572	3600
8	3629	3657	3685	3714	3742	3770	3799	3827	3856	3884	3912	3941	3969	3997	4026	4054
9	4082	4111	4139	4167	4196	4224	4252	4281	4309	4337	4366	4394	4423	4451	4479	4508
10	4536	4564	4593	4621	4649	4678	4706	4734	4763	4791	4819	4848	4876	4904	4933	4961
11	4990	5018	5046	5075	5103	5131	5160	5188	5216	5245	5273	5301	5330	5358	5386	5415
12	5443	5471	5500	5528	5557	5585	5613	5642	5670	5698	5727	5755	5783	5812	5840	5868
13	5897	5925	5953	5982	6010	6038	6067	6095	6123	6152	6180	6209	6237	6265	6294	6322
14	6350	6379	6407	6435	6464	6492	6520	6549	6577	6605	6634	6662	6690	6719	6747	6776
15	6804	6832	6860	6889	6917	6945	6973	7002	7030	7059	7087	7115	7144	7172	7201	7228

*To convert pounds and ounces to grams, multiply the pounds by 453.6 and the ounces by 28.35; add the totals.
To convert grams into pounds and decimals of a pound, multiply the grams by 0.0022.
To convert grams into ounces, divide the grams by 28.35 (16 oz = 1 lb).

APPENDIX F

Recommended Energy Intake for Age

Age (yr)	REE* (kcal/kg/day)	Average Energy Needs (kcal/kg/day)	(kcal/day)
Infants			
0.0-0.5	53	108	650
0.5-1.0	56	98	850
Children			
1-3	57	102	1300
4-6	48	90	1800
7-10	40	70	2000
Males			
11-14	32	55	2500
15-18	27	45	3000
Females			
11-14	28	47	2200
15-18	25	40	2200
Pregnancy			
First trimester			+0
Second and third trimesters			+300
Lactation			
			+500

Modified from Food Nutrition Board, National Research Council: *Recommended dietary allowances,* ed 10, Washington, DC, 1989, National Academy Press.

*REE, Resting energy expenditure (based on Food and Agricultural Organization [FAO] equations).

APPENDIX G

Vital Signs for Normal Values

| Table G-1 | **Blood Pressure Levels by Percentiles of Height: Boys, 1 to 17 Years** |

Systolic BP (mmHg) by Percentile of Height

Age (yr)	Percentiles Height*→ BP†↓	5%	10%	25%	50%	75%	90%	95%
1	90th	94	95	97	98	100	102	102
	95th	98	99	101	102	104	106	106
2	90th	98	99	100	102	104	105	106
	95th	101	102	104	106	108	109	110
3	90th	100	101	103	105	107	108	109
	95th	104	105	107	109	111	112	113
4	90th	102	103	105	107	109	110	111
	95th	106	107	109	111	113	114	115
5	90th	104	105	106	108	110	112	112
	95th	108	109	110	112	114	115	116
6	90th	105	106	108	110	111	113	114
	95th	109	110	112	114	115	117	117
7	90th	106	107	109	111	113	114	115
	95th	110	111	113	115	116	118	119
8	90th	107	108	110	112	114	115	116
	95th	111	112	114	116	118	119	120
9	90th	109	110	112	113	115	117	117
	95th	113	114	116	117	119	121	121
10	90th	110	112	113	115	117	118	119
	95th	114	115	117	119	121	122	123
11	90th	112	113	115	117	119	120	121
	95th	116	117	119	121	123	124	125
12	90th	115	116	117	119	121	123	123
	95th	119	120	121	123	125	126	127
13	90th	117	118	120	122	124	125	126
	95th	121	122	124	126	128	129	130
14	90th	120	121	123	125	126	128	128
	95th	124	125	127	128	130	132	132
15	90th	123	124	125	127	129	131	131
	95th	127	128	129	131	133	134	135
16	90th	125	126	128	130	132	133	134
	95th	129	130	132	134	136	137	138
17	90th	128	129	131	133	134	136	136
	95th	132	133	135	136	138	140	140

BP, Blood pressure.
*Height percentile determined by standard growth curves.
†Blood pressure percentile determined by a single measurement.

Diastolic BP (mmHg) by Percentile of Height

Age (yr)	Percentiles Height*→ BP†↓	5%	10%	25%	50%	75%	90%	95%
1	90th	50	51	52	53	54	54	55
	95th	55	55	56	57	58	59	59
2	90th	55	55	56	57	58	59	59
	95th	59	59	60	61	62	63	63
3	90th	59	59	60	61	62	63	63
	95th	63	63	64	65	66	67	67
4	90th	62	62	63	64	65	66	66
	95th	66	67	67	68	69	70	71
5	90th	65	65	66	67	68	69	69
	95th	69	70	70	71	72	73	74
6	90th	67	68	69	70	70	71	72
	95th	72	72	73	74	75	76	76
7	90th	69	70	71	72	72	73	74
	95th	74	74	75	76	77	78	78
8	90th	71	71	72	73	74	75	75
	95th	75	76	76	77	78	79	80
9	90th	72	73	73	74	75	76	77
	95th	76	77	78	79	80	80	81
10	90th	73	74	74	75	76	77	78
	95th	77	78	79	80	80	81	82
11	90th	74	74	75	76	77	78	78
	95th	78	79	79	80	81	82	83
12	90th	75	75	76	77	78	78	79
	95th	79	79	80	81	82	83	83
13	90th	75	76	76	77	78	79	80
	95th	79	80	81	82	83	83	84
14	90th	76	76	77	78	79	80	80
	95th	80	81	81	82	83	84	85
15	90th	77	77	78	79	80	81	81
	95th	81	82	83	83	84	85	86
16	90th	79	79	80	81	82	82	83
	95th	83	83	84	85	86	87	87
17	90th	81	81	82	83	84	85	85
	95th	85	85	86	87	88	89	89

Table G-2 — *Blood Pressure Levels by Percentiles of Height: Girls, 1 to 17 Years*

		Systolic BP (mmHg) by Percentile of Height						
Age (yr)	Percentiles Height*→ †BP↓	5%	10%	25%	50%	75%	90%	95%
1	90th	97	98	99	100	102	103	104
	95th	101	102	103	104	105	107	107
2	90th	99	99	100	102	103	104	105
	95th	102	103	104	105	107	108	109
3	90th	100	100	102	103	104	105	106
	95th	104	104	105	107	108	109	110
4	90th	101	102	103	104	106	107	108
	95th	105	106	107	108	109	111	111
5	90th	103	103	104	106	107	108	109
	95th	107	107	108	110	111	112	113
6	90th	104	105	106	107	109	110	111
	95th	108	109	110	111	112	114	114
7	90th	106	107	108	109	110	112	112
	95th	110	110	112	113	114	115	116
8	90th	108	109	110	111	112	113	114
	95th	112	112	113	115	116	117	118
9	90th	110	110	112	113	114	115	116
	95th	114	114	115	117	118	119	120
10	90th	112	112	114	115	116	117	118
	95th	116	116	117	119	120	121	122
11	90th	114	114	116	117	118	119	120
	95th	118	118	119	121	122	123	124
12	90th	116	116	118	119	120	121	122
	95th	120	120	121	123	124	125	126
13	90th	118	118	119	121	122	123	124
	95th	121	122	123	125	126	127	128
14	90th	119	120	121	122	124	125	126
	95th	123	124	125	126	128	129	130
15	90th	121	121	122	124	125	126	127
	95th	124	125	126	128	129	130	131
16	90th	122	122	123	125	126	127	128
	95th	125	126	127	128	130	131	132
17	90th	122	123	124	125	126	128	128
	95th	126	126	127	129	130	131	132

BP, Blood pressure.
*Height percentile determined by standard growth curves.
†Blood pressure percentile determined by a single measurement.

Diastolic BP (mmHg) by Percentile of Height

Age (yr)	Percentiles Height*→ †BP↓	5%	10%	25%	50%	75%	90%	95%
1	90th	53	53	53	54	55	56	56
	95th	57	57	57	58	59	60	60
2	90th	57	57	58	58	59	60	61
	95th	61	61	62	62	63	64	65
3	90th	61	61	61	62	63	63	64
	95th	65	65	65	66	67	67	68
4	90th	63	63	64	65	65	66	67
	95th	67	67	68	69	69	70	71
5	90th	66	66	66	67	68	68	69
	95th	69	70	70	71	72	72	73
6	90th	67	67	68	69	69	70	71
	95th	71	71	72	73	73	74	75
7	90th	69	69	69	70	71	72	72
	95th	73	73	73	74	75	76	76
8	90th	70	70	71	71	72	73	74
	95th	74	74	75	75	76	77	78
9	90th	71	72	72	73	74	74	75
	95th	75	76	77	78	78	78	79
10	90th	73	73	73	74	75	76	76
	95th	77	77	77	78	79	80	80
11	90th	74	74	75	75	76	77	77
	95th	78	78	79	79	80	81	81
12	90th	75	75	76	76	77	78	78
	95th	79	79	80	80	81	82	82
13	90th	76	76	77	78	78	79	80
	95th	80	80	81	82	82	83	84
14	90th	77	77	78	79	79	80	81
	95th	81	81	82	83	83	84	85
15	90th	78	78	79	79	80	81	82
	95th	82	82	83	83	84	85	86
16	90th	79	79	79	80	81	82	82
	95th	83	83	83	84	85	86	86
17	90th	79	79	79	80	81	82	82
	95th	83	83	83	84	85	86	86

Table G-3 — *Age-Specific Heart Rates, Birth to 15 Years*

Age	2%	Mean	98%
<1 day	93	123	154
1-2 days	91	123	159
3-6 days	91	129	166
1-3 wk	107	148	182
1-2 mo	121	149	179
3-5 mo	106	141	186
6-11 mo	109	134	169
1-2 yr	89	119	151
3-4 yr	73	108	137
5-7 yr	65	100	133
8-11 yr	62	91	130
12-15 yr	60	85	119

Table G-4 — *Age-Specific Respiratory Rates, Birth to 18 years*

Age (yr)	Boys	Girls	Age (yr)	Boys	Girls
0-1	31 ± 8	30 ± 6	9-10	19 ± 2	19 ± 2
1-2	26 ± 4	27 ± 4	10-11	19 ± 2	19 ± 2
2-3	25 ± 4	25 ± 3	11-12	19 ± 3	19 ± 3
3-4	24 ± 3	24 ± 3	12-13	19 ± 3	19 ± 2
4-5	23 ± 2	22 ± 2	13-14	19 ± 2	18 ± 2
5-6	22 ± 2	21 ± 2	14-15	18 ± 2	18 ± 3
6-7	21 ± 3	21 ± 3	15-16	17 ± 3	18 ± 3
7-8	20 ± 3	20 ± 2	16-17	17 ± 2	17 ± 3
8-9	20 ± 2	20 ± 2	17-18	16 ± 3	17 ± 3

From Illif A, Lee V: *Child Dev* 23:240, 1952.

APPENDIX H

Abbreviations and Symbols for Laboratory Tests

Table H-1	*Prefixes Denoting Decimal Factors*

Prefix	Symbol
mega	M
kilo	k
hecto	h
deka	da
deci	d
centi	c
milli	m
micro	μ
nano	n
pico	p
femto	f

Table H-2	*Abbreviations*

Ab	absorbance
AI	angiotensin I
AU	arbitrary unit
cAMP	cyclic adenosine 3', 5' monophosphate
cap	capillary
CH^{50}	dilution required to lyse 50% of indicator RBC; indicates complement activity
CHF	congestive heart failure
CKBB	brain isoenzyme of creatine kinase
CKMB	heart isoenzyme of creatine kinase
CNS	central nervous system
conc.	concentration
Cr.	creatinine
d	diem, day, days
F	female
g	gram
hr	hour, hours
Hb	hemoglobin
HbCO	carboxyhemoglobin
Hgb	hemoglobin
hpf	high-power field
HPLC	high-performance liquid chromatography
IFA	indirect fluorescent antibody
IU	International Unit of hormone activity

Continued

Table H-2	*Abbreviations*—cont'd
L	liter
M	male
MCV	mean corpuscular volume
mEq/L	milliequivalents per liter
min	minute, minutes
mm^3	cubic millimeter; equivalent to microliter (μl)
mmHg	millimeters of mercury
mo	month, months
mol	mole
mOsm	milliosmole
MW	relative molecular weight
Na	sodium
nm	nanometer (wavelength)
Pa	pascal
pp	postprandial
RBC	red blood cell(s); erythrocyte(s)
RIA	radioimmunoassay
RID	radial immunodiffusion
RT	room temperature
s	second, seconds
SD	standard deviation
std.	standard
therap.	therapeutic
U	International Unit of enzyme activity
V	volume
WBC	white blood cell(s)
WHO	World Health Organization
wk	week, weeks
yr	year, years

Table H-3	*Abbreviations for Specimens*
S	serum
P	plasma
(H)	heparin
(LiH)	lithium heparin
(E)	EDTA
(C)	citrate
(O)	oxalate
W	whole blood
U	urine
F	feces
CSF	cerebrospinal fluid
AF	amniotic fluid
(NaC)	sodium citrate
(NH$_4$H)	ammonium heparinate

Table H-4	*Symbols*
>	greater than
≥	greater than or equal to
<	less than
≤	less than or equal to
±	plus/minus
≅	approximately equal to

APPENDIX I

Weights and Measures

Table I-1	*Measures of Capacity: Apothecaries' (Wine) Measures*			
Minims	**Fluid Drams**	**Fluid Ounces**	**Gills**	**Pints**
1	0.0166	0.002	0.005	0.0013
60	1	0.125	0.0312	0.0078
480	8	1	0.25	0.0625
1920	32	4	1	0.25
7680	128	16	4	1
15360	256	32	8	2
61440	1024	128	32	8

Table I-2	*Measures of Capacity: Metric Measure*			
Microliter	**Milliliter**	**Centiliter**	**Deciliter**	**Liter**
1	—	—	—	—
10^3	1	—	—	—
10^4	10	1	—	—
10^5	100	10	1	—
10^6	10^3	100	10	1
10^7	10^4	10^3	100	10
10^8	10^5	10^4	10^3	100
10^9	10^6	10^5	10^4	10^3
10^{12}	10^9	10^8	10^7	10^6

1 liter = 2.113363738 pints (Apothecaries').

Quarts	Gallons	Cubic Inches	Equivalents Milliliters	Cubic Centimeters
—	—	0.00376	0.06161	0.06161
0.0039	—	0.22558	3.6967	3.6967
0.0312	0.0078	1.80468	29.5737	29.5737
0.125	0.0312	7.21875	118.2948	118.2948
0.5	0.125	28.875	473.179	473.179
1	0.25	57.75	946.358	946.358
4	1	231	3785.434	3785.434

Dekaliter	Hectoliter	Kiloliter	Megaliter	Equivalents (Apothecaries' Fluid)
—	—	—	—	0.01623108 min
—	—	—	—	16.23 min
—	—	—	—	2.7 fl dr
—	—	—	—	3.38 fl oz
—	—	—	—	2.11 pts
1	—	—	—	2.64 gal
10	1	—	—	26.418 gals
100	10	1	—	264.18 gals
10^5	10^4	10^3	1	26418 gals

Table I-3   *Measures of Length: Metric Measure*

Micrometer	Millimeter	Centimeter	Decimeter	Meter	Dekameter	Hectometer	Kilometer	Megameter	Equivalents
1	0.001	10^{-4}	—	—	—	—	—	—	0.000039 in
10^3	1	10^{-1}	—	—	—	—	—	—	0.03937 in
10^4	10	1	—	—	—	—	—	—	0.3937 in
10^5	100	10	1	—	—	—	—	—	3.937 in
10^6	1000	100	10	1	—	—	—	—	39.37 in
10^7	10^4	1000	100	10	1	—	—	—	10.9361 yd
10^8	10^5	10^4	1000	100	10	1	—	—	109.3612 yd
10^9	10^6	10^5	10^4	1000	100	10	1	—	1093.6121 yd
10^{10}	10^7	10^6	10^5	10^4	1000	100	10	—	6.2137 m
10^{12}	10^9	10^8	10^7	10^6	10^5	10^4	1000	1	621.370 m

| Table I-4 | | Conversion Tables: Avoirdupois—Metric Weight | | | | |

Ounces	Grams	Ounces	Grams	Pounds	Grams	Kilograms
1/16	1.772	7	198.447	1 (16 oz)	453.59	
1/8	3.544	8	226.796	2	907.18	
1/4	7.088	9	255.146	3	1360.78	1.36
1/2	14.175	10	283.495	4	1814.37	1.81
1	28.350	11	311.845	5	2267.96	2.27
2	56.699	12	340.194	6	2721.55	2.72
3	85.049	13	368.544	7	3175.15	3.18
4	113.398	14	396.893	8	3628.74	3.63
5	141.748	15	425.243	9	4082.33	4.08
6	170.097	16 (1 lb)	453.59	10	4535.92	4.54

| Table I-5 | | Conversion Tables: Metric—Avoirdupois Weight | | | |

Grams	Ounces	Grams	Ounces	Grams	Pounds
0.001 (1 mg)	0.000035274	1	0.035274	1000 (1 kg)	2.2046

| Table I-6 | | Conversion Tables: Apothecaries'—Metric Weight | | | |

Grains	Grams	Grains	Grams	Scruples	Grams
1/150	0.0004	2/5	0.03	1	1.296 (1.3)
1/120	0.0005	1/2	0.032	2	2.592 (2.6)
1/100	0.0006	3/5	0.04	3 (1 dram)	3.888 (3.9)
1/90	0.0007	2/3	0.043	**Drams**	**Grams**
1/80	0.0008	3/4	0.0	1	3.888
1/64	0.001	7/8	0.057	2	7.776
1/60	0.0011	1	0.065	3	11.664
1/50	0.0013	1½	0.097 (0.1)	4	15.552
1/48	0.0014	2	0.12	5	19.440
1/40	0.0016	3	0.20	6	23.328
1/36	0.0018	4	0.24	7	27.216
1/32	0.002	5	0.30	8 (1 oz)	31.103
1/30	0.0022	6	0.40	**Ounces**	**Grams**
1/25	0.0026	7	0.45	1	31.103
1/20	0.003	8	0.50	2	62.207
1/16	0.004	9	0.60	3	93.310
1/12	0.005	10	0.65	4	124.414
1/10	0.006	15	1.00	5	155.517
1/9	0.007	20 (1 scruple)	1.30	6	186.621
1/8	0.008	30	2.00	7	217.724
1/7	0.009			8	248.828
1/6	0.01			9	279.931
1/5	0.013			10	311.035
1/4	0.016			11	342.138
1/3	0.02			12 (1 lb t)	373.242

Table I-7	Conversion Tables: Metric—Apothecaries' Weight				
Milligrams	Grains	Grams	Grains	Grams	Equivalents
1	0.015432	0.1	1.5432	10	2.572 drams
2	0.030864	0.2	3.0864	15	3.858 drams
3	0.046296	0.3	4.6296	20	5.144 drams
4	0.061728	0.4	6.1728	25	6.430 drams
5	0.077160	0.5	7.7160	30	7.716 drams
6	0.092592	0.6	9.2592	40	1.286 oz
7	0.108024	0.7	10.8024	45	1.447 oz
8	0.123456	0.8	12.3456	50	1.607 oz
9	0.138888	0.9	13.8888	100	3.215 oz
10	0.154320	1.0	15.4320	200	6.430 oz
15	0.231480	1.5	23.1480	300	9.644 oz
20	0.308640	2.0	30.8640	400	12.859 oz
25	0.385800	2.5	38.5800	500	1.34 lb
30	0.462960	3.0	46.2960	600	1.61 lb
35	0.540120	3.5	54.0120	700	1.88 lb
40	0.617280	4.0	61.728	800	2.14 lb
45	0.694440	4.5	69.444	900	2.41 lb
50	0.771600	5.0	77.162	1000	2.68 lb
100	1.543240	10.0	154.3240		

Table I-8	Conversion Tables: Apothecaries'—Metric Liquid Measure				
Minims	Milliliters	Fluid Drams	Milliliters	Fluid Ounces	Milliliters
1	0.06	1	3.70	1	29.57
2	0.12	2	7.39	2	59.15
3	0.19	3	11.09	3	88.72
4	0.25	4	14.79	4	118.29
5	0.31	5	18.48	5	147.87
10	0.62	6	22.18	6	177.44
15	0.92	7	25.88	7	207.01
20	1.23	8 (1 fl oz)	29.57	8	236.58
25	1.54			9	266.16
30	1.85			10	295.73
35	2.16			11	325.30
40	2.46			12	354.88
45	2.77			13	384.45
50	3.08			14	414.02
55	3.39			15	443.59
60 (1 fl dr)	3.70			16 (1 pt)	473.17
				32 (1 qt)	946.33
				128 (1 gal)	3785.32

Table I-9	Conversion Tables: Metric—Apothecaries' Liquid Measure				
Milliliters	Minims	Milliliters	Fluid Drams	Milliliters	Fluid Ounces
1	16.2315	1.35	30	1.01	
2	32.5	10	2.71	40	1.35
3	48.7	15	4.06	50	1.69
4	64.9	20	5.4	500	16.91
5	81.1	25	6.76	1000 (1 L)	33.815
		30	71		

Table I-10	Conversion Tables: U.S. and British—Metric Length		
Inches	Millimeters	Centimeters	Meters
1/25	1.00	0.1	0.001
1/8	3.18	0.318	0.00318
1/4	6.35	0.635	0.00635
1/2	12.70	1.27	0.0127
1	25.40	2.54	0.0254
12 (1 foot)	304.80	30.48	0.3048

APPROXIMATE APOTHECARY EQUIVALENTS

These *approximate* dose equivalents represent the quantities usually prescribed, under identical conditions, by physicians using, respectively, the metric system or the apothecary system of weights and measures. In labeling dosage forms in both the metric and the apothecary systems, if one is the approximate equivalent of the other, the approximate figure shall be enclosed in parentheses.

When prepared dosage forms such as tablets, capsules, and pills are prescribed in the metric system, the pharmacist may dispense the corresponding *approximate* equivalent in the apothecary system, and vice versa, as indicated in the following table.

For the conversion of specific quantities in converting pharmaceutical formulas, equivalents must be used. In the compounding of prescriptions, the exact equivalents, rounded to three significant figures, should be used.

Table I-11	*Liquid Measure*

Metric	Approximate Apothecary Equivalents	Metric	Approximate Apothecary Equivalents
1000 ml	1 quart	3 ml	45 minims
750 ml	11/2 pints	2 ml	30 minims
500 ml	1 pint	1 ml	15 minims
250 ml	8 fluid ounces	0.75 ml	12 minims
200 ml	7 fluid ounces	0.6 ml	10 minims
100 ml	11/2 fluid ounces	0.5 ml	8 minims
50 ml	13/4 fluid ounces	0.3 ml	5 minims
30 ml	1 fluid ounce	0.25 ml	4 minims
15 ml	4 fluid drams	0.2 ml	3 minims
10 ml	2½ fluid drams	0.1 ml	1½ minims
8 ml	2 fluid drams	0.06 ml	1 minims
5 ml	11/4 fluid drams	0.05 ml	3/4 minim
4 ml	1 fluid drams	0.03 ml	1/2 minim

Table I-12	*Weight*

Metric	Approximate Apothecary Equivalents	Metric	Approximate Apothecary Equivalents
30 g	1 ounce	30 mg	1/2 grain
15 g	4 drams	25 mg	3/8 grain
10 g	2½ drams	20 mg	1/3 grain
7.5 g	2 drams	15 mg	1/4 grain
6 g	90 grains	12 mg	1/5 grain
5 g	75 grains	10 mg	1/6 grain
4 g	60 grains (1 dram)	8 mg	1/8 grain
3 g	45 grains	6 mg	1/10 grain
2 g	30 grains (1/2 dram)	5 mg	1/12 grain
1.5 g	22 grains	4 mg	1/15 grain
1 g	15 grains	3 mg	1/20 grain
750 mg	12 grains	2 mg	1/30 grain
600 mg	10 grains	1.5 mg	1/40 grain
500 mg	7½ grains	1.2 mg	1/50 grain
400 mg	6 grains	1 mg	1/60 grain
300 mg	5 grains	800 µg	1/80 grain
250 mg	4 grains	600 µg	1/100 grain
200 mg	3 grains	500 µg	1/120 grain
150 mg	2½ grains	400 µg	1/150 grain
125 mg	2 grains	300 µg	1/200 grain
100 mg	1½ grains	250 µg	1/250 grain
75 mg	1½ grains	200 µg	1/300 grain
60 mg	1 grain	150 µg	1/400 grain
50 mg	3/4 grain	120 µg	1/500 grain
40 mg	2/3 grain	100 µg	1/600 grain

The above *approximate* dose equivalents have been adopted by the *United States Pharmacopeia* and the *National Formulary,* and these dose equivalents have the approval of the federal Food and Drug Administration.

APPENDIX J

National Health and Educational Resources

The Web sites listed here do not imply endorsement. An attempt has been made to list important and informative health resources, but as with any electronic site, locations may change; therefore data need to be reviewed for correctness and the date the data were updated.

GOVERNMENT WEB SITES AND CLEARINGHOUSES

Administration for Children and Families, Office of Head Start
www.acf.dhhs.gov/programs/hsb
Centers for Disease Control and Prevention (CDC)
www.cdc.gov
Child Welfare Information Gateway
www.childwelfare.gov
ERIC Education Resources Information Center
www.eric.ed.gov
Healthfinder: Your Guide to Reliable Health Information (US DHHS)
www.healthfinder.gov
Health Resources and Services Administration Information Center (US DHHS)
http://ask.hrsa.gov
Healthy People 2010
www.healthypeople.gov
National Center for Education Statistics (NCES)
www.nces.ed.gov
National Center for Health Statistics (NCHS)
www.cdc.gov/nchs
National Clearinghouse for Alcohol and Drug Information (NCADI)
http://ncadi.samhsa.gov
National Diabetes Information Clearinghouse (NDIC)
www.niddk.nih.gov/health/diabetes/ndic.htm
National Dissemination Center for Children with Disabilities (NICHCY)
www.nichcy.org
National Health Information Center (NHIC)
www.health.gov/nhic
National Heart, Lung, and Blood Institute (NHLBI)
www.nhlbi.nih.gov
National Institute of Arthritis and Musculoskeletal and Skin Diseases (NIAMS)
www.nih.gov/niams
National Institute of Child Health and Human Development
www.nichd.nih.gov
National Institute on Deafness and Other Communication Disorders (NIDCD)
www.nidcd.nih.gov
National Institute of Diabetes and Digestive and Kidney Diseases (NIDDK)
www2.niddk.nih.gov

National Institutes of Health (NIH)
    www.nih.gov
National Lead Information Center
    www.epa.gov/lead
National Library of Medicine (NLM)
    www.nlm.nih.gov
National Mental Health Information Center
    http://mentalhealth.samhsa.gov
National Organization for Rare Disorders (NORD)
    www.rarediseases.org
Occupational Safety and Health Administration (OSHA)
    www.osha.gov
The Internet for School Nurses
    www.ohsu.edu/library/ref/schoolnurse
U.S. Department of Education (DOE)
    www.ed.gov/index.jsp
U.S. Department of Health and Human Services (DHHS)
    www.os.dhhs.gov
U.S. Food and Drug Administration (FDA)
    www.fda.gov

ORGANIZATIONS

Alliance for Technology Access (ATA)
    www.ataccess.org
American Academy of Allergy, Asthma, and Immunology (AAAAI)
    www.aaaai.org
American Academy of Child and Adolescent Psychiatry (AACAP)
    www.aacap.org
American Academy of Pediatrics (AAP)
    www.aap.org
American Brain Tumor Association (ABTA)
    www.abta.org
American Diabetes Association (ADA)
    www.diabetes.org
American Foundation for the Blind (AFB)
    www.afb.org
American Heart Association—National Center (AHA)
    www.americanheart.org
American Lung Association (ALA)
    www.lungusa.org
American Occupational Therapy Association (AOTA)
    www.aota.org
American Physical Therapy Association (APTA)
    www.apta.org
American Psychological Association (APA)
    www.apa.org
American School Health Association (ASHA)
    www.ashaweb.org
American Speech-Language-Hearing Association (ASHA)
    www.asha.org
Angelman Syndrome Foundation
    www.angelman.org
Anxiety Disorders Association of America (ADAA)
    www.adaa.org

The Annie E. Casey Foundation: Helping Vulnerable Kids and Families Succeed
    www.aecf.org/kidscount
Aplastic Anemia and MDS International Foundation
    www.aamds.org
Autism Society of America
    www.autism-society.org
Brain Injury Association (BIA)
    www.biausa.org
Center for Health and Health Care in Schools
    www.healthinschools.org/home.asp
Childhood Apraxia of Speech Association of North America (CASANA)
    www.apraxia-kids.org
Children and Adults with Attention-Deficit/Hyperactivity Disorder (CHADD)
    www.chadd.org
Children's Environmental Health Network (CEHN)
    www.cehn.org
Children's Tumor Foundation
    www.ctf.org
Chronic Fatigue and Immune Dysfunction Syndrome Association of America
(CFIDS)
    www.cfids.org/youth.asp
Cleft Palate Foundation (CPF)
    www.cleftline.org
Council of Chief State School Officers
    www.ccsso.org
Council for Exceptional Children (CEC)
    www.cec.sped.org
Cross Cultural Health Care Program (CCHCP)
    www.xculture.org
Easter Seals Disability Services
    www.easter-seals.org
Epilepsy Foundation
    www.epilepsyfoundation.org
FACES: The National Craniofacial Association
    www.faces-cranio.org
Family Voices: Speaking on Behalf of Children and Youth with Special Health
Care Needs
    www.familyvoices.org
Father's Network
    www.fathersnetwork.org
Food Allergy and Anaphylaxis Network (FAAN)
    www.foodallergy.org
Foundation for Ichthyosis and Related Skin Types (FIRST)
    www.scalyskin.org
The Future of Children
    www.futureofchildren.org
Global School Net: Linking Kids Around the World
    www.globalschoolnet.org
Great Schools: The Parents' Guide to K-12 Success
    www.schwablearning.org
Hydrocephalus Association
    www.hydroassoc.org
Immunization Action Coalition (IAC)
    www.immunize.org
International Dyslexia Association (IDA)
    www.interdys.org

Learning Disabilities Association of America (LDA)
www.ldanatl.org
Leukemia and Lymphoma Society (formerly Leukemia Society of America)
www.leukemia-lymphoma.org
Little People of America (LPA)
www.lpaonline.org
March of Dimes Birth Defects Foundation (MOD)
www.marchofdimes.com
Mental Health America
www.nmha.org
Muscular Dystrophy Association (MDA)
www.mdausa.org
National Alliance on Mental Illness (NAMI)
www.nami.org
National Assembly on School-Based Health Care
www.nasbhc.org
National Association of Pediatric Nurse Practitioners (NAPNAP)
www.napnap.org
National Association of State Boards of Education
www.nasbe.org
National Association of School Nurses (NASN)
www.nasn.org
National Association of School Nurses for the Deaf (NASND)
www.nasnd.org/index.htm
National Association of State Directors of Special Education
www.nasdse.org
National Brain Tumor Foundation (NBTF)
www.braintumor.org
National Council of State Boards of Nursing
https://www.ncsbn.org/index.htm
National Down Syndrome Congress (NDSC)
www.ndsccenter.org
National Eating Disorders Association
www.nationaleatingdisorders.org
National Federation for the Blind (NFB)
www.nfb.org
National Fragile X Foundation (FXF)
www.nfxf.org
National Organization for Albinism and Hypopigmentation (NOAH)
www.albinism.org
National Organization on Fetal Alcohol Syndrome (NOFAS)
www.nofas.org
National Resource Center for Paraprofessionals (NRCP)
www.nrcpara.org
National Reye's Syndrome Foundation (NRSF)
www.reyessyndrome.org
National Sleep Foundation (NSF)
www.sleepfoundation.org
Obsessive Compulsive Foundation (OCF)
www.ocfoundation.org
Osteogenesis Imperfecta Foundation (OI Foundation)
www.oif.org
Parents Helping Parents (PHP)
www.php.com

Prader-Willi Syndrome Association (PWSA)
   www.pwsausa.org
Society for Adolescent Medicine (SAM)
   www.adolescenthealth.org
Special Olympics
   www.specialolympics.org
Spina Bifida Association (SBA)
   ww.sbaa.org
Stuttering Foundation
   www.stutterhelp.org
Tourette's Syndrome Association (TSA)
   www.tsa-usa.org
Tuberous Sclerosis Alliance
   www.tsalliance.org
United Cerebral Palsy (UCP)
   www.ucp.org
Vestibular Disorders Association (VEDA)
   www.vestibular.org
Williams Syndrome Association (WSA)
   www.williams-syndrome.org
World Health Organization (WHO)
   www.who.int/en/

GLOSSARY

Acanthosis nigricans A velvety hyperpigmentation found on the neck, axillae, and groin that is probably the skin manifestation of severe and chronic hyperinsulinemia. Associated with obesity and type 2 diabetes.

Agonist Any agent with a certain cellular affinity that produces a predictable response.

Agranulocytosis An acute febrile condition in which production of white blood cells is severely depressed. Symptoms include chills, swollen neck, sore throat, and prostration; sometimes with local ulceration of rectum, mouth, and vagina. May be side effects of certain medications or to radiation therapy. Also known as *granulocytopenia*.

Amenorrheic Not having menstruation.

Amygdala A nucleus of tissue found at the base of the temporal lobe, which is one of several structures of the limbic system and regulates aspects of emotional behavior.

Anovulatory Inability of the ovaries to produce, mature, or release eggs.

Antagonists Any agent that competes or exerts a negative action to that of a receptor site or another action.

Anthropometry Science of measuring the height, weight, and size of various parts of the human body, such as skinfolds. Ability to compare proportions for normal and atypical findings.

Antibody Develops in reaction to bacteria, virus, and to other antigenic (foreign to the body) substances. An antibody is specific to an antigen.

Asthenia Loss of strength and energy; weakness.

Atopy Genetic predisposition for development of an IgE (immunoglobulin E)-mediated response to common allergens. Determined by a skin test.

Autoimmunity Abnormal condition in which one's body acts against its own tissue constituents.

Autosomal dominant disorder If one parent is a carrier and the other is normal, there is a 50% chance a child will inherit the trait.

Autosomal recessive disorder Both parents must be carriers for their child to have the disease; if their child inherits the gene from only one parent, he or she will be a carrier. If the child inherits the gene from both parents, he or she will have the disease.

Bacteria Simple one-celled organism and the most plentiful of pathogens. Most bacteria do not cause disease.

Beta-blockers Drugs that block the response to epinephrine/ norepinephrine, slowing the heart rate and decreasing cardiac output; they cause bronchoconstriction, thus increasing airway resistance in asthmatics.

Bioavailability The level of activity or quantity of administered drug or other substance that becomes available for use by the targeted cells.

Blepharitis An inflammatory condition of the lash follicles and glands of the eyelids, characterized by redness, swelling, and crusting of dried mucus. Ulcerative blepharitis is caused by bacteria; and nonulcerative blepharitis is caused by seborrhea, psoriasis, or an allergic response.

Bolus feeding A concentrated mass of food or pharmaceutical preparation given by mouth, nasogastric tube, or gastrostomy feeding methods over a short period.

Celiac sprue/celiac disease An inborn error of metabolism that affects the ability to hydrolyze peptides contained in gluten. Gluten is found in barley, wheat, and oats. Gluten-free substitutes are rice and corn; vitamin or mineral deficiencies can be fulfilled with oral preparations.

Chelation therapy Using a chelating agent to bind with a metal in the body so that the metal loses its toxic effect. Procedure used in lead poisoning.

Cholelithiasis Formation or presence of calculi (gallstones) in the gallbladder. Factors that increase the probability of gallstones include female gender, increased age, obesity, and a positive family history.

Chorionic villus sampling Chorionic villus sampling (CVS) is a procedure used for prenatal diagnosis in the first trimester of pregnancy by withdrawing a chorionic villi sample from the fetal membranes. CVS tests for similar range of abnormalities as an amniocentesis. The advantage of CVS is that the results are obtained much earlier in pregnancy (8 to 12 weeks). CVS carries a risk of complications, as does amniocentesis.

Chromatin-positive nuclei Description of the nuclei of cells that have characteristics of the normal female but also may be present in some chromosomal abnormalities (e.g., Klinefelter's syndrome).

Chromosomal analysis An analysis of the chromosome, which is the threadlike structure in the nucleus of the cell that functions as the transmission of genetic information.

Clinodactyly A congenital anomaly of the hand marked by lateral or medial bending of one or more fingers or toes.

Coarctation of the aorta A congenital anomaly in which there is localized narrowing of the aorta. Symptoms include headaches, dizziness, fainting, nosebleeds, and muscle cramps during exercise secondary to tissue anoxia. Murmur may or may not be present. Surgical correction is recommended for even a minor defect.

Computed tomography In computed tomography (CT), the CT scan functions as a diagnostic tool; also known as *computed axial tomography* or *CAT scan*. A rotating camera is used to film the head or other body parts, taking images from numerous x-ray beams going through the body and converting the information into a three dimensional picture of the body part. The x-ray image is defined by various shades of gray delineated by the tissue density.

Congenital adrenogenital hyperplasia Congenital adrenogenital hyperplasia (CAH) is a category of autosomal recessive disorders that results in virilization of female fetuses.

Convolutions Rolled or twisted together, with one part over the other.

Copropraxia Involuntarily making obscene gestures; a rare characteristic of Tourette's Syndrome.

Coprolalia   Involuntary vocalizing obscene or other socially unacceptable words or phrases. Associated with Tourette's Syndrome.

Cortex   The outer layer of a structure or other body organ as identified from the internal matter. In the brain, the gray matter of the cerebellum and cerebral hemispheres is where most neurons are found. Cortic means "cortex" or "bark."

Coryza   An acute inflammation of the nasal mucous membrane with a profuse discharge from the nostrils.

Cushing's Syndrome   A hormonal disorder secondary to excessive levels of cortisol due to the body's overproduction of cortisol or taking too much cortisol or other steroid hormones.

Cyclothymic disorder   Cycle of moods from hypomania to depression, but not severe enough to meet the criteria for major depressive disorder. Must be of at least 1 year duration in children and adolescents.

Cytotoxic   Describes a drug or agent that damages or destroys tissue cells.

Demineralization   The process of removing minerals, in the form of mineral ions, from dental enamel. Precursor of caries. It is another term for dissolving of the enamel.

Desquamation   A normal process of shedding of epithelium elements, mainly the skin, in fine sheets or scales; peeling.

Dopamine   Primarily an inhibitory catecholamine. An important part of the brain's reward and pleasure system, causing feelings of euphoria. Roles include regulation of conscious movement and mood and affects management of hormonal balance and the immune system via the pituitary gland.

Dysfluency   Disruption of the normal pattern of speech for the individual's developmental age (e.g., stuttering, prolonged sounds, word substitution).

Dyspareunia   Unusual pain during sexual intercourse.

Ectoderm, mesoderm, and endoderm   The three *embryonic germ layers:* the *ectoderm,* or outer layer, which gives rise to the nervous system (brain and spinal cord) and epidermis; the *mesoderm,* or middle layer, which gives rise to the connective tissue, muscle, skeleton, and other structures; and the *endoderm,* or inner layer, which is the source of the epithelium of the digestive tract and its derivatives.

Effusion   The escape of fluid, usually into a body cavity. In the middle ear, the disorder otitis media, an accumulation of fluid present in the middle ear space, decreases the mobility of the eardrum.

Electromyogram   The electromyogram (EMG) measures electrical activity in a skeletal muscle by putting on surface electrodes or inserting electrode needles into the muscle and displaying the activity on an oscilloscope.

Endoscopy   Visualization of the interior organs and cavities of the gastrointestinal tract with a flexible instrument called an *endoscope.*

Epiphyseal   The enlarged distal and proximal ends of a large bone.

Exanthem   A wide rash secondary to viral or bacterial infections or drug reaction, most commonly antibiotics.

Functional magnetic resonance imaging   Functional magnetic resonance imaging (fMRI) is a diagnostic tool that uses the same technology as an MRI by adding to the basic anatomical picture. It measures the areas with the highest oxygen level in the brain that indicate the part of the brain used as the individual does different tasks or reacts to different stimuli. Particular areas of brain activity use larger concentrations of oxygen, which correspond to brighter areas in the color image created by this technique.

Fungus   Single or multicelled organism that reproduces by spores present in soil, air, or water.

Gamma aminobutyric acid   Gamma aminobutyric acid (GABA) is an inhibitor. Aggression and violence are associated with low levels of GABA, together with low levels of serotonin. Passive behavior is associated with high levels of GABA and serotonin.

Genital tubercle   A small eminence or nodule on the skin that is larger than a papule.

Glia/glial   A neural cell that provides support and nutrition. It is a non-neuron because it is not involved in the networking process. The Greek translation for glia is "glue."

Gonad   A sex gland; the ovary in the female and the testis in the male.

Health care provider   A health care provider (HCP) is any health care professional who has the ability to assess and diagnose health, provide treatment, and prescribe medication.

Helminthic   Referring to a parasitic worm.

Hydronephrosis   Distension of the kidney secondary to structural or functional changes in the urinary tract that obstruct normal urine flow, sometimes leading to renal dysfunction (obstructive nephropathy). May be due to kidney stone in ureter, tumor, or edema from urinary tract infection.

Hyperconvex fingernails   Nails that have an extreme curve outward.

Hypogonadism   Insufficiency in the secretory activity of the ovary or testis. May be primary or secondary (e.g., caused by a hypothalamus-pituitary disorder).

Hypopituitarism   Decreased activity of the pituitary gland, resulting in excessive deposits of fat and persistence of adolescent characteristics.

Icteric phase   A jaundice phase caused by an abnormal amount of bilirubin in the blood.

Ig   Abbreviation for *immunoglobulin*. Antibodies in the serum and external secretions of the body. They are formed in the spleen, bone marrow, and all lymphoid tissues, except the thymus, in response to a specific antigen. IgA, IgD, IgE, IgG, and IgM are all abbreviations for their respective immunoglobulin letters; and IgF is an abbreviation for insulin-like growth factors.

Interphalangeal   Situated or occurring between the phalanges (the bones of the fingers or toes); relating to an interphalangeal joint.

Keratin   A constituent of the epidermis, hair, nails, horny tissues, and enamel of the teeth.

Keratitis   An inflammation of the cornea.

Laparotomy   A surgical incision into the peritoneal cavity under general or regional anesthesia, usually for exploration.

Leptin   A protein hormone that provides the body with an indication of nutritional status and helps regulate body weight, metabolism, and reproductive function. Leptin's effects on body weight occur through effects on hypothalamic centers that control feeding behavior and hunger, body temperature, and energy expenditure.

Leukopenia Abnormal decrease in white blood cells to below 5000 per cubic millimeter.

Limbic system Term that refers to subcortical and cortical structures of the brain that are associated with emotions and feelings; such as, sadness, anger, fear, and sexual arousal; structures of the limbic system include the cingulate gyrus, hippocampal gyrus, uncus, and amygdala.

Live-attenuated Decreasing the virulence of a pathogenic microorganism for its host by increasing virulence for a new host; a basis for live vaccine development.

Lordosis An abnormal anterior concavity of the lumbar spine.

Macule A small flat discoloration or blemish that is skin level (e.g., freckle, certain rashes).

Maculopapular A rash consisting of both macules and papules.

Magnetic resonance imaging Magnetic resonance imaging (MRI) is a diagnostic tool sometimes called *nuclear magnetic resonance imaging (NMR)*. It creates a magnetic field around the brain by using a large magnet and radio waves. A three-dimensional computer image of the brain/body part results as the cells respond to the radio waves. The image is made when the tissues with high concentrations of water (such as fat) appear light and bone (with less water) appears dark. A high-level software system, computerized tomography (CT) converts the image data into a 3-D picture.

Melatonin A hormone secreted by the pineal gland, especially in response to darkness, that has been linked to the regulation of diurnal rhythms. An over-the-counter supplement is often taken to regulate sleep patterns and is claimed to have anti-aging properties.

Metabolic syndrome A cluster of conditions that include: abdominal obesity, abnormal cholesterol levels, increased blood pressure, elevated triclycerides and blood sugar. This puts one at risk for diabetes, heart disease, and stroke.

Micrognathia Small, underdeveloped jaw, especially the mandible.

Myalgias Pain in one or more muscles, usually diffuse.

Myelin A fatty substance that forms a covering around some axons, is composed mainly of protein and phospholipids, and acts like an electrical insulator by helping to speed the conduction of nerve impulses.

Myelination The production of myelin surrounding an axon; also called the *myelin sheath*.

Neocortex The six-layered cortex that covers most of the cerebral hemispheres in the brain.

Neuraxis The spinal cord and brain, central nervous system, and a point of reference for given directions within the nervous system.

Neuron The basic nerve cell of the nervous system. Neurons are identified by the direction in which they send impulses. *Sensory neurons* send information towards the spinal cord and the brain, whereas *motor neurons* send information from the brain and spinal cord toward muscles and glandular tissue. Each neuron has one axon and one or more dendrites.

Neurotransmitter A chemical involved in the transmission of nerve impulses between synapses. *Excitatory impulses* decrease the negativity potential, thus increasing transmission of impulses between synapses. *Inhibitory impulses* increase the negativity potential, thus decreasing neural transmission.

Noradrenergic Released by the sympathetic nervous system and not subject to voluntary control. A vasoconstrictor relaxes the muscle wall, raises blood pressure, dilates eyes, and initiates the fight-or-flight response.

Nucleus accumbens A structure in the middle of the brain.

Oligohydramnios An abnormal condition in which there is a very small amount or an absence of amniotic fluid.

Orthostatic blood pressure Measurement of blood pressure while in a standing position.

Papillae A small nipple projection or extension from tissue or fibers.

Papilledema Swelling of the optic disc caused by increased intracranial pressure. Vision is usually normal.

Papule A solid raised skin lesion that is 1 cm or less in diameter (e.g., nonpustular acne/pimple).

Parasite Multicellular animal that attacks specific tissues or organs and competes with host for nutrients.

Paresthesias Feelings of numbness or tingling that are subjective and may change with posture, edema, rest, activity, or an underlying disorder. Sometimes called *acroparesthesia* when felt in the extremities.

Parotitis Inflammation of one or both of the parotid salivary glands. Infectious or epidemic parotitis is known as *mumps*.

Pectus excavatum An abnormal formation of the chest in which the sternum is depressed. Also called *funnel chest*. Surgical correction may be necessary if the pectus excavatum interferes with breathing and is often sought for cosmetic reasons.

Philtrum The natural groove of the upper lip, extending to the nose. The groove is usually smooth or nonexistent in persons with fetal alcohol syndrome.

Photophobia Atypical sensitivity to light, especially by the eyes; is found in certain conditions (albinism) and is a symptom of various diseases and disorders (e.g., measles, encephalitis, Reiter's syndrome).

Pilosebaceous units Well-developed sebaceous glands with miniature hairs.

Polyhydramnios Excess amount of amniotic fluid, indicating a problem in the pregnancy. Also called *hydramnios*. See oligohydramnios.

Positron emission tomography Positron emission tomography (PET) functions as a research tool more than as a diagnostic one. A radioactive chemical compound marker is injected into the blood stream. The compound attaches to glucose molecules, giving off gamma rays, which translate as color images onto a computer screen. PET produces a clear picture of the brain areas working the hardest; however, it does not have the same fine resolution as a fMRI.

Primordial The most primitive or underdeveloped state, such as those cells formed during the early stages of embryonic development.

Prepuce   A fold of skin that forms a retractable sheath; foreskin of the penis or the fold around the clitoris.

Prognathia   One or both jaws, mandible and maxilla, project forward.

Pyoderma   A purulent skin disease (e.g., impetigo).

Reye's syndrome   Disease affecting all organs of the body, most harmful to the brain and the liver. Always follows another illness and associated with taking aspirin or other salicylates. Can affect all ages but primarlily occurs in children.

Serotonin   Primarily an inhibitory monoamine. Plays a role in the regulation of mood, control of eating, arousal, perception of pain, and in sleep. It appears to be related to dreaming.

Sinovaginal bulbs   Endodermal outgrowths that fuse to become the opening of the vagina.

Spermatogenesis   Process of development of spermatozoa.

Stridor   A harsh, shrill sound usually heard on inspiration in laryngeal obstruction.

Subacute   A disease in which clinical symptoms are not apparent.

Subluxation   An incomplete separation of the articular surfaces of a joint.

Superior colliculus   A nucleus in the midbrain that controls saccadic eye movement. The superior colliculus is also responsible for turning the head and eyes to see a stimulus that is heard or felt.

Synapse   The space between two neurons across which nerve impulses, that either *inhibit* or *continue* the impulse, are transmitted.

Synovial membrane   The connective-tissue membrane lining the articular capsules that surround freely moving joints. It secretes thick synovial fluid that normally lubricates the joint; but, when an injury occurs, an excess amount may accumulate, causing pain.

Temporomandibular joint   The temporomandibular joint (TMJ) is the joint between the temporal bone of the skull and the mandible of the jaw that includes the condyloid process and allows for the opening, closing, protrusion, retraction, and lateral movement of the mandible.

Tenesmus   Persistent ineffectual spasms of the bladder or rectum accompanied by a desire to empty the bladder or bowel.

Torticollis   An abnormal tipping of the head to one side caused by muscle contractures on that side of the neck. May be congenital or acquired. Treatment depends on the cause and includes physical therapy, heat, immobilization, or surgery.

Toxigenicity   There are differences in virulence because of growth rate differences and the ability to produce the toxin. When the organism reproduces at an increased rate, it may be able to probe further into its host, producing still greater amounts of the toxin.

Trichotillomania   Repetitive behaviors to the body, such as pulling out hair, scratching, and drawing blood to the skin.

Tricyclic antidepressants   Tricyclic antidepressants (TCAs) are a group of drugs that are useful in a wide range of disorders, including enuresis, panic disorder, social phobia, bulimia, narcolepsy, attention deficit disorder (ADD) with or without hyperactivity, and migraine headaches.

Ultrasonography   Assessment of the deep structures within the body by measuring and recording the reflection of pulsed sound waves.

Vasculitis   An inflammatory condition of the blood vessels characteristic of particular systemic diseases.

Velopharyngeal insufficiency   Incomplete closure of the oral cavity beneath the nasal passages, as found in cleft palate, allowing regurgitation of food through the nose. It impairs speech and is usually corrected with surgery.

Vesicles   A small sac that contains liquid, such as a blister.

Virilization   Masculinization.

Virus   The smallest form of organism causing disease; also the toughest.

X-linked recessive   Inheritance in which an abnormal recessive gene on the X chromosome results in a carrier state in females and characteristics of the condition in males.

INDEX

A

AAAAI. *See* American Academy of Allergy, Asthma, and Immunology
AABR. *See* Automated auditory brainstem response
AACAP. *See* American Academy of Child and Adolescent Psychiatry
AAI. *See* Atlantoaxial instability
AAOS. *See* American Academy of Orthopedic Surgeons
AAP. *See* American Academy of Pediatrics
AAS. *See* American Association of Suicidology
ABAS-II. *See* Adaptive Behavior Assessment System, Second Edition
Abbreviations, 593t-594t
  usage. *See* Specimens
Abdominal anorchia, 413
Abdominal pain, first aid, 511
ABI. *See* Auditory brainstem implant
ABR. *See* Auditory brainstem response
Abrasions/lacerations, 375
Absence seizures (petit mal), 265, 297
  characteristics, 266-267
Abstinence, usage, 417t
ABTA. *See* American Brain Tumor Association
Abusable gases, inhalants, 345
Acanthosis nigricans, 620
Accommodation, definition, 77
Accommodative esotropia, 55
Acetylcholine, actions, 333b
Achenbach System of Empirically Based Assessment (ASEBA), 529
Achondroplasia, presence. *See* Boys; Girls
Acid-fast bacillus, impact. *See* Tuberculosis
ACIP. *See* Advisory Committee on Immunization Practices
Acne cosmetica, cause, 395
Acne fulminans, 392
Acne vulgaris, 391-393
  characteristics, 391-392
  definition, 391
  differential diagnosis, 392
  etiology, 391
  health concerns/emergencies, 392
  management/treatment, 392-393
  medications, 392-393
  student education, 392
Acoustic feedback, 96
Acquaintance assault, 373
Acquaintance rape. *See* Nonstranger rape
Acquired, definition, 77
Acquired immunodeficiency syndrome (AIDS), 239-244
  asymptomatic infection, 240-241
  blood exposure, 239, 240
  characteristics, 239-241
  contracting, fear, 371
  definition, 239
  development stages, 239
  etiology, 239

Acquired immunodeficiency syndrome (AIDS) *(Continued)*
  health concerns/emergencies, 241-242
  impact, 242
  information, 244
  management/treatment, 242-243
  perinatal transmission, 239, 240
  primary infection, 240
  sexual contact, 239, 240
  transmission, modes, 239-240
Acquired nystagmus, 61-62
ACS. *See* Acute chest syndrome
Acuity
  definition, 77
  level. *See* Visual acuity
Acute chest syndrome (ACS), 166-167
Acute conditions, 110
Acute diarrhea. *See* Shigellosis
Acute otitis media (AOM), 105-106
Acute rheumatic fever (ARF), 147
ADA. *See* American Diabetes Association
ADAA. *See* Anxiety Disorders Association of America
Adam's forward bend test, 263
Adapted physical education, definition, 457
Adaptive Behavior Assessment System, Second Edition (ABAS-II), 530
ADD. *See* Attention-deficit disorder
ADDA. *See* Attention Deficit Disorder Association
Adderall, usage. *See* Attention deficit-hyperactivity disorder
ADHD. *See* Attention deficit-hyperactivity disorder
Administration for Children and Families, Office of Head Start (web site), 603
Adolescence (13 to 19 years), 31-34. *See also* Early adolescence; Late adolescence; Middle adolescence
  brain findings, 31
  television viewing, excess, 479
Adolescent idiopathic scoliosis, 264
Adolescents
  depression, 325
  gender developmental characteristics, 35
  relationship. *See* School start time
  sleep, requirement, 473
  SM characteristics, 367-368
  stress reaction, 498
Adolescents Never Suicide When Everyone Responds (ANSWER), web site, 369
Adolescent-specific issues, 389
  general conditions, 391-403
Adolescent suicide, causes, 367
Adolescent Training and Learning To Avoid Steroids (ATLAS), 351
Adventitious, definition, 103
Advisory Committee on Immunization Practices (ACIP), recommendations, 126
AEPS-II. *See* Assessment, Evaluation, Progress, and Systems, Second Edition
Aerosol sprays, risks, 394t
AFB. *See* American Foundation for the Blind

Page numbers followed by *f* indicate figures; by *t,* tables; and by *b,* boxes.